RESPIRATORY CARE CERTIFICATION GUIDE

RESPIRATORY CARE CERTIFICATION GUIDE

James R. Sills, M.Ed., C.P.F.T., R.R.T.

Director, Respiratory Care Programs
Rock Valley College
Rockford, Illinois

SECOND EDITION

Original illustrations by
Sandra Hogan
Rock Valley College
Rockford, Illinois

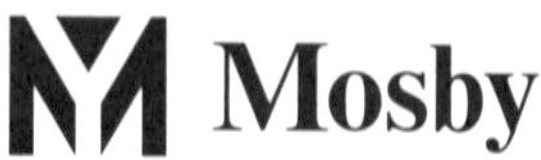

St. Louis Baltimore Berlin Boston Carlsbad Chicago London Madrid
Naples New York Philadelphia Sydney Tokyo Toronto

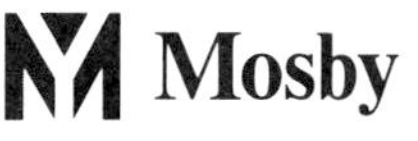

Dedicated to Publishing Excellence

Editor: James Shanahan
Developmental Editor: Jennifer Roche
Project Manager: Nancy Baker
Designer: Sheilah Barrett
Manufacturing Supervisor: Kathy Grone

SECOND EDITION

Printed in the United States of America
Composition by The Clarinda Company
Printing/binding by Maple Vail

Mosby-Year Book, Inc.
11830 Westline Industrial Drive
St. Louis, MO 63146

Library of Congress Cataloging-in-Publication Data

Sills, James R.
Respiratory care certification guide / James R. Sills ; original illustrations by Sandra Hogan. —2nd ed.
p. cm.
Includes bibliographical references and index.
ISBN 0-8151-7515-9
1. Respiratory therapy—Examinations, questions, etc. I. Title.
[DNLM: 1. Respiratory Therapy. WB 342 S584r 1993]
RC735.I5S58 1993
616.2′0046—dc20
DNLM/DLC
for Library of Congress 94-8962
CIP

94 95 96 97 98 CL/MY 9 8 7 6 5 4 3 2 1

FOREWORD

Jim Sills' *Respiratory Care Certification Guide* provides both educators and students an outstanding resource that covers all the basic areas of knowledge, skills, and professional attributes that are identified by the National Board for Respiratory Care (NBRC) as essential for respiratory therapy technicians. Every 5 years the NBRC conducts a national job analysis in order to develop a comprehensive inventory of tasks performed by the technician. Based on this survey, the NBRC's examinations are then designed to test for only the important (or essential) job functions, eliminating differences in practice resulting from geographic region and institutional size. In addition, the Joint Review Committee for Respiratory Therapy Education recommends that the basic competency goal be based on the NBRC's comprehensive task survey.

Because Jim Sills' textbook is based on the most objective and extensive research available in the field of respiratory care, the material presented serves as an excellent guide for both the student and the educator. While it is not the intent of this book to exclude important subjects or tasks that may (or should) also be a vital part of a respiratory care program (e.g., cardiopulmonary anatomy and physiology, microbiology, mathematics/algebra, chemistry, or specific community needs such as various hemodynamic skills), it does provide the basic core curriculum that should be understood and performed by all technicians for their success on the NBRC's exams and in their profession.

By focusing this textbook around the NBRC's job survey and comprehensive task inventory and, importantly, writing in a clear and precise manner, Jim Sills has made an outstanding and valuable contribution to the field of respiratory care. When you are uncertain about what the "state-of-the-art" is regarding the practice of technicians, read this book.

Terry Des Jardins, M.Ed., R.R.T.
Parkland College
Department of Respiratory Care
Champaign, Illinois

PREFACE TO FIRST EDITION

This textbook came about in my attempt as an educator to prepare students as thoroughly as possible for working as technicians and for passing the Entry Level Exam. Gaining and keeping rewarding employment and earning the Certified Respiratory Therapy Technician credential are important milestones in their lives. Because the content of the exam is based on a national survey conducted by the National Board for Respiratory Care (NBRC) to determine a technician's professional duties, preparation for the exam and to work in any respiratory care department are simultaneous goals. Graduates of any program who have a thorough understanding of what is expected of them on a national level will have the mobility to move wherever the best opportunity presents itself.

Our students purchase a variety of textbooks, since a particular book may only cover some subjects well. Unfortunately, some necessary subjects are not well covered in any current respiratory care textbook. I have attempted to write a standard textbook that presents *all* of the subject areas deemed essential by the NBRC.

James R. Sills, M.Ed., C.P.F.T., R.R.T.

PREFACE TO SECOND EDITION

This book is designed to do two things. First and foremost, it covers in detail *every* item listed by the National Board for Respiratory Care in its 1993 Examination Content Outline for the Entry Level Exam. This should help any student or graduate who is preparing for the examination. Second, it has been updated to reflect current practices, errors in the first edition have been corrected, and confusing areas have been clarified.

James R. Sills, M.Ed., C.P.F.T., R.R.T.

This book is dedicated to my wife Deb and our children Rachael and David, who make my life full and complete; our dog Amber, who keeps me company when I work at home; my parents; and Carl Hammond, who taught me respiratory care.

Words to live by:

Hope for the best but plan for the worst.

The journey of 1000 miles begins with a single step.

INTRODUCTION FOR STUDENTS AND EDUCATORS

This text is designed to cover in detail all of the knowledge areas, skills, and professional attitudes required of technicians by the National Board for Respiratory Care (NBRC). The NBRC made this extensive list available through the Examination Content Outline (released to all Respiratory Care Programs in August 1993); only the areas listed on this outline will appear on the Entry Level Exams given from July 1994 to March 1995. (The first edition of this book covered the NBRC's July 1987 Examination Content Outline.)

The sections in this text are designed to progress logically from patient assessment, to infection control, and through the various floor therapies to mechanical ventilation. Patient assessment is reinforced with all of the specific therapies and procedures because it is the cornerstone of appropriate care. Each section is followed by a series of self-assessment questions to help the student judge understanding.

Almost every heading that is used in this text is followed by two alphanumeric codes. The first (in parentheses) is the NBRC code for that subject found in the Examination Content Outline. The user may wish to refer to the outline for specific wording used by the NBRC. My choice of words is a paraphrasing of their's. Occasionally a heading will appear without an NBRC code after it. Sometimes these headings are added in because they are vital in order to understand what the NBRC is testing for. This background information will not, in itself, be tested, but the information must be understood to grasp what will be tested. Other non-NBRC coded headings are added because the information has appeared on one or more of the Entry Level Exams but is not specifically listed on the Examination Content Outline. (The student must understand that at times the NBRC used rather broad language.)

The second code [in brackets] is the NBRC code for the difficulty level of the questions that will be used to test the examinee's understanding of the material. R stands for Recall. Ap stands for Application. An stands for Analysis. See the Introduction for Examinees for a more detailed explanation, if needed.

It is important to also understand what this text does *not* discuss. The student and educator must look elsewhere for textbooks on human anatomy and physiology, microbiology, mathematics/algebra, chemistry, or any other areas that may be important background information for the technician student. It is certainly important for the student to have a solid understanding of these areas to which he or she may add understanding of the science of respiratory care. These subjects are not presented in this text because they will not be tested by the NBRC on the Entry Level Exam.

Although cardiopulmonary pathologic and abnormal conditions are not specifically listed on the Examination Content Outline, the NBRC has added a few questions on these areas to past Entry Level Exams. It is beyond the scope of this text to specifically address the various cardiopulmonary pathologic conditions. Some discussion of pathologic processes is included in the general discussion of each section as they relate to the treatment or procedure that the Respiratory Therapy Technician would perform. It is recommended that the student study the major types of adult and infant disease states and abnormal conditions.

INTRODUCTION FOR EXAMINEES

A graduate of a technician or therapist program preparing for the Entry Level Exam can use this text to help focus on what needs to be studied. Just as important, it will help in understanding what will *not* be on the exam. That is not to say that other learning is not important—just that it will not be on the Entry Level Exam. Therapist program graduates will likely find that some topics they have studied will only be tested on the Advanced Practitioners Examinations.

Almost every heading used in this text is followed by alphanumeric codes. The first (in parentheses) is the NBRC code for that subject found in the August 1993 Examination Content Outline. The user may wish to refer to the outline for specific wording used by the NBRC. (See the *NBRC Horizons*, July/August 1993.) My choice of words is a paraphrasing of their's. Occasionally a heading will appear without an NBRC code after it. Sometimes headings are added in because they are vital in order to understand what the NBRC is testing for. This background information will not, in itself, be tested, but the information must be understood to grasp what will be tested. Other non-NBRC coded headings are added because the information has appeared on the Entry Level Exam, but is not specifically listed on the Examination Content Outline. You must understand that at times the NBRC used rather broad language. For example, although cardiopulmonary pathologic and abnormal conditions are not specifically listed on past Examination Content Outline, the NBRC has added a few questions on these areas to past Entry Level Exams. It is beyond the scope of this text to specifically address the various cardiopulmonary pathologic conditions. Some discussion of pathologic processes is included in the general discussion of each section as they relate to the treatment or procedure that the Respiratory Therapy Technician would perform. It is recommended that you study the major types of adult and infant disease states and abnormal conditions.

The second code [in brackets] is the NBRC code for the difficulty level of the questions that will be used to test your understanding of the material. R stands for Recall. Ap stands for Application. An stands for Analysis. You will find that the NBRC asks questions at these three different levels of difficulty.

Entry Level Exam

The Entry Level Exam is made up of 140 questions. You will have 3 hours to complete it, which works out to 1 minute, 17 seconds per question. Pace yourself to be at about question 50 after 1 hour and question 100 after 2 hours. If you have difficulty with a question, put a check mark by it on the answer sheet and move on.

Go back to these near the end of the third hour. Do not leave any blank spaces on the answer sheet. A passing score is 75% or greater. However, you could get less than 105 questions correct and still pass, because the Application and Analysis questions are weighted more heavily than the Recall ones (see below.) Examinees passing the exam will be awarded the Certified Respiratory Therapy Technician (C.R.T.T.) credential by the National Board for Respiratory Care.

The actual content of a given examination is a closely guarded secret. Several exams are usually maintained at a given time by the NBRC with others in production. Old exams are retired. Not everyone will be taking the same exam even at the same test site. The best way to prepare is to know the types of things that may be tested and how the test is constructed. There are three difficulty levels to the questions:

Recall [R]

Recall refers to remembering factual information that was previously learned. "Identify" would be a commonly used action verb in these types of questions. You may be asked to identify specific facts, terms, methods, procedures, principles, or concepts.

Prepare for these types of questions by studying the full range of factual information, equations, etc., seen in respiratory care practice. These types of questions are on the lowest order of difficulty. You either know the answer or you do not; there is little to ponder more deeply. It is very important to have a solid understanding of the factual basis of respiratory care in order to do well in this and the next two categories of questions.

Application [Ap]

Application refers to being able to use factual type information in real clinical situations that may be new to you. "Apply," "classify," and "calculate" would be commonly used action verbs in these types of questions. You may be asked to apply laws, theories, concepts, and/or principles to new, practical clinical situations. Calculations may have to be performed. Charts and graphs, such as seen in pulmonary function testing, may need to be used.

These types of questions are on higher order of difficulty than the Recall [R] types. Critical thinking must be applied to the factual information in order to answer these questions.

Analysis [An]

Analysis refers to being able to separate a patient care problem into its component parts or elements in order to evaluate the relationship of the parts or elements to the whole problem. "Evaluate," "compare," "contrast," "revise," and/or "select" would be commonly used action verbs in these types of questions. You may be questioned about revising a patient care plan or evaluating therapy.

These types of questions require the highest level of critical thinking. You may have to recall previously learned information, apply it to a patient care situation, and make a judgment as to the best way to care for the patient.

You will find that the NBRC uses two different types of questions on the exam in these three ways:

One Best Answer

This type of question has a stem (the question) followed by four possible answers coded A, B, C, and D. You must select the *best* answer from among those presented. Only one is clearly best even though other possible answers may be good. Carefully read the stem to make sure that you do not misunderstand the clear intent of the question. Controversial issues may be questioned. The use of "should" in the stem will clue you in to the need to select the answer that would be selected by the majority of practitioners.

Some questions may be worded in such a way that you will need to exclude a *false* answer. In other words, three answers are correct and one is incorrect. The use of "except" will clue you in to this type of question.

Multiple True-False

This type of question has a stem (the question) followed by four or five possible answers coded with Roman numerals I, II, III, IV, and V; then four combinations of the answers coded by letters A, B, C, and D. The stem may ask you to include all true statements or all false statements in the final answer. You must select the letter that represents the correct combination of answers.

There should not be any controversial answers offered. They are all either clearly correct or incorrect. That is the key to selecting the best answer. Read each possible answer as separate from the others. It is suggested that you mark each possible answer as true or false. Next, find the final answer from among those offered. Even if you do not find a final answer that included all of the answers that you selected, you will be able to find the best answer through the process of eliminating the final answers offered that you know are incorrect.

Situational Sets

This involves the use of a patient care scenario that may include the patient's history, vital signs, blood gas values, pulmonary function results, etc. Three to five questions follow that ask you about patient and/or equipment management. These questions are the "one best answer" or "multiple true-false" types as discussed above. However, because of the amount of information that is offered and the critical thinking that is required, these questions are categorized as being at the Application [Ap] or Analysis [An] level of difficulty.

It is important to carefully read the scenario to fully understand the information. Then, after reading a related question, refer back to the scenario for information that will help you pick the best answer. Do this for each question and also refer to the prior questions for information that may help you with the current one.

General Suggestions for Exam Preparation

1. Begin studying about 2 months before the exam. Pace yourself so that everything can be covered in the time that you have. Avoid "cramming" a few days before the examination; this test will demand more than the simple recall of facts.

2. Study the most important and heavily tested areas first. Work down to the less important areas.

3. Focus on the areas where you are weakest, especially if they are heavily tested.

4. Arrive at the city where the test will be given the evening before the exam. Make a practice drive from your motel to the test site and where you will park. Check the time required and add more for morning traffic.

5. Eat a good dinner. Avoid alcohol, even if you are nervous, so you have a clear head in the morning.

6. Do not cram for the exam back at the motel. If you are not prepared by now, a few more hours will not really help. If necessary, brush up on a few test areas.

7. Set the alarm to get up in plenty of time to be ready. Get a good night's sleep. Avoid sleeping pills.

8. Eat a good breakfast to get you through to lunch. Minimize caffeine intake. You will have plenty of adrenaline running through your system to keep you awake while taking the test!

9. Attempt to relax with the self-confidence that comes from knowing that you are well prepared.

Relative Weights of the Various Tested Areas on the Entry Level Exam

I have attempted to analyze the content of each of the 140 questions on versions II, III, and IV of the Self-Assessment Entry Level Exam that represents the 1987 NBRC Examination Content Outline. Each question has been placed into one of the sections on p. xv. The numbers of questions and percentages are averages and may not be followed exactly on other versions of the Entry Level Exam taken by examinees. However, the relative weights can offer some guidance as to what content is relatively more important or less important. Study time can be spent accordingly.

The major revisions found between the 1987 and 1993 Examination Content Outlines are the addition of more infection control items and the deletion of all items related to pumonary rehabilitation and home care. This table reflects these changes. It is my assumption that the increased number of questions on infection control will be about the same as the number deleted on rehabilitation and home care. This is because the NBRC has written that, overall, the examinations encompassing the August 1993 Examination Content Outline will not be greatly changed from previous versions.

Sections		**Questions**	**Percentage**
1	Patient Assessment	25	18%
2	Infection Control	6	4%
3	Blood Gases	8	6%
4	Pulmonary Function Testing	7	5%
5	Oxygen Therapy	15	11%
6	Hyperinflation Therapy	3	2%
7	Aerosol Therapy	7	5%
8	Pharmacology	6	4%
9	Postural Drainage Therapy	4	3%
10	Cardiopulmonary Resuscitation (Emergency Care)	6	4%
11	Airway Management	8	6%
12	Suctioning the Airway	4	3%
13	Intermittent Positive Pressure Breathing (IPPB)	6	4%
14	Mechanical Ventilation	32	23%
	Miscellaneous pulmonary conditions or diseases	3	2%
	TOTAL	**140**	**100%**

It is my opinion that the content of Sections 1, 3, and 4 must be thoroughly understood. This information is questioned directly and also incorporated into questions covering all of the other sections. The content in Section 14 is the most heavily questioned of all.

James R. Sills, M.Ed., C.P.F.T., R.R.T.

IMPORTANT ADDRESSES AND PHONE NUMBERS

For information on the examination process contact the following:

National Board for Respiratory Care
8310 Nieman Rd
Lenexa, KS 66214
(913) 599–4200

For information on purchasing self-assessment examinations contact the following:

Applied Measurement Professionals
11015 W. 75th Terrace, Suite 110
Shawnee Mission, KS 66214
(913) 268–6362

For information on accredited respiratory therapy technician educational programs contact the following:

Joint Review Committee for Respiratory Therapy Education
1701 W. Euless Blvd
Suite 200
Euless, TX 76039
(817) 283–2835

For information on state credentialing requirements contact the following:

American Association for Respiratory Care
11030 Ables Lane
Dallas, TX 75229
(214) 234–AARC

CONTENTS

1 Patient Assessment

Module A. Review the patient's chart for the following data and recommend the following diagnostic procedures based on the current information:

1. Review the patient's history, results of the physical examination, and current vital signs. (IA1a) [R]

Patient History

Review the complete, initial patient history that has been written up by the physician(s) and nurse(s). The following points should be noted:

1. Date of history taking
2. Patient data: name, age, sex, race, and occupation
3. Primary complaints
4. Secondary complaints
5. Present illness history and symptoms
6. Family history
7. Medical history of cardiopulmonary disease(s)

The medical history is most important for understanding the patient's problem(s) and developing the care plan. Fig. 1-1 shows a possible flow diagram for questions to ask the patient. (Dyspnea is discussed in detail in Module C 5.)

It is important to obtain a *brief* history before beginning therapeutic procedures. Determine how the patient has been doing since the last treatment. Has there been a change in dyspnea, cough and secretions, chest pain, etc? This will help guide therapy as effectively as possible.

After the medical history is completed, the patient should be placed into one of the following four categories:

A. Crisis/acute onset of illness (Fig. 1-2).

- Examples: trauma, heart attack, allergic reaction, aspiration of a foreign body, pneumothorax, pulmonary embolism, and some pneumonias.

B. Intermittent but repeated illness (Fig. 1-3).

- Examples: asthma, chronic bronchitis, congestive heart failure, angina pectoris, myasthenia gravis, and some pneumonias.

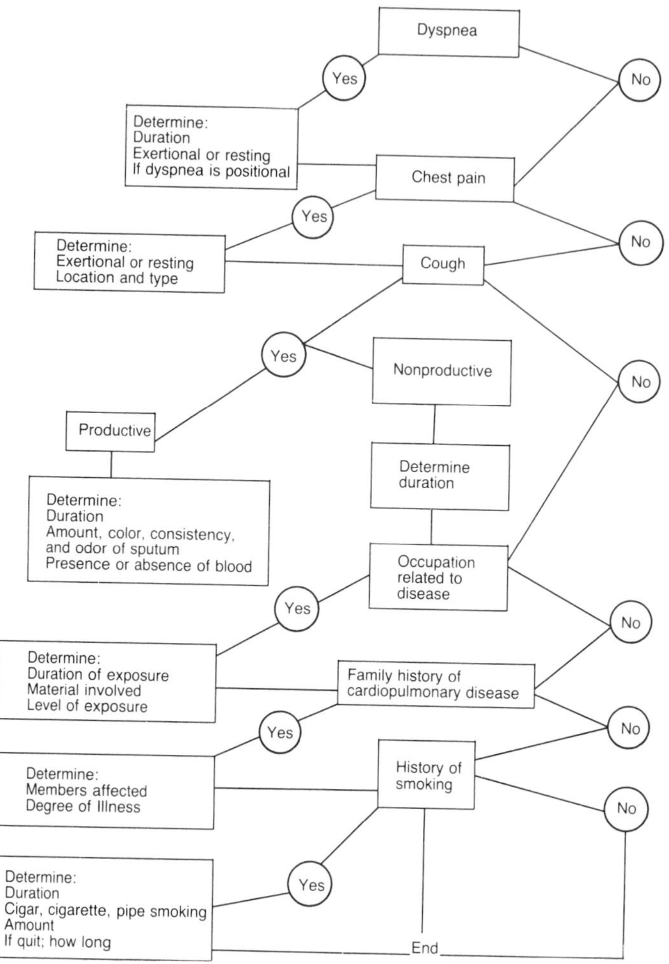

Fig. 1-1 Flow diagram for obtaining pertinent patient history. (From DiPietro JS, Mustard MN: *Clinical guide for respiratory care practitioners.* Norwalk, CN, Appleton & Lange, 1987. Used by permission.)

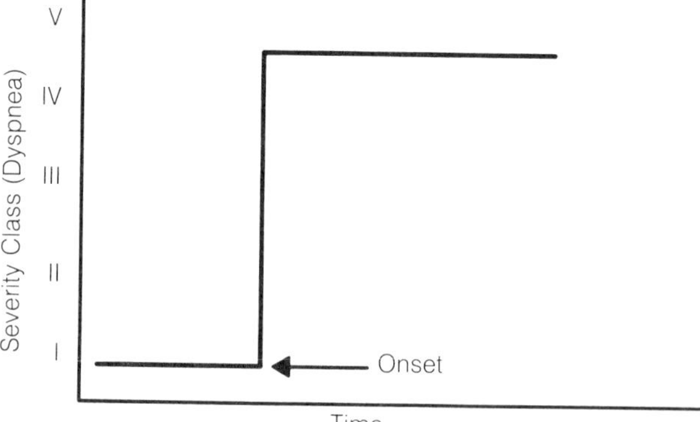

Fig. 1-2 Crisis/acute onset of illness. The sudden onset of the patient's illness can be seen. Quick, effective action may be needed. A thorough patient history may have to be delayed until the patient is stabilized. If the problem is correctable, and the proper care is given, the patient may return to his or her previous state of health. (From Burton GG: Patient assessment procedures, in Barnes TA (ed): *Respiratory Care Practice.* Chicago, Mosby, 1988. Used by permission.)

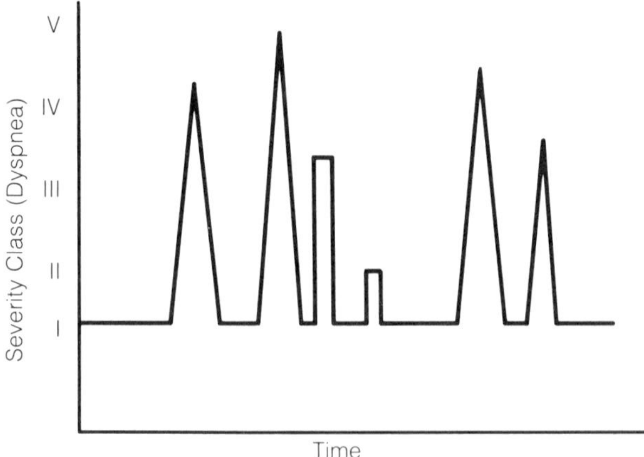

Fig. 1-3 Intermittent but repeated illness. Note that there are a series of sudden illnesses that appear to be of the crisis/acute onset type. However, the patient is relatively symptom free and healthy between these episodes. The patient quickly improves with the proper treatment. (From Burton GG: Patient assessment procedures, in Barnes TA (ed): *Respiratory Care Practice.* Chicago, Mosby, 1988. Used by permission.)

C. Progressive worsening (see Fig. 1-4).

- Examples: congestive heart failure, chronic bronchitis, emphysema, upper respiratory tract infection leading to bronchitis and/or pneumonia.

D. Mixed patterns/multiple problems (see Fig. 1-5).

- Examples: chronic obstructive lung disease and cystic fibrosis complicated by mucus plugging and/or infection, mixes of congestive heart failure and chronic lung disease, mixes of neuromuscular and lung disease, mixes of renal failure, and congestive heart failure with chronic lung disease.

Physical Examination

Review the results of the physical examinations performed by physician(s), nurse(s), and respiratory therapists. Review the following organ systems:

1. Pulmonary
2. Cardiovascular
3. Neuromuscular
4. Renal

The following are details of specific examination procedures.

Current Vital Signs

Review the current vital signs in the patient's chart. Compare them with the admission vital signs and what you observe in the patient now. Look for a change in pattern that would suggest a worsening or improvement in the patient.

Temperature

The textbook "normal" oral body temperature is 98.6° F (37° C). It is normal for there to be some range from 96.5 to 99.5° F (35.8 to 37.4° C). Make sure the patient has not eaten any hot or cold foods recently or been smoking before taking the temperature.

A rectal or core temperature is commonly taken in very sick patients because it is

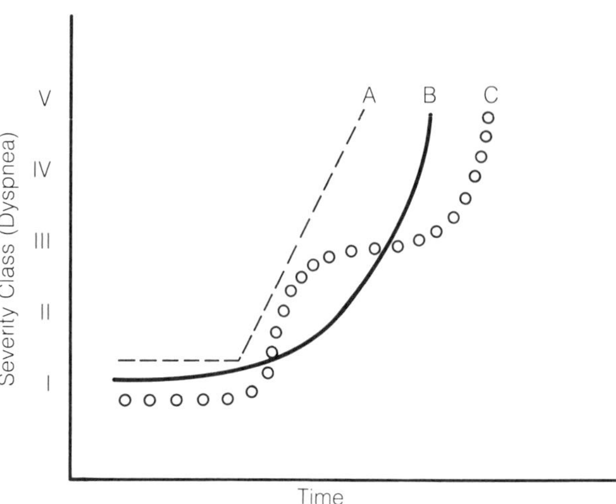

Fig. 1-4 Progressive worsening. The patient's history shows a long period of worsening symptoms that are now rather severe. Note that there may be a number of variations in the pattern. (From Burton GG: Patient assessment procedures, in Barnes TA (ed): *Respiratory Care Practice*. Chicago, Mosby, 1988. Used by permission.)

more accurate and reliable. The normal rectal temperature is 97.5 to 100.4° F (36.4 to 38° C). It is normal to see some, but less variance here.

Axillary temperatures are used as a last resort in stable patients. These run 1° F less than oral temperatures and are less accurate and reliable.

The variations in temperature noted above depend on the time of day, activity level, and, in women, menstrual cycle. For example, it is normal to see a lower body temperature when a person is a deep asleep.

An oral temperature of over 99.4° F or 37.4° C in a patient with a history of respiratory disease indicates a fever. Typically, it could be caused by atelectasis or a pulmonary or systemic infection. The infection could be either bacterial, viral, or fungal in origin. The *Streptococcus pneumoniae* organism (also known as *Pneumococcus* or *Diplococcus*) is known to cause a high fever with rigor (shaking chills) at onset. Patients are commonly treated to keep the fever below 103° F if possible.

In general, a rectal temperature below 97° F (36° C) is considered hypothermic. There are some procedures, such as open heart surgery, during which a patient's temperature is brought down to reduce metabolism and oxygen needs. The rectal temperature must be kept above 90° F (32° C) to prevent cardiac dysrhythmias occurring from the cold.

Healthy children tend to run a slightly higher temperature than adults. Premature neonates have less ability than children and adults to regulate body temperature and can

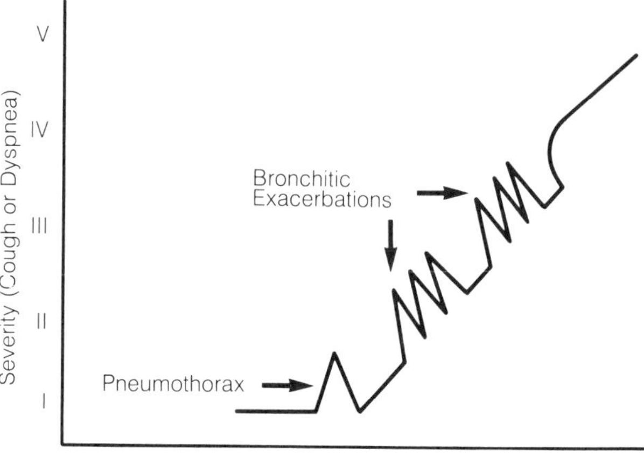

Fig. 1-5 Mixed patterns/multiple problems. These may be some of the most challenging patients to deal with because it may be difficult to tell which problem worsened first. You then have to determine which problem to treat first because it is the most dangerous to the patient. The patient may return to his or her previous state of health after proper treatment. (From Burton GG: Patient assessment procedures, in Barnes TA (ed): *Respiratory Care Practice*. Chicago, Mosby, 1988. Used by permission.)

easily become hypothermic. Special attention must be paid to keeping them at normal body temperature.

The other vital signs will be discussed.

2. Review the admission orders and the current respiratory care orders. (IA1b) [R]

Physician orders must have the patient's name, date, time, complete and proper orders for each therapeutic procedure, and the physician's signature.

Example:

Patient's name: Jane Doe (Note: Confirm the patient's identification number in the chart.)

Date: January 30, 1991.

Time: 2:30 P.M.

Order 1: 35% oxygen by venturi-type mask. Keep on the patient at all times.

Order 2: Nebulize 0.5 ml of 1% Bronkosol with 3 ml of normal saline by a hand-held nebulizer for 15 minutes or until empty every 3 hours.

Order 3: Perform percussion and postural drainage to the lower portion of the right lower lobe every 4 hours while awake.

Fred Jones, M.D.

Verbal orders from the physician to the nurse or respiratory therapist must follow hospital guidelines and include the above. Incomplete, improper, or questionable orders must be confirmed by calling the physician for clarification or correction.

3. Review the progress notes for the patient. (IA1c) [R]

Review the physician's, nurses', and respiratory therapist's patient progress notes before seeing the patient and beginning the therapeutic procedure. Look for any cardiopulmonary or other organ system changes that will have an impact on the patient's ability to take the treatment. You may need to revise the therapy, get different equipment, or seek help.

Check for new patient care orders if the physician notes a change in the patient's care plan.

Decreased hemoglobin and hematocrit values indicate that the patient is anemic. This patient has less oxygen carrying capacity, which places more stress on the heart during exercise. Hypoxemia from a cardiopulmonary abnormality places this patient at great risk.

Increased hemoglobin and hematocrit values indicate that the patient is polycythemic. Usually this is a response to chronic hypoxemia from chronic obstructive pulmonary disease (COPD). This patient is also at risk. The thickened blood causes an increased afterload for the heart to pump against. These patients are also more prone to have blood clots.

When reviewing the white blood cell (WBC) count analysis, look for an elevated count as a sign of the body's reaction to a bacterial infection. The laboratory report may note a left shift in the types of WBCs. This would indicate that the body is releasing immature WBCs in an attempt to combat the acute, serious bacterial infection. A pulmonary infection is often identified by an increase in sputum that is thick, is changed in color from the normal clear or white to yellow or green, and/or has a putrid smell.

In the neonate, the most useful indicator of bacterial infection is neutropenia, that is, when the neutrophil count is less than 7800 in the first 60 hours of life or less than 1750 afterward. Initially, the average normal neutrophil count is 11,000.

Patients with acquired immunodeficiency syndrome (AIDS) or other immunodeficiencies may show a low or normal WBC count while having a bacterial infection.

4. Review the results of the patient's pulmonary function tests and arterial blood gas analysis. (IA1d) [R, Ap]

See Section 3 for the details of blood gases.

See Section 4 for the details of pulmonary function values.

In general, it is important to look for these values before seeing the patient. They can give much information about the seriousness of the patient's condition.

When working with a patient, if it is believed that important information can be gained by these tests, they should be suggested. Write suggestions and their justifications in the respiratory care progress notes area so that the physician will see them. If possible, also directly relay suggestions to the physician, nurse, or next shift's therapist so that they can be investigated.

5. Review the patient's chest x-ray findings. (IA1e) [R, Ap]

Findings reported in the patient's chart may be interpreted as follows:

a. Air is present in the pleural space—pneumothorax.

b. Air is present in the pericardial space—pneumopericardium.

c. Air is present below the diaphragm—pneumoperitonium.

d. Air is present in the soft tissues (usually axilla and neck)—transcutaneous emphysema.

e. White areas in the lungs—consolidation, fluid in the lungs from pneumonia, or congestive heart failure with pulmonary edema.

f. White coloration in the pleural space—fluid in the pleural space.

g. Ground glass appearance in the lungs—neonatal respiratory distress syndrome in premature infants with generalized atelectasis.

h. Intestine found in the chest with a flat abdomen—congenital diaphragmatic hernia in the newborn or traumatic diaphragmatic rupture.

i. Raised hemidiaphragm(s)—atelectasis.

j. Flattened hemidiaphragms with wide rib spacings—hyperinflation from chronic obstructive lung disease or asthma.

Chest x-ray films should be recommended in the following situations:

a. After an endotracheal tube has been placed or repositioned.

b. When a pneumothorax is suspected. That is, the patient may show one or more of the following: sudden chest pain with an increase in dyspnea and shortness of breath, absent breath sounds over a lung field, tracheal deviation, asymetrical chest movement, and/or air in the soft tissues.

c. After a chest tube has been placed in the pleural space to remove air or fluids.

d. Hemoptysis (bloody sputum).

6. View the patient's chest x-ray film to find the position of the endotracheal or tracheostomy tube. (IB5) [R, Ap]

These findings would be interpreted as follows:

a. Endotracheal tube tip positioned in the trachea above the carina and below the larynx—the tube is properly placed.

b. Endotracheal tube tip positioned in the right mainstem bronchus—the tube is down too far and needs to be pulled back into the trachea.

c. Tracheostomy tube is in mid-line with the trachea, above the carina, and below the larynx—the tube is properly placed.

7. Review the results of monitoring the following respiratory parameters: (IA1f1) [R, Ap]

a. Review the patient's respiratory rate.

The respiratory rate (*f* for frequency) is the number of breaths the patient takes in a minute. The number is counted by looking at or feeling the chest and/or abdominal movements. The normal rate varies with age, as seen in Table 1-1. It is assumed that the patient is resting but awake and has a normal temperature and metabolic rate. A respiratory rate that is above or below normal should be a cause for alarm.

Hyperthermia (fever), acidemia, hypoxemia, fear, anxiety, and pain will cause a patient to breathe more rapidly. Hypothermia, alkalemia, hyperoxia in the patient breathing on hypoxic drive, sedation, and coma will cause a patient to breathe more slowly.

It must be remembered that even in healthy people there is considerable variation in the respiratory rate. It is best to consider the respiratory rate along with the patient's tidal volume and minute volume in order to have a more complete impression of how the patient is breathing.

Carefully measure the respiratory rate of any patient with cardiopulmonary disease or with a respiratory rate outside of the normal range. The rate should be checked as often as needed to monitor the patient's condition.

b. Review the patient's tidal volume.

The tidal volume (V_T) is the volume of gas breathed out with each respiratory cycle. It should be appropriate for the patient's size and metabolic rate. (See Section 4 for more detail.)

A tidal volume that is too shallow will not allow for the exhalation of enough carbon dioxide (causing acidemia) or inhalation of enough oxygen (causing hypoxemia). Atelectasis can also occur. A tidal volume that is too large will blow off too much carbon dioxide and cause alkalemia. The tidal volume should be evaluated by itself and along with the patient's respiratory rate and minute volume.

Carefully measure the tidal volume of any patient who has unstable cardiopulmonary disease, neuromuscular disease that affects the patient's breathing, or any other condition that may affect the patient's ability to breathe. The tidal volume should be measured as often as needed to monitor the patient's condition.

c. Review the patient's minute volume.

The minute volume ($\dot{V}_E$) is the volume of gas exhaled in 1 minute. It should be appropriate for the patient's size and metabolic rate. (See Section 4 for more detail.) The minute volume is the product of the patient's respiratory rate and tidal volume.

Table 1-1. Normal Resting Respiratory Rates

Age (yr)	Male	Female
0-1	31 ± 8	30 ± 6
1-2	26 ± 4	27 ± 4
2-3	25 ± 4	25 ± 3
5-6	22 ± 2	21 ± 2
9-10	19 ± 2	19 ± 2
13-14	19 ± 2	18 ± 2
15-16	17 ± 3	18 ± 3
17-18	16 ± 3	17 ± 3
Older	16 ± 3	17 ± 3

From Eubanks DH, Bone RC: *Comprehensive Respiratory Care,* ed 2. St Louis, Mosby, 1990. Used by permission.

The minute volume should be evaluated by itself and along with the patient's respiratory rate and tidal volume. This is because the minute volume can be normal even though the breathing rate and tidal volume are abnormal.

Example:

Normal patient: $f = 12$, tidal volume $= 500$ ml
minute volume $= 12 \times 500$ ml $= 6000$ ml
Tachypneic patient: $f = 24$, tidal volume $= 250$ ml
minute volume $= 24 \times 250$ ml $= 6000$ ml
Bradypneic patient: $f = 6$, tidal volume $= 1000$ ml
minute volume $= 6 \times 1000$ ml $= 6000$ ml

These may be somewhat extreme examples, but they show the need to evaluate all three breathing parameters at the same time.

A low minute volume may result in hypoventilation with carbon dioxide retention, acidemia, hypoxemia, and atelectasis. A high minute volume may result in hyperventilation and alkalemia.

Recommend a minute volume measurement in any patient with cardiopulmonary disease, neuromuscular disease that affects the patient's breathing, or any condition that may affect the patient's ability to breathe.

d. Review the patient's inspiratory time to expiratory time ratio.

This is the ratio of the patient's inspiratory time to expiratory time. It varies considerably depending on the patient's respiratory rate and pulmonary condition. See Module D, 12, for details and graphs.

e. Review the patient's maximum inspiratory pressure.

The maximum inspiratory pressure (MIP) is the amount of vacuum that a patient can create against an obstruction. Some authors refer to this test as the negative inspiratory force (NIF). It is a measurement of the strength of the patient's inspiratory muscles of respiration. (See Section 4 for more detail.)

This test is commonly ordered for patients who are weakened by a neuromuscular disease, having mechanical ventilation discontinued, or having mechanical ventilation initiated. Recommend a maximum inspiratory pressure for any patient who has an abnormal respiratory rate, tidal volume, and/or minute volume; appears abnormally weak and fatigued, or who has a worsening neuromuscular disease.

f. Review the maximum expiratory force.

The maximum expiratory force (MEF) is the amount of positive pressure that a patient can generate when blowing out against an obstruction. It is a measure of the strength of the patient's expiratory muscles of respiration. (See Section 4 for more detail.) The test would be indicated in patients with the same kinds of conditions as discussed with the maximum inspiratory force test.

g. Review the patient's vital capacity.

The vital capacity (VC) is the maximum amount of air that the patient can breathe out after the lungs have been completely filled. (See Section 4 for more detail.) It is necessary for the patient to have an adequate vital capacity in order to be able to cough out secretions. An adequate vital capacity is also needed in order to open up atelectatic areas.

Recommend a vital capacity measurement in any patient with excessive secretions. A vital capacity measurement is also needed in any patient who is being weaned off of a mechanical ventilator, for whom mechanical ventilation is being considered, or who has a worsening neuromuscular condition.

h. Pulse oximetry (Sp_{O_2}). (IA1f2) [R, Ap]

Pulse oximetry is a noninvasive measurement of the saturation of hemoglobin with oxygen by use of a pulse oximeter device. It is a fast and simple way to find out if the patient is adequately oxygenated. (See Section 3 for more detail.) Suggest pulse oximetry in any patient (except those with known or suspected carbon monoxide poisoning) who has clinical signs or symptoms of hypoxemia, recently been given supplemental oxygen, or had a change in the delivered oxygen percentage. Usually an Sp_{O_2} of 90% or greater is desired.

8. Review the results of monitoring the following hemodynamic parameters: (IA1g) [R, Ap]

a. Review the patient's blood pressure.

The blood pressure (BP) is the result of the pumping ability of the left ventricle (made up of the heart rate and stroke volume), arterial resistance, and blood volume. Normal blood pressure is caused by all three factors being in balance against each other. If one factor is abnormal, the other two have some ability to compensate. For example, if the patient has lost a lot of blood, the body attempts to maintain blood pressure by increasing the arterial resistance and increasing the heart rate.

Normal Blood Pressures:

Adult: 120/80 mm Hg
Infant to a child of less than 10 years: 60-100/20-70 mm Hg

As with the other vital signs, there is some variation of blood pressure among individuals. It is important to know what the patient's normal blood pressure is in order to compare it with the current value. Carefully measure the blood pressure in any patient who has cardiopulmonary disease or a history of hypotension or hypertension.

Hypotension in the adult is a systolic blood pressure of less than 80 mm Hg. Recommend a blood pressure measurement in any patient who has a history of hypotension, appears to be in shock, has lost a lot of blood, has a weak pulse, shows mental confusion, is unconscious, or has low urine output.

Hypertension in the adult is a systolic blood pressure of 140 mm Hg or greater and/or a diastolic blood pressure of 90 mm Hg or greater. Carefully measure the blood pressure of any patient with a history of hypertension, bounding pulse, or symptoms of a stroke (mental confusion, headache, and sudden weakness or partial paralysis). Fear, anxiety, and pain will also cause the patient's blood pressure to temporarily rise.

b. Review the results of the patient's heart/pulse rate.

The heart/pulse rate (HR) is the number of heartbeats per minute. It can be counted by listening to the heart tones with a stethoscope or by feeling any of the common sites where an artery is easy to locate. (See Module E for more detail.) Table 1-2 shows the normal pulse rates based on age. It is assumed that the patient is alert but resting when the pulse is counted. Carefully measure the heart/pulse rate in any patient with cardiopulmonary disease or any of the aforementioned conditions for hypotension or hypertension.

Table 1-2. Normal Pulse Rates According to Age

Age	Beats per Min
Birth	70-170
Neonate	120-140
1 yr	80-140
2 yr	80-130
3 yr	80-120
4 yr	70-115
Adult	60-100

From Eubanks DH, Bone RC: *Comprehensive Respiratory Care*, ed 2. St Louis, Mosby, 1990. Used by permission.

Module B. Talk to the patient in layman's (nonmedical) terms whenever possible to achieve the best results from the treatment or procedure. (IIIA1) [R, Ap]

Avoid using technical and medical terms except if the patient has a medical background or tells you that he or she wants to know the specifics of what you are doing. Generally, it is best to describe the procedure in layman's terms that do not demean the intelligence of the patient.

Describe the procedure in steps rather than tell about the whole process from beginning to end. Demonstrate each step for the patient. Ask the patient for any questions; answer them or redemonstrate. Coach the patient to perform the step; correct any problems. Describe and demonstrate the next step until the procedure is completed.

Module C. *Interview* the patient to answer the following questions:

1. What is the patient's level of consciousness? (IB4a) [R, Ap, An]

One common way to evaluate a patient's level of consciousness is to categorize him or her as alert, stuporous, semicomatose, or comatose as follows:

a. *Alert.* This is the normal mental state. The patient is conscious or can be fully awakened from sleep by calling his or her name. The patient can voluntarily ask logical questions and answer questions logically. The conversation is relevant to the topic under discussion. The patient's movements and actions are willful and purposeful.

Example of a Conversation:

Introduce yourself, your department, and what you are there for, as usual.

Ask the patient, "Are you Mr. Jones?" or "What is your name?" He should answer your question in an appropriate way.

Ask, "Can I see your wristband for identification?" He should show it to you.

Tell him, "I am here to draw a sample of blood to check your oxygen level. Can I feel the pulse in your left wrist?" He should offer his left wrist to you.

Mr. Jones asks, "Is it going to hurt a lot? The last one was hard to get!"

b. *Stuporous/very lethargic.* The patient is sleepy or seems to be in a trance. He or she can be aroused to respond with willful, purposeful movements and actions but the patient may be slow. The patient may not respond to questions in a totally appropriate way.

Example of a Conversation:

Introduce yourself, your department, and what you are there for, as usual.
Ask the patient, "Are you Mr. Jones?" or "What is your name?" No answer.
Ask again more loudly, "Are you Mr. Jones?" No answer.
Say more loudly and with a gentle shaking of the shoulder, "Mr. Jones!"
He becomes more alert, looks at you, and asks, "Who are you?"

c. *Semicomatose.* The patient does not perform requested movements or actions. The patient will not answer questions in an appropriate way. He or she will respond defensively to pain. For example, if the right arm is pinched, it will be withdrawn.

Posturing of semicomatose patients includes the following:

1. Decerebrate—legs are extended; arms are extended and rotated either inward or outward.
2. Decorticate—legs are extended; arms are flexed, and the forearms may be rotated either inward or outward.
3. Opisthotonic—legs, arms, and neck are extended, and the body is arched forward.

d. *Comatose/coma.* The patient has no spontaneous-oriented responses to the environment. Pain causes no defensive movement, but there may be an increase in the heart and respiratory rates.

Another common way to evaluate a patient's level of consciousness is to make use of the Glasgow coma scale. With this scale of 3 to 15, the larger the total number, the more normal the patient. A score of 15 is achieved in a patient normally awake and alert; a

Table 1-3. Glasgow Coma Scale

Test Parameter	Response	Score*
Eyes		
Open	Spontaneously	4
	To verbal command	3
	To pain	2
	No response	1
Best motor response		
To verbal command	Obeys command	6
Moves arms to painful stimulus of knuckles against sternum	Localizes pain	5
	Flexion—withdrawal	4
	Flexion—abnormal movement (decorticate rigidity)	3
	Extension—abnormal movement (decerebrate rigidity)	2
	No response	1
Best verbal response (may arouse by painful stimulus if necessary)		
	Oriented and converses	5
	Disoriented and converses	4
	Inappropriate words used	3
	Incomprehensible sounds	2
	No response	1

From *Apache II: A Severity of Disease Classification System.* ICU Research Unit, Washington, DC; product information from Upjohn, Kalamazoo, MI.
*The total is obtained by adding the scores in all three areas. The range is 3 to 15.

score of 3 would be found in an unresponsive patient. See Table 1-3 for details of the scale.

2. Is the patient oriented to time, place, and person? (IB4b) [R, Ap]

a. *Time.* Ask the patient, "Do you know what day of the week it is? Do you know what the date is?" (The patient must be able to see a calendar.) "Do you know what time it is?" (The patient must be able to see a clock.) If the patient can answer these questions, he or she is oriented to time. If not, inform and show him or her. Tell the patient that you will return at a certain time. Ask the same questions when you return.

b. *Place.* Ask the patient, "Do you know where you are?" If the patient knows, he or she is oriented to place. If not, inform the patient of the hospital's name and nursing care unit. Tell the patient that you will return at a certain time. Ask the same question when you return.

c. *Person.* Ask the patient, "Do you know who the President (or the physician) is?" If not, inform the patient. Tell the patient who you are and what your job is. When you return for your next treatment ask the patient if he remembers who you are and what you do. If the patient remembers who the President (or the physician) is and your name or job, he or she is oriented to person.

Orienting the stuporous/very lethargic patient to person, place, and time may help to get him or her to cooperate more in his or her care. Pain-relieving and sedative drugs, stroke, injury to or edema of the brain, and other illnesses may cause disorientation.

3. What is the patient's emotional state? (IB4c) [R, Ap, An]

A number of authors have approached this subject from varying points of view. Table 1-4 represents a presentation of a patient's reaction to chronic illness. Substitute "respiratory care practitioners" for "nurses" as needed.

A patient's statements and actions that indicate the *disbelief* stage of adaptation include the following:

- "I don't have that." (Fill in the disease or condition.)
- "There is nothing really wrong with me."

Table 1-4. Teaching-Learning Process in Adaptation to Chronic Illness

Stages of Adaptation	Patient's Behavior	Nurse's Behavior	Nurse's Facilitation of the Teaching-Learning Process
Disbelief	Denial of threatening condition to protect self and conserve energy: Refuses to accept diagnosis. May claim to have something else. May behave so as to avoid the issue. May seem to accept diagnosis but avoid feeling about it.	Allows patient to deny illness as he needs to. Functions as noncritical listener: Accepts patient's statements of how he feels. Helps clarify patient's statements. Does not point out reality.	Orients all teaching to the present, not to tomorrow or next week. Teaches as she does other nursing activities. Assesses patient's level of anxiety. Assures patient that he is safe and being observed carefully. Explains all procedures and activities to the patient. Gives clear, concise explanations. Coordinates activities to include rest periods.

Stages of Adaptation	Patient's Behavior	Nurse's Behavior	Nurse's Facilitation of the Teaching-Learning Process
Developing awareness	Uses anger as a defense against being dependent and against guilt about being sick.	Listens to patient's expressions of anger and recognizes them for what they are. Explores own feelings about illness and helplessness. Does not argue with patient. Gives dependable care with an attitude that it is necessary.	Does not give anxious patient long lists of facts. Continues development of trust and rapport through good physical care. Orients teaching to present. Explains symptoms, care, and treatment in terms of the fact that they are necessary *now*. Does not mention long-range care needs.
Reorganization	Accepts increased dependence and reorganizes relationships with significant others. Patient's family may also use denial while they adapt to what patient's illness means to them.	Establishes climate in which family and friends can express feelings about patient's illness. Does not solve patient's problems, but helps build communication so that patient and family can work together to solve problems.	Assures family that patient is all right and safe. Uses clear, concise explanations. Does not argue about need for care.
Resolution	Acknowledges changes seen in self. Identifies with others with same problem.	Encourages expression of feelings, including crying. Understands own feelings of loss.	Brings groups of patients with same illness together for group discussions. Has recovered patient visit patient. Teaches patient what he wants to learn (or perceives he needs to learn) first.
Identity change	Defines self as an individual who has undergone change and is now different. "There are limits to my life because I have a disease."	Understands own feelings about patient's becoming independent again.	Realizes that as patient's own perceived needs are met, more mature (more progressive) needs will surface. Is prepared to answer patient's questions as they arise.
Successful adaptation	Can live comfortably or resignedly with himself as a person who has a specific condition.	Initiates closure of nurse-patient relationship.	Has helped develop a relationship with the patient in which the nurse is a guide that the patient can consult when he wishes.

From Kenner CV, Guzzetta CE, Dossey BM: *Critical Care Nursing: Body-Mind-Spirit*. Boston, Little, Brown, 1981. Used by permission.

- "The laboratory results are wrong."
- "The equipment is faulty."
- "The doctor/nurse/therapist is incompetent."
- Refusal to take medications.
- Refusal to take treatments or follow other physician orders.

A patient's statements and actions that indicate the *developing awareness* state of adaptation include the following:

- "The doctor/nurse/therapist doesn't know what he/she is doing."
- "It's all their fault."
- "Why is this happening to me?"
- The patient is angry about his or her illness.
- The patient may strike out verbally or physically at staff members.
- Some patients who do not get angry will withdraw into a depression and wish to be left alone.

A patient's statements and actions that indicate that he or she is progressing from the *reorganization* to the *successful adaptation* stage include the following:

- "I'll never be able to do that again." (Fill in the activity.)
- "I have to get on with my life."
- "At least I'm still alive and can do this for myself."
- The patient may be sad and cry often.
- The patient may invent a nickname for his/her defect or diseased body part.
- The patient accepts the disability and focuses on his or her abilities.
- The patient works with family and others in planning for the future.

4. What is the patient's ability to cooperate? (IB4d) [R, Ap]

You should be able to judge the patient's ability to cooperate. It should be based on his or her responses to your questions on level of consciousness; orientation to time, place, and person; and emotional state. An alert patient should be able to understand and follow directions. He or she should be able to take an effective treatment or cooperate in a procedure. On the other hand, if the patient truly refuses the treatment or procedure, it should not be forced. Contact the patient's nurse and/or physician about the refusal. The physician must then decide what to do.

An alert but fearful or anxious patient may be unable to fully cooperate until he or she is calmed by understanding who you are, what you are there to do, and why the treatment or procedure is important. Try to reassure the patient in order to improve cooperation.

If the patient appears alert but does not follow what you are saying, check to see whether he or she is deaf or does not speak English. An effective way to communicate must be found. Writing materials, a picture board, or a sign language interpreter will be needed with a deaf patient. A native language translator will be needed with a patient who does not speak English.

The stuporous/very lethargic patient may be aroused by talking more loudly or by gentle shaking. He or she may or may not be able to cooperate fully. The practitioner may have to modify the treatment plan or how it is given to compensate for the patient's lack of cooperation.

Pain relievers and sedatives may make a normal, alert patient seem stuporous. If the patient has not been medicated, check with the nurse or physician to see what may have recently changed in the patient's condition.

A semicomatose patient may present the greatest problems in providing treatment or performing a procedure. These patients will not cooperate in any way. Additionally, some of their involuntary body posturings make correct positioning impossible. You will likely have to modify your equipment or procedure because of the patient's inability to cooperate.

A comatose patient will not cooperate in any procedure or treatment but is unlikely

Table 1-5. Severity of Dyspnea in Evaluating Permanent Impairment

Class I	Class II	Class III	Class IV	Class V
Dyspnea only on severe exertion ("appropriate" dyspnea)	Can keep pace with person of same age and body build on the level without breathlessness, but not on hills or stairs	Can walk a mile at own pace without dyspnea, but cannot keep pace on the level with a normal person	Dyspnea present after walking about 100 yd on the level or upon climbing one flight of stairs	Dyspnea on even less activity or even at rest

From Burton GG: Practical physical diagnosis in respiratory care, in Burton GG, Hodgkin JE (eds): *Respiratory Care: A Guide to Clinical Practice,* ed 2. Philadelphia, Lippincott, 1984. Used by permission.

to fight against you either. You will have to modify your equipment or procedure because of the patient's inability to cooperate.

It is important to treat all patients with dignity no matter what their level of consciousness. Talk to every patient the same way. Explain who you are, what you are there to do, and why the treatment or procedure is important for the patient.

5. Does the patient complain of dyspnea and/or orthopnea? (IB4e) [R, Ap]

Dyspnea is the patient's subjective feeling of shortness of breath (SOB) or labored breathing. This is normal after vigorous exercise but abnormal when seen in a resting patient. Orthopnea is the condition in which a patient must sit erect or stand in order to breathe comfortably. Lying flat causes dyspnea.

Table 1-5 classifies the degrees of dyspnea, and Table 1-6 lists different kinds of dyspnea, including orthopnea. Only class I is normal dyspnea (on severe exertion). Classes

Table 1-6. Causes of Dyspnea Related to Preferred Body Position

Kind of Dyspnea	Clinical Correlations
Orthopnea (must sit up to breathe; often occurs at night as paroxysmal nocturnal dyspnea)	Congestive heart failure
Obstructive sleep apnea (periodically stops breathing, particularly when lying on back)	Obesity—obstructive sleep apnea syndromes
Emphysematous habitus	COPD*
Platypnea	Pleural effusion, dyspnea associated with various body positions
Orthodeoxia	Pulmonary fibrosis, dyspnea is improved when patient is lying flat

From Burton GG: Patient assessment procedures, in Barnes TA (ed): *Respiratory Care Practice.* Chicago, Mosby, 1990. Used by permission.
*COPD, Chronic obstructive pulmonary disease

II to V are progressively severe and limiting for the patient. Any orthopnea is abnormal, and the more the patient must sit up to breathe, the more limited the patient.

Ask the patient the following kinds of questions to evaluate dyspnea:

- "How far can you walk before you feel SOB?"
- "How many flights of stairs can you climb before you become SOB?"
- "How far can you walk when walking as fast as your spouse?"
- "Is there anything you do that makes the SOB *worse?*"
- "Is there anything you do that makes the SOB *better?*"
- "How long does the SOB last after you stop to rest?"
- "Is the SOB worse at any particular time of the *day?*"
- "Is the SOB worse at any particular time of the *year?* "

Ask the following kinds of questions to evaluate the patient's orthopnea:

- "Do you wake up at night with shortness of breath?"
- "Does your nighttime SOB get better after you sit up on the side of your bed or in a chair?"
- "Do you get SOB when lying down to take a nap?"
- "Do you use extra pillows behind your head and back to help you not get SOB at night or during a nap?"
- "How many pillows do you need to keep you from getting SOB at night or when taking a nap?"

6. What is the patient's sputum production like? (IB4f) [R, Ap]

A. Time of maximum and minimum expectoration. Interview the patient to determine the following:
   1. Time of maximum expectoration. Ask the patient, "When do you cough up the most? For example, is it in the morning; after eating spicy foods; after a breathing treatment; after smoking, work, or other exposure to dusts; etc."
   2. Time of minimum expectoration. Ask the patient, "When do you cough up the least? For example, during certain nonallergic seasons of the year, after a breathing treatment, after consuming milk or milk products, etc."

B. Quantity. Some practioners prefer to know of a specific amount such as a teaspoon, tablespoon, 10 ml, etc. Others prefer to use subjective measures such as "a little" or "a lot." Interview the patient to determine the following:
   1. How the quantity of sputum relates to the times of maximum and minimum expectoration and the patient's life-style. Ask the patient, "Is there anything that you do that increases or decreases the amount you cough out?" For example, the patient states that he coughs up 20 ml after breathing treatments but can cough up nothing after eating a bowl of ice cream.
   2. Whether the amount coughed up changes in a cyclical way? Ask the patient, "Do you cough up the most in the mornings or at night? Is there a work or life-style habit that changes how much you cough up? Is there a seasonal allergic condition that influences your asthma and sputum production?"

C. Adhesiveness of the sputum. Interview the patient to determine the following:
   1. "Are there times of the day or things that you do in the day that seem to result in your secretions becoming thicker or thinner?"
   2. "Do your medications (like acetylcysteine) make the secretions easier to cough out?"
   3. "Are there foods that make your secretions easier to cough out?"

7. What is the patient's work of breathing. (IB4g) [R, Ap, An]

Work of breathing refers to the patient's subjective feeling of how easy or difficult it is to breathe. A person at rest should feel no difficulty in breathing. During vigorous exercise a person should be aware that he or she is working harder than normal to breathe. This is to be expected. After recovering from exercise the work of breathing should again be easy.

Patients with acute or chronic lung disease will feel that they are breathing with some difficulty. If bronchospasm or secretions have increased, the patient will tell you that his or her work of breathing has worsened. If medications such as bronchodilators and/or mucolytics are effective, the patient should feel that his or her breathing is easier.

Module D. Determine the patient's complete respiratory condition in the following ways by *observation:*

1. Evaluate the patient's general appearance. (IB1a) [R, Ap]

Start by inspecting the patient quickly from head to toe including how he or she is dressed and found in the room. Ideally, this is done without the patient knowing that he or she is being observed. The patient who is not suffering from cardiopulmonary disease should be able to lie flat in bed or on either side without any breathing difficulty. The patient should appear to breathe comfortably without any undue effort. The patient with one-sided lung disease may prefer to lie with the good side down. This might be the case with lobar pneumonia, pleurisy, or broken ribs. The patient with severe airway obstruction as seen with asthma, bronchitis, or emphysema will tend to sit up in a chair or on the edge of the bed and use locked arms and shoulders for support. This enables the patient to use accessory muscles (Fig. 1-6). The patient with orthopnea will not want to lie down flat because of the resulting SOB. This is commonly seen in patients with congestive heart failure and pulmonary edema.

2. Determine if the patient is cyanotic. (IB1e) [R, Ap]

Cyanosis is an abnormal blue or ashen gray coloration of the skin and mucus membranes. It is most easily seen in white persons by looking at the lips and nail beds. It can be seen in darker-pigmented people by looking at the inner portion of the lip, the inner portion of the lower eyelid, or the nail beds. Commonly, it is said to be caused by hypoxemia and that the more bluish a patient's color the more hypoxemic he or she is. This is often the case, but cyanosis is *not* an accurate measurement of a patient's oxygenation.

Cyanosis occurs when more than 5 volumes percent (vol%) of hemoglobin is desaturated. This happens whenever an insufficient amount of oxygen is delivered to the skin and other tissues to meet its metabolic needs (as in cardiopulmonary arrest). However, there are three fairly common clinical situations during which cyanosis is not a good observational tool to judge the patient's oxygen level. First, an anemic patient may be hypoxic but not cyanotic. This could happen there was not enough hemoglobin to desaturate 5 vol%. Second, a polycythemic patient may appear cyanotic even though the patient is not hypoxic. This would be seen if there was more than 5 vol% of desaturated hemoglobin despite an acceptable Pa_{O_2}. Third, a patient in shock may have a normal Pa_{O_2} but be cyanotic because the blood pressure is low and not delivering the oxygen to the tissues. To be safe, a patient with cyanosis should have a blood gas sample drawn for Pa_{O_2} measurement or pulse oximetry performed for Sp_{O_2} measurement to evaluate oxygenation.

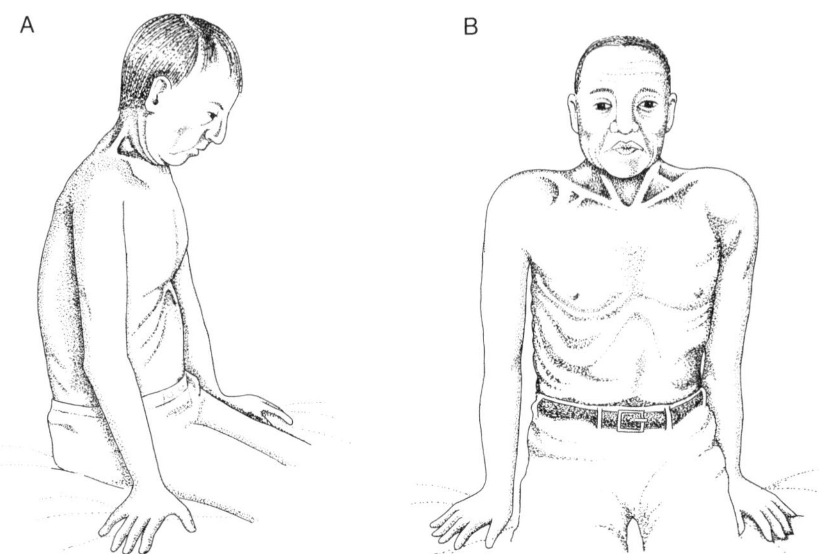

Fig. 1-6 Typical postures seen in patients using accessory muscles of respiration. In both postures, the shoulders are locked so that the accessory muscles can be used more effectively. (**A,** From Burton GG: Practical physical diagnosis in respiratory care, in Burton GG, Hodgkin JE (eds): *Respiratory Care,* ed 2. Philadelphia, Lippincott, 1984. **B** from Barriascout JR: Chest physical therapy and related procedures, in Burton GG, Hodgkin JE (eds): *Respiratory Care,* ed 2. Philadelphia, JB Lippincott, 1984. Used by permission.)

3. Determine if the patient is diaphoretic. (IB1c) [R, Ap]

Diaphoresis is profuse sweating. It is normally seen after vigorous exercise. You would expect to see a patient sweating after a stress test or even an oxygen-assisted walk. Diaphoresis in a patient who is resting in bed is a sign of serious trouble. When the body is severely stressed, it releases adrenaline into the blood stream. Diaphoresis is one many bodily effects caused by the release of adrenaline. Similar sweating may be seen if a large enough dose of epinephrine is given. (See Section 7—Pharmacology—for a more complete discussion of adrenaline/epinephrine.)

Diaphoresis is a nonspecific sign of serious cardiopulmonary difficulties. It may be seen any time the patient is in shock and/or hypoxemic. Patients suffering from a myocardial infarct are commonly diaphoretic. The practitioner should promptly evaluate the diaphoretic patient's pulse, respiratory rate, blood pressure, and arterial blood gases.

4. Determine if the patient has nasal flaring. (IB1l) [R, Ap]

Nasal flaring is a dilation of the nares on inspiration. A person breathing comfortably should have little or no nasal flaring. A person who is exercising vigorously may have it. It is abnormal to see nasal flaring in a patient who is resting in bed, and it is a sign of increased work of breathing. The patient is attempting to reduce airway resistance by dilating the nares. Patients of any age will have nasal flaring when experiencing an increased work of breathing, but it is most commonly seen in the premature newborn (Fig. 1-7).

Nasal flaring is not specific to any disease or condition. Examples of conditions during which nasal flaring is seen include infant respiratory distress syndrome, adult respiratory distress syndrome, or any condition in which pulmonary compliance is decreased or airway resistance is increased.

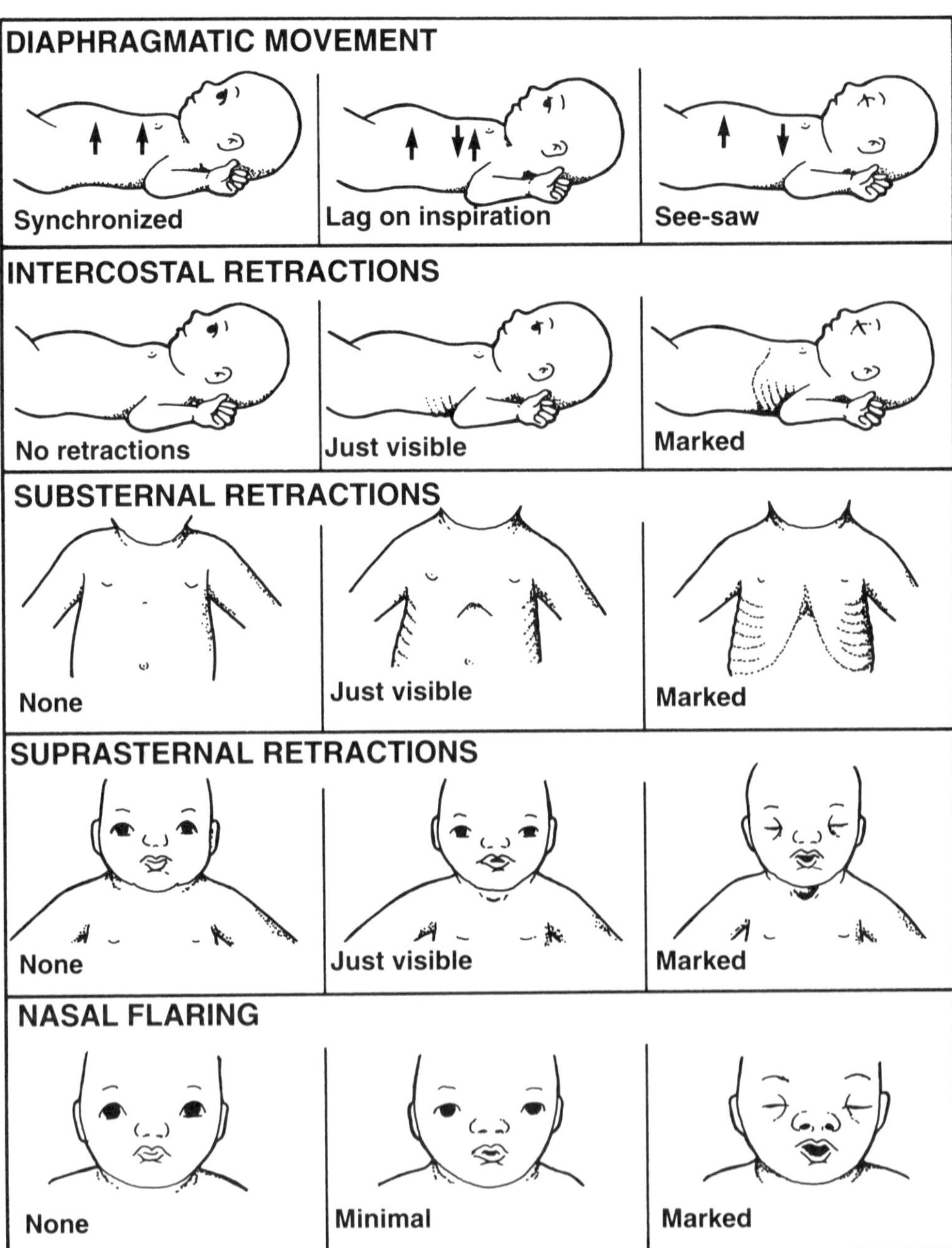

Fig. 1-7 Physical indications of labored breathing.

5. Determine if the patient has clubbing of the fingers. (IB1d) [R, Ap]

Clubbing of the fingers (also known as digital clubbing) is an abnormal thickening of the ends of the fingers. It can also occur in the toes. The key finding is an angle of more than 160 degrees between the top of the finger and the nail when seen from the side. Clinically, you will notice both a lateral and an anterioposterior thickening of the ends of

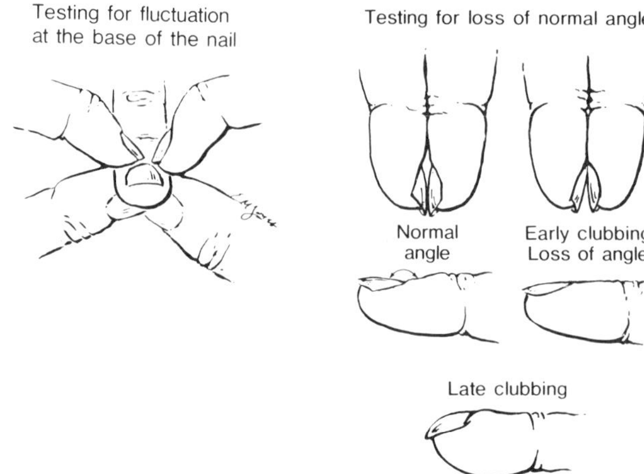

Fig. 1-8 Signs of and test for clubbing. (From Lehrer S: *Understanding Lung Sounds.* Philadelphia, WB Saunders, 1984. Used by permission.)

the fingers. See Fig. 1-8 for a comparison of normal to clubbed fingers. The finger and toenail beds may be cyanotic.

The underlying cause is not completely understood but at least in part seems to be chronic hypoxemia. This results in arteriovenous anastomosis with thickening of the tissues. The list of diseases in which clubbing is seen includes chronic obstructive pulmonary disease (COPD), bronchogenic carcinoma, bronchiectasis, sarcoidosis, and infective endocarditis.

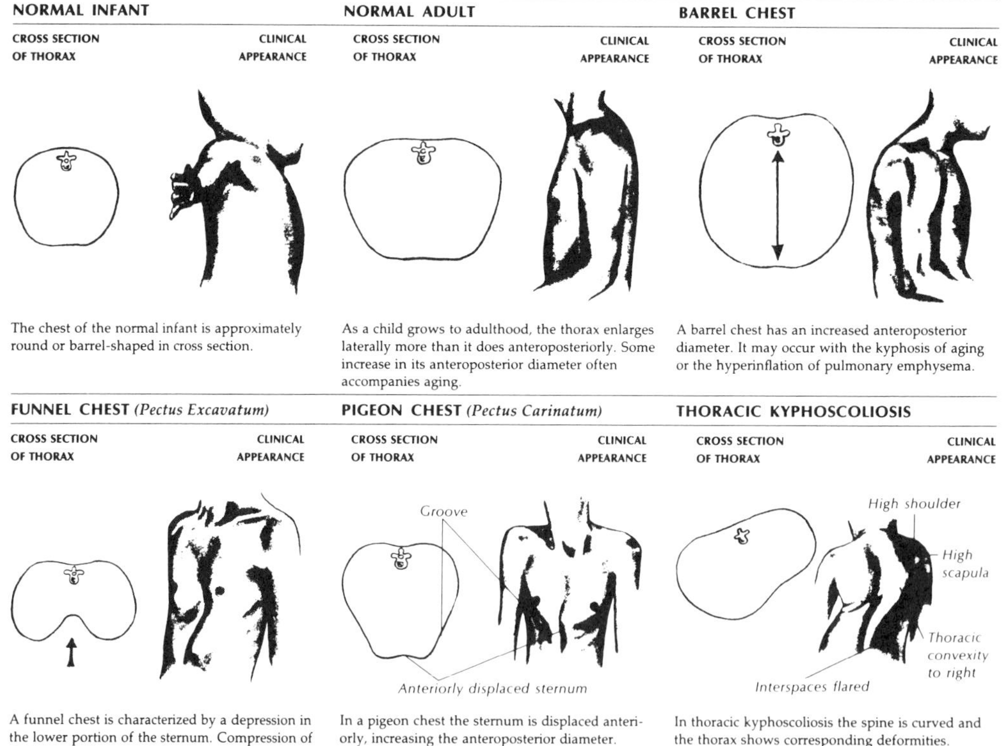

Fig. 1-9 Deformities of the thorax. (From Bates B: *A Guide to Physical Examination and History Taking,* ed. 4. Philadelphia, Lippincott, 1987. Used by permission.)

6. Determine if the patient has peripheral edema. (IB1b) [R, Ap]

Peripheral edema is seen when fluid leaks from the capillary bed into the tissues. It is most commonly seen in the ankles and feet or along the back when the patient is lying supine in bed. You measure the extent of the edema by pressing a finger into the tissues. Normal skin will spring back, whereas edematous skin will be pitted. The pitting edema is graded as plus 1 for 1 mm, plus 2 for 2 mm, etc., of indentation. Obviously, the deeper the pitting, the more peripheral edema the patient has.

Peripheral edema is most commonly seen in patients with congestive heart failure or those who have a fluid overload. Patients with septicemia will often have peripheral edema because the blood-borne pathogen (usually staphylococci) will cause abnormal capillary leakage.

7. Determine the shape of the patient's chest. (IB1f) [R, Ap]

The patient should be sitting up straight or standing erect when being examined for chest configuration. Look at the patient from the front, back, and both sides to see the symmetry. See Fig. 1-9 for the appearance of a normal infant's and adult's chest, barrel

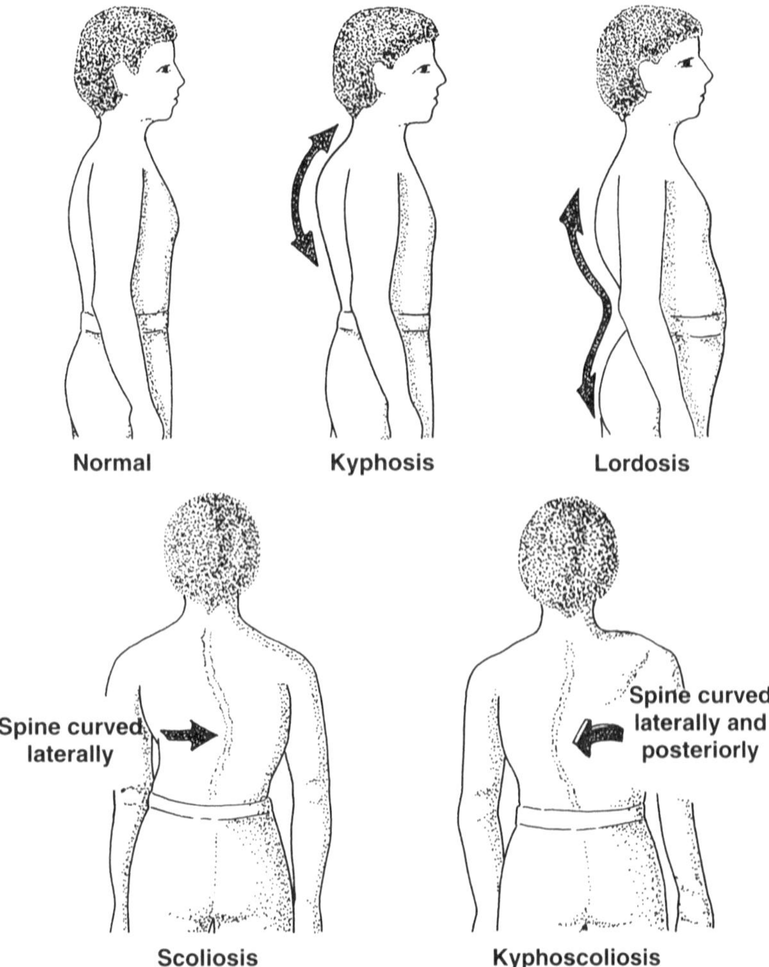

Fig. 1-10 Normal and abnormal spinal curves.

chest, funnel chest, pigeon chest, and thoracic kyphoscoliosis. Fig. 1-10 shows variations on curvature of the spine. Kyphosis is an exaggerated anterioposterior (AP) curvature of the upper portion of the spine. Lordosis is an exaggerated AP curvature of the lower portion of the spine. Scoliosis is either a right or left lateral curvature of the spine. Kyphoscoliosis is either a right or left lateral curvature combined with an AP curvature of the spine.

8. Determine if the patient has asymmetrical chest movement when breathing. (IB1j) [R, Ap, An]

A normal infant and adult will have symmetrical chest movement when breathing at rest or during exercise. All breathing efforts are best observed when the patient is shirtless. In females, it may be necessary to observe only the uncovered back to judge chest movement. Any kind of asymmetrical chest movement is abnormal. The asymmetrical movement may be from an abnormality of the chest wall or abdomen or from a pulmonary disorder.

Thoracic Scoliosis or Kyphoscoliosis.—Refer to Fig. 1-10 which shows the back view of these patients. The scoliosis patient would tend to have more chest movement on the right side because of the right spinal curvature. The left side of the chest and left lung would inflate more than the right if the spine curved to the left. These same findings would be seen in a patient with kyphoscoliosis.

Flail Chest.—The flail segment will move in the opposite direction from the rest of the chest (also known as paradoxical movement). That is, with inspiration, the flail segment will move inward while the rest of the chest moves outward, and during expiration the flail segment will move outward as the rest of the chest moves inward. As the ribs heal, the segment will stabilize and move with the rest of the chest.

Pneumothorax.—The side with the collapsed lung will not move as much as the chest wall over the normal lung (Fig. 1-11).

Atelectasis/Pneumonia.—The side with the atelectasis or pneumonia will not move as much as the chest wall over the normal lung (Fig. 1-11).

9. Determine if the patient has intercostal and/or sternal retractions when breathing. (IB1k) [R, Ap]

Intercostal retractions are noticed when the soft tissues between the ribs are drawn inward during inspiration as the chest wall moves outward (Fig. 1-7). Suprasternal retractions are noticed when the soft tissues *above* the sternum are drawn inward during an inspiration as the chest wall moves outward. Substernal retractions are noticed when the soft tissues *below* the sternum are drawn inward during an inspiration as the chest wall moves outward (see Fig. 1-7 for both).

A person who is breathing at rest should not have any retractions. That same person may have some minor retractions during vigorous exercise. Retractions of any kind are abnormal in any patient of any age who is resting in bed. Retractions are commonly seen in conditions where the airway resistance is increased or the lung compliance is decreased. Both will increase a patient's work of breathing. The patient must generate a more negative intrathoracic pressure to breathe, and as a result the various soft tissues are drawn inward during inspiration. Conditions in which this is seen include infant respiratory distress syndrome, adult respiratory distress syndrome, pulmonary edema, pneumonia, asthma, bronchitis, and emphysema.

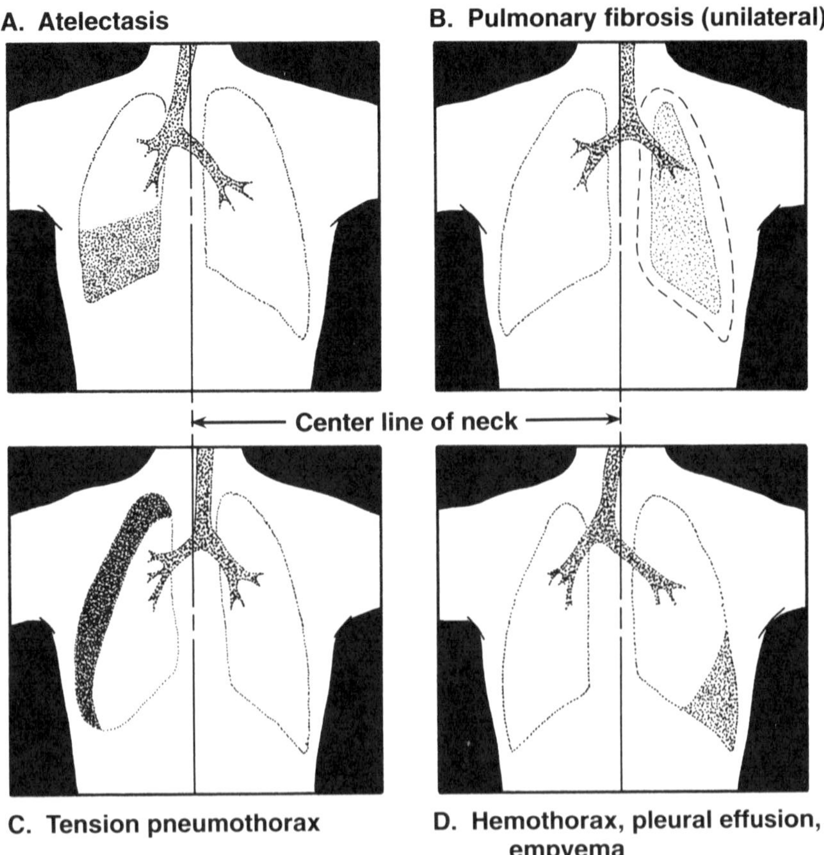

Fig. 1-11 A-D, Conditions causing tracheal deviation and asymmetrical chest movement. (Simulated chest x-ray findings.) The normal lung will expand more than the abnormal one during inspiration.

10. Determine if the patient uses accessory muscles when breathing. (IB1i) [R, Ap]

Accessory muscles of respiration should not be needed during passive, resting breathing. They may be used when breathing vigorously during exercise. A dyspneic patient will likely use them even when resting. The accessory muscles of inspiration are the intercostals, scalenes, sternocleidomastoids, trapezius, and rhomboids. The abdominal muscles are used during active expiration. The easiest accessory muscles of inspiration to observe in action are the sternocleidomastoids from the front and side of the patient and the trapezius from the back of the patient (Fig. 1-12).

Accessory muscle use in a patient who is resting should make you realize that the work of breathing is greatly increased. The finding is not specific for any one condition but is commonly seen in a patient with emphysema (Fig. 1-6).

11. Determine if the patient has diaphragmatic movement when breathing. (IB1g) [R, Ap]

Normally, an adult's diaphragm moves downward several centimeters toward the abdomen during inspiration as the chest wall moves outward. This is seen when the abdomen protrudes as its contents are forced forward. The chest and abdomen should rise and

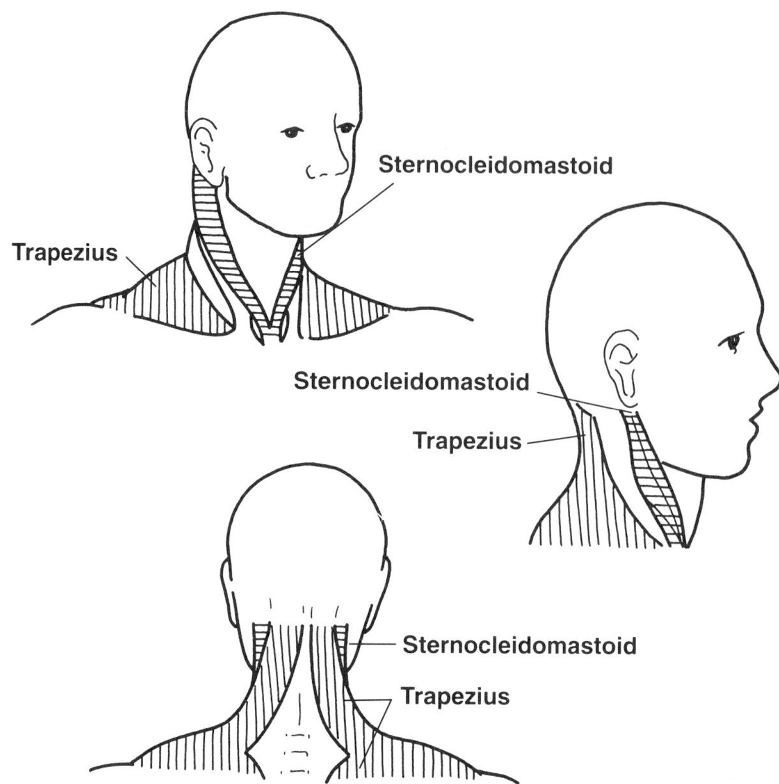

Fig. 1-12 The sternocleidomastoid and trapezius accessory muscles of respiration.

fall together during quiet and vigorous breathing efforts. There are two conditions in which this normal chest and abdominal movement does not occur.

Patients with emphysema, severe air trapping, and a barrel chest have diaphragms that are depressed and flat rather than domed because of the air that is trapped in the lungs. On inspiration, the diaphragm still contracts but is unable to displace the abdominal contents down to permit air to be drawn into the lungs. You will notice that these patients do not have the expected abdominal movement during inspiration. These patients will use the accessory muscles of inspiration to assist breathing.

Second is any condition in which the airway resistance is increased or lung compliance is decreased. The greater negative intrathoracic pressure needed to draw the tidal volume into the lungs can cause the chest wall to collapse inward as the abdominal contents are displaced outward. The result is a kind of "seesaw" or paradoxical movement relationship between the chest wall and abdomen. On inspiration the chest wall may move inward as the abdomen moves outward. This is most commonly seen in infant respiratory distress syndrome because the premature neonate's rib cage is relatively compliant when compared with the stiff lungs (Fig. 1-7).

12. Determine the patient's breathing pattern. (IB1h) [R, Ap]

The various respiratory patterns can be identified by their characteristic respiratory rate, respiratory cycle, and tidal volume as follows:

A. Eupnea (normal breathing). See Fig. 1-13.
   1. Normal respiratory rate for the age of the patient (see Table 1-1).
   2. Normal respiratory cycle. When timing the flow of air into and out of the lungs, the inspiratory: expiratory (I/E) ratio is 1:1.5 to 1:2. A pause of vari-

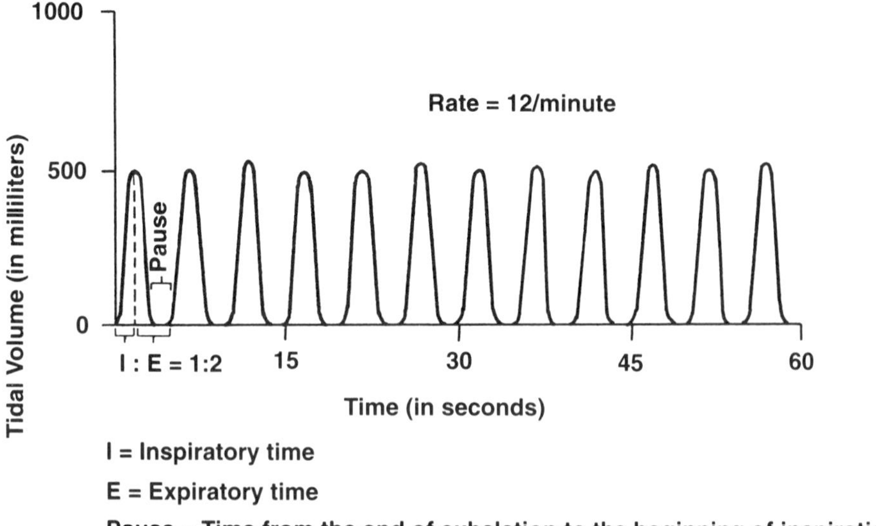

Fig. 1-13 Eupnea.

able time will follow exhalation of the tidal volume. This will change the true I/E ratio to 1:2 to 1:4.

3. Tidal volume normal for the size of the patient. (Tidal volume is discussed earlier in this section and in Section 4. Fig. 1-13 and the other figures relate to an average adult.) Inspiration is achieved without the use of accessory muscles of inspiration; exhalation is passive.

B. Hypopnea (shallow breathing). See Fig. 1-14.
   1. Respiratory rate usually somewhat slower than normal.
   2. Normal respiratory cycle.
   3. Tidal volume decreased for the size of the patient.
   4. Possible causes: deep sleep, sedation, coma, hypothermia, alkalemia, restrictive lung disease.
   5. May be combined with bradypnea.

C. Hyperpnea (deep breathing). See Fig. 1-15.
   1. Respiratory rate may be normal or somewhat faster.
   2. Normal respiratory cycle.
   3. Tidal volume increased for the size of the patient.

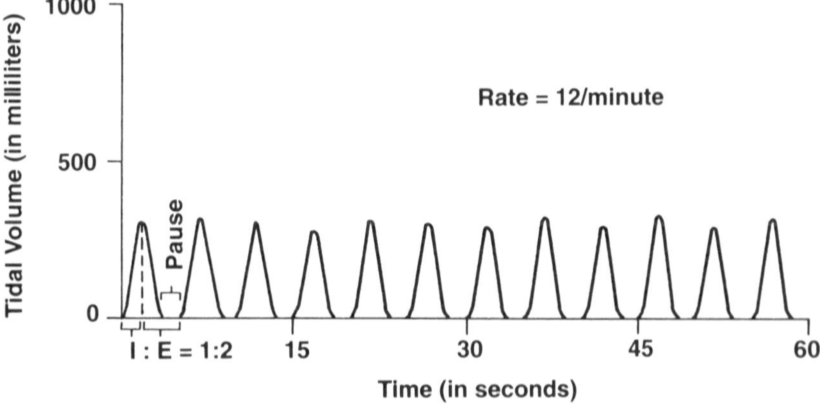

Fig. 1-14 Hypopnea.

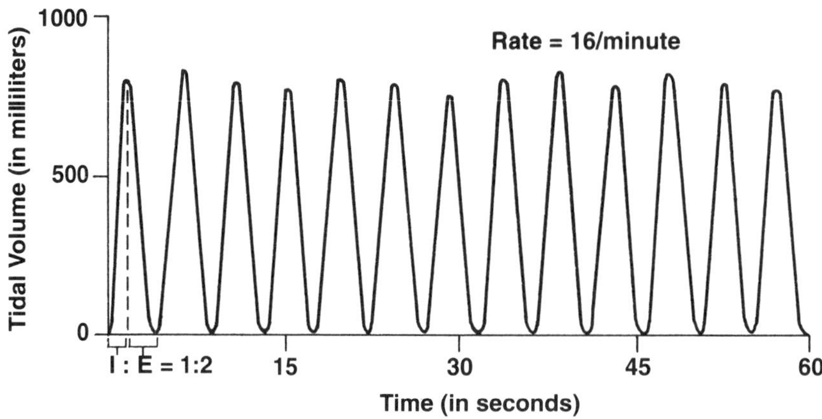

Fig. 1-15 Hyperpnea.

4. Possible causes: acidemia, fever, pain, fear, anxiety, increased intracranial pressure.
5. May be combined with tachypnea.

D. Bradypnea (slow breathing). See Fig. 1-16.
1. Slower-than-normal respiratory rate.
2. Expiration may be longer than normal as a result of a longer pause.
3. Tidal volume may be decreased for the size of the patient.
4. Possible causes: deep sleep, sedation, coma, hypothermia, alkalemia.
5. May be combined with hypopnea.

E. Tachypnea (rapid breathing). See Fig. 1-17.
1. Faster than the normal respiratory rate.
2. Inspiration may be faster than normal with the help of inspiratory accessory muscles. Expiration may be shorter than normal, and expiratory accessory muscles may be used to force the air out faster. The pause seen in eupnea will be gone. The I/E ratio may be 1:2 or less.
3. Tidal volume may be increased for the size of the patient.
4. Possible causes: acidemia, fever, pain, anxiety, increased intracranial pressure.
5. May be combined with hyperpnea.

F. Obstructed inspiration (Fig. 1-18).
1. Normal to slower respiratory rate.

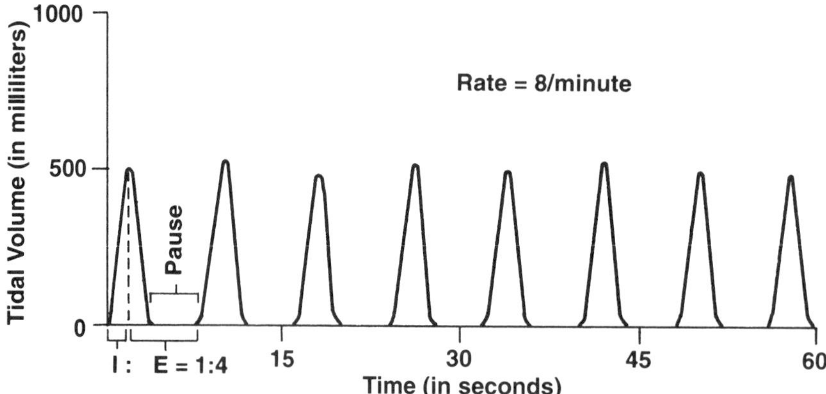

Fig. 1-16 Bradypnea.

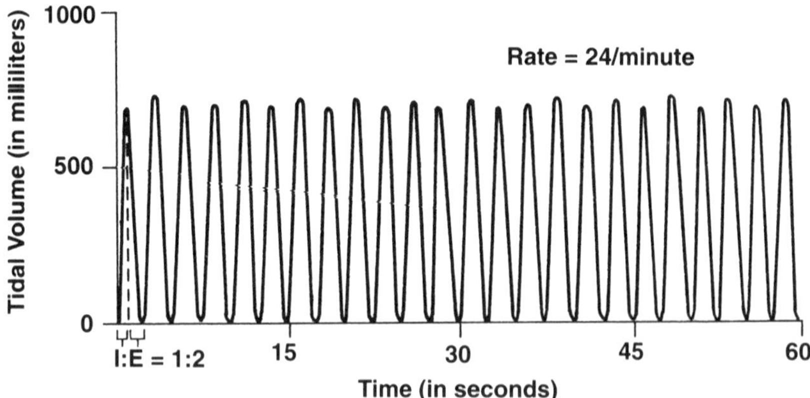

Fig. 1-17 Tachypnea.

2. Inspiratory time will be equal to or longer than expiratory time. Inspiration will be aided by use of the inspiratory accessory muscles. Expiration will be passive.
3. Tidal volume may be normal, larger, or smaller than normal depending on how the patient adapts to the increased work of breathing. It is most common to see a slower rate with a larger tidal volume.
4. Possible causes: croup, epiglottitis, foreign body aspiration with partial airway obstruction, postextubation laryngeal edema, airway tumor, or airway trauma.

G. Obstructed expiration (Fig. 1-19).
1. Normal to slower respiratory rate.
2. Expiratory time will be longer than normal. Accessory muscles of inspiration and expiration may be used.
3. Tidal volume may be normal or decreased for the size of the patient.
4. Possible causes: asthma, emphysema, bronchitis, cystic fibrosis, bronchiectasis, airway tumor, or airway trauma.

H. Kussmaul's respiration (rapid, large breaths). See Fig. 1-20.
1. Faster-than-normal rate.
2. I/E ratio will approach 1:1. Both inspiratory and expiratory accessory muscles may be used.
3. Tidal volume will be increased for the size of the patient.
4. Probable cause: acidemia (pH 7.2 to 6.95) from diabetic ketoacidosis.

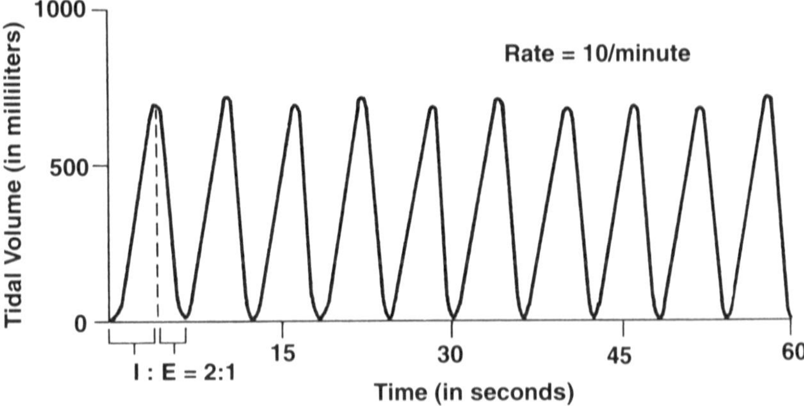

Fig. 1-18 Obstructed inspiration.

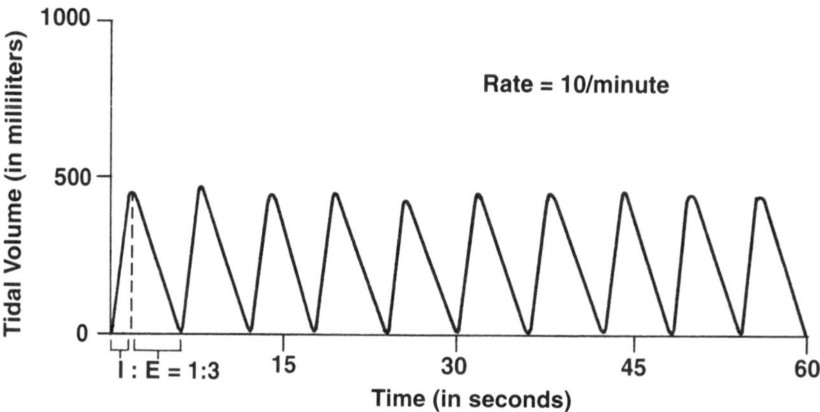

Fig. 1-19 Obstructed expiration.

I. Cheyne-Stokes respiration (waxing and waning tidal volumes). See Fig. 1-21.
   1. The respiratory rate varies from normal or faster and may have short periods of apnea.
   2. The respiratory cycle is normal or approximates it except if the patient has periods of apnea.
   3. The tidal volumes "wax and wane" over a variable time cycle. A 20-second cycle is fairly common. There may be periods of apnea between the decreased tidal volumes.
   4. Possible causes: head injury, stroke, increased intracranial pressure, or congestive heart failure.

J. Biot's respiration (unpredictably variable). See Fig. 1-22.
   1. The respiratory rate will vary from rapid to short periods of apnea.
   2. The respiratory cycle will vary considerably.
   3. Tidal volume will vary from shallow to large.
   4. Possible causes: head injury, brain tumor, increased intracranial pressure.

K. Apnea (cessation of breathing at the end of exhalation). See Figs. 1-23 and 1-24.
   1. Apnea that lasts long enough to result in hypoxemia, bradycardia, and hypotension must be treated aggressively. Artificial respiration, with or without supplemental oxygen, must be started immediately.
   2. It is important to evaluate the patient's previous breathing pattern to deter-

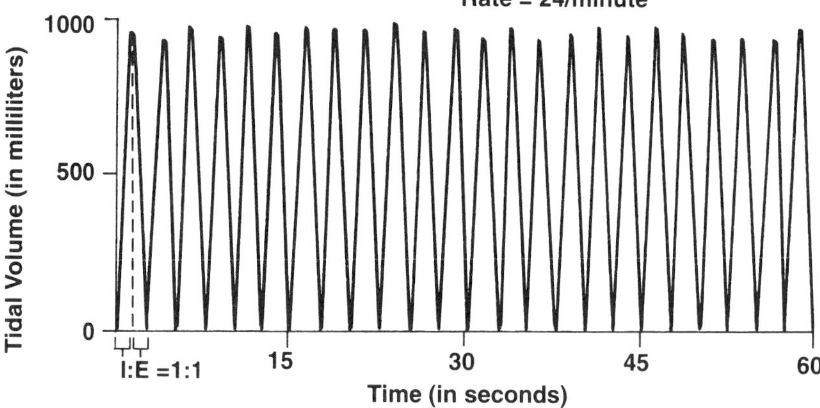

Fig. 1-20 Kussmaul.

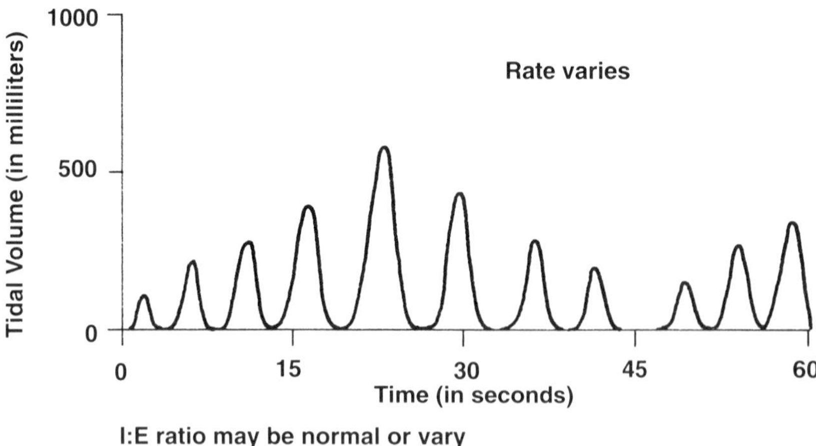

Fig. 1-21 Cheyne-Stokes.

mine the cause of the apnea. Normal breathing followed by apnea might lead you to consider causes of heart attack, stroke, or upper airway obstruction. An abnormal breathing pattern followed by apnea might lead you to consider the cause(s) of the original abnormal breathing.

3. Evaluate the previous tidal volume variation for the same reasons as above.
4. Possible causes: airway obstruction, heart attack, stroke, or head injury.

13. Determine the kind of cough the patient has. (IB1m) [R, Ap]

Normal Cough

A normal cough has four parts: (1) a deep inspiration is taken in, (2) the epiglottis and vocal cords close to keep the air trapped in the lungs, (3) the abdominal and other expiratory muscles contract to raise the air pressure in the lungs, and (4) the epiglottis and vocal cords open to allow the compressed air to explosively escape and remove any mucus or foreign matter. All components must work individually and in a coordinated manner for the patient to have an effective cough. The following are possible variations used by patients who for some reason cannot cough normally.

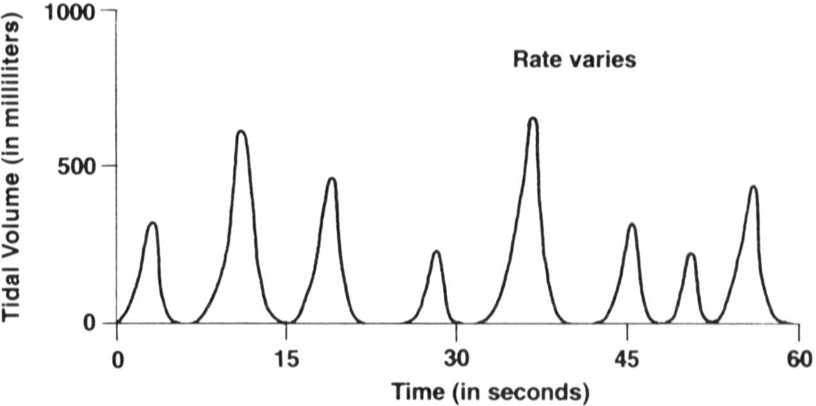

Fig. 1-22 Biots.

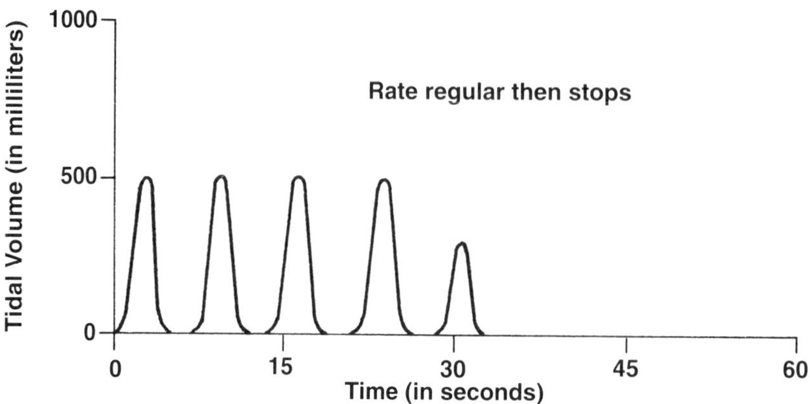

Fig. 1-23 Apnea after normal breathing.

Serial Cough

All actions of a normal cough take place except that the patient performs a series of smaller coughs rather than a single large one. This method of coughing may be used by postoperative patients who have too much abdominal or thoracic pain to cough normally. As the pain lessens, the patient should be able to cough normally.

Midinspiratory Cough

All actions of a normal cough take place except that the patient does not take as deep a breath. This is sometimes used by patients with emphysema and bronchitis to help prevent airway collapse when they cough.

Huff Cough

This is used by patients with artificial airways. They cannot close their epiglottis and vocal cords, so they can only take a large breath and blow out with as much force as possible. It is still an effective way to remove watery secretions.

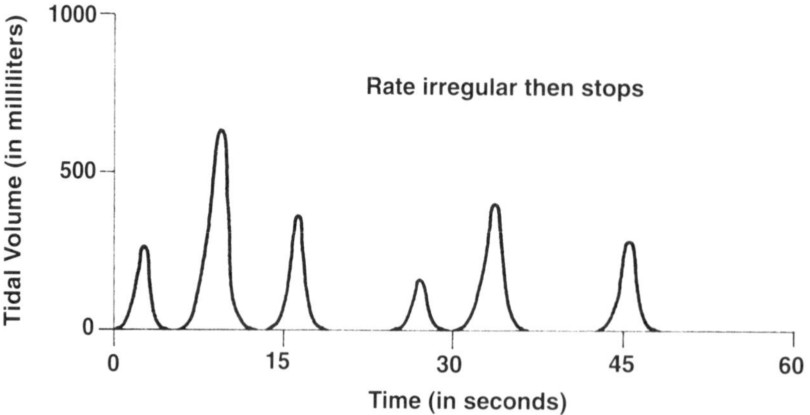

Fig. 1-24 Apnea after Biot's breathing.

Assisted Cough

This patient needs direct help from the practitioner. The patient is given a deep breath by means of intermittent positive pressure breathing (IPPB) machine or manual ventilator. Then the practitioner helps the patient blow the air out quickly by pushing on the abdominal area to move the diaphragm up. This procedure is limited to conscious patients with neuromuscular defects who cannot cough effectively on their own.

14. Determine the quantity and qualities of the patient's sputum. (IB1n) [R, Ap]

Quantity

Normally a person is not aware of mucus production. The mucociliary escalator moves mucus toward the throat where it is unconsciously swallowed. Normally mucus is uninfected and clear or white.

Typically, infections causing bronchitis or pneumonia result in the production of large amounts of mucus. The patient will report coughing and spitting it up. This mix of mucus from the lungs and saliva from the mouth is sputum. Any increase in mucus or sputum production, to the extent that the patient is aware of it, is abnormal.

As mentioned earlier, some practioners prefer to use subjective measurements of sputum production such as "a little," "medium amount," or "copious." Objective measurements such as teaspoon, tablespoon, or 5, 10, 15, etc., ml are preferred to quantify production. A marked measuring cup is needed to do this.

Note any changes in the amount of sputum that the patient is producing. This is best done in a timed manner such as production per hour or per shift. It is also wise to correlate sputum production with breathing treatments or other procedures that may increase or decrease its production or clearance.

Qualities of the Sputum

Homogeneity is best determined by letting a sputum sample stand in a test tube for several hours so that it will stratify. This is an important test in the patient with a pulmonary infection. Normal sputum will separate into a relatively thin surface layer of gel from the goblet cells that float on a lower layer of water (sol) from the bronchial glands. Dehydration reduces the water content of the sputum, thus making it more viscous and more difficult to expectorate. Patients with COPD tend to produce more gel from the goblet cells. This also makes the sputum more viscous and difficult to cough out. The patient with a pulmonary infection will have more viscous sputum because it will contain dead bacterial cells, dead white blood cells, and cellular debris from the infected lung tissues. These cells will settle over time to the bottom of a sputum sample and create a third layer of sediment.

See Fig. 1-25 for how this layering would look in the sputum from a patient who has a pulmonary infection that eventually clears up. See Table 1-7 for other details on sputum characteristics.

Module E. Determine the patient's complete respiratory condition in the following ways by *palpation:*

1. Determine the patient's pulse rate, rhythm, and force. (IB2a) [R, Ap]

The heart rate is most commonly counted by palpating the following locations: carotid, femoral, radial, and brachial arteries and apical pulse of the heart (see Fig. 1-26).

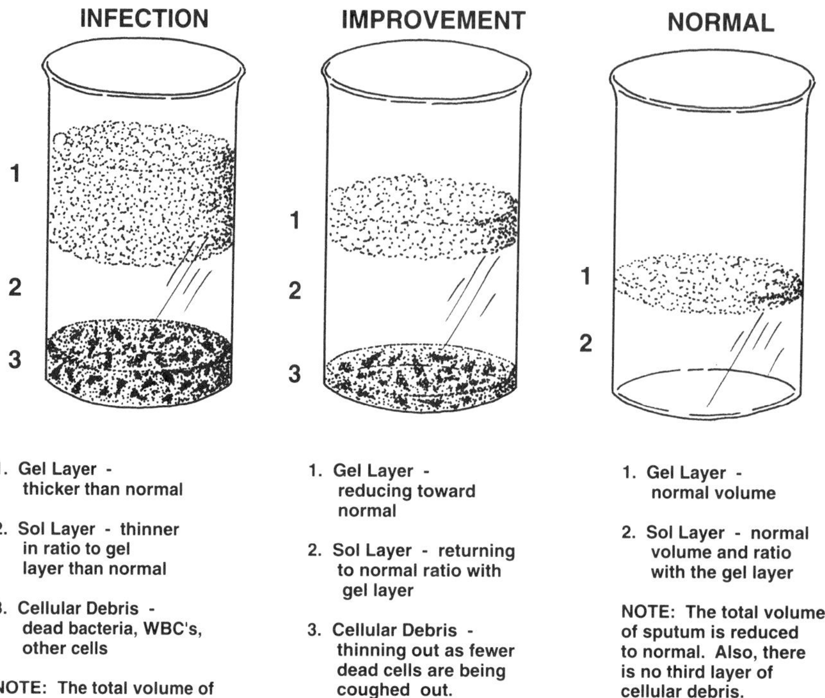

Fig. 1-25 Evaluation of the homogeneity of sputum in the infected patient.

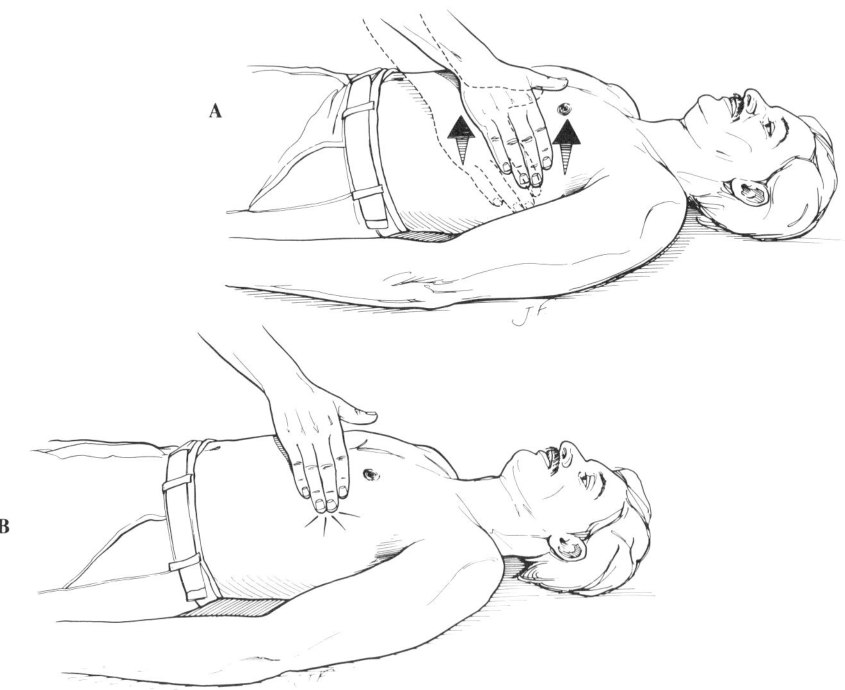

Fig. 1-26 Determining the position of the apical pulse. **A,** Technique for locating the apical pulse by palpation. **B,** Location of the apical pulse. (From Eubanks DH, Bone RC: *Comprehensive Respiratory Care,* ed 2. St. Louis, Mosby, 1990. Used by permission.)

Table 1-7. Sputum Characteristics

Sputum Type	Color	Contents	Illnesses	Odor
Bloody (hemoptysis)	Red	Blood	Bronchogenic carcinoma; pulmonary hemorrhage; lung abscess; TB; pulmonary infarction	Typically none
Frothy or bubbly	Clear or pink	Water, plasma proteins, red blood cells	Pulmonary edema	Typically none
Mucoid	Clear or white	Water, complex sugars, glycoproteins, some cellular debris	Asthma; chronic bronchitis	Typically none
Mucopurulent	Light to medium yellow	Decreased water and complex sugars, increased cellular debris and causative organisms (if applicable). Organisms are usually aerobes	Chronic and acute bronchitis	Typically none, but may exist depending on organism
Purulent	Dark yellow or green	Decreased water, greatly increased cellular debris and causative organisms that are usually aerobes, complex sugars	Bronchiectasis; lung abscess; pneumonia	Depending on organism, along with clearance of mucus; also may be foul tasting to the patient. Odor usually not offensive
Purulent (fetid)	Dark yellow or green	Decreased water, may contain some blood, greatly exaggerated cellular debris and causative organisms that frequently are anaerobes, complex sugars	Bronchiectasis; lung abscess; cystic fibrosis	Offensive odor

From DiPietro JS, Mustard MN: *Clinical Guide for Respiratory Care Practitioners*. Norwalk, Conn, Appleton & Lange, 1987. Used by permission.

Other arterial sites such as the temporal, dorsalis pedis, and posterior tibial can be used but are more difficult to find (see Fig. 1-27). The pulse should be counted for a minimum of 30 seconds, with 1 minute being the most accurate.

Palpating a pulse at any of the aforementioned sites reveals the timing between the heart beats. This rhythm is normally regular in people who are at rest or exercising at a steady level. The rhythm is felt and mentally timed as the pulse rate is counted. The time period between beats should be about the same.

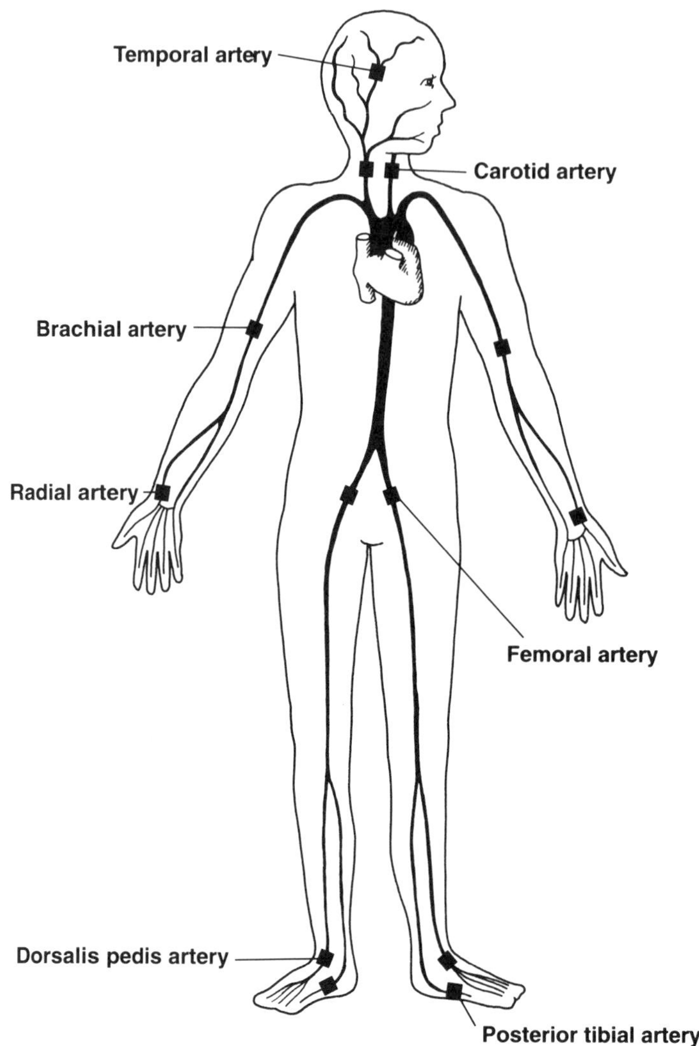

Fig. 1-27 Arteries and pulse points.

The respiratory effort may have some influence on the rhythm. Fairly common in children and sometimes in adults, the heart rhythm and rate speed up on inspiration and slow down on expiration. This sinus arrhythmia is not really abnormal. It is caused when the negative intrathoracic pressure during inspiration draws blood more quickly into the thorax and heart. The opposite may be true during mechanical ventilation with a high peak pressure or mean airway pressure. Then the heart rhythm and rate may slow down during inspiration and speed up during expiration. In any other case, an irregular rhythm would indicate some sort of cardiac problem. An electrocardiogram would be needed to help determine the specific cause.

The force of the pulse is an indicator of the strength of the heart's contraction and blood pressure. Normally each heartbeat should be felt with the same amount of force. The clinical experience of feeling the pulses of many patients with normal blood pressure and without heart disease will lead to the development of a sense of touch for a "normal" heart's force of contraction.

A "thready" or variable force felt with each heartbeat is usually a sign of heart disease. Atrial fibrillation is an example of an irregular heart rhythm that results in an irregular force. The irregular rate and rhythm cause variable volumes of blood to be pumped with each contraction. A large volume of blood will be felt as a strong pulse, while a small volume of blood will be felt as a weak pulse.

A "bounding" or greater-than-normal force felt with each beat is usually a sign of hypertension. In either case, for safety's sake, blood pressure should be measured and compared with the patient's previous blood pressure to see if there has been a change.

2. Determine if the patient has asymmetrical chest movements when breathing. (IB2b) [R, Ap, An]

Normally the lungs and chest move together in symmetry throughout the respiratory cycle. Asymmetrical chest wall movement during an inspiration would indicate a lung or chest wall problem. If the patient does not have an abnormal chest wall configuration, the problem has to be in the lungs. Less air is getting into the affected lung area(s), so the chest wall does not move out as far as the chest wall over the normal lung. This is a nonspecific finding of lung disease but would be seen in pneumonia, bronchial or lung tumor, and pneumothorax.

The hands should be placed over the chest to assess the patient for asymmetrical chest movement (Fig. 1-28). The thumbs should touch at the end of expiration. The patient is then instructed to breathe in deeply as asymmetrical movement is looked for and felt. Panels A and B of Fig. 1-28 show the movement of the anterior apical lobes, panels C and D show the movement of the anterior middle and lower lobes, panels E and F show the movement in the posterior lower lobes, and panels G and H show the movement of the costal margins.

3. Determine if the patient has palpable rhonchi indicating secretions in the airway. (IB2c) [R, Ap, An]

Palpable rhonchi are also known as tactile fremitus and are noticed when vibrations from airway secretions can be felt through the chest wall as the patient breathes. They are abnormal since they indicate that the patient has a significant secretion problem. Palpable rhonchi would not be detected in a patient with clear airways. Having the patient cough or suctioning the airway to remove secretions will result in the reduction or complete elimination of palpable rhonchi. Remember that an airway that is completely occluded by a mucus plug or foreign body will *not* reveal palpable rhonchi because there is no airflow. Breath sounds would also be absent in this area.

Fig. 1-29 shows different methods of detecting palpable rhonchi; some practitioners may prefer to use their fingertips as in panels A and B, while others prefer the edge of the open or closed hand as in panels C and D. It is important to assess all areas of the patient's chest for palpable rhonchi to detect their exact location(s). Panels E and F show that this should be done over both lung fields to compare their symmetry as well as their anterior and posterior differences.

4. Determine if the patient has crepitus. (IB2e) [R, Ap]

Crepitus (also known as crepitation) is the sound heard when an area with subcutaneous emphysema is gently pressed. The sound is a dry crackling-like "Rice Krispies in milk." A stethoscope can be used to help focus the sound to the exact location. In extreme instances, the unaided ear will detect the sound. As the fingers of one hand are sequentially pressed into the affected area, the subcutaneous air will be felt to move away from the pressure points.

Subcutaneous emphysema is air under the skin that has leaked from a damaged lung. The skin will appear puffy or edematous and is most commonly seen in the tissues on the side of the leaking lung. The pressurized air will dissect through the tissues following the path of least resistance and will most likely be found under the skin in the axilla, neck, chest wall, and breast. In extreme cases, air will be found under the skin through out the body.

While not dangerous, crepitus is a serious finding because it indicates that the patient has a pulmonary air leak. It may be accompanied by pneumothorax, pneumomediastinum, and/or pulmonary interstitial emphysema. A chest x-ray examination should be done immediately if the crepitation is a new finding.

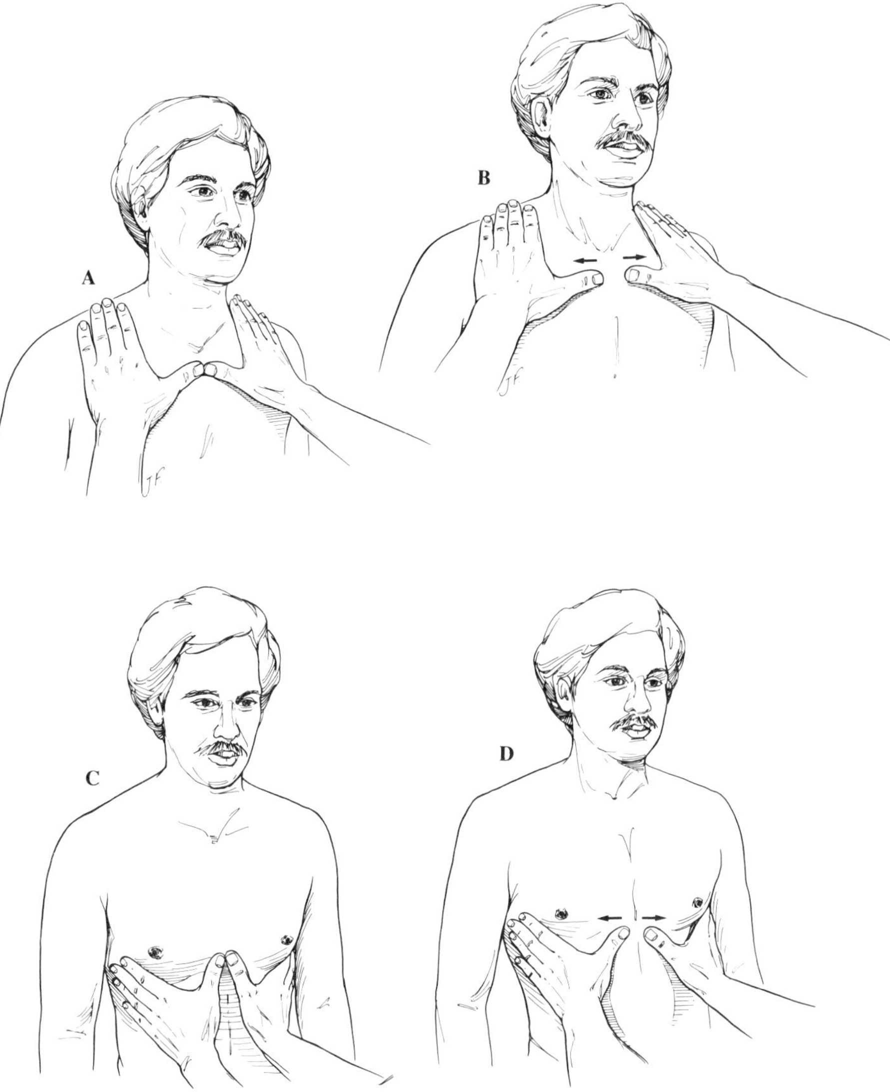

Fig. 1-28 Palpation to access symmetrical chest movements. **A,** Hand position over the apical lobes during expiration. **B,** Apical movement during inspiration. **C,** Hand position over anterior middle and lower lobes during expiration. **D,** Middle and lower lobe movement during inspiration. **E,** Hand position over the posterior middle lobes during expiration. **F,** Movement of the posterior middle lobes during inspiration. **G,** Hand position to check for movement of the costal margins during expiration. **H,** Costal movement during inspiration. (From Eubanks DH, Bone RC: *Comprehensive Respiratory Care,* ed 2. St. Louis, Mosby, 1990. Used by permission.)

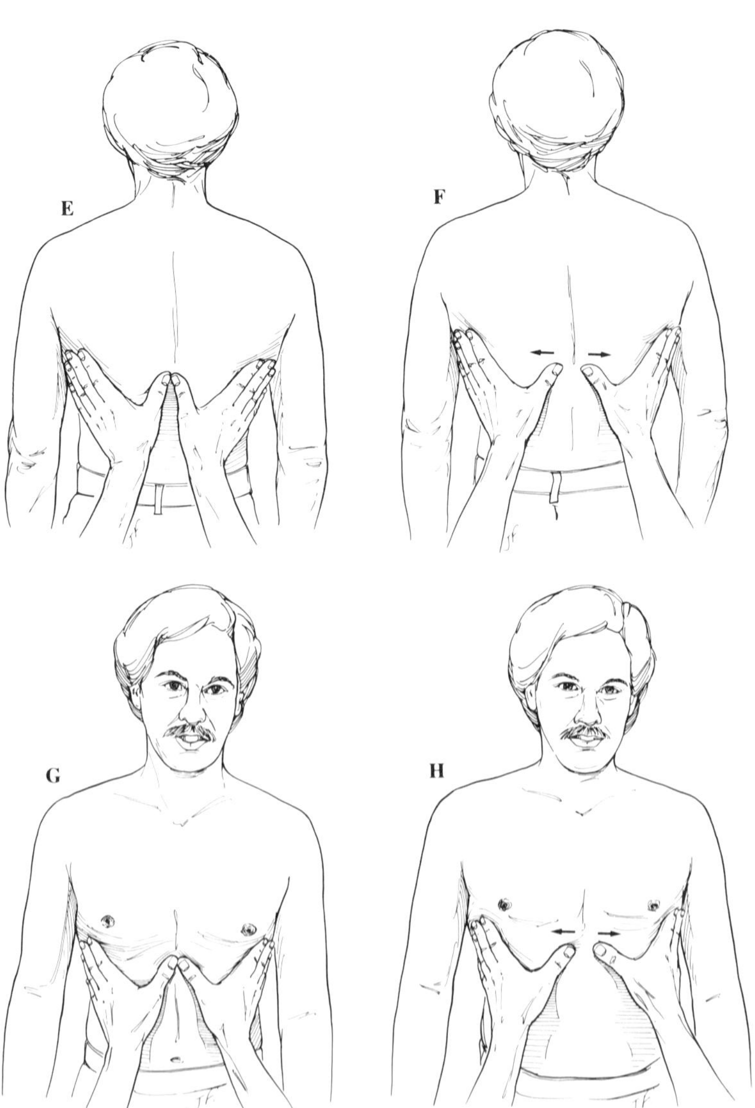

Fig. 1-28 (cont.).

Module F. Determine the patient's complete respiratory condition in the following ways by *auscultation:*

1. Determine if the patient has bilaterally normal breath sounds. (IB3a) [R, Ap]

Because the assessment of breath sounds is such an important part of the diagnosis, it must be performed under the best of circumstances. The following procedures are recommended for the best results:

a. Use the diaphragm side of the stethoscope. Hold it flat and stationary against the patient's chest. It should be held against skin. Chest hair should be moistened or shaved to avoid the confusing background noise.

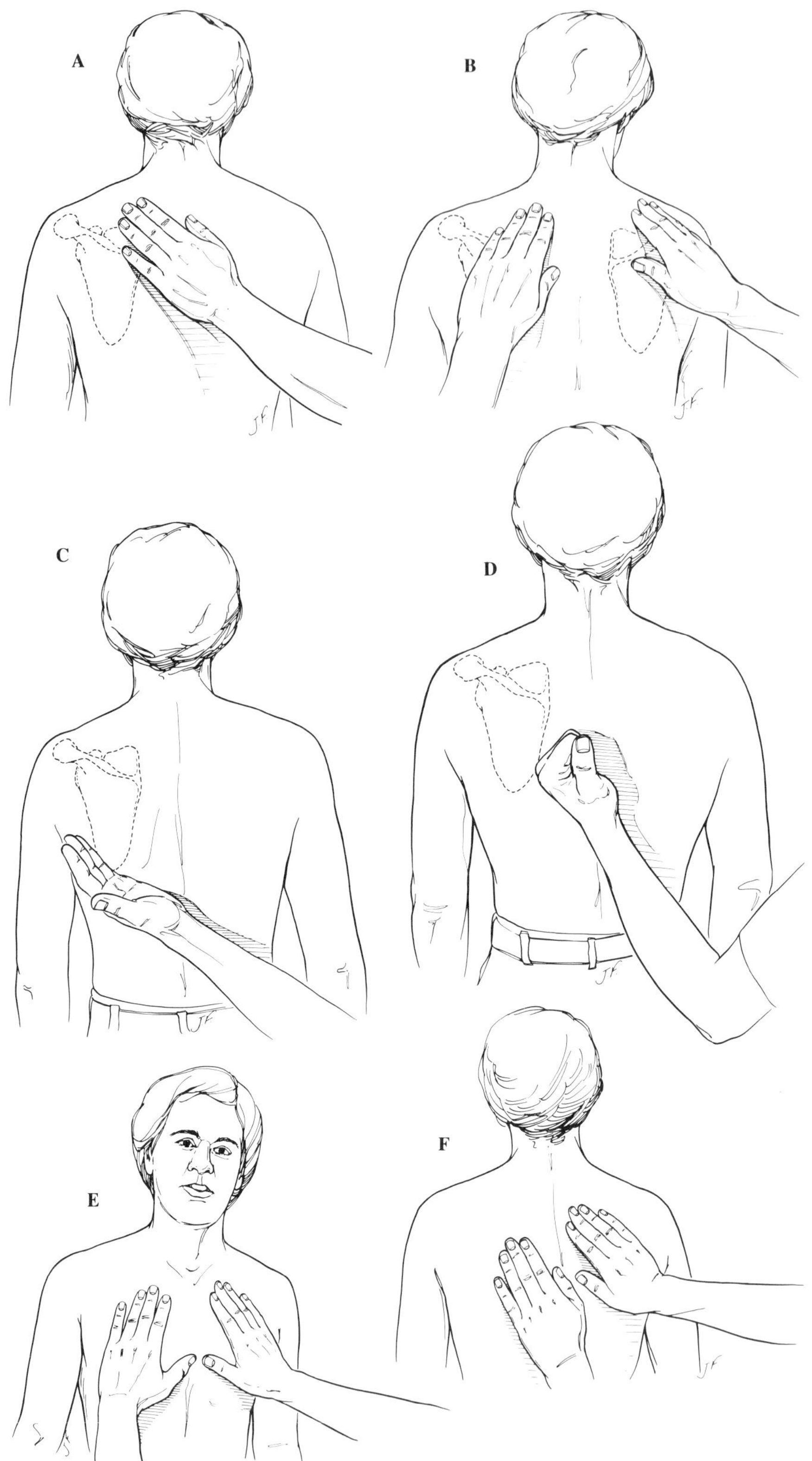

Fig. 1-29 A-D, Techniques for feeling palpable rhonchi/tactile fremitus. **E** and **F,** Anterior and posterior placement of hands to detect bilateral changes in palpable rhonchi/tactile fremitus. (From Eubanks DH, Bone RC: *Comprehensive Respiratory Care,* ed 2. St. Louis, Mosby, 1990. Used by permission.)

b. The room should be quiet. The patient should be instructed to breathe in and out deeply through the mouth as you listen.

c. The patient should be sitting upright if at all possible so that the anterior and posterior aspects of the chest can be auscultated. Have the patient roll his or her shoulders forward when listening to the posterior portion of the chest to better hear the lung areas beneath the scapulae. Roll the patient from side to side, if needed, to listen to the posterior lung areas in a patient who is unable to sit up.

d. A symmetrical system of listening must be used so that both lung fields can be compared. See Fig. 1-30, A–C for posterior, anterior, and lateral auscultation positions. Note that both lungs are compared in the upper, middle, and lower lobe areas from the anterior and posterior positions. This enables the practitioner to localize any problem area and compare it with normal areas. Repeated examination will reveal whether the patient's condition has changed in any way.

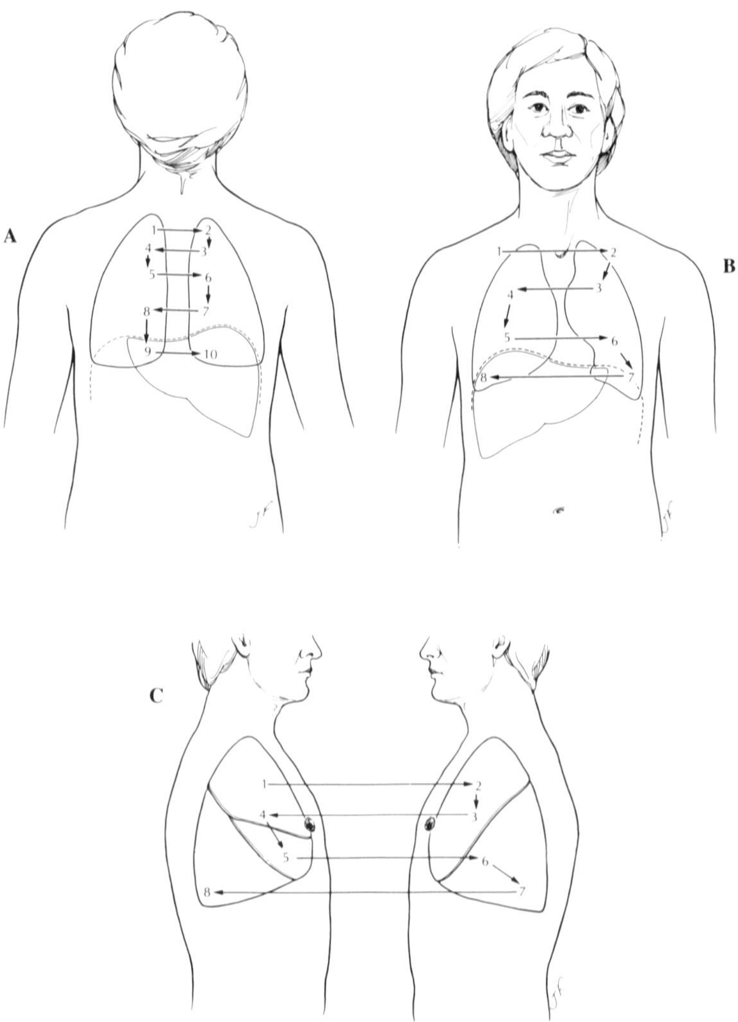

Fig. 1-30 A-C, Auscultation positions on the chest. (From Eubanks DH, Bone RC: *Comprehensive Respiratory Care,* ed 2. St. Louis, Mosby, 1990. Used by permission.)

A number of different words and phrases have been used to describe normal (and abnormal) breath sounds. This can lead to considerable confusion if all practitioners are not using the same terminology. It is most important to be concerned about the sound that is heard and what it represents rather than the words used to label the sound.

The Joint Pulmonary Nomenclature Committee of the American College of Chest Physicians and the American Thoracic Society has recommended the following two terms:

a. *Normal.* These are also called vesicular (Eubanks and Bone), alveolar (Burton, 1984), and normal vesicular (Lehrer, 1984). These normal breath sounds would be heard over all areas of normally ventilated lungs. See the areas marked by the *x* 's in Fig. 1-31 and the shaded areas in Fig. 1-32. Normal breath sounds have been variously described as "leaves rustling," "like a gentle breeze," etc. These faint sounds are made as air is moved through the small airways of the lungs during the breathing cycle. They should be heard equally in all lung fields. The inspiratory-to-expiratory phase ratio is about 3:1. The inspiratory sound is louder than the expiratory sound, and there is no pause between inspiration and expiration. See Fig. 1-33 and Table 1-8 for a graphic representation and other information about normal/vesicular breath sounds.

b. *Bronchial.* These are also called tubular (Eubanks and Bone), tracheal (Burton, 1984), and tracheobronchial (Wilkins et al.). These normal breath sounds would be heard over the trachea and main bronchi. See the areas marked by the shaded circle over the larynx and shaded rectangle over the midchest area in Fig. 1-31 and the circles over the trachea in Fig. 1-32. Bronchial breath sounds have been described as being louder, harsher, and higher pitched than normal. They have a uniform pitch on inspiration and expiration and a distinct pause in the transition of flow. The I/E ratio is about 1:1.5.

Table 1-8. Normal Breath Sounds

Breath Sound	Graphic Representation*	Location	Quality	I/E Ratio
Vesicular		Areas other than trachea and large airways	Lower pitched and less loud than other normal breath sounds, breezy sounding	3:1
Tracheal		Over trachea	Loudest and highest pitched of the normal breath sounds, harsh and tubular	5:6
Bronchial		Over larger airways	Loud and high pitched but less loud and lower pitched than tracheal sounds, hollow sounding	2:3
Bronchovesicular		Near large airways	Moderately loud, lower pitch than bronchial sounds of vesicular and bronchial breath sounds	1:1

From DiPietro JS, Mustard MN: *Clinical Guide for Respiratory Care Practitioners.* Norwalk, Conn, Appleton & Lange, 1987. Used by permission.

*

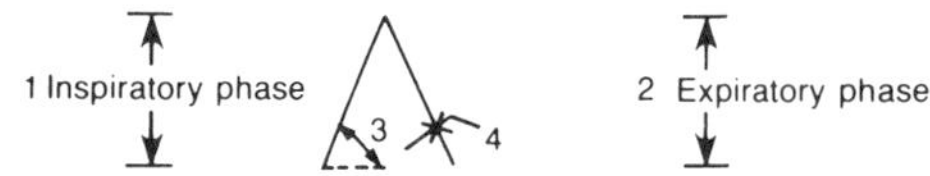

1, Graphic representation of inspiration. Line length represents duration. 2, Graphic representation of expiration. Line length represents duration. 3, Graphic representation of the pitch of the breath sound, as demonstrated by the angle. 4, Line thickness, graphically representing the amplitude of the breath sound.

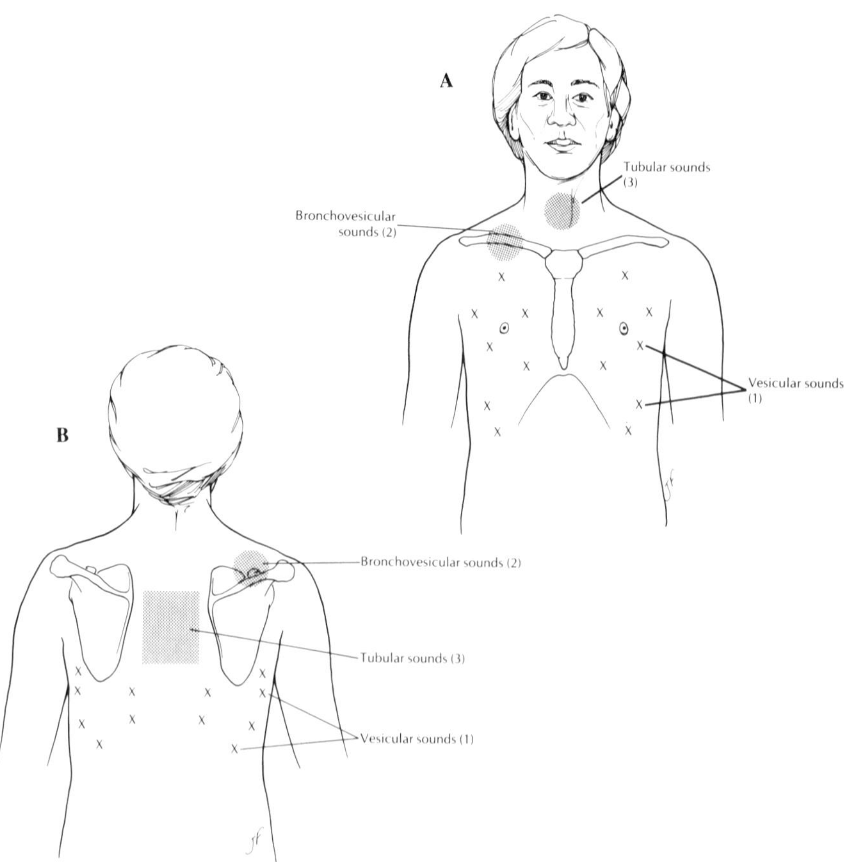

Fig. 1-31 A and **B,** Placement of stethoscope to hear normal breath sounds. (From Eubanks DH, Bone RC: *Comprehensive Respiratory Care,* ed 2. St. Louis, Mosby, 1990. Used by permission.)

Lehrer and Wilkins et al. describe a *tracheal* breath sound that is normally heard over the laryngeal area. It is loud and high pitched. The I/E ratio is about 1:1, and there is a distinct pause between the phases. This normal sound heard in the larynx will be contrasted later with the abnormal sound of stridor. See Fig. 1-33 and Table 1-8 for a graphic representation and other information about bronchial/tubular/tracheal breath sounds.

Bronchial breath sounds are abnormal if heard in any other areas except those mentioned previously. When bronchial sounds are heard over areas that should be normally vesicular, it is a sign of consolidation or atelectasis with a patent airway.

Eubanks and Bone, Burton, Lehrer, and Wilkins et al. describe the following third breath sound as normal:

c. *Bronchovesicular.* Eubanks and Bone and Burton (1984) say that this sound is heard normally over the right supraclavicular area because large bronchi are relatively close to the surface. See the area marked by the shaded circle over the right clavical in Fig. 1-31. Lehrer says that this sound is heard normally anteriorly between the first and second intercostal spaces and posteriorly between the scapula. (Note that Eubanks and Bone call the sound in this location tubular.) See the area with triangles in Fig. 1-32.

The sound is a cross between bronchial and vesicular. It is more muffled than bronchial but louder than vesicular and has the same pitch throughout inspiration and expiration. The I/E ratio is about 1:1. See Fig. 1-33 and Table 1-8 for a graphic representation and other information about bronchovesicular breath sounds.

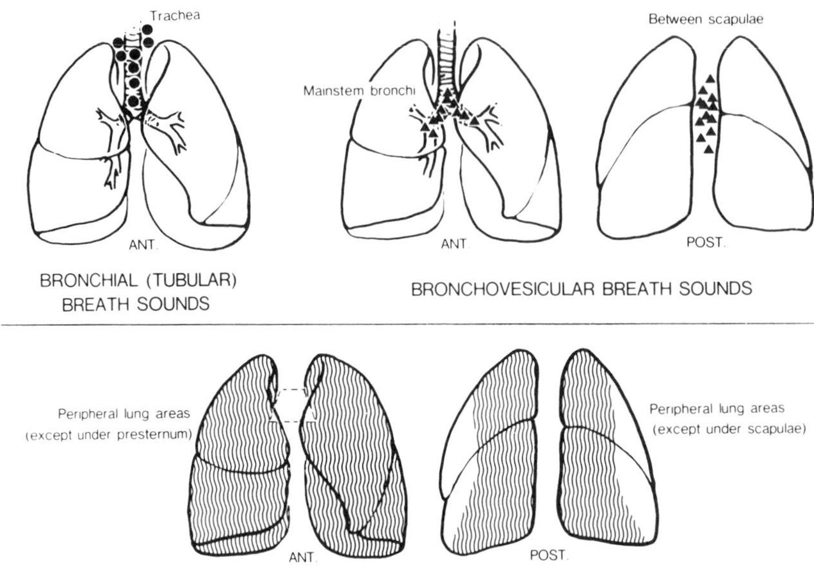

Fig. 1-32 Breath sounds over the normal chest. (From Lehrer S: *Understanding Lung Sounds.* Philadelphia, WB Saunders, 1984. Used by permission.)

Bronchovesicular breath sounds are abnormal if heard in any other areas except those mentioned. When bronchovesicular sounds are heard over areas that should be normally vesicular, it is a sign of partial consolidation or atelectasis with a patent airway.

2. Determine if the patient has increased, decreased, absent, or unequal breath sounds. (IB3b) [R, Ap]

This discussion will be limited to variations in normal vesicular breath sounds. The abnormal appearance of bronchial and bronchovesicular breath sounds was discussed ear-

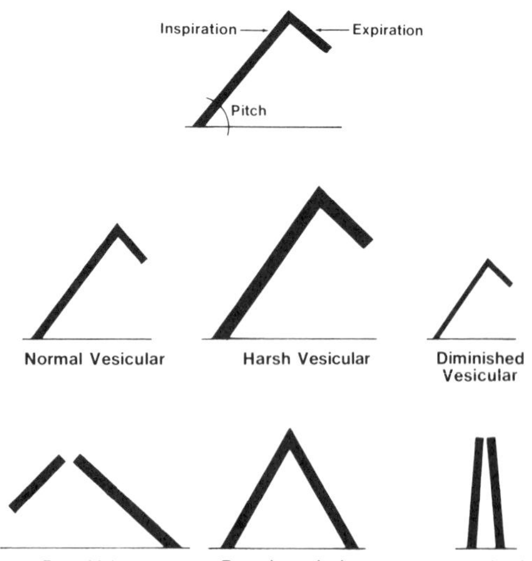

Fig. 1-33 Graphic representation of normal breath sounds patterns. (From Lehrer S: *Understanding Lung Sounds.* Philadelphia, WB Saunders, 1984. Used by permission.)

lier. Table 1-9 lists some common conditions with breath sounds and other physical findings.

a. Increased normal vesicular breath sounds:

- Found most often in children and in debilitated adults because their thinner chest walls transmit the sounds better.

b. Decreased normal vesicular breath sounds:

- Most commonly caused by a pleural effusion, hemothorax, or empyema because of fluid between the lung and the stethoscope (see Fig. 1-11,D).
- Pulmonary fibrosis caused by decreased air flow (see Fig. 1-11,B).
- Emphysema caused by decreased airflow.
- Pleural thickening caused by dampening from the thicker pleural tissues.

c. Absent normal vesicular breath sounds:

- Pneumothorax as a result of the lung being forced away from the chest wall (see Fig. 1-11,C).
- Atelectasis because no air moves into the collapsed area (see Fig. 1-11,A).
- Endotracheal tube placed into a bronchus instead of the trachea. In this case, the right bronchus is most commonly intubated so that the breath sounds are absent over the left lung.
- Large pleural effusion, etc.
- Very obese patient.

Table 1-9. Physical Findings in Some Common Pulmonary Disorders

Disorder	Inspection	Palpation	Percussion	Auscultation
Bronchial asthma (acute attack)	Hyperinflation Use of accessory muscles	Impaired expansion Decreased fremitus	Hyperresonance Low diaphragms	Prolonged expiration Wheezes
Pneumothorax (complete)	Lag on affected side	Absent fremitus	Hyperresonant or tympanitic	Absent breath sounds
Pleural effusion (large)	Lag on affected side	Decreased fremitus Trachea and heart shifted away from affected side	Dullness or flatness	Absent breath sounds
Atelectasis (lobar obstruction)	Lag on affected side	Decreased fremitus Trachea and heart shifted toward affected side	Dullness or flatness	Absent breath sounds
Consolidation (pneumonia)	Possible lag or splinting on affected side	Increased fremitus	Dullness	Bronchial breath sounds Bronchophony Pectoriloquy

From Hinshaw HC, Murray JF: *Diseases of the Chest,* ed 4. Philadelphia, WB Saunders, 1980, p 23. Used by permission.

d. Unequal normal vesicular breath sounds:

- Pneumonia, consolidation, or atelectasis that decreases airflow into a segment or lobe.
- Foreign body or tumor in a bronchus that decreases airflow to the distal portion of the lung.
- Spinal or thoracic deformity that reduces airflow to the underlying lung.

We are once again faced with the task of trying to make sense of a variety of terms and phrases that have been coined over the years to describe abnormal/adventitious breath sounds. The Joint Pulmonary Nomenclature Committee of the American College of Chest Physicians and the American Thoracic Society suggest terms that do not necessarily match the terms listed below by the National Board of Respiratory Care (NBRC). The common features of the various phrases and terms will be presented. Primary authors like Eubanks and Bone,[1] Burton,[2] Lehrer,[3] and Wilkins et al.[4] can be referred to for more details. Fig. 1-34 and Tables 1-9 to 1-13 should be referred to extensively to help understand the various abnormal breath sounds.

3. Determine if the patient has rhonchi (wheezing) or rales (crackles). (IB3c and d) [R, Ap]

Rhonchi

Rhonchi (also known as wheeze and rhonchus) have the following features or characteristics:

- They are continuous sounds.
- They are more commonly heard on expiration than inspiration.
- Low-pitched, polyphonic expiratory sounds are commonly associated with secretions in the airways. Coughing or tracheal suctioning will often cause these sounds to be modified or eliminated. Common pulmonary conditions include asthma, bronchitis, pneumonia, or any other secretion-causing problem. Common terms for these sounds include rhonchus, sonorous rhonchus, low-pitched wheeze, sonorous wheeze, and polyphonic wheeze.

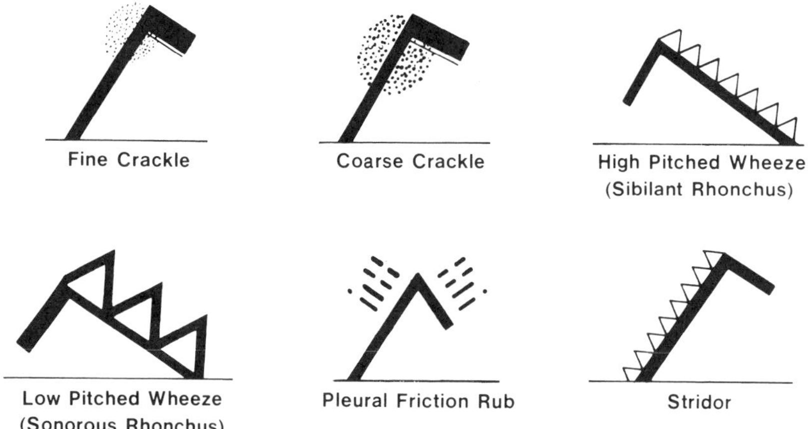

Fig. 1-34 Graphic representation of abnormal breath sounds patterns. (From Lehrer S: *Understanding Lung Sounds.* Philadelphia, WB Saunders, 1984. Used by permission.)

Table 1-10. Adventitious Sounds

Acoustic Characteristics	Time-Expanded Waveform	Recommended Term	ACCP† Report	Current British Usage	Other Terms	Some Common Clinical Associations
Discontinuous, interrupted, explosive sounds—loud, duration of about 10 ms. Low in pitch: initial deflection width averaging 1.5 ms.		Coarse crackle	Rale	Crackle	Bubbling rales, coarse crepitations	Pulmonary edema, resolving pneumonia
Discontinuous, interrupted, explosive sounds—less loud than above and of shorter duration. They average less than 5 ms in duration and are lower in pitch.		Fine crackle	Rale	Crackle	Fine crepitations	Interstitial fibrosis
Continuous sounds—longer than 250 ms, high-pitched dominant frequency of 400 Hz or more; a hissing sound.		Wheeze	Sibilant rhonchus	High-pitched wheeze	Sibilant rale, musical rale	Airway narrowing
Continuous sounds—longer than 250 ms, low-pitched, dominant frequency about 200 Hz or less; a snoring sound.		Rhonchus	Sonorous rhonchus	Low-pitched wheeze		Sputum production

From Burton GG: Practical physical diagnosis in respiratory care, in Burton GG, Hodgkin JE (eds): *Respiratory Care,* ed 2. Philadelphia, Lippincott, 1984. Used by permission.
†ACCP, American College of Chest Physicians.

Table 1-11. Adventitious Breath Sounds*

Crackling	Short, burst of noise, primarily in I	Popping of bubbles and/or opening of small airways	Local to pathology—mostly at bases	Fibrosis, CHF, pulmonary edema, alveolar proteinosis, peripneumonic
Fibrotic	High frequency (like hair rubbing together)			
Peripneumonic and CHF	Medium frequency			
Pulmonary edema	Low frequency (both I and E)			
Wheeze	Prolonged sound—E more than I but can be both; often musical. The higher pitched are from smaller airways	Air currents at point of airway bifurcation	Local to pathology	Airway constriction
Rub	Low pitched, duration is very specific—often at end inspiration	Pleural surfaces rubbing together	Local to pathology	Pleural inflammation or mass

From Eubanks DH, Bone RC: *Comprehensive Respiratory Care*, ed 2. St Louis, Mosby, 1988. Used by permission.
**I*, Inspiration; *E*, expiration; *CHF*, congestive heart failure.

- High-pitched, monophonic expiratory sounds are commonly associated with closure of the small airways. Coughing or tracheal suctioning is unlikely to eliminate these sounds. Common pulmonary conditions include asthma, emphysema, congestive heart failure, foreign body aspiration, airway tumor, asbestosis, and interstitial fibrosis. Common terms for these sounds include wheeze, high-pitched wheeze, sibilant rhonchus, sibilant rale, and monophonic wheeze.

Table 1-12. Common Features of Lung Crackles in Chronic Bronchitis, Bronchiectasis, and Interstitial Fibrosis

Feature	Chronic Bronchitis	Bronchiectasis	Interstitial Fibrosis
Inspiratory crackles			
Usual timing	Early in inspiration	Early and middle of inspiration	Late in inspiration
Usual number	Usually few	Usually moderate	Can be profuse
Effect of cough	Unchanged	Temporarily reduced	Unchanged
Effect of position	Unchanged	Unchanged	Modified or undetectable
Volume/intensity	Faint	Loud	Moderately loud
Pitch	Low	Low	High
Transmission to the mouth	Yes	Yes	No
Expiratory crackles	May be present	Usually present	May be present

*Modified from Nath AR, Capel LH: *Thorax* 1980; 35:694.

Table 1-13. Changes in Lung Sounds With Pulmonary Disease

Lung Disease	Breath Sounds	Adventitious Lung Sound
Pneumonia	Bronchial or absent	Inspiratory crackles
Atelectasis	Harsh/bronchial	Late-inspiratory crackles
Pneumothorax	Absent	None
Emphysema	Diminished	Early-inspiratory crackles
Chronic bronchitis	Normal	Wheezes and crackles
Pulmonary fibrosis	Harsh	Inspiratory crackles
Congestive heart failure	Diminished	Inspiratory crackles
Pleural effusion	Diminished	None
Asthma	Diminished	Wheezes

*Wilkins RL, Hodgkin JE, Lopez B: *Lung Sounds, Practical Guide.* St Louis, Mosby, 1988. Used by permission.

Rales (Crackles)

These have the following features or characteristics:

- They are discontinuous sounds.
- They are more commonly heard on inspiration than expiration.
- They are caused by the sudden opening of collapsed airways.
- They are heard as a repeated sound during the same phase of the respiratory cycle.
- Early inspiratory crackles are heard in patients with obstructive lung diseases such as chronic bronchitis, bronchiectasis, asthma, and emphysema. A patient with bronchitis or bronchiectasis may have some clearing of the sounds after coughing or tracheal suctioning. Common terms for these sounds include course crackle, rale, bubbling rale, and course crepitation.
- Late inspiratory crackles are heard in patients with restrictive lung diseases such as interstitial fibrosis and asbestosis. These sounds do not clear with coughing or suctioning. Common terms for these sounds include fine crackle, rale, crackle, and fine crepitations.
- The Joint Pulmonary Nomenclature Committee states that rales and crackles mean the same thing. However, the term *rales* is used by some to describe the sound heard in the lungs of patients with congestive heart failure and pulmonary edema. These sounds will clear with the correction of the pulmonary edema.

4. Determine if the patient has any stridor. (IB3e) [R, Ap]

- Stridor is heard as a harsh, monophonic, high-pitched inspiratory sound over the larynx. (It is not the normal tracheal sound.)
- Stridor can often be heard without a stethoscope.
- Common pediatric conditions include acute epiglottitis, laryngotracheobronchitis (croup), and laryngomalacia (congenital stridor).
- Common adult conditions include postextubation laryngeal edema and laryngeal tumor.
- When stridor is heard on inspiration and expiration, it is commonly caused by an aspirated foreign body, tracheal stenosis, or a laryngeal tumor.
- Severe stridor is a respiratory emergency because the airway may rapidly close completely.

5. Determine the patient's blood pressure. (IB3f) [R, Ap]

A general discussion of blood pressure is found in Module A, 8, a. The practitioner must be practiced in the skill of measuring the blood pressure on any patient. Measuring the blood pressure is indicated in any situation when you believe that there is a significant increase or decrease from the patient's normal value. The patient's blood pressure should be approximately the same in either arm or either leg.

The practitioner should have experience taking blood pressures with either a mercury column or aneroid-type sphygmomanometer. The mercury types are limited in that the mercury column must be kept in a stable, upright position to be accurate. For that reason the aneroid type is preferred for patient transport or when exercising.

The arm (or leg) cuff must be the right size for the patient. They come in different sizes for adults and pediatric patients. Fig. 1-35 shows blood pressure being taken on the right arm with an aneroid-type sphygmomanometer. Note that the air bladder is positioned to close the brachial artery when the bladder is inflated. Also note that the diaphragm of the stethoscope is positioned over the brachial artery so that the returning blood flow sounds can be heard. The first distinct sound to be heard indicates systolic pressure, while the last distinct sound to be heard indicates diastolic pressure. Clinical practice is needed to accurately determine blood pressure.

This ends the general discussion on patient assessment that may be tested on the entry level examination to earn the certified respiratory therapy technician (CRTT) credential. The NBRC may ask *direct* questions on the aforementioned patient assessment techniques. It may also *incorporate* this information into questions that cover other patient care procedures or techniques to be covered in the following sections.

The following Modules are presented in their entirety and relate to this section as well sections 3 to 14. To save space and avoid unnecessary repetition, they will *not* be reprinted after each of these succeeding sections. However, they should be reviewed in terms of how they relate to the procedures or techniques that have just been presented.

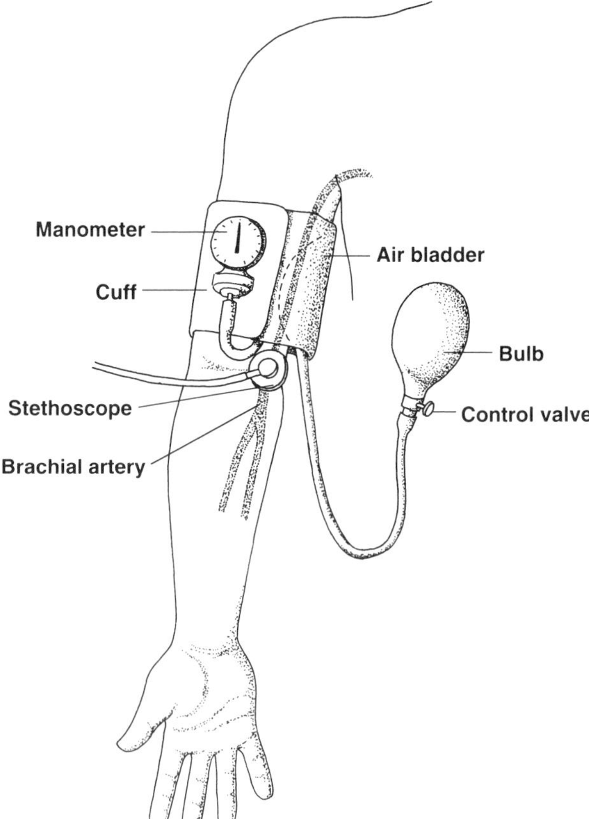

Fig. 1-35 Blood pressure measurement with an anaeroid sphygmomanometer. (From Eubanks DH, Bone RC: *Comprehensive Respiratory Care,* ed 2. St. Louis, Mosby, 1990. Used by permission.)

Module G. Determine and continue to monitor how the patient responds to the treatment or procedure. (IIIE)

1. **Determine the patient's vital signs and record them in the chart. (IIIE1) [R, Ap]**
2. **Monitor the patient's heart rhythm. (IIIE2) [R, Ap]**
3. **Auscultate the patient's breath sounds and record any changes. (IIIE4) [R, Ap]**
4. **Recommend a chest x-ray examination, as needed, to help determine the patient's condition. (IA2b) [R, Ap]**
5. **Perform bedside spirometry. (IIIE13) [R, Ap]**
6. **Ask about the patient's feelings toward the treatment or procedure and write it in the chart. (IIIE6) [R, Ap]**

Module H. Evaluate the physician's orders and the patient's respiratory care plan; make any recommendations or changes, as needed.

1. **Determine the treatment/procedural goal(s) after reviewing the orders and respiratory care plan. (ID1) [R, Ap, An]**
2. **Evaluate how appropriate the orders, respiratory care plan, and goal(s) are for the patient's disease or condition. (ID2) [R, Ap, An]**
3. **Make any recommendations to the respiratory care plan you believe are appropriate based on existing or new information. (ID3) [R, Ap, An]**
4. **Participate in developing the respiratory care plan. (ID4) [R, Ap]**

These four items relate to the respiratory care practitioner being involved with the patient care team of the physician, nurse, and others in deciding how to best care for the patient. Be prepared to use the information contained in this section and the rest of the text to help you make decisions on how to care for your patients. The NBRC will ask questions that relate to what would be the best recommendations for care. The following steps are necessary in the respiratory care plan for any patient:

a. Determine an expected outcome or goal(s).
b. Develop a plan to achieve success.
c. Decide how to measure the patient's achievement of the goal.
d. Plan a time-line to measure the patient's progress.
e. Document the patient's response to care and the final outcome.

Module I. Modify the treatment or procedure and recommend any changes in the patient's respiratory care plan depending on the response.

1. **Recommend to change how long a treatment or procedure should be given to a patient. (IIIF9b) [R, Ap, An]**
2. **Stop the treatment or procedure if the patient has an adverse reaction to it. (IIIF1) [R, Ap, An]**
3. **Recommend to cancel the physician's order for a treatment or procedure because of the patient's adverse reaction to it. (IIIF9a) [R, Ap, An]**

Module J. Record any treatment(s) and/or procedure(s) on the patient's chart and communicate with the other members of the health care team.

1. Record any treatment(s) and/or procedure(s) performed, including the date, time, frequency of therapy, medication, and ventilatory data. (IIIA2a) [R, Ap]

2. Record and evaluate the patient's objective response to the treatment(s) and/or procedure(s), including:

a. Record the following vital signs: heart rate and rhythm, respiratory rate, and blood pressure. (IIIA2b1) [R, Ap]

b. Record the patient's breath sounds. (IIIA2b2) [R, Ap]

c. Record the type of cough the patient has and the nature of the sputum. (IIIA2b3) [R, Ap]

d. Record any adverse reactions the patient had to the treatment(s) and/or procedure(s). (IIIA2b4) [R, Ap, An]

e. Record and evaluate the patient's subjective feelings and reaction to the treatment(s) and/or procedure(s). (IIIA2b4) [R, Ap]

3. Recheck any math work and make note of incorrect data. (IIIA2c) [R, Ap, An]

If an error is made in charting, it must be corrected. Do this by drawing a single mark through the error, then write out the correct information. Some prefer that the error be further clarified by writing in "error" next to it and adding your initials. *Never* erase or use any covering material over an error.

4. Establish contact with other members of the health care team about significant clinical information regarding the patient. (IIIA2d) [R, Ap]

Inform the patient's nurse and/or physician and the supervising therapist if any serious problem occurs with the patient. Routine communication should occur between these people or any other care giver as needed.

5. Establish contact with other members of the health care team about scheduling and coordinating patient care to avoid time conflicts. (IIIA2e) [R, Ap]

Some of the more common scheduling problems are related to eating times and when the patient must go to another department such as radiology or physical therapy. Some of our procedures such as giving aerosolized medications and performing chest physiotherapy should be performed before eating.

Remember, Modules G, H, I, and J as well as all the earlier material relate to all the procedures and techniques presented in sections 3 to 14. The NBRC may test you on any of this information.

BIBLIOGRAPHY

Aloan CA: *Respiratory Care of the Newborn, a Clinical Manual.* Philadelphia, Lippincott, 1987.

Barrascout JR: Chest physical therapy and related procedures, in Burton GG, Hodgkin JE (eds): *Respiratory Care,* ed 2. Philadelphia, Lippincott, 1984.

Bates B: *A Guide to Physical Examination and History Taking,* ed 4. Philadelphia, Lippincott, 1987.

Bennington JL (ed): *Saunders Dictionary & Encyclopedia of Laboratory Medicine and Technology*. Philadelphia, WB Saunders, 1984.

Burton GG: Patient assessment procedures, in Barnes TA (ed): *Respiratory Care Practice*. Chicago, Mosby, 1988.

Burton GG: Practical physical diagnosis in respiratory care, in Burton GG, Hodgkin JE (eds): *Respiratory Care*, ed 2. Philadelphia, Lippincott, 1984.

Daily EK, Schroeder JS: *Techniques in Bedside Hemodynamic Monitoring*, ed 4. St Louis, Mosby, 1989.

Des Jardins TR: *Cardiopulmonary Anatomy & Physiology: Essentials for Respiratory Care*. Albany, NY, Delmar Publishers, 1988.

DiPietro JS, Mustard MN: *Clinical Guide for Respiratory Care Practitioners*. Norwalk, Conn, Appleton & Lange, 1987.

Eubanks DH, Bone RC: *Comprehensive Respiratory Care*, ed 2. St Louis, Mosby, 1990.

Hudak CM, Gallo BM, Lohr T: *Critical Care Nursing*. Philadelphia, Lippincott, 1973.

Kenner CV, Guzzetta CE, Dossey BM: *Critical Care Nursing: Body-Mind-Spirit*. Boston, Little, Brown, 1981.

Lehrer S: *Understanding Lung Sounds*. Philadelphia, WB Saunders, 1984.

Nath AR, Capel LH: Lung crackles in bronchiectasis. *Thorax* 1980; 35:694.

Tilkian SM, Conover MB, Tilkian AG: *Clinical Implications of Laboratory Tests*. St Louis, Mosby, Inc., 1983.

White GC: *Basic Clinical Lab Competencies for Respiratory Care*. Albany, NY, Delmar Publishers, 1988.

Wilkins RL, Hodgkin JE, Lopez B: *Lung Sounds: A Practical Guide*. St Louis, Mosby, 1988.

Wilkins RL, Hodgkin JE: History and physical examination of the respiratory patient, in Burton GG, Hodgkin JE (eds): *Respiratory Care*, ed 3. Philadelphia, JB Lippincott, 1991.

SELF-STUDY QUESTIONS

1. You have finished charting on your patient when you notice that you made an error. You should do which of the following?
   A. Tell the patient so that he will tell the physician the next day.
   B. Tell the nurse so that she will tell the physician.
   C. Tell the nurse so that she will chart the correct information.
   D. Place a line through the error, initial it, and write in the correct information.
   E. Have your supervisor chart the correct information.

2. In listening to your patient's lungs you notice that she has bronchial breath sounds in her right lower lobe. These would indicate which of the following?
   A. She has normal lungs.
   B. She has a pneumothorax.
   C. She has a consolidation in her right lower lobe.
   D. She has a pleural effusion in her left lower lobe.
   E. She has a pleural effusion in her right lower lobe.

3. You are called to start a new aerosolized medication treatment. On reading the physician's order you notice that the drug dosage is outside the normal department guidelines. You should do which of the following?
   A. Give the treatment as ordered.
   B. Contact the physician to confirm that the order is indeed correct.

C. Give the treatment as ordered and leave a note in the chart asking for clarification for the next treatment.
D. Have the nurse rewrite the order.
E. Have your supervisor rewrite the order.

4. You are called to the emergency room to help care for a patient who was in a car accident and has chest injuries, which include broken ribs. While palpating her neck you feel a crackling, popping sound. What is the most likely cause of this sound?
   A. She has a laryngeal tumor.
   B. There is blood in the back of her throat.
   C. She has aspirated a tooth.
   D. The endotracheal tube is in the right bronchus.
   E. She has an air leak from her lung.

5. You are called to help in the evaluation of a new 55-year-old male patient. You notice the following signs and symptoms: oral temperature of 104.5° F, diaphoresis, respiratory rate of 22, the use of accessory muscles of respiration, and palpable rhonchi in the right lower lobe. You would suspect the following to be the diagnosis:
   A. Bacterial pneumonia
   B. Heart attack
   C. Pneumothorax
   D. Viral pneumonia
   E. Stroke

6. The normal resting pulse rate in an adult is:
   A. 120-140
   B. 80-140
   C. 80-130
   D. 80-120
   E. 60-100

7. A patient who has become argumentative about his care since being told of the diagnosis of cancer and threatens to hit the nurse and therapist should be evaluated for:
   A. Language barrier problems
   B. Medication imbalance
   C. Emotional state
   D. Marital difficulties
   E. Hypoxemia

8. To help determine your patient's level of consciousness you might ask the following questions:
   I. "Do you know what day this is?"
   II. "Can I see your identification wristband?"
   III. "Do you know where you are?"
   IV. "How are you feeling today?"
   V. "Do you know who the president is?"
   A. I only
   B. II and IV only
   C. III only
   D. V only
   E. I and III only

9. To help you determine if your patient has orthopnea you would ask the following:
   A. "How many flights of stairs can you climb before you become short of breath?"
   B. "Do you know who the governor is?"

C. "Do you need to use extra pillows behind your head and back to keep from getting short of breath when you sleep?"
D. "Are there any particular foods that seem to make it harder for you to cough up your secretions?"
E. "Do you know which hospital you are in?"

10. In observing your infant patient's chest configuration you notice that it is the same size in both the anterioposterior and lateral dimensions. This would indicate to you that the patient has:
   A. A normal chest
   B. Kyphoscoliosis
   C. Funnel chest/pectus excavatum
   D. Pulmonary emphysema with air trapping
   E. Lordosis

11. In examining your patient you notice that she has bronchial breath sounds in her right lower lobe and her trachea is shifted to the right. These signs would indicate to you that she has which condition?
   A. Right-sided pneumothorax
   B. Right-sided atelectasis
   C. Left-sided pneumothorax
   D. Left-sided hemothorax
   E. Left-sided pneumonia

12. In palpating your patient for symmetrical chest movements you notice that his left side does not move as much as his right side. This sign could indicate to you that he has what conditions?
   I. Emphysema
   II. Congestive heart failure
   III. Left-sided pneumonia
   IV. Left-sided pneumothorax
   V. Right-sided pneumonia
   A. I and II only
   B. III and IV only
   C. IV and V only
   D. II only
   E. V only

13. You are called to the emergency room to help evaluate a pediatric patient. Upon entering the room you observe the patient's breathing and can hear a harsh, high-pitched sound on inspiration. Which of the following is true?
   A. The breath sounds are tracheal and are normal.
   B. The breath sounds are bronchovesicular and not normal.
   C. The breath sounds are stridor and indicate a respiratory emergency.
   D. The breath sounds are bronchial and indicate a respiratory emergency.
   E. The breath sounds are bronchovesicular and are normal.

14. You are called to evaluate a patient's breathing pattern. You notice that the patient's tidal volumes go from small to large to small and then stop for 10 seconds before starting up again. The pattern repeats itself. This patient's breathing pattern would best be called:
   A. Eupnea
   B. Obstructed expiration
   C. Kussmaul's respiration
   D. Cheyne-Stokes respiration
   E. Tachypnea

15. A patient with hypopnea would show all of the following *except:*
    A. Unpredictably variable respiratory cycle
    B. Normal respiratory cycle
    C. Small tidal volumes
    D. Normal to somewhat slower respiratory rate
    E. Deep sleep

Answer Key:

1. D; 2. C; 3. B; 4. E; 5. A; 6. E; 7. C; 8. B; 9. C; 10. A; 11. B; 12. B; 13. C; 14. D; 15. A.

2 Infection Control

Module A. Follow established infection control procedures to minimize the patient's risk of getting a hospital-acquired (nosocomial) infection. (IIIA3) [R, Ap]

Handwashing

Handwashing is probably the single most important procedure that can be performed to reduce the spread of infection. Respiratory care practitioners should wash their hands before and between each patient contact. The following handwashing times are recommended:

1. When coming on duty.
2. When hands are obviously soiled or after contamination by blood or other patient body fluids.
3. Before contact about the face and mouth of patients. This is especially important if the patient has an artificial airway.
4. Before setting up equipment or pouring medicines.
5. On leaving an isolation area or handling contaminated articles from an isolation area.
6. After handling soiled dressings, sputum containers, urinals, bedpans, catheters, etc.
7. After personal use of the toilet.
8. After using your hands to cover your mouth when coughing.
9. After blowing or wiping the nose.
10. Before eating.
11. Before serving food.
12. Upon completion of duty.

The most common bacterial organism spread by personal contact is *Staphylococcus aureus*. Suspect personal contact whenever a patient gets a Staphylococcal infection.

Universal Precautions

Universal precautions are used to prevent the transmission of blood or body fluid pathogens by assuming that *all* patients are infected. Barriers such as gloves and masks and other procedures are used to prevent contact with body fluids. This approach to patient care has been adopted because of the concern of health care workers and the public that the human immunodeficiency virus (HIV), hepatitis B, or other deadly pathogens can be spread unknowingly by these contacts. Table 2-1 includes specific universal precaution guidelines established by the Centers for Disease Control (CDC) and the Occupational Health and Safety Administration (OSHA).

Respiratory Care Equipment and Procedures

The following general guidelines are recommended to minimize the spread of infection by equipment and procedures. Follow the manufacturer's specific guidelines when applicable.

1. Each patient should have his/her own equipment.
2. Disposable equipment should be discarded after patient use.
3. Reusable equipment should undergo high-level disinfection or be sterilized between patients.
4. Equipment, oxygen masks, breathing circuits, etc. should be changed every 24 hours.
5. Sterile water should be used for procedures, and the unused portion should be discarded after 24 hours.

Table 2-1. Universal Precautions to Prevent the Spread of Infection

Exclusion from Patient Contact:

1. Any health care worker with exudative skin lesions should not work in the direct care of patients.

Barriers:

1. Gloves should be worn under these conditions: during direct contact with blood, body fluids, secretions, mucus membranes, wounds; when handling all items or surfaces contaminated by blood or body fluids; when performing venipuncture or handling intravenous catheters or monitoring devices.
2. Gloves must be changed between patients or if the gloves become torn or punctured as with a needlestick injury.
3. Hands should be washed immediately after the gloves are removed. The hands or any other body areas must be washed immediately if contaminated by blood or other body fluid.
4. Masks, eye goggles, or face shields should be worn when performing a procedure that may lead to the splashing or splattering of blood, secretions, or body fluids.
5. Gowns or aprons should be worn as discussed in item 4.
6. Contaminated masks, goggles, face shields, gowns, and aprons should be removed and disposed of properly.
7. Contaminated worker uniforms should be left at the hospital for cleaning.

Needle and Instrument Precautions:

1. Care should be taken when handling needles and sharp instruments.
2. Used needles and sharp instruments should be placed into puncture-resistant containers for proper disposal. Reusable needles should be placed into a puncture-resistant container for transport.
3. No attempt should be made to manually recap needles, remove them from the syringe, or bend or cut them. (Needle covering systems or pushing the needle into a rubber cube are widely used. These should only require the use of one hand without any touching of the needle itself.)

Patient Specimens:

1. Blood and body fluids should be placed into leakproof, sturdy plastic bags for transportation to the laboratory.
2. The laboratory requisition form should be placed on the outside of this bag.

Cardiopulmonary Resuscitation:

1. Mouth-to-mouth breathing should be avoided even though there is no evidence that saliva transmits HIV infection.
2. Mouth-to-valve mask resuscitators and manual resuscitators (bag-valve) should be readily available to ventilate patients.

6. Add water to reservoir systems immediately before using.
7. Discard any unused water in a reservoir system before filling it again.
8. Drain and discard any water collected in tubing. Do *not* drain it back into the reservoir.
9. Medications should be stored under the conditions set by the manufacturer. Medications that appear abnormal should be discarded. Medications should be discarded on the expiration date.
10. Unused portions of medications should be discarded after 24 hours.
11. Sterile syringes should be used when measuring medications.
12. Sterile suction catheters should be used and sterile gloves worn whenever the patient's airway is suctioned.

Patient Isolation Categories

The following are general guidelines and specific diseases or conditions established by the CDC for the seven types of patient isolation categories. Additionally, hospitals may establish extra standards and post them at the door to the patient's room.

Strict Isolation

1. Private room—mandatory; door must be kept closed.
2. Gowns—must be worn by all persons entering the room.
3. Masks—must be worn by all persons entering the room.
4. Hands—must be washed before leaving the room.
5. Gloves—must be worn by all persons entering the room.
6. Articles—must be discarded, or double-bagged and labeled before being sent to Central Service for disinfection or sterilization.

Diseases:

1. Diphtheria.
2. Pneumonic plague.
3. Varicella (chickenpox).

Contact Isolation

1. Private room—mandatory; door must be kept closed. Generally, patients with the same condition can share a room.
2. Gowns—must be worn if hand contamination is likely.
3. Masks—must be worn if close patient contact is likely.
4. Hands—must be washed before leaving the room.
5. Gloves—must be worn if infected material will be touched.
6. Articles—must be discarded, or double-bagged and labeled before being sent to Central Service for disinfection or sterilization.

Diseases:

1. Major wound or burn infection if draining fluid or pus and not covered by a bandage
2. Newborn and child diseases such as laryngotracheobronchitis (croup), bronchitis, influenza, viral bronchitis and pneumonia, gonococcal conjunctivitis, disseminated herpes simplex, impetigo

3. Staphylococcal pneumonia
4. Group A streptococcal pneumonia
5. Multiple antibiotic resistant bacterial infection

Respiratory Isolation

1. Private room—indicated. Generally, patients with the same condition can share a room.
2. Gowns—not necessary.
3. Masks—must be worn if close patient contact is likely.
4. Hands—must be washed before leaving the room.
5. Gloves—not necessary but recommended if contact will be made with secretions.
6. Articles—must be discarded, or double-bagged and labeled before being sent to Central Service for disinfection or sterilization.

Diseases:

1. *H influenzae* pneumonia in children
2. Mumps
3. Pertussis
4. Epiglottitis
5. Meningococcal pneumonia
6. Rubella
7. Meningitis

Tuberculosis (AFB) Isolation

1. Private room—mandatory with special ventilation and air filtration; door must be kept closed. Generally, patients with the same condition can share a room.
2. Gowns—not necessary unless health care worker's clothing can become contaminated.
3. Masks—high-efficiency particulate air (HEPA) filtered mask required until the patient is not contagious.
4. Hands—must be washed before leaving the room.
5. Gloves—not necessary but recommended if contact will be made with secretions.
6. Articles—not usually a cause of contamination. Contaminated articles, however, must be discarded, or double-bagged and labeled before being sent to Central Service for disinfection or sterilization.

Diseases:

1. *Mycobacterium tuberculosis* confirmed by a positive sputum smear results; chest x-ray findings suggest active disease probable.
2. Laryngeal tuberculosis.

Enteric Isolation

1. Private room—not needed unless the patient shows poor hygiene with fecal material or contaminates the room with infective material. Generally, patients with the same condition can share a room.

2. Gowns—not necessary unless health care worker's clothing can become contaminated.
3. Masks—not necessary.
4. Hands—must be washed before leaving the room.
5. Gloves—must be worn by all persons having direct contact with infected material.
6. Articles—contaminated articles must be discarded, or double-bagged and labeled before being sent to Central Service for disinfection or sterilization.

Diseases:

1. Encephalitis
2. Viral meningitis
3. Type A viral hepatitis
4. Cholera
5. Viral pericarditis or myocarditis
6. Gastrointestinal infections such as amebic dysentery, gastroenteritis from *E. Coli*, salmonellae, or shigellae bacteria; necrotizing enterocolitis

Drainage/Secretion Precautions

1. Private room—not needed.
2. Gowns—not necessary unless health care worker's clothing can become contaminated.
3. Masks—not necessary.
4. Hands—must be washed before leaving the room.
5. Gloves—must be worn by all persons having direct contact with infected material.
6. Articles—contaminated articles must be discarded, or double-bagged and labeled before being sent to Central Service for disinfection or sterilization.

Diseases:

1. Minor, limited wound or burn infections
2. Gas gangrene
3. Conjunctivitis
4. Chlamydia infection
5. Infected decubitus ulcer

Blood/Body-Fluid Precautions

1. Private room—not needed unless the patient shows poor hygiene with infective material or contaminates the room with infective material. Generally, patients with the same condition can share a room.
2. Gowns—not necessary unless health care worker's clothing can become contaminated.
3. Masks—not necessary.
4. Hands—must be washed before leaving the room.
5. Gloves—must be worn by all persons having direct contact with infected material.
6. Articles—contaminated articles must be discarded, or double-bagged and labeled before being sent to Central Service for disinfection or sterilization.

7. Health care workers must take care to avoid needlestick injuries. Use universal precautions with needles and blood.
8. Any spilled blood must be cleaned up with a disinfecting agent.

Diseases:

1. Any patient suspected or known to have HIV or to have the acquired immunodeficiency syndrome (AIDS).
2. Hepatitis B, non-A, or non-B
3. Malaria
4. Yellow fever
5. Colorado tick fever

Module B. Decontaminate respiratory care equipment.

Decontamination is the process of disassembling, washing to remove debris, rinsing, and disinfecting or sterilizing used patient care equipment. The process will result in the equipment being free of any pathogens so that it can be used with another patient. Obviously, once disinfected, the equipment must be aseptically reassembled and stored for future use.

1. Choose the appropriate agent and method for disinfection and sterilization. (IIA15a) [R, Ap]

Disinfection

Disinfection is a procedure that significantly reduces the microbial contamination of the equipment that has been processed. All disinfection processes destroy the vegetative form (the cell) of pathogenic organisms. This includes the vast majority of respiratory system pathogens. However, a few bacillus-type bacteria are difficult to kill because they have a particularly tough cell wall or have spores for reproduction. Spores are analogous to seeds in that they will grow into bacteria under the right conditions and are resistant to drying, heat, and many chemicals that will kill the bacterial cell. So, a spore-forming organism may be able to reproduce itself after the cells have been killed. Obviously, disinfection can only be used on equipment that is *not* contaminated by spore-forming bacteria. It is important, if possible, to know what pathogen has infected the patient so that the appropriate disinfection (or sterilization) method can be used on the contaminated equipment. As will be noted, some disinfecting agents will kill different kinds of organisms, depending on the length of time that they are exposed.

Another consideration in selecting the appropriate disinfection method is how the equipment will be used in patient care. Equipment or instruments that do not directly touch the patient are classified as "noncritical" (low risk of spreading infection) and can undergo low-level disinfection (for example, an electrocardiograph machine). Low-level disinfectants are agents capable of killing some vegetative bacteria, fungi, and lipophilic viruses. Equipment or instruments that touch surface mucus membranes and the skin but do not penetrate them are listed as "semicritical" and must undergo high-level disinfection (for example, larygoscope blades and a bronchoscope). Agents that kill all microorganisms except bacterial spores are classified as high-level disinfectants.

A third consideration in choosing the best disinfection method is the type of equipment that needs to be decontaminated. Certain processes and agents can only be used on certain types of equipment. Table 2-2 lists the various ways to disinfect reuseable patient care equipment decontaminated in the hospital.

Table 2-2. Methods of Disinfection

Method	Conditions	Microbes Effective Against					Comments
		Bacteria	Tuberculosis	Spores	Viruses	Fungi	
Pasteurization	Complete immersion in water heated to 70° C (170° F) for 30 min.	Yes	Yes	No	Yes	Yes	Used with rubber and many plastics used in respiratory care, especially those that are sensitive to a high temperature. **Avoid use** with any item that cannot be immersed or will be damaged at this temperature.
Glutaraldehyde Solutions							
Alkaline gluteraldehyde (Cidex, Cidex 7, Sporicidin)	Complete immersion for 10 min.	Yes	Yes	No	Yes	Yes	Used with rubber and many plastics used in respiratory care, especially those that are heat sensitive. Care must be taken to thoroughly rinse items after being disinfect. **Avoid use** with any item that cannot be immersed or will absorb the solution.
Acid gluteraldehyde (Sonacide)	Complete immersion for 20 min.	Yes	Yes	No	Yes	Yes	Used with rubber and many plastics used in respiratory care, especially those that are heat sensitive. Care must be taken to thoroughly rinse items after being disinfected. **Avoid use** with any item that cannot be immersed or will a absorb the solution.

(Continued)

Table 2-2 (cont.).

Method	Conditions	Microbes Effective Against					Comments
		Bacteria	Tuberculosis	Spores	Viruses	Fungi	
Alcohols (70% ethyl or 90% isopropyl)	Complete immersion for several minutes or pooling of the alcohol on the equipment.	Yes	Yes	No	Lipophilic only	Yes	Used with metallic or plastic surfaces of large pieces of equipment that cannot be disinfected by any other means. May also be used with most plastics. **Avoid use** with any item that cannot be immersed or will absorb or be damaged by the alcohol.
Iodines (iodine or iodophore with 70% ethyl alcohol)	Complete immersion for several minutes or pooling of the solution on the equipment.	Yes	Yes	No	Yes	Yes	Used with metallic or plastic surfaces of large pieces of equipment that cannot be disinfected by any other means. May also be used with most plastics. **Avoid use** with any item that cannot be immersed or will absorb or be damaged by the alcohol.

Sterilization

Sterilization is a procedure that destroys all living microbial organisms and renders them unable to reproduce. All sterilization procedures destroy the vegetative forms and spores of all microscopic organisms. Examples of spore-forming bacteria include *Bacillus anthracis* (anthrax), and members of the Clostridia genus *C. botulinum* (botulism), *C. tetanis* (tetanus), and *C. perfringens* (gas gangrene). Any equipment or instruments that penetrate body tissue are listed as "critical" (high risk of spreading infection) and must be sterilized before use on another patient (for example, a surgical scalpel). As discussed, the method of sterilization will depend on the type of equipment under consideration. Table 2-3 lists the various methods of sterilization for reuseable supplies and patient care equipment decontaminated in the hospital.

2. Disinfect or sterilize respiratory care equipment. (IIA15b)[R, Ap]

As discussed, the choice of whether to disinfect or sterilize equipment depends on how it is used clinically, the type of pathogen involved, and from what the equipment is made. Most respiratory pathogens are not spore-formers so low-level or high-level disinfection is acceptable. Either a gluteraldehyde solution or pasteurization is used in most departments for disinfecting plastic masks, hoses, etc.

Any department that processes its own equipment must have adequate facilities to do so. There must be a "dirty" area where contaminated equipment is brought for disassembly, scrubbing of secretions or blood, and rinsing. From there it is either placed into the gluteraldehyde solution or pasteurizing machine. After that, it is taken to a "clean" area to be rinsed, dried, reassembled, and placed into plastic bags for storage. Care must be taken not to recontaminate the equipment during this procedure. Items that must be sterilized are usually just processed through the "dirty" area before being sent to the Central Supply Department. There the equipment is sterilized based on the criteria shown in Table 2-3.

3. Monitor the sterilization process to ensure its effectiveness. (IIA15c)[R]

Surveillance is used to describe the monitoring of equipment to be sure that the disinfection or sterilization process was successful and that in-use equipment is not a source of patient contamination. Processing indicators are used to ensure that disinfection or sterilization was done correctly. Examples include special tapes used to hold wrapping around packages of equipment being autoclaved or placed into ethylene oxide. These tapes turn color when the autoclave has reached the proper temperature or the correct concentration of ethylene oxide has been reached. Besides showing the user that the package was processed correctly, it identifies sterile from unsterile, wrapped packages.

Another example is a biologic indicator placed into the wrapped package before it is sterilized. These biologic indicators are bacterial spores that are only killed if the required conditions are met. After the equipment and spores have been sent through the sterilization process, the spores are placed into conditions favorable for growth. If no growth occurs, they are dead. It can then be concluded that no other living organisms survived.

Equipment that is held in storage or being used in patient care is also randomly sampled for contamination. There are three ways that a sample is taken for culturing of possible organisms. The first involves a sterile swab being wiped onto an equipment surface. It is then rubbed over a plate of growth medium or placed into a tube of liquid broth. The second is used to check inside lengths of tubing. It requires pouring a liquid broth through the tube and into a sterile container. The third involves sampling the aerosol that a nebulizer produces. Usually, a hose is attached to the outlet of the nebulizer. The

Table 2-3. Methods of Sterilization

Method	Conditions	Comments
Steam autoclave	Autoclave chamber with an internal steam pressure of 15 lb per sq in, 121° C, 15 min.	Used with glass, cloth, bandages, unsharpened stainless steel instruments. **Avoid use** with many plastics used in respiratory care, rubber, dextrose solutions, sharpened stainless steel instruments, electrical devices or machines.
Dry heat	Autoclave chamber at 160-180° C, 2 hr use.	Used with glass, sharpened stainless steel instruments. **Avoid use** with many plastics used in respiratory care, rubber, dextrose solutions, electrical devices or machines.
Ethylene oxide gas	Specific guidelines vary considerably depending on the manufacturer of the chamber and the supplies or equipment being sterilized. In general, a gas concentration of 800-100 mg/L must be kept for 3-4 hr at 50% to 100% relative humidity and 49-57° C. Great care must be taken to predry all items before gassing and properly aerate them after sterilization.	Used with heat-sensitive and moisture-sensitive items like many plastics used in respiratory care. **Avoid use** with supply pouches or plastic films such as aluminum foil; nylon, thermoplastic resin (Saran), Mylar, cellophane polyamide, polyester, or polyvinylidene films that are penetrated by the gas. *PVC that has been previously sterilized by the manufacturer with gamma radiation.
Gluteraldehyde solutions Alkaline gluteraldehyde (Cidex, Cidex 7, Sporicidin)	Complete immersion. Cidex products for 10 hr; Sporicidin for 6 hr and 45 min.	Used with rubber and many plastics in respiratory care, especially those that are heat sensitive. Care must be taken to thoroughly rinse items after being cleaned. **Avoid use** with any item that cannot be immersed or will absorb the solution.
Acid gluteraldehyde (Sonacide)	Complete immersion for 1 hr at 60° C.	Used with rubber and many plastics used in respiratory care, especially those that are heat sensitive. Care must be taken to thoroughly rinse items after being cleaned. **Avoid use** with any item that cannot be immersed or will absorb the solution.

*PVC, Polyvinyl choloride.

other end of the hose is connected to a funnel that is attached to a culture plate where the droplets impact. In all three examples, the growth of any organism in the growth medium indicates a form of contamination. The laboratory then determines if the organism is pathogenic. If it is, measurements will need to be taken to improve the disinfection or sterilization process.

BIBLIOGRAPHY

American Respiratory Care Foundation: Guidelines for disinfection of respiratory care equipment used in the home. *Respir Care* 1988; 33:801-808.

Ayerst Laboratories, New York, New York, product information.

Bennington JJ: *Saunders Dictionary & Encyclopedia of Laboratory Medicine and Technology*. Philadelphia, WB Saunders, 1984.

Couperus JJ, Elder HA: Infectious disease aspects of respiratory therapy. In Burton GG, Hodgkin JE (eds): *Respiratory Care*, ed 2. Philadelphia, Lippincott, 1984.

Eubanks DH, Bone RC: *Comprehensive Respiratory Care*, ed 2. St. Louis, Mosby, 1990.

Guidelines for the prevention of nosocomial infections, *AARTimes*, September 1983, 49-52.

Scanlan CL, St. Hill H: Principles of infection control. In Scanlan CL, Spearman CB, Sheldon RL (eds): *Egan's Fundamentals of Respiratory Care*, ed 5. St. Louis, Mosby, 1990.

The Sporicidin Company, Washington, DC, product information.

Surgikos, Arlington, Texas, product information.

Washington JA: Infectious disease aspects of respiratory therapy. In Burton GG, Hodgkin JE, Ward JJ (eds): *Respiratory Care*, ed 3. Philadelphia, Lippincott, 1991.

SELF-STUDY QUESTIONS

1. Handwashing should be performed:
   - I. When coming on duty.
   - II. After obtaining a sputum sample.
   - III. After using the toilet.
   - IV. Before eating.

   A. I only
   B. II only
   C. III only
   D. II and III only
   E. I, II, III, and IV

2. You are about to refill a patient's nebulizer for an aerosol mask when you notice that the water bottle is dated as having been opened two day ago. You would procede to:
   A. Refill the nebulizer.
   B. Throw away the water.
   C. Refill the nebulizer but throw away any remaining water.
   D. Ask the nurse if she wants to use the water for a wound irrigation.
   E. Call your supervisor for advice.

3. Which of the following precautions should be taken with a patient in respiratory isolation:
   - I. Private room.
   - II. Gowns must be worn by all persons entering the room.
   - III. Gowns are not necessary.
   - IV. Articles contaminated with secretions must be disinfected or discarded.
   - V. Masks must be worn by all persons who will be in close personal contact with the patient.

   A. I, III, IV, and V only
   B. I, II, and IV only
   C. V only
   D. I and IV only
   E. IV only

4. The patient with new, major burns is placed into the following type of isolation:
   A. Strict
   B. Contact
   C. Respiratory
   D. Enteric
   E. Drainage

5. Plastic oxygen masks and tubing can be disinfected by all of the following methods except:
   A. Pasteurization
   B. 70% ethyl alcohol
   C. Ethylene oxide
   D. Iodine

6. The best method of sterilizing a contaminated Bird Mark 7 IPPB unit is:
   A. 10 hour soak in Cidex 7
   B. Steam autoclave
   C. Iodine
   D. Ethylene oxide
   E. 20 min soak in Sonacide

7. You suspect that several large volume jet nebulizers are the cause of an outbreak of pneumonia in the recovery room. To determine if the in-use nebulizers are contaminated, which method of surveillance would you recommend?
   A. Check if the ethylene oxide tape turned color after the units were sterilized.
   B. Swab the air intake ports on the nebulizers.
   C. Sample the aerosol droplets from each nebulizer.
   D. Check the Cidex they were soaked in for contamination.
   E. Add liquid broth to the water in the reservoir jar and then pour the solution into a sterile container. Check for bacterial growth.

Answer Key:

1. E; 2. B; 3. A; 4. B; 5. C; 6. D; 7. C.

3 Blood Gases

Module A. Make a recommendation for arterial puncture to obtain a blood sample for analysis. (IA2b)[R, Ap]

Note: Throughout this section and in all other sections, the common phrase "arterial blood gas" (ABG) will be used when discussing drawing a sample of blood from a patient's artery for the purposes of determining the arterial pressures of oxygen and carbon dioxide, acid-base status (pH), and related values. (The entry level examination will not specifically test you on mixed venous blood gas values.)

There are three broad, general indications for this recommendation:

1. To check a patient's oxygenation status (Pa_{O_2}).
2. To check a patient's acid-base status (pH).
3. To check a patient's ventilation status (Pa_{CO_2}).

A number of authors have written extensively on these and other indications. No attempt will be made to include every possible indication; broad areas will be listed with some common examples. It is very important to evaluate the patient's vital signs and physical condition as described in Section 1 to help determine if an ABG determination is indicated.

- A. Cardiac failure
  1. Congenital defect
  2. Heart attack (myocardial infarct)
  3. Congestive heart failure with or without pulmonary edema
- B. Chronic obstructive pulmonary disease (COPD)
  1. Asthma
  2. Emphysema
  3. Bronchitis
  4. Bronchiectasis
- C. Any pneumonia causing hypoxemia
- D. Trauma
  1. Broken ribs
  2. Flail chest
  3. Pneumothorax
  4. Hemothorax
  5. Upper airway trauma

E. Ventilatory failure
   1. Overdosage of sedatives or pain relievers
   2. Stroke or head (brain) injury
   3. Spinal cord injury
   4. Neuromuscular diseases such as myasthenia gravis or Guillain-Barré syndrome

F. Airway obstruction
   1. Foreign body aspiration
   2. Laryngotracheobronchitis (croup)
   3. Epiglottitis

G. Miscellaneous
   1. Smoke inhalation
   2. Carbon monoxide poisoning
   3. Near drowning
   4. Infant respiratory distress syndrome (IRDS)/hyaline membrane disease
   5. Adult respiratory distress syndrome (ARDS)
   6. The patient does not have an indwelling arterial line
   7. A shunt or $P(A-a)O_2$ calculation must be made
   8. Cardiopulmonary resuscitation

Module B. Obtain an arterial blood sample.

1. Get the appropriate blood gas sampler. (IIA7f)[R, Ap]

Generally, this involves selecting a prepackaged, sterile blood gas kit that contains the following:

1. Variety of short-bevel needles: 23-24 gauge for radial or dorsalis pedis puncture and a 22 gauge for brachial or femoral puncture.
2. 3 ml syringe. Many kits will have the syringe prepared with heparin as an anticoagulant.
3. If needed, liquid sodium or lithium heparin with a 1000 U/ml concentration.

If a blood gas kit is not available, an appropriate individual needle, 3 or 5 ml syringe, and liquid sodium or lithium heparin will have to be obtained. These should be available at any nursing station or from the respiratory care department.

Using sterile technique, screw the selected needle onto the syringe. If the syringe does not contain heparin it will have to be added. Do this by aspirating liquid heparin through the needle into the syringe. Coat the inside of the syringe with heparin by tipping the needle up, pulling the plunger back, and pushing the plunger forward to squirt the excess heparin out the needle. This assures that the needle and dead space of the needle are filled with heparin, and the inside of the syringe is coated.

2. Perform an arterial puncture to obtain a blood sample for analysis. (IIIE9)[R, Ap]

There are a number of possible variations in the technique. The following is a general but thorough listing of the steps and any important related information.

A. Check for a valid physician order.

B. Check the patient's chart for pertinent information on supplemental oxygen being used and bleeding disorders such as hemophilia.

   It is important to check the patient's clotting time because a hematoma will result if extra time is not spent holding the puncture site. The normal activated partial thromboplastin time (APTT or PTT) is 16 to 25 seconds. The normal prothrombin time (PT) is 11 to 16 seconds. If the patient is receiving coumarin (Coumadin), the PT will be significantly increased; heparin therapy may prolong the PT slightly. Be prepared to hold the site for longer than normal if the APPT or PT times are increased or the patient is receiving either of these medications.

C. Collect necessary equipment:
   1. Ice-water in a cup.
   2. A 3-5 ml glass or plastic syringe.
   3. The syringe and needle.
   4. An anticoagulant, if needed.
   5. Seventy percent isopropyl alcohol and/or iodophor swabs to clean the puncture site. A sterile 4 by 4 inch gauze pad to hold over the puncture site to aid in clotting.
   6. A seal for the needle or syringe to prevent room air contamination.
   7. Clean gloves to protect both of the practitioner's hands from any contact with spilled blood. Eyeglasses or goggles may be worn.

D. Introduce yourself and your department to the patient. Explain what you are there to do. Gain the patient's confidence so that there will be full cooperation.

E. Select the puncture site. The following choices are listed in order from most to least favorable: radial, brachial, dorsalis pedis, and femoral (see Fig. 1-27). If the radial site is selected, try to puncture the left wrist if the patient is right-handed or vice versa.

F. If the radial or pedal sites are selected, the *modified Allen's test* must be performed to ensure that there is adequate collateral flow in case the artery should become clotted because of the procedure.
   1. Radial artery site. See Fig. 3-1 for the basic procedure. Circulation to the hand is stopped by pressing both the radial and ulnar arteries closed. Releasing the pressure over the ulnar artery should result in the hand flushing within 10 to 15 seconds. This is a *positive* test result and proves that the ulnar artery has adequate circulation to the hand. Do not confuse this with a positive Allen's test, which would indicate poor circulation through the ulnar artery. The key point is that if the hand flushes when the ulnar artery is released, there is good flow through it; radial puncture is safe to perform. If the hand does not flush within 15 seconds of the release of the ulnar artery, the circulation is inadequate, and the radial artery of that wrist must *not* be punctured. Another site must be evaluated for puncture.
   2. Dorsalis pedis artery site. Press down on the dorsalis pedis artery to occlude it. Press on the nail of the great toe so that it blanches. Release the pressure on the nail and watch for a rapid return of color. This *positive* test finding confirms that there is good blood flow through the posterior tibial and lateral plantar arteries. So it is safe to draw a sample from the site. A slow return of blood flow indicates poor circulation; another site must be chosen.

G. Prepare the equipment and the puncture site by using sterile technique.
   1. Wash your hands.
   2. If necessary, draw up the heparin solution, flush the syringe with it, and discard the excess.
   3. If a radial or brachial site is selected, the joint should be hyperextended with a folded towel to help stabilize it.
   4. Clean the site by wiping the area with an alcohol and/or iodophor swab in a widening spiral motion that starts at the desired puncture site.
   5. Put on your gloves and eyeglasses or goggles.
   6. Some prefer to anesthetize the puncture site with a 0.8- to 1.0-ml injection of 2% lidocaine (Xylocaine) into the skin. Others believe that this is unnecessary because the injection will cause pain by itself.

A

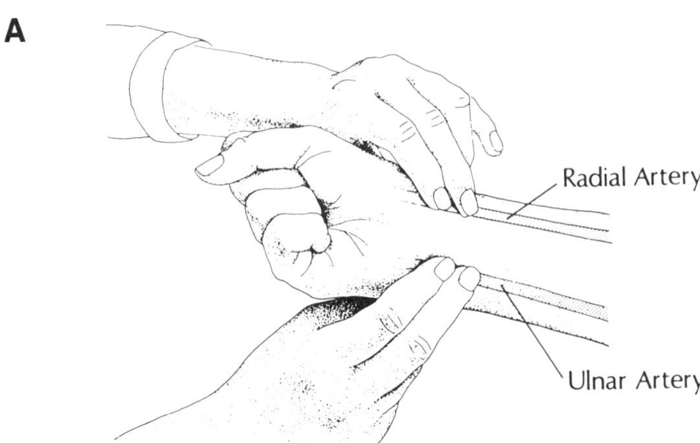

B

C

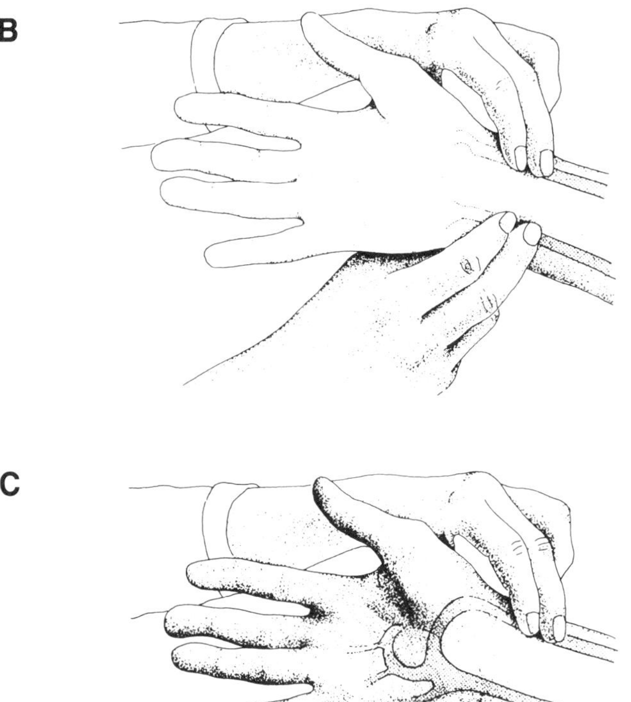

Fig. 3-1 The modified Allen's test. **A,** The hand is clenched into a tight fist and pressure is applied to the radial and ulnar arteries. **B,** The hand is opened (but not fully extended); the palm and fingers are blanched. **C,** Removal of the pressure on the ulnar artery should result in flushing of the entire hand. (From Shapiro BA, Harrison RA, Cane RD, et al: *Clinical Application of Blood Gases,* ed 4. Chicago, Mosby, 1989. Used by permission.)

H. Draw the blood sample.
   1. Hold the syringe like a pencil. The radial and dorsalis pedis arteries should be entered from a 45-degree angle; the brachial and femoral arteries should be entered from a 90-degree angle (Fig. 3-2). Use the first two fingers of your free hand to palpate the pulse and hold the artery still. The bevel of the needle should be up as it enters the skin.
   2. The needle should enter the skin quickly to minimize pain. Carefully advance the needle into the artery. A pulsatile flow is seen with each heart beat. If unsuccessful, withdraw the needle to the skin, change the angle as needed, and reinsert into the artery.

3. Withdraw 2 to 4 ml of blood before removing the needle.
4. Press the sterile gauze onto the puncture site for 2 to 5 minutes. Check the site to ensure that clotting has occurred. Hold longer if needed. An assistant may help with this and step 5.
5. While holding the site, seal the needle, roll the syringe to mix the heparin, and place the syringe in the ice water. (Failure to put the blood sample in ice water will result in a decrease in the Pao_2 value, an increase in the $Paco_2$ value, and a decrease in the pH value. Some department protocols say to

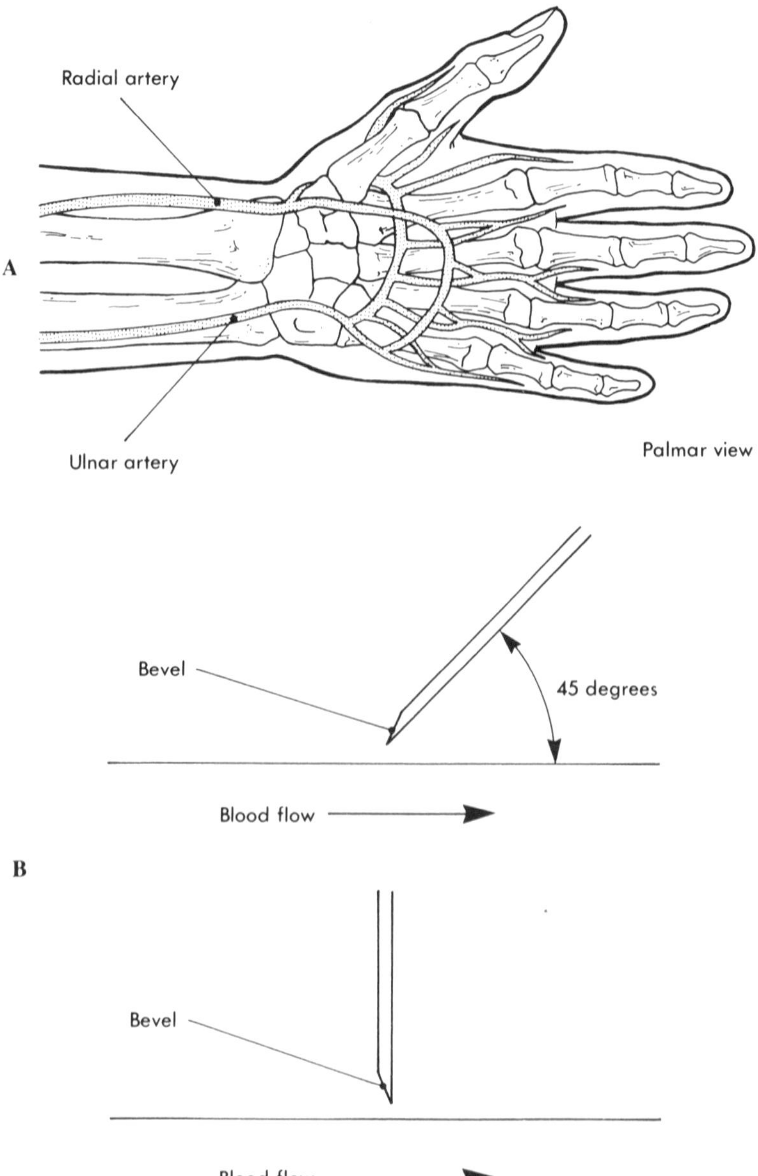

Fig. 3-2 A, Radial arterial position in the lower arm and wrist. **B,** Bevel and needle positioning for radial arterial puncture and other arterial punctures, respectively. (From Lane EE, Walker JF: *Clinical Arterial Blood Gas Analysis.* St. Louis, Mosby, 1987. Used by permission.)

leave the needle unsealed and uncapped to minimize the risk of accidental technician puncture. This is to reduce the risk of spreading hepatitis or acquired immunodeficiency syndrome [AIDS].)

6. Label the syringe with the patient's name, oxygen percentage, and temperature if abnormal. Some departments may also add the patient's age and position when the sample was drawn because of the effects they may have on oyxgenation.
7. Have the sample analyzed as soon as possible.

Module C. Analyze arterial blood.

1. Select the appropriate blood gas analyzer. (IIA7f)[R, Ap]

The blood gas values of Pa_{O_2}, Pa_{CO_2}, and pH are typically obtained from a standard blood gas analyzer. Instrumentation Laboratory (IL) and Ciba Corning Diagnostics Corporation are two well-known manufacturers. Every hospital has a least one blood gas analyzer and it is often kept in the respiratory care department where practitioners are responsible for performing blood gas analysis. If not, the analyzer will be found in the clinical laboratory. These standard units are acceptable for all patient care situations *except* when carbon monoxide poisoning is known or suspected. A standard blood gas analyzer is unable to measure carboxyhemoglobin. A CO oximeter is needed to measure the patient's level of carboxyhemoglobin in carbon monoxide cases.

2. Put the equipment together, make sure that it works properly, and identify any problems with it. (IIB7f)[R, Ap]
3. Perform blood gas analysis. (ICl1)[R, Ap, An]

pH Electrode

a. Electrode design and basic function.

The modern pH electrode has existed since the mid-1950s and is usually referred as the Sanz electrode after its principal inventor. It consists of a reference electrode half-cell and a measuring electrode half-cell, which are connected through a KCl salt bridge and a voltimeter for displaying any electrical flow. The basic principal behind the pH analyzer is its ability to measure the voltage (potential for electrical flow) between two different solutions. This is based on the different hydrogen ion (H^+) concentrations between the solutions that reflect their relative pHs. The *reference electrode* is usually composed of a mercury bead and mercurous chloride (calomel). It is immersed in a KCl solution. This produces a constant voltage as long as the temperature is kept stable. The *measuring electrode* is usually composed of a silver-silver chloride substance. It is immersed in a solution with a pH of 6.840 that fills a glass or plastic chamber. The blood sample, of unknown pH, is placed in a separate measuring chamber called a cuvette. These two chambers are separated by a special glass membrane that contains metals and sodium ions (Na^+) thus making it pH sensitive. Both chambers are kept at a stable 37° C temperature. See Figs. 3-3 and 3-4 for graphic representations of the pH electrode. When blood or a quality control material is introduced into the cuvette there is the potential for hydrogen ions to replace the sodium ions in the pH-sensitive glass if the two pHs are different. The replacement is proportional to the difference in the two pHs.

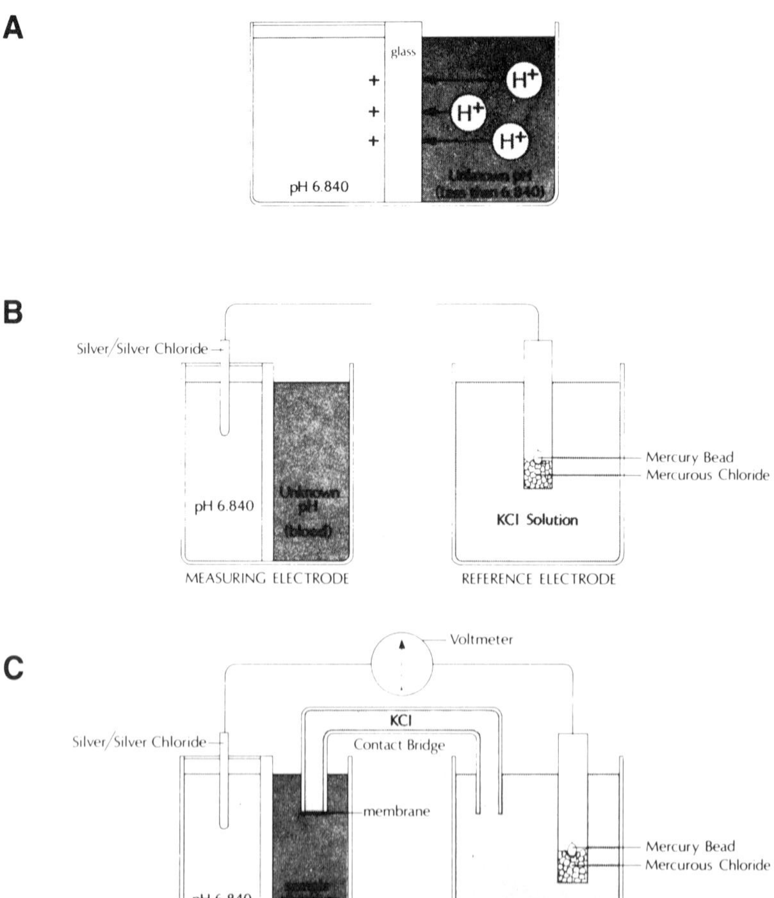

Fig. 3-3 Key components of the pH electrode. **A,** A voltage develops across the pH-sensitive glass when there is a difference in the hydrogen ion concentration between the two solutions. **B,** Two separate half-cells are used for the measuring electrode and the reference electrode. **C,** The addition of a KCl contact bridge and voltmeter completes the electrical circuit and enables the pH of the patient's blood sample to be measured. (From Shapiro BA, Harrison RA, Cane RD, et al: *Clinical Application of Blood Gases,* ed 4. Chicago, Mosby, 1989. Used by permission.)

b. One-point calibration.

Note: These and the following guidelines are based on Clinical Laboratory Improvement Act (CLIA) standards or widely reported industry standards. The various brands and models of blood gas analyzers may have different frequency of calibration requirements, depending on their Food and Drug Association (FDA) approved manufacturers' studies.

a. Should be done before every sample is analyzed if one-point calibration is not automatically performed every 30 minutes.

b. Performed with the near-normal quality control material of 7.384 ± .005 pH used to set the balance potentiometer.

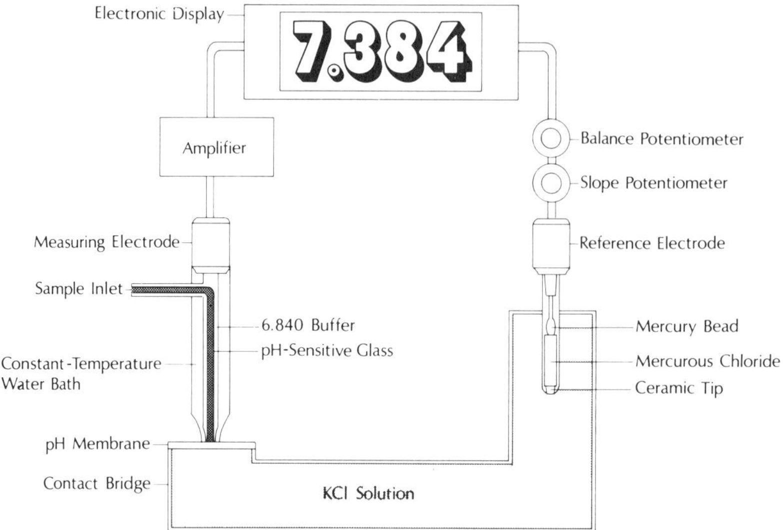

Fig. 3-4 A schematic illustration of a modern, ultramicro pH electrode. (From Shapiro BA, Harrison RA, Cane RD, et al: *Clinical Application of Blood Gases,* ed 4. Chicago, Mosby, 1989. Used by permission.)

c. Recommended every 30 minutes.

d. Should be rechecked after a suspicious pH result; the blood sample should then be rerun.

c. Two-point calibration.

a. Should be done at least once every 8 hours when patient samples are being analyzed.

b. Recommended every 25 patient samples.

c. Performed with the slope potentiometer set with a quality control material or 6.840 ± .005 pH (this is the same pH as the reference electrode solution).

d. Performed with the balance potentiometer set with a quality control material of 7.384 ± .005 pH.

d. Three-point calibration.

a. Should be done at least every 6 months on existing equipment.

b. Should be done done whenever a new electrode is put into use.

c. Covers the physiologic range to confirm linearity: quality control materials of 6.840 ± .005, 7.384 ± .005, and 7.874 ± .005 pH are used.

P_{CO_2} Electrode

a. Electrode design and basic function.

The P_{CO_2} electrode is a modified pH electrode. This was first designed in the mid-1950s by Stowe and further perfected by Severinghaus. Accordingly, these units are now referred to as Severinghaus electrodes or sometimes as Stowe-Severinghaus electrodes. In Fig. 3-5, the electrode is depicted in cross section. It has a reference half-cell and measuring half-cell that are both made of silver-silver chloride. They are enclosed within pH sensitive glass, which is inside a lucite jacket and electrically connected by an electrolyte contact bridge. A nylon spacer separates the tip of the electrode containing the measuring half-cell from a bicarbonate solution (HCO_3^-). The blood sample is introduced into a cuvette heated to 37° C. It is separated from direct contact with the bicarbonate solution by a thin silicon elastic (Silastic) or polytetrafluoroethylene (Teflon) membrane.

The principle of operation is based on the amount of CO_2 found in the blood sample that diffuses through the membrane. The CO_2 chemically combines with the bicarbonate solution to change the pH of the solution by the release of H^+. This H^+ change creates a voltage difference between the measuring and reference half-cells that is proportional to the amount of CO_2 found in the patient's blood sample.

b. One-point calibration.

a. Should be done before every sample is analyzed if one-point calibration is not automatically performed every 30 minutes.
b. Performed with 5% ± .03% CO_2 used to set the balance potentiometer
c. Recommended every 30 minutes.
d. Should be rechecked after a suspicious P_{CO_2} result; the blood sample should then be rerun.

The CO_2 can be directly in contact with the electrode, tomometered with an aqueous material or blood, or premixed in aqueous buffers, assayed liquids, or fluorocarbon-based emulsion.

The predicted P_{CO_2} value at this CO_2% is calculated with this formula: (Note: The solving of this equation has been tested on a past written registry exam when blood gas analysis was listed as a therapist skill. It may now be tested on the entry level examination. Remember that more than one carbon dioxide percentage can be used.)

$$P_{CO_2} = (P_B - P_{H_2O}) \times \% \, CO_2$$

Where:
P_{CO_2} = Predicted PCO_2 in mm Hg
P_B = Barometric pressure at the institution where the analysis is being performed
P_{H_2O} = Water vapor pressure based on the patient's temperature; 47 mm Hg at 37° C/98.6° F
$\% \, CO_2$ = Percentage of CO_2 (also listed as $F\,CO_2$)

Example for 1-point (balance) potentiometer calibration at sea level:

$$P_{CO_2} = (P_B - P_{H_2O}) \times \% \, CO_2$$

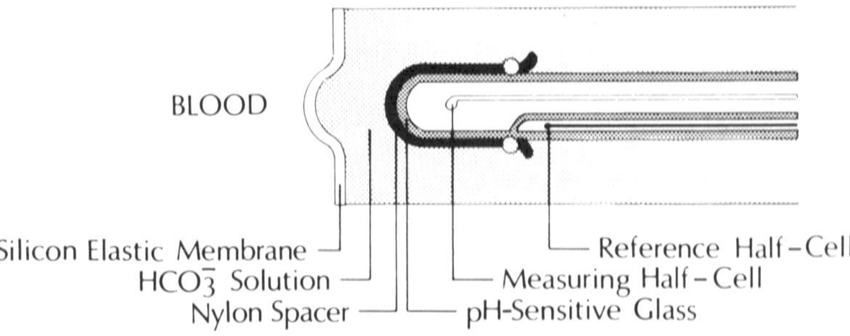

Fig. 3-5 Schematic illustration of the modern P_{CO_2} electrode. (Note that the space between the silicon membrane and the nylon spacer is greatly enlarged for clarity.) (From Shapiro BA, Harrison RA, Cane RD, et al: *Clinical Application of Blood Gases,* ed 4. Chicago, Mosby, 1989. Used by permission.)

Where:
P_{CO_2} = Predicted P_{CO_2} in mm Hg
P_B = 760 mm Hg
P_{H_2O} = 47 mm Hg
% CO_2 = 5%

Therefore:
P_{CO_2} = (760 − 47) × .05
= (713) × .05
= 35.65 or 36 mm Hg. Therefore, set the P_{CO_2} control at 36 mm Hg.

c. Two-point calibration.

a. Should be done at least once every 8 hours when patient samples are being analyzed.
b. Recommended every 25 patient samples.
c. Performed with 10% ± .03% CO_2 to set the slope potentiometer.
d. Performed with 5% ± .03% CO_2 to set the balance potentiometer.

d. Three-point calibration.

a. Should be done at least every 6 months on existing equipment.
b. Should be done done whenever a new electrode is put into use.
c. Covers the physiologic range to confirm linearity; three P_{CO_2} values between 0 and 80 mm Hg should be determined.
d. Room air or a gas cylinder containing 0% ± .03% CO_2 can be used to set the 0 point

P_{O_2} Electrode

a. Electrode design and basic function.

This unit is completely different from the others mentioned and was developed in the late 1950s by Clark and, thus, is usually called a Clark electrode. It is also sometimes known as a polarographic electrode because of the basis of its operation, as will be discussed. Fig. 3-6 is a drawing of key features of the unit. It consists of a silver anode and a platinum wire cathode that runs to the tip of the plastic jacket. A phosphate-KCl buffer solution surrounds the silver anode. The tip of the electrode is covered by a membrane made of either polypropylene or polyethylene. This thin membrane separates the blood-filled cuvette from direct contact with the electrode but allows oxygen molecules to slowly diffuse through to contact the platinum wire cathode. The whole unit is heated to 37° C. The term polarographic comes from the addition of about −0.7 volts to the cathode to make it slightly "polarized" or negative compared with the anode. This is needed to ensure that oxygen is rapidly chemically reduced (gains electrons) at the cathode. This creates an electrical current that is directly proportional to the number of reduced oxygen molecules. See Fig. 3-7 for a schematic drawing of the chemical reaction in the Clark/polarographic electrode.

It must be understood that the P_{O_2} being measured is derived from oxygen that is dissolved in the plasma. It does not come from the hemoglobin found in the erythrocytes (red blood cells). The reported value for the saturation of oxygen in the hemoglobin (Sa_{O_2}) is calculated using a mathematical table. Under normal conditions, the calculated Sa_{O_2} value is the same or close to the true Sa_{O_2} value.

Carbon monoxide poisoning is the only commonly seen clinical situation during

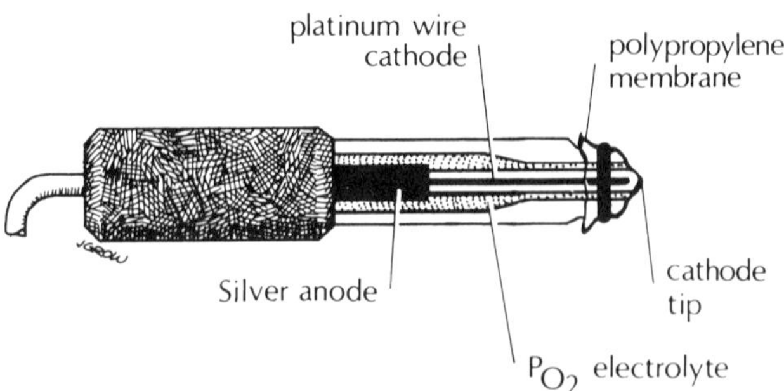

Fig. 3-6 Schematic illustration of the Clark electrode. (From Shapiro BA, Harrison RA, Cane RD, and Templin R: *Clinical Application of Blood Gases,* ed 4. Chicago, Mosby, 1989. Used by permission.)

which a calculated saturation can be incorrectly high. If carbon monoxide poisoning is suspected or known, the patient's blood sample should be analyzed on a CO oximeter unit. This is discussed later in this section. A pulse oximeter unit also should not be used to measure Spo_2 in these patients. Currently available oximeters are only able to evaluate functional hemoglobin. The nonfunctional carboxyhemoglobin will be ignored and the clinician will be given a saturation value for only the remaining functional oxyhemoglobin. Pulse oximeters and the interpretation of their values will be discussed in detail.

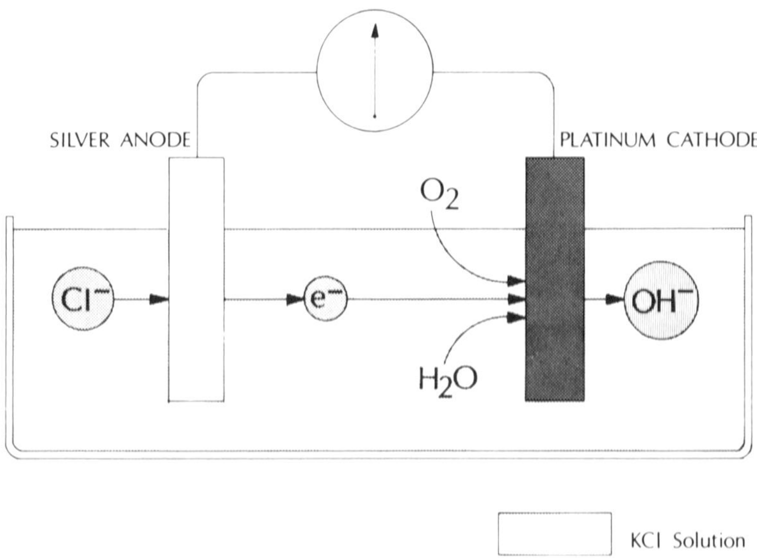

Fig. 3-7 The basic principle of the Clark/polarographic electrode, showing the required chemical reactions. The chloride ion from the KCl solution reacts with the silver anode to form silver chloride. This is an oxidation reaction that releases electrons. Oxygen will use these electrons (a reduction reaction) to chemically react with the water in the solution, and the platinum cathode to release OH^- (hydronium) ions. This produces an electrical flow that is proportional to the oxygen concentration and displayed on the amp meter as Po_2. (From Shapiro BA, Harrison RA, Cane RD, et al: *Clinical Application of Blood Gases,* ed 4. Chicago, Mosby, 1989. Used by permission.)

b. Blood gas factor

The blood gas factor relates to the phenomenon that when a given percentage of oxygen is directly introduced into the electrode a higher reading is found than when the same oxygen percentage is tonometered with blood before being introduced into the electrode. If oxygen is directly used to calibrate the electrode, this results in an understatement of the patient's PO_2 value of 2% to 15%. Since the blood gas factor is progressively greater as the PO_2 value increases, there is probably no need to make an adjustment to any patient results that are less than 100 mm Hg. However, if results of over 150 mm Hg are anticipated, as in a shunt study, the factor should be taken into account. This can be done in two ways. First, the electrode can be three-point calibrated with a higher oxygen percentage as will be described. Second, the blood gas factor can be calculated and the patient's values adjusted mathematically.

c. One-point calibration.

a. Should be done before every sample is analyzed if one-point calibration is not automatically performed every 30 minutes.

b. Performed with 12% ± .03% O_2 used to set the balance potentiometer; some analyzers are designed to use 20% ± .03% O_2 from a gas cylinder or draw room air (20.95% oxygen) into the unit.

c. Recommended every 30 minutes.

d. Should be rechecked after a suspicious PO_2 result; the blood sample should then be rerun.

The O_2 can be directly in contact with the electrode, tomometered with an aqueous material or blood, or pre-mixed in aqueous buffers, assayed liquids, or fluorocarbon-based emulsion as discussed.

The predicted PO_2 values at these O_2% are calculated with this formula: (Note: The solving of this equation has been tested on a past written registry exam when blood gas analysis was listed as a therapist skill. It may now be tested on the entry level exam. Remember that more than one oxygen percentage can be used.)

$$PO_2 = (P_B - PH_2O) \times \%\ O_2$$

Where:

PO_2 = Predicted PO_2 in mm Hg
P_B = Barometric pressure at the institution where the analysis is being performed
PH_2O = Water vapor pressure based on the patient's temperature; 47 mm Hg at 37° C/98.6° F
% O_2 = percentage of O_2 (also listed as F O_2)

Example for 1-point (balance) potentiometer calibration at sea level using *12% oxygen:*

$$PO_2 = (P_B - PH_2O) \times \%\ O_2$$

Where:

PO_2 = predicted PO_2 in mm Hg
P_B = 760 mm Hg
PH_2O = 47 mm Hg
% O_2 = 12%

Therefore:

$$\begin{aligned} Po_2 &= (760 - 47) \times .12 \\ &= (713) \times .12 \\ &= 85.56 \text{ or } 86 \text{ mm Hg; Set the } Po_2 \text{ control at } 86 \text{ mm Hg.} \end{aligned}$$

d. Two-point calibration.

a. Should be done at least once every 8 hours when patient samples are being analyzed.

b. Should be done whenever readjustment of 1-point calibration is greater than 3 mm Hg.

c. Recommended every 25 patient samples.

d. Performed with 0% ± .03% O_2 to set the slope potentiometer.

e. Performed with 12% ± .03% O_2 to set the balance potentiometer; some analyzers are designed to use 20% ± .03% O_2 from a gas cylinder or draw room air (20.95% oxygen) into the unit.

e. Three-point calibration.

a. Should be done at least every 6 months on existing equipment.

b. Should be done whenever a new electrode is put into use.

c. Should be done to compensate for the blood gas factor and confirm linearity whenever the Po_2 value could be over 150 mm Hg, assuming that the balance point is set on room oxygen content; the third point should be set on 100% ± .03% O_2 from a gas cylinder.

Miscellaneous Topics

a. Calibration gas cylinders.

It should be noted that for economic reasons the low-percentage oxygen and carbon dioxide gases are placed together in one cylinder and the high-percentage oxygen and carbon dioxide gases are placed together in a second cylinder. Table 3-1 summarizes the normal precision of the electrodes discussed and the gases used in their calibration. A cylinder containing 100% oxygen and 0% carbon dioxide could be used for 3-point calibration.

b. Temperature correction.

Temperature correction refers to mathematically adjusting a patient's Pao_2, $Paco_2$, and pH values because his or her temperature is not 37° C. It should be recalled that blood gas analyzers are calibrated at 37° C since it is normal body temperature. If the patient has a fever, the oxygen and carbon dioxide partial pressures in the blood will be greater than those found during the blood gas analysis. Conversely, the hypothermic patient will have lower oxygen and carbon dioxide partial pressures in the blood than those found during the blood gas analysis. The pH value will shift in the opposite direction as the Pco_2 value. Usually, this small shift in values is ignored. However, since some physicians may specify that their patient's blood gases be temperature corrected, the patient's temperature should be listed on the blood gas slip. It is a simple mathematical process to temperature correct the blood gas results. Most modern analyzers will perform it automatically when programmed to do so.

Remember to flush the electrode membrane after each use, if possible, to prevent protein buildup. If this occurs, the response time is longer than normal. Rerun the cali-

Table 3-1. Electrode Precision and Calibration Gases

Electrodes:
- pH ± 0.01 unit
- P_{CO_2} ± 2% (approximately ± 1 mm Hg at 40 mm Hg)
- P_{O_2} ± 3% (approximately ± 2.5 mm Hg at 80 mm Hg)
- If the P_{O_2} is over 150 mm Hg P_{O_2}, the precision is approximately ± 10% unless 3-point calibration is performed.

Calibration gases:
- "low" gas: 0% oxygen, 5% carbon dioxide (both ± .03%), balance nitrogen
- "high" gas: 12% or 21% oxygen, 10% carbon dioxide (both ± .03%), balance nitrogen
- Suggested 3-point gases: 100% oxygen, 0% carbon dioxide (both ± .03%)

bration for any of the electrodes and reanalyze the sample if you are suspicious of the result. If the electrode will not calibrate close to the reference buffer solutions or gases, it should not be used.

Module D. Interpret the arterial blood gas results in order to determine how the patient is responding to respiratory care.

A number of authors have written extensively on how to interpret arterial blood gases. Individuals preparing for the entry level examination must find a system of interpretation that works best for him or her. After reviewing a number of works, the author has found the system proposed by Shapiro to be both practical and relatively easy to understand. Most of the following discussion and tables are based on this system. This does not mean that if you have learned another system you are at any disadvantage for taking the NBRC's examinations.

The NBRC examination will include questions that are specifically on blood gas interpretation. It will also include blood gas results in other questions that relate to any respiratory care technique or procedure. The examinee must be proficient in blood gas interpretation to do well on the entry level examination!

Assessment of Oxygenation

Hypoxemia/hypoxia can be rapidly life-threatening. Because of this, it is most authors' opinion that it should be the first blood gas value to be interpreted. Table 3-2 shows the normal Pa_{O_2} values for the newborn, child to adult, and the aged when room air (21% oxygen) is inhaled at sea level. These values will decrease progressively as the altitude increases. However, under most clinical conditions this is not a factor (unless you work in a hospital in Denver or another Rocky Mountain city).

A general rule is that any patient is seriously hypoxemic if the Pa_{O_2} is less than 60 mm Hg on room air. See Table 3-3 for guidelines on judging the seriousness of hypoxemia. Once hypoxemia is recognized, it must be corrected. The most obvious way is to give supplemental oxygen. The clinician must realize that oxygen alone will not correct the hypoxemia if the patient is hypoventilating (increased Pa_{CO_2}), has heart failure, or is unable to carry or make use of the oxygen. See Table 3-3 for the guidelines on giving supplemental oxygen so as to not undersupply or oversupply what the patient needs. In general, try to keep the patient's Pa_{O_2} between 60 and 100 mm Hg.

Table 3-4 lists general guidelines for the relationship between inspired oxygen and Pa_{O_2}. However, since most patients receiving respiratory care do not have normal lung physiology, it can be anticipated that their Pa_{O_2} values will not increase as expected in

Table 3-2. Age-based Acceptable Pa_{O_2} Levels When Breathing Room Air (21% Oxygen) at Sea Level

Age	Pa_{O_2} (mm Hg)
Newborn	
Acceptable range	40-70
Child to Adult	
Normal	97
Acceptable range	>80
Hypoxemia	<80
Aged (yr)	
60	>80
70	>70
80	>60
90	>50

Adapted from Shapiro BA, Harrison RA, Cane RD, et al: *Clinical Application of Blood Gases,* ed 4. Chicago, Mosby, 1989.

the face of increased inspired oxygen. Shapiro et al.[1] suggest the following formula for determining whether the patient will be hypoxemic on room air: "If Pa_{O_2} is less than $FI_{O_2} \times 5$, the patient can be assumed to be hypoxemic on room air."

Fig. 3-8 shows a normal oxyhemoglobin dissociation curve. The saturation value is important to know because it shows how much hemoglobin is saturated with oxygen. It is best to directly measure the saturation on a CO oximeter–type blood gas analyzer. Calculated saturation values can be misleadingly high if the patient has inhaled carbon monoxide. There are several points of correlation between the Sa_{O_2} and the Pa_{O_2} as shown in Fig. 3-8.

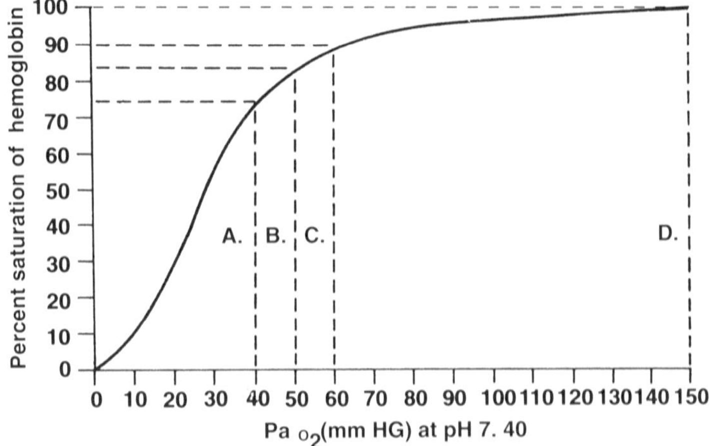

Fig. 3-8 The oxygen (oxyhemoglobin) dissociation curve plots the relationship between hemoglobin saturation (y-axis) and plasma Pa_{O_2} (x-axis). **A,** 75% saturation and a Pa_{O_2} of 40 mm Hg are normally seen in venous blood. **B,** 85% saturation and a Pa_{O_2} of 50 mm Hg are the minimal levels that should be allowed in a *chronically* hypoxemic patient. **C,** 90% saturation and Pa_{O_2} of 60 mm Hg are the minimal levels that should be allowed in an *acutely* hypoxemic patient. **D,** Hemoglobin in the pulmonary capillaries adjacent to normal alveoli will become 100% saturated when the Pa_{O_2} reaches 150 mm Hg. (Adapted from Lane EE, Walker JF: *Clinical Arterial Blood Gas Analysis.* St. Louis, Mosby, 1987.)

Sa_{O_2} (%)	Pa_{O_2} (mm Hg)	Comment
100	150	Hemoglobin is fully saturated.
90	60	The patient who is *acutely* ill with cardiopulmonary disease should not be allowed to have the oxygenation values fall below these levels.
85	50	The patient who is *chronically* ill with cardiopulmonary disease should not be allowed to have the oxygenation values fall below these levels.
75	40	These are the normal mixed venous blood gas values as obtained from a pulmonary artery (Swan-Ganz) catheter. It is possible to obtain similar values from an attempted arterial puncture that sampled venous blood. If these values are obtained from a true arterial sample, the patient is in serious trouble. Fast action must be taken to correct this life-threatening hypoxemia.

Table 3-3. Evaluation of Hypoxemia

Hypoxemia	Pa_{O_2}
Conditions: room air is inspired; the patient is <60 yr	
Mild†	<80 mm Hg
Moderate†	<60 mm Hg
Severe†	<40 mm Hg
Conditions: supplemental oxygen is inspired; the patient is <60 yr	
Uncorrected	Less than room air acceptable limit
Corrected	Within the room air acceptable limit; <100 mm Hg
Excessively corrected	>100 mm Hg; less than the minimal level predicted in Table 3-4

Adapted from Shapiro BA, Harrison RA, Cane RD, et al: *Clinical Application of Blood Gases,* ed 4. Chicago, Mosby, Inc, 1989.

†Subtract 1 mm Hg of oxygen to limits of mild and moderate hypoxemia for each year over 60. A Pa_{O_2} <40 mm Hg indicates severe hypoxemia in any patient at any age.

Table 3-4. General Relationship Between Inspired Oxygen Percentage and Pa_{O_2}

Oxygen (%) or Fi_{O_2}	Minimal Predicted Pa_{O_2} (mm Hg)*
30	150
40	200
50	250
60	300
70	350
80	400
90	450
100	500

Adapted from Shapiro BA, Harrison RA, Cane RD, et al: *Clinical Application of Blood Gases,* ed 4. Chicago, Mosby, Inc, 1989.

*Note: This is for estimation purposes. It is not as accurate as calculating the patient's $P(A-a)_{O_2}$.

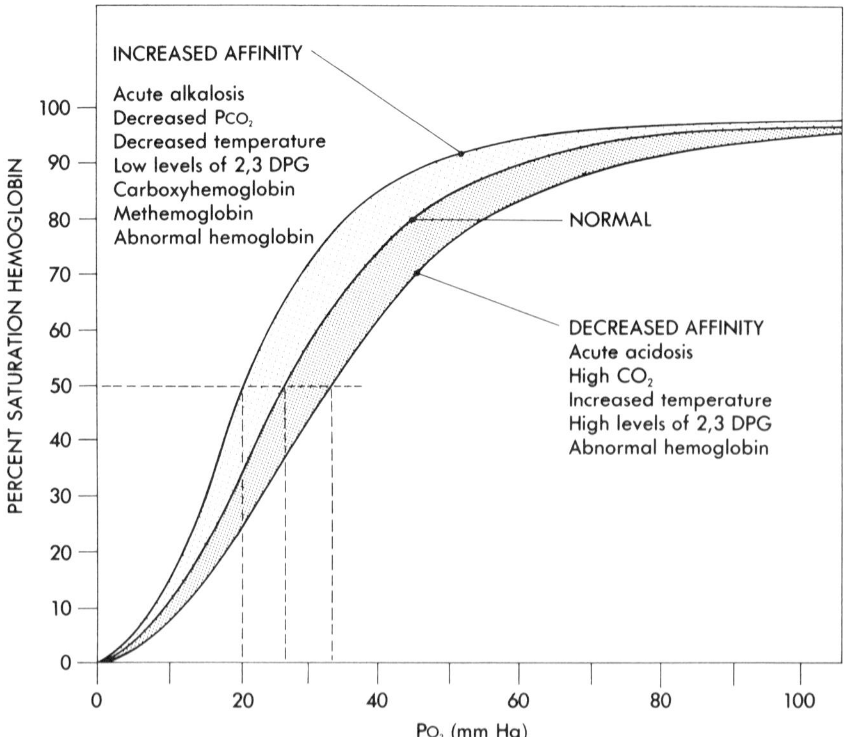

Fig. 3-9 Conditions associated with altered affinity of hemoglobin for O_2. P_{50} is the Pao_2 at which hemoglobin is 50% saturated, normally 26.6 mm Hg. A lower than normal P_{50} represents increased affinity of hemoglobin for O_2; a high P_{50} is seen with decreased affinity. Note that variation from normal is associated with decreased (low P_{50}) or increased (high P_{50}) availability of O_2 to tissues *(dotted lines)*. The shaded area shows the entire oxyhemoglobin dissociation curve under the same circumstances. (From Lane EE, Walker JF: *Clinical Arterial Blood Gas Analysis.* St. Louis, Mosby, 1987. Used by permission.)

Fig. 3-9 shows a number of factors that can influence the oxyhemoglobin dissociation curve and how oxygen loads onto and unloads from hemoglobin. In a patient with normal oxygenation these factors are not clinically significant. However, when the Pao_2 is less than 60 mm Hg and the Sao_2 is less than 90%, these factors can become an important consideration. As can be seen in the Fig. 2-4, a left-shifted oxyhemoglobin dissociation curve results in a lower Pao_2 at any given saturation. This would result in even less oxygen being delivered to the tissues.

Assessment of Carbon Dioxide and pH

The pH is the next most important value to interpret because extreme acidemia/acidosis and alkalemia/alkalosis can be life-threatening. The carbon dioxide value is important to interpret because it has a direct effect upon the pH and indirectly affects the oxygen level. A high or low $Paco_2$ level, by itself, is not life-threatening.

Table 3-5 shows normal values for pH and $Paco_2$ and the acceptable ranges around the mean or average. Table 3-6 shows the most widely acceptable therapeutic ranges for pH and $Paco_2$. Values that fall outside of these ranges present a progressively greater risk to the patient.

Table 3-7 shows the definitions of Shapiro et al.[1] for alkalemia and acidemia from a respiratory cause. Strictly speaking, a pH greater than 7.4 is alkalemia, and a pH less

Table 3-5. Normal Laboratory Ranges for $Paco_2$ and pH

Measurement	Mean	SD	2 SD*
$Paco_2$	40	38-42 mm Hg	35-45 mm Hg
pH	7.40	7.38-7.42	7.35-7.45

Adapted from Shapiro BA, Harrison RA, Cane RD, et al: *Clinical Application of Blood Gases,* ed 4. Chicago, Mosby, 1989.
**SD,* Standard deviation.

Table 3-6. Acceptable Clinical Ranges for $Paco_2$ and pH

$Paco_2$	30-50 mm Hg*
pH	7.30-7.50

Adapted from Shapiro BA, Harrison RA, Cane RD, et al: *Clinical Application of Blood Gases,* ed 4, Chicago, Mosby, Inc, 1989.
*This is the range for patients with an acute change. It does not apply to patients with long-standing disease such as COPD. These patients may have $Paco_2$ values greater than 50 mm Hg.

Table 3-7. Naming Unacceptable Values for $Paco_2$ and pH

$Paco_2 > 50$ mm Hg	Respiratory acidosis/alveolar hypoventilation/ventilatory failure
pH < 7.30	Acidemia
$Paco_2 < 30$ mm Hg	Respiratory alkalosis/alveolar hyperventilation
pH > 7.50	Alkalemia

Adapted from Shapiro BA, Harrison RA, Cane RD, et al: *Clinical Application of Blood Gases,* ed 4. Chicago, Mosby, Inc, 1989.

than 7.4 is acidemia. Also, a $Paco_2$ less than 40 mm Hg would cause a respiratory alkalosis, and a $Paco_2$ greater than 40 mm Hg would cause a respiratory acidosis. However, Shapiro and colleagues[1] would argue that such narrow values are clinically unnecessary.

Table 3-8 shows the relationship between $Paco_2$ and pH. An *acute* change in the patient's ventilation will cause the following when starting from a $Paco_2$ of 40 mm Hg:

a. If the $Paco_2$ increases by 20 mm Hg, the pH will decrease by 0.10 units.
b. If the $Paco_2$ decreases by 10 mm Hg, the pH will increase by 0.10 units.

From this it can be seen that the body is better able to compensate with metabolic buffers for a respiratory acidosis than a respiratory alkalosis. Changes inside or outside of these values will be from *chronic* respiratory conditions and/or metabolic conditions.

Metabolic effects are evaluated by interpreting either the bicarbonate (HCO_3^-) value or base excess/base deficit (BE/BD) value. Both will reveal whether there is any metabolic effect on the pH. Normal values are as shown:

- HCO_3^-: 24 mEq/L.
- BE/BD: 0 mEq/L; ±1 mEq/L is often listed as the normal range.

Values indicating metabolic acidosis of a primary or secondary nature are as follows:

Table 3-8. Approximate Relationships Between Pa_{CO_2}, pH and Bicarbonate

Pa_{CO_2} (mm Hg)	pH	Bicarbonate/HCO_3^- (mEq/L)
80	7.20	28
60	7.30	26
40	7.40	24
30	7.50	22
20	7.60	20

Adapted from Shapiro BA, Harrison RA, Cane RD, et al: *Clinical Application of Blood Gases,* ed 4. Chicago, Mosby, 1989.

- Bicarbonate greater than 24 mEq/L.
- BE greater than 0 or greater than plus 1 mEq/L.

Values indicating metabolic acidosis of a primary or secondary nature are as follows:

- Bicarbonate less than 24 mEq/L.
- BE less than 0 or less than minus 1 mEq/L. Some laboratories report this as a base deficit (BD) or negative base excess.

Tables 3-9 to 3-11 show definitions of terms and classifications of the various acid-base states. This is a complex subject because of all the variables. The reader should

Table 3-9. Clinical Terminology for Arterial Blood Gas Measurements

Clinical Terminology	Clinical Findings
Respiratory acidosis/alveolar hypoventilation/ ventilatory failure	$Pa_{CO_2} > 50$ mm Hg
Acute ventilatory failure	$Pa_{CO_2} > 50$ mm Hg; pH <7.30
Chronic ventilatory failure	$Pa_{CO_2} > 50$ mm Hg; pH 7.30-7.40
Respiratory alkalosis/alveolar hyperventilation	$Pa_{CO_2} < 30$ mm Hg
Acute alveolar hyperventilation	$Pa_{CO_2} < 30$ mm Hg; pH >7.50
Chronic alveolar hyperventilation	$Pa_{CO_2} < 30$ mm Hg; pH 7.40-7.50
Acidemia	pH < 7.40
Acidosis	Pathophysiologic condition in which the patient has a significant base deficit (plasma bicarbonate below normal)
Alkalemia	pH greater than 7.40*
Alkalosis	Pathophysiologic condition in which the patient has a significant base excess (plasma bicarbonate above normal)

Adapted from Shapiro BA, Harrison RA, Cane RD, et al: *Clinical Application of Blood Gases,* ed 4. Chicago, Mosby, Inc, 1989.

*Some authors prefer wider limits such as 7.35 to 7.45 or 7.30 to 7.50.

Table 3-10. Evaluation of Ventilatory and Metabolic Effects on Acid-Base Status

Evaluation of Pa_{CO_2}	
>50 mm Hg	Respiratory acidosis/alveolar hypoventilation/ ventilatory failure
30-50 mm Hg	Acceptable alveolar ventilation
<30 mm Hg	Respiratory alkalosis/alveolar hyperventilation
Evaluation of Pa_{CO_2} in conjunction with pH*	
Acceptable alveolar ventilation (Pa_{CO_2} 30-50 mm Hg)	
pH >7.50	Metabolic alkalosis
pH 7.30-7.50	Acceptable ventilatory and metabolic acid-base status
pH <7.30	Metabolic acidosis
Alveolar hypoventilation (Pa_{CO_2} >50 mm Hg)	
pH >7.40	*Partially compensated* metabolic alkalosis
pH 7.30-7.40	*Chronic* ventilatory failure
pH <7.30	*Acute* ventilatory failure
Alveolar hyperventilation (Pa_{CO_2} <30 mm Hg)	
pH >7.50	*Acute* alveolar hyperventilation
pH 7.40-7.50	*Chronic* alveolar hyperventilation
pH 7.30-7.40	*Compensated* metabolic acidosis
pH <7.30	*Partially compensated* metabolic acidosis

Adapted from Shapiro BA, Harrison RA, Cane RD, et al: *Clinical Application of Blood Gases,* ed 4. Chicago, Mosby, 1989.
*Note: Some authors use a more narrow pH range for these classifications.

study these tables and practice their application on arterial blood gases from real-life situations.

As stated earlier, there are other systems for interpreting blood gases. All are probably satisfactory for interpretation purposes and preparing for the entry level examination.

Table 3-11. Primary Blood Gas Classifications

Condition	Pa_{CO_2}	pH	Bicarbonate	Base Excess
Ventilatory imbalance				
Acute alveolar hypoventilation	I*	D*	N*	N
Chronic alveolar hypoventilation	I	N	I	I
Acute alveolar hyperventilation	D	I	N	N
Chronic alveolar hyperventilation	D	N	D	D
Metabolic imbalance				
Uncompensated acidosis	N	D	D	D
Partially compensated acidosis	D	D	D	D
Uncompensated alkalosis	N	I	I	I
Partially compensated alkalosis	I	I	I	I
Compensated acidosis or alkalosis	I or D	N	I or D	I or D

Adapted from Shapiro BA, Harrison RA, Cane RD, et al: *Clinical Application of Blood Gases,* ed 4. Chicago, Mosby, 1989.
**I*, increased; *D*, decreased; *N*, normal range.

Table 3-12. Normal Hemoglobin Values for Adults

Total hemoglobin (THb)	Men: 13.5-18.0 g/dl* Women: 12.0-16.0 g/dl 15.0 g/dl is often listed as an average for both
Oxyhemoglobin (O_2Hb) (arterial sample)	94%-100% of THb (reported as SaO_2 of 94% to 100%)
Carboxyhemoglobin (COHb)	Nonsmokers: less than 1.5% (0.225 g/dl) of THb Smokers: 1.5%-10% of THb
Methemoglobin (MetHB) O_2 content (arterial sample)	0.5%-3% (0.75-0.45 g/dl) of THb 15-23 vol/dl

*g/dl is grams per deciliter and is sometimes listed as g/100 ml.

Module E. Interpret the results of CO oximetry blood gas analysis. (IC3)[R, Ap]

The CO oximeter-type blood gas analyzer gives values for oxyhemoglobin (O_2Hb), reduced hemoglobin (RHb), carboxyhemoglobin (COHb), and methemoglobin (MetHb)/sulfhemoglobin (SHb). Each of these hemoglobin moities can be displayed in terms of grams per deciliter, percentage of the whole, and added together for a total hemoglobin (THb). See Table 3-12 for the normal adult hemoglobin values. The amount of carboxyhemoglobin and methemoglobin should be subtracted from the total hemoglobin to find the amount of functional hemoglobin. Any increase in the carboxyhemoglobin and/or methemoglobin level above those listed is abnormal and results in even less normal hemoglobin to carry oxygen. The patient who suffers from carbon monoxide poisoning is at greatest risk. A COHb level of 30% saturation or greater can be fatal. By subtraction, the O_2Hb (Sao_2) level can be no greater than 70% with a resulting Pao_2 of less than 40 mm Hg.

Calculate the amount of functional hemoglobin and saturation in the following way:

Example for a patient with normal COHb and MetHb levels:

15.0 gm total Hb
−.225 gm COHb
14.775 gm
−.15 gm MetHb
14.625 gm functional Hb

100% potential saturation of oxyhemoglobin in arterial blood
−1.5% saturation of COHb
98.5%
−1.5% saturation of MetHb
97% saturation of arterial blood (Sao_2 of 97%)

Example for a patient with an elevated COHb and a normal MetHb level:

15.0 gm total Hb
−3.0 gm COHb
12.0 gm
−.15 gm MetHb
11.85 gm functional Hb

100% potential saturation of oxyhemoglobin in arterial blood
−20% saturation of COHb
80%
−1.5% saturation of MetHb
78.5% saturation of arterial blood (Sa_{O_2} of 78.5%)

Module F. Pulse oximetry.

1. Check the patient's chart for previous pulse oximetry (Sp_{O_2}) results. (IAlf2)[R, Ap]

The general indication for pulse oximetry is whenever a patient's oxygenation must be monitored, except when there is carbon monoxide poisoning. An Sp_{O_2} of 90% or greater indicates that the patient is adequately oxygenated. Past values should be compared with current readings to follow the patients progress or response to treatment.

2. Make a recommendation to perform pulse oximetry. (IA2d)[R, Ap]

Pulse oximetry is indicated in the following situations: during anesthesia and intraoperative monitoring of oxygenation, postoperatively when the patient is still sedated, when the patient is receiving sedatives or analgesics that can blunt the airway protective reflexes, during bronchoscopy, during a sleep study, and when the effectiveness of oxygen therapy is being evaluated.

3. Get an appropriate pulse oximeter and related equipment. (IIA7g)[R, Ap]

All pulse oximeters will report an Sp_{O_2} percentage on a light emitting diode (LED) display. Many newer units will also display the patient's pulse rate. More expensive units will print out a copy of Sp_{O_2} percentage and pulse rate to be placed into the patient's chart if it is required. There are a variety of sensors that will fit the feet and/or hands of infants, and adult's fingers, the bridge of the nose, forehead, and ear lobe. Choose a sensor that is designed to fit the site that is selected.

4. Put the equipment together, make sure that it works properly, identify and fix any problems with it. (IIB7g)[R, Ap]

Follow the manufacturer's suggestions for the set up. The newer pulse oximetry systems will visually display the strength of the pulse so that the best place for the probe can be found.(See Fig. 3-10.) Keep bright light out of the patient site and transducer. See Table 3-13 for common sources of error and their solutions. Figs. 3-11 to 3-14 show how to apply the different probes in the pulse oximetry systems to the various sites.

5. Perform pulse oximetry on your patient. (IC2a and IIIE3)[R, Ap]

Pulse oximetry has gained wide acceptance because it offers a way to continuously and noninvasively monitor a patient's oxygenation by following the percent of hemoglobin saturated with oxygen. The reported Sp_{O_2} % is the percent of oxyhemoglobin. Manufacturers of ear and pulse oximeters include Biochem International, Inc., Catalyst Research, CritiCare Research, Medical Graphics Corporation, Nonin Medical, Inc., Ohmeda, and SensorMedics Corporation, among others.

Pulse oximetry makes practical use of two physical principles. The first is spectrophotometry, which is used to analyze the transmission of two wavelengths of light through

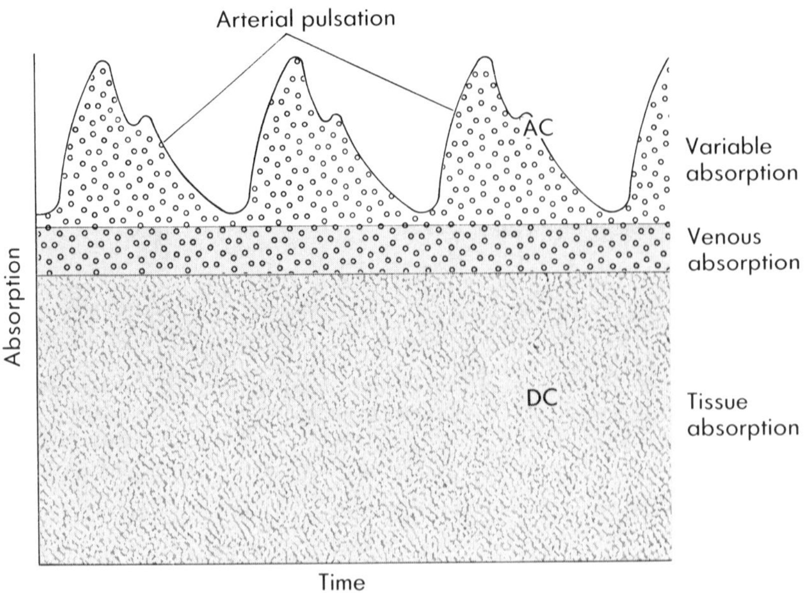

Fig. 3-10 Pulse oximetry signal strength. The strong surge of blood through the artery with each heartbeat results in variable absorption of the light emitted by the pulse oximeter. Venous and tissue absorption of light is stable when the heart is at rest. This absorption difference is used to find the patient's artery and measure the heart rate. (*AC* refers to variable absorption, *DC* to stable absorption.) (From Rupple G: *Manual of Pulmonary Function Testing*, ed 6. St. Louis, Mosby, 1994. Used by permission.)

the blood and body tissues. One wavelength is 660 nm and the other is between 920 and 940 nm, depending on the manufacturer. The 660 nm wavelength can be seen as red and is preferentially absorbed by O_2Hb. The 920 to 940 nm wavelength is not visible since it is in the infrared range. It is preferentially absorbed by reduced Rhb.

The second principle is plethysmography. It is used to find and then evaluate the

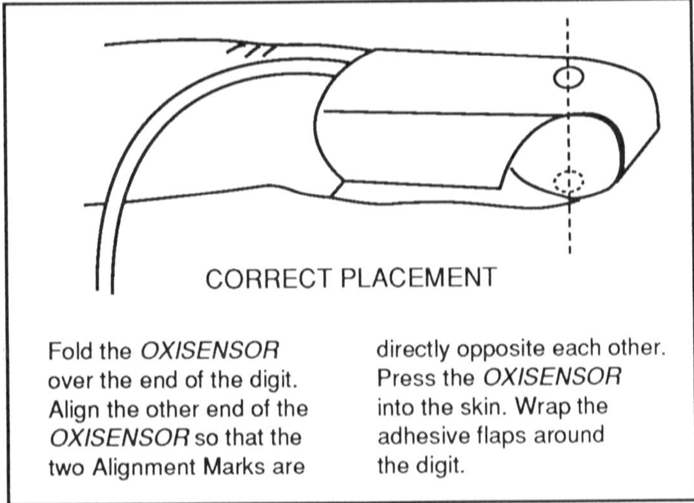

Fig. 3-11 Pulse oximetry transducer placed on a finger. (Courtesy of Nellcor, Inc.)

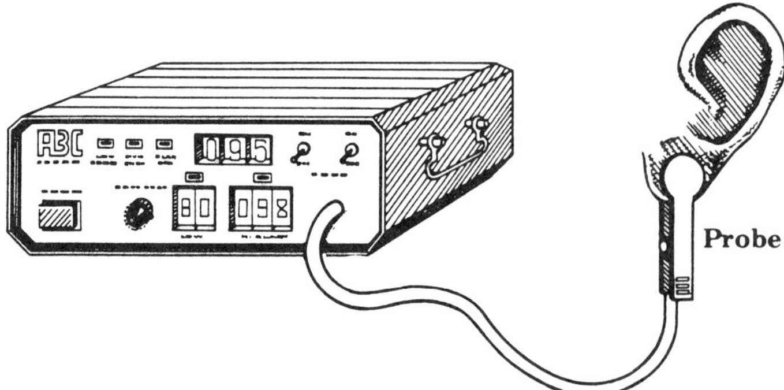

Fig. 3-12 Pulse oximeter unit with transducer placed on the ear lobe. (From Pilbeam SP: *Mechanical Ventilation—Physiological and Clinical Applications,* ed 2. St. Louis, Mosby, 1992. Used by permission.)

amplitude of the arterial pulse waveform. See Fig. 3-10 for the plethysmographic arterial waveform. When the pulse oximeter sensor is placed on a patient site, the fingertip for example, the two wavelengths of light shine through the blood, tissues, and bone within the finger. See Fig. 3-11 for the proper placement. It is important that the sending LED and receiving (photodiode) sensors be opposite each other. Most units have a signal strength display that indicates when the photodiode is receiving a strong signal, and the patient's pulse has been detected. The microprocessor is designed to detect a baseline level of light absorption by the tissues and venous blood, containing more RHb, as well as the light absorption of arterial blood, containing more O_2Hb. It can then compare the absorptions of the two wavelengths to determine the level of saturated oxyhemoglobin. This is displayed as saturation by pulse oximetry, or Spo_2. (Do not be confused by some authors who use the abbreviations Sao_2 or $Stco_2$ [saturation of transcutaneous oxygen] for pulse oximetry.)

It must be realized that because pulse oximetry samples only two wavelengths of light, the technology is unable to recognize the presence or quantity of the nonfunctional hemoglobin species of COHb and MetHb. Pulse oximetry can only recognize the saturation of functional oxyhemoglobin. Patients with carbon monoxide poisoning or an ele-

Table 3-13. Sources of Error in Pulse Oximetry

Source of Error	Remedy
Light interference: xenon lamp, fluorescent light, infrared (bilirubin) light	Cover the probe with an opaque wrap
Low perfusion: low blood pressure, hypothermia, vasoconstricting drugs	Use ear lobe, bridge of nose, or forehead instead of finger or toe; discontinue use if still unreliable
Motion artifact	Secure the probe site; ensure that the Spo_2 reading is synchronized with the heart rate
Darkly pigmented patient	Use lightly pigmented site such as tip of finger or toe; Spo_2 value may overestimate Pao_2; discontinue use if still unreliable
Artificial or painted finger nails	Remove acrylic nails, remove black, blue, green, metallic, or frosted nail polish; use a different site
Venous pulsation read as an arterial pulsation	Loosen a tight sensor; change the finger sensor site every 2-4 hours; loosen the cause of a tourniquet-like effect
Vascular dyes that cause low Spo_2 readings (methylene blue, indigo carmine, indocyanine green)	Do not use pulse oximetry

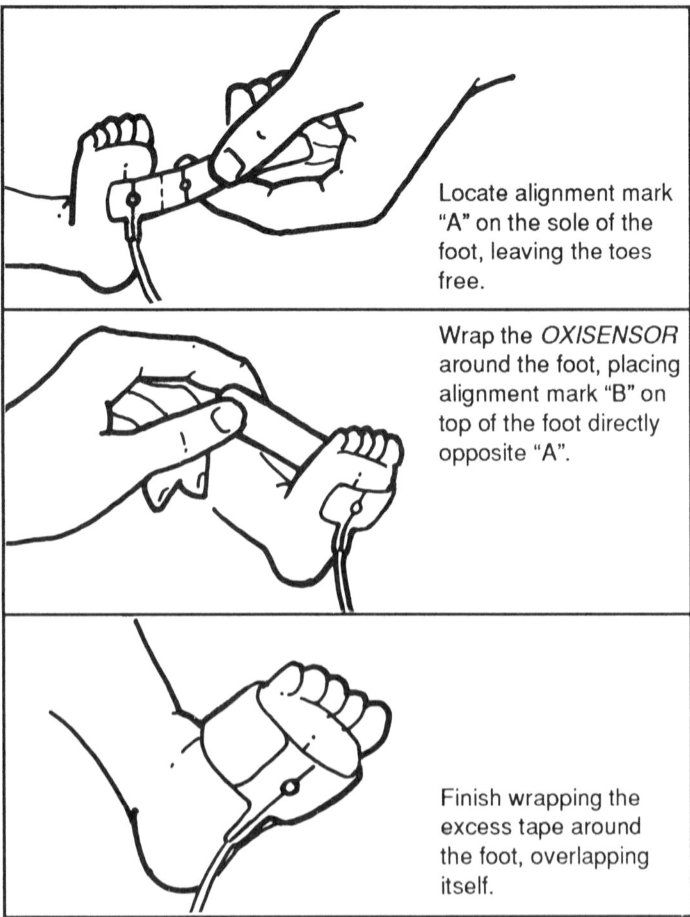

Fig. 3-13 Pulse oximetry transducer placed on an infant's foot. (Courtesy of Nellcor, Inc.)

vated MetHb value should not have pulse oximetry used to evaluate oxygenation because it will give an incorrect high reading. Instead, an ABG should be drawn and sent off to be passed through a CO oximeter for a complete fractional hemoglobin analysis. Even healthy persons have small amounts of COHb and MetHB. For this and other technical reasons, manufacturers report the following Spo_2 values for general accuracy at one standard deviation (1SD) for a general population: ±2% from 100% to 70% saturation, and ±3% from 70% to 50% saturation. For example, 68% (1SD) of the patients who have a Spo_2 value of 90% will have a true saturation in the range of 88% to 92% on CO oximetry. The other 32% of the patients with an Spo_2 value of 90% would have an even wider range of true saturation. Because of these limitations, the following clinical guidelines have been made by a number of authors:

1. Do not use pulse oximetry on patients with significant levels of COHb or MetHB.
2. If in doubt about abnormal hemoglobins, analyze an ABG through a CO oximeter and compare the true Sao_2 with the Spo_2 from pulse oximetry. Pulse oximetry can be used if the correlation of values is within 4%.
3. Question the Spo_2 value when the displayed heart rate is different from the actual heart rate.
4. Do not use pulse oximetry when the Spo_2 reading is less than 70% because the values tend to be erroneously high.

5. Pulse oximetry can be used on a term neonate or one that is 1500 grams or larger. Smaller neonates should have oxygenation measured by a transcutaneous oxygen monitor. This is because it is too easy to hyperoxygenate a small neonate when small changes in saturation can result in wide swings in Po_2. The risk of retinopathy of prematurity (formerly called retrolental fibroplasia) from hyperoxia is too great in the small neonate.

Table 3-14 lists common clinical ranges for Spo_2 values. For the aforementioned reasons, the minimum safe values are 2% higher than the corresponding Sao_2 value by CO oximetry. It is important that the patient have good pulsatile blood flow to the measurement site in order to get an accurate reading. Shock, vasoconstricting drugs such as tolazoline and dopamine, and poor local perfusion to the site can result in unreliable readings. Severe anemia, carbon monoxide poisoning, excessive amounts of methemoglobin, and excessive movement of the site can also result in unrealiable readings. Avoid bony areas like joints.

The new pulse oximetry systems have become popular because they are relatively small can be hand carried easily. Many systems will provide a heart rate and print it out along with the Spo_2 value. Nellcor and Novametrix are manufacturers. Saturation can be measured with a variety of transducers at the following sites:

a. Adult- and infant-sized sensors are available for the index finger, great toe, and any other finger that it fits well. There is a reusable finger clip or a disposable adhesive type of sensor. See Fig. 3-11.

b. Adult sensor that clips over the ear lobe. See Fig. 3-12.

c. Neonatal sized disposable adhesive sensors are available to fit around the foot, hand, or Achilles tendon. See Fig. 3-13.

d. Adult sensors for the bridge of the nose. This site must be cleansed of oils with an acetate/alcohol solution. Patients who are immobile or anesthetized, vasoconstricted, and breathing through the mouth are best suited for this type. See Fig. 3-14.

e. Reflectance sensors for the forehead. The two wavelengths of light shine through the skin and blood vessels, bounce off of the skull, and are received by the photodiode. The site must be cleansed of oils with an acetate/alcohol solution. Patients who are immobile, anesthetized, or vasoconstricted are best suited for this type.

Table 3-14. Recommended Clinical Ranges for True Sao_2 Values, Spo_2 Values*, and Their Correlation With Pao_2 Values

	Sao_2	Spo_2	Approximate Pao_2
Adult			
Acute hypoxemia	90%-95%	92%-95%†	60-95 torr
Chronic hypoxemia	85%-90%	87%-92%	50-60 torr
Neonate‡			
Less than 1500 gm in the first week of life	about 97%	92%-96%	60-70 torr
Greater than 1500 gm or after the first week of life	90%-96%	90%-96%	50-70 torr
Greater than one month of age with chronic lung disease	85%-90%	87%-92%	50-60 torr

*Based on the patient having normal COHb and MetHb levels. Elevated level(s) will result in an erroneously high Spo_2 reading and unsuspected hypoxemia.

†Black patients should have an Spo_2 of 95% maintained to ensure adequate oxygenation. Melanin can partially block light from passing through the skin.

‡The clinical goal with most neonates is to prevent both hypoxemia, defined as a Pao_2 of less than 45 torr, and hyperoxemia, defined as a Pao_2 of greater than 90 torr.

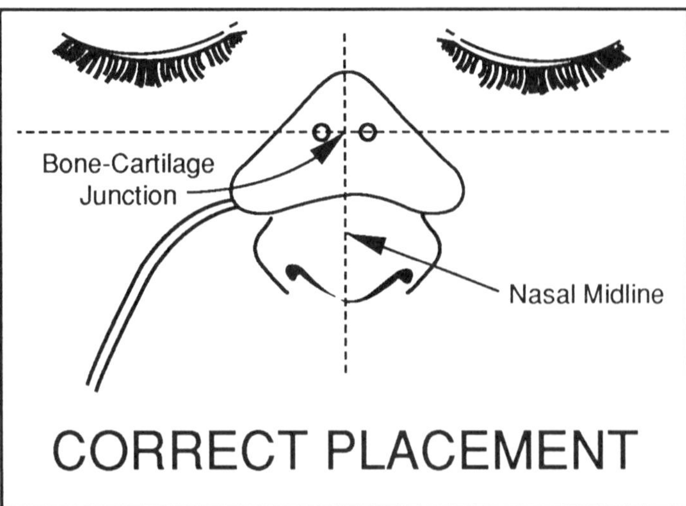

Fig. 3-14 Pulse oximetry transducer placed over the bridge of an adult's nose. (Courtesy of Nellcor, Inc.)

6. Interpret your patient's ear or pulse oximetry value. (IC1a)[R, Ap]

The previously healthy patient who has cardiopulmonary failure should have the Spo_2 value kept at 92% or greater to ensure adequate oxygenation. The patient with chronic obstructive pulmonary disease can probably tolerate a Spo_2 value of as low as 87%. The neonate should have the Spo_2 kept between 92% to 96%. Saturations below these values indicate hypoxemia in most patients.

Note the site where the saturation was measured. This is especially important in neonates who may have congenital heart defects. A higher saturation in the right fingers or right ear lobe compared with the rest of the body is seen with a patent ductus arteriosus. A higher saturation in the fingers and ear lobes as compared with the toes is seen with a coarctation of the aorta.

The patient with carbon monoxide poisoning should not be evaluated with a pulse oximeter because the units are unable to distinguish oxyhemoglobin from carboxyhemoglobin. Only the functional hemoglobin will be read and a higher than true O_2Hb saturation will be reported. These patients should only be evaluated for oxygenation by an arterial blood gas that is analyzed in a CO oximeter blood gas analyzer.

Module G. Patient assessment

Review, as needed, Section 1 for anything that might explain how the patient's condition will have an impact on blood gas results. Specifically, there are three factors that should be taken into account. First, the patient's oxygenation status cannot be accurately interpreted without knowing the inspired oxygen percentage. It is important to make sure that the patient is inspiring the correct percentage of oxygen. He or she should be breathing in this percentage for at least fifteen minutes before the blood sample is drawn. This will allow enough time for stabilization. Second, the patient's tidal volume, respiratory frequency, and minute volume have a direct effect on the $Paco_2$ and, because of that, on the pH. See Table 3-15 for examples. The patient with a dead space-producing disease, may have an elevated minute volume and *not* blow off as much carbon dioxide as expected. Third, pain from the puncture is subjective. If done properly, it should be no worse than the pain from a venous puncture. If a patient complains of intense pain, the

Table 3-15. Normal Resting Breathing Relationship Between Minute Volume and $Paco_2$*

Minute Volume	Approximate $Paco_2$ (mm Hg)
Normal	40
Twice normal	30
Quadruple normal	20
Half normal	50
One quarter normal	60

*It is assumed that the patient has a normal amount of anatomic dead space and a normal ventilation to perfusion ratio.
Modified from Shapiro BA, Harrison RA, Cane RD et al: *Clinical Application of Blood Gases*, ed 4. St. Louis, Mosby, 1989.

procedure should be stopped. Another site may need to be selected. Injecting a small amount of lidocaine into the site before the actual puncture will reduce any pain.

Shapiro et al. do not believe that there is any significant change in the blood gas values if patients either hold their breath or hyperventilate during the puncture. However, a stable patient who is breathing steadily leaves no room for doubt about this. Try to gain your patients' confidence so that they are as calm as possible during the procedure.

This ends the general discussion on blood gases. Remember, the entry level examination will include *direct* questions regarding this material. The examination will also *incorporate* blood gas values into questions that relate to techniques or procedures covered in the following sections.

BIBLIOGRAPHY

AARC Clinical Practice Guideline: Pulse oximetry. *Respir Care* 1991; 36:1406-1409.

Bennington JL: *Saunders Dictionary & Encyclopedia of Laboratory medicine and Technology*. Philadelphia, WB Saunders, 1984.

Bickford L, Bickford C, Hodgkin JE: Methodology of arterial blood gas analysis, in Burton GC, Hodgkin JE (eds): *Respiratory Care: A Guide to Clinical Practice*, ed 2. Philadelphia, Lippincott, 1984.

Bohn DJ: Ask the expert, *The Respiratory Tract*, February 1988,9.

Blanchette T: Appropriate use of pulse oximetry. RT, *J Respir Care Pract* 1991; 3:35-40.

Blanchette T, Dziodzio J, Harris K: Pulse oximetry and normoximetry in neonatal intensive care. *Respiratory Care* 1991; 36:25-32.

Federal Government Releases CLIA '88 Final Regulations. *AARC Times*, April 1992, 76-86.

Fell WL: Sampling and measurement of blood gases, in Lane EE, Walker JF (eds): *Clinical Arterial Blood Gas Analysis*. St. Louis, Mosby, 1987.

Jubran A, Tobin MJ: Reliability of pulse oximetry in titrating supplemental oxygen therapy in ventilator-dependent patients. *Chest* 1990; 97:1420.

Levitzky MG, Cairo JM, Hall SM: *Introduction to Respiratory Care*. Philadelphia, WB Saunders, 1990.

McPherson SP: *Respiratory Therapy Equipment*, ed 4. St. Louis, Mosby, 1990.

Mohler JG, Collier CR, Brandt W, et al: Blood gases, in Clausen JL (ed): *Pulmonary Function Testing Guidelines and Controversies*. Orlando, Grune & Stratton, 1984.

*Moran RF: CLIA regulations, part I: the cure might be worse than the disease. *AARCTimes*, November 1990, 41-43, 50-51.

Moran RF: CLIA regulations, part II: an analysis of some technical requirements. *AARCTimes*, December 1990, 25-32.

Nelson CM, Murphy EM, Bradley JK, et al: Clinical use of pulse oximetry to determine oxygen prescriptions for patients with hypoxemia. *Respir Care* 1986; 31:673-680.

Peters JA, Hodgkin JE, Collier CA: Blood gas analysis and acid-base physiology, in Burton GG, Hodgkin JE, Ward JJ (eds): *Respiratory Care: A Guide to Clinical Practice*, ed 3. Philadelphia, Lippincott, 1991.

Plunkett PF: Blood gas interpretation, in Barnes TA (ed): *Respiratory Care Practice*. Chicago, Mosby, 1988.

Nellcor Incorporated, Hayward, California, product information on Oxi sensors.

Ruppel G: *Manual of Pulmonary Function Testing*, ed 5. St. Louis, Mosby, 1991.

Salyer JW: Pulse oximetry in the neonatal intensive care unit. *Respir Care* 1991; 36:17-20.

Shapiro BA, Harrison RA, Walton JR: *Clinical Application of Blood Gases*, ed 3. Chicago, Mosby, 1982.

Shapiro BA, Harrison RA, Cane RD, et al: *Clinical Application of Blood Gases*, ed 4. Chicago, Mosby, 1989.

Sills JR: *Respiratory Care Certification Guide*. St. Louis, Mosby, 1991.

Sonnesso G: Are you ready to use pulse oximetry. Nursing 1991; August: 60-64.

Tilkian SM, Conover MB, Tilkian AG: *Clinical Implications of Laboratory Tests*, ed 3. St. Louis, Mosby, 1983.

Uhing M, Dziedzic K: Pulse oximetry in neonatal management. *Respir Management* 20:116-120.

Welch JP, DeCesare R, Hess D: Pulse oximetry: instrumentation and clinical applications. *Respir Care* 1990; 35:584-601.

Yelderman M, New W: Evaluation of pulse oximetry. *Anesthesiology* 1983; 59:349-352.

*__Note:__ A copy of the final CLIA regulations can be purchased with a check for $3.50 sent to: Government Printing Office, Attn.: New Order, P.O. Box 371954, Pittsburg, PA 15250-7954. Be sure to request stock #069-001-0042-4 Final Clinical Laboratory Regulations, February 28, 1992.

SELF-STUDY QUESTIONS

1. Before drawing a blood gas sample from the radial artery, you should perform which test of adequate perfusion?
   A. Allen's test
   B. Modified Allen's test
   C. Measure a blood pressure
   D. A−aDO$_2$
   E. Bishop's test

2. A patient is brought into the emergency room after being rescued from a home fire. She is unconscious and has facial burns. The physician believes that she is suffering from smoke inhalation. What would you recommend as the best way to evaluate her oxygenation status?
   A. Arterial blood gases analysed through a CO oximeter
   B. Pulse oximetry
   C. Arterial blood gases analysed through a standard blood gas analyzer
   D. Transcutaneous oxygen monitor

3. You are ordered to draw a blood sample from your patient's radial artery. You test for adequate circulation by having the patient make a fist and putting pressure over his ulnar and radial arteries. The patient's hand is then opened, and pressure is released from the ulnar artery. His hand color returns within 15 seconds. This would indicate:

A. The patient's radial circulation is adequate.
B. The patient's radial circulation is not adequate.
C. The patient's ulnar circulation is adequate.
D. The patient's ulnar circulation is not adequate.
E. A and C

4. You are working in the intensive care unit when you notice that an arterial blood sample has been sitting out for 10 minutes. It was not put in ice water. You could expect the blood gas analysis to be affected in which way?
   I. Increased Pao_2
   II. Increased $Paco_2$
   III. Decreased Pao_2
   IV. Decreased $Paco_2$
   V. Increased pH
   VI. Decreased pH
   A. I, II, VI
   B. III, IV, V
   C. I, II, V
   D. II, III, VI
   E. III, IV, VI

5. You would recommend an arterial puncture to obtain a sample for blood gas analysis under which of the following conditions:
   I. To measure the patient's Pao_2 after a change in his inspired oxygen.
   II. Suspected carbon monoxide poisoning.
   III. To measure the patient's $Paco_2$ after a change in his minute volume.
   IV. The patient has been admitted into the emergency room with a tension pneumothorax.
   V. During a cardiopulmonary resuscitation attempt.
   A. I
   B. I, III
   C. II, IV
   D. V
   E. All of the above

6. Current safety guidelines for the protection of the technician drawing the arterial blood gas include:
   I. Wash your hands before drawing the sample.
   II. Put a glove on the hand used to draw the sample.
   III. Put a glove on the hand with which you will feel the pulse.
   IV. Put gloves on both hands.
   V. Wear eyeglasses or goggles.
   A. IV, V
   B. I, V
   C. II
   D. III
   E. IV

7. A 50-year-old patient has a Pao_2 of 72 mm Hg when breathing room air. You would interpret this as:
   A. Normal for a person of his age
   B. Mild hypoxemia
   C. Moderate hypoxemia
   D. Severe hypoxemia
   E. None of the above

8. Your patient had a Pao_2 of 53 mm Hg on room air. He was then given a 30% oxygen mask. His Pao_2 is 85 mm Hg with the extra oxygen. You would interpret this as:
   A. Normal
   B. Uncorrected hypoxemia
   C. Corrected hypoxemia
   D. Excessively corrected hypoxemia
   E. None of the above

9. Which of the following will shift the oxyhemoglobin dissociation curve to the right and in effect decrease the hemoglobin's affinity for oxygen?
   I. Acute acidosis
   II. Acute alkalosis
   III. High carbon dioxide
   IV. Low carbon dioxide
   V. Increased temperature
   VI. Decreased temperature
   A. II, III, VI
   B. I, IV, V
   C. II, III, V
   D. IV, VI
   E. I, III, V

10. An acute rise in $Paco_2$ from 40 to 50 mm Hg would result in the following change in pH:
   A. Rise of 0.10 units
   B. Fall of 0.05 units
   C. Rise of 0.25 units
   D. Fall of 0.10 units
   E. Rise of 0.05 units

11. An acute drop in $Paco_2$ from 40 to 30 mm Hg would result in the following change in pH:
   A. Rise of 0.10 units
   B. Fall of 0.05 units
   C. Rise of 0.25 units
   D. Fall of 0.10 units
   E. Rise of 0.05 units

12. Interpret the following blood gas drawn when the patient was breathing in 40% oxygen: Pao_2, 54 mm Hg; Sao_2, 87%; pH 7.37; $Paco_2$ 62 mm Hg; bicarbonate, 38 mEq/L; and base excess, +11 mEq/L.
   I. Corrected hypoxemia
   II. Uncorrected hypoxemia
   III. Metabolic alkalosis
   IV. Compensated respiratory acidosis
   V. Metabolic acidosis
   A. I, IV
   B. I, III
   C. II, V
   D. I, V
   E. II, IV

13. Interpret the following blood gas drawn when the patient was breathing in 35% oxygen; Pao_2, 66 mm Hg; Sao_2, 90%; pH 7.29; $Paco_2$, 37 mm Hg; bicarbonate, 17 mEq/L; and base excess, −8 mEq/L.
   I. Corrected hypoxemia
   II. Uncorrected hypoxemia

III. Compensated metabolic acidosis
IV. Uncompensated metabolic acidosis
V. Compensated respiratory acidosis
A. II, IV
B. I, IV
C. II, V
D. I, III
E. II, III

14. Interpret the following blood gas drawn when the patient was breathing in 21% oxygen: Pa_{O_2}, 117 mm Hg; Sa_{O_2}, 98%; pH 7.57; Pa_{CO_2}, 20 mm Hg; bicarbonate, 24 mEq/L; and base excess, +1 mEq/L.
I. Normal oxygenation
II. Excessively corrected hypoxemia
III. Uncompensated respiratory alkalosis
IV. Uncompensated metabolic acidosis
V. Combined respiratory and metabolic alkalosis
A. II, III
B. I, V
C. II, V
D. I, III
E. I, IV

15. Interpret the following blood gas drawn when the patient was breathing in 60% oxygen: Pa_{O_2}, 72 mm Hg; Sa_{O_2}, 84%; pH 7.18; Pa_{CO_2}, 50 mm Hg; bicarbonate, 18 mEq/L; and base excess, −10 mEq/L.
I. Uncorrected hypoxemia
II. Corrected hypoxemia
III. Uncorrected respiratory acidosis
IV. Uncorrected metabolic acidosis
V. Combined metabolic and respiratory acidosis
A. I, V
B. II, V
C. II, III
D. I, III
E. II, IV

16. Interpret the following blood gas drawn when the patient was breathing in 24% oxygen: Pa_{O_2} 57 mm Hg; Sa_{O_2}, 91%; pH 7.45; Pa_{CO_2}, 22 mm Hg; bicarbonate, 16 mEq/L; and base excess, −6 mEq/L.
I. Corrected hypoxemia
II. Uncorrected hypoxemia
III. Compensated respiratory alkalosis
IV. Uncompensated respiratory alkalosis
V. Combined metabolic and respiratory acidosis
A. I, III
B. I, IV
C. II, III
D. II, V
E. II, IV

17. Interpret the following blood gas drawn when the patient was breathing in 21% oxygen: Pa_{O_2}, 58 mm Hg; Sa_{O_2}, 87%; pH 7.35; Pa_{CO_2}, 50 mm Hg; bicarbonate, 25 mEq/L; and base excess, +1 mEq/L.

I. Moderate hypoxemia
II. Severe hypoxemia
III. Uncompensated metabolic acidosis
IV. Uncompensated respiratory acidosis
V. Compensated metabolic alkalosis

A. I, IV
B. II, IV
C. I, V
D. II, III
E. I, III

Answer Key:

1. B; 2. A; 3. C; 4. D; 5. E; 6. A; 7. B; 8. C; 9. E; 10. B; 11. A; 12. E; 13. B; 14. D; 15. B; 16. C; 17. A.

4 Pulmonary Function Testing

Module A. Perform the following types of bedside spirometry.

1. Measure and interpret the patient's tidal volume at the bedside. (IC1b and IIIE13) [R, Ap]

The tidal volume (V_T) is the volume of gas breathed out with each respiratory cycle. See Section 1, Module A, 7, b, for the general discussion. It is important to realize that individual tidal volumes are rarely identical. Normally there is some variation. (See Fig. 4-1 for several different tidal volumes before and after a nonforced [slow] vital capacity.) For that reason it is recommended that the tidal volumes be accumulated for a minute (giving you a minute volume) and the respiratory rate counted. An average tidal volume is found by dividing the minute volume by the respiratory rate. The average, predicted tidal volume for a resting, afebrile, alert adult should be about 3 to 4 ml/lb or 6 to 9 ml/kg.

For example, the predicted tidal volume range of a 154-lb (70-kg) patient would be calculated as follows:

a. 3 to 4 ml/lb × 154 lb = 462 to 616 ml
b. 6 to 9 ml/kg × 70 kg = 420 to 630 ml

It is recommended that the patient be allowed to relax before the test is performed so that the measured volume is accurate and not enlarged because of any undue stress or excitement. Keeping the instructions and demonstration simple and easy to follow will help reduce the patient's anxiety. Some patients will not tolerate a full minute's tidal volume measurement. In that case, measure the accumulated tidal volumes for as long as possible, and divide by the number of respirations to obtain the average.

A tidal volume that is larger or smaller than expected for the patient's size requires further evaluation. A small tidal volume may be seen in patients who have low metabolic rates, are asleep or in a coma, have neuromuscular diseases that make them unable to breathe deeply, or are alkalotic. A large tidal volume will be seen in patients with high metabolic rates, fever, dead space–producing diseases, increased intracranial pressure, or acidotic conditions.

2. Measure and interpret the patient's inspiratory-to-expiratory ratio at the bedside. (IC1d and IIIE13) [R, Ap]

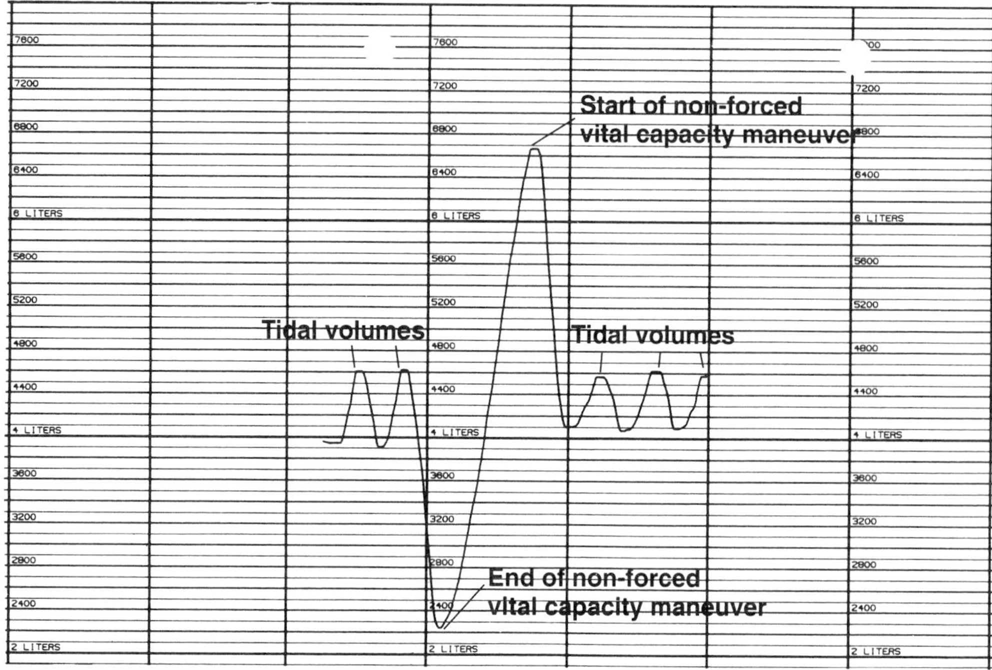

Fig. 4-1 Tracing of tidal volumes and nonforced vital capacity.

The inspiratory-to-expiratory (I/E) ratio can be simply measured at the bedside with a stopwatch. Again, make sure that the patient is relaxed and breathing in the normal pattern to get an accurate timing. Measure several of the patient's inspiratory times and expiratory times to figure an average for each. A spirometer that gives a printout will be needed if a more complete analysis of the patient's breathing pattern is needed. See Section 1, Module D, 12, for a detailed presentation on various breathing patterns and the resulting I/E ratios.

The National Board of Respiratory Care NBRC is known to test the examinee's ability to calculate 1, the inspiratory time (TI) and expiratory time (TE) from a given I/E ratio and respiratory rate or 2, the I/E ratio from a given TI and TE. These examples should help.

A. Calculate the patient's inspiratory time and expiratory time when the I/E ratio is 1:2 and the respiratory rate is 12/min.
   1. $\frac{60 \text{ sec/min}}{12 \text{ breaths/min}} = 5 \text{ sec/respiratory cycle}$
   2. $\frac{5 \text{ sec/respiratory cycle}}{3 \text{ parts of I and E}} = 1.66 \text{ seconds for one part}$
   3. Inspiratory time = 1 part = 1.66 seconds
   4. Expiratory time = 2 parts = 3.32 seconds

B. Calculate the patient's I/E ratio when the inspiratory time is 0.3 seconds and expiratory time is 0.9 seconds.
   1. $I/E = \frac{I}{E} = \frac{0.3 \text{ sec}}{0.9 \text{ sec}}$
   2. $\frac{I}{E} = \frac{1}{3}$ (The I/E ratio is 1:3.)

3. Measure and interpret the patient's minute volume at the bedside. (IC1c) [R, Ap]

The minute volume ($\dot{V}_E$) is the volume of gas exhaled in 1 minute. See Section 1, Module A, 7, c, for the general discussion. The minute volume is usually a more stable value than are individual tidal volumes. As discussed, it is found by adding up the accumulated tidal volumes for a minute. A simple hand-held spirometer such as that made by the Fraser-Harlake Company is often used to accumulate the tidal volume breaths. If the patient cannot perform the test for a minute, do it for 30 seconds, and double the value. The predicted range for a minute volume in a resting, afebrile, alert adult should be 5 to 10 l/min.

The wide range is found in part because it is made up of two factors: tidal volume and respiratory rate. It is possible for either one or both of these factors to be normal, abnormally high, or abnormally low. For these reasons, the minute volume must be evaluated along with the tidal volume and respiratory rate to reach any conclusion about the patient's condition.

Examples from Section 1:

Normal patient: f = 12, tidal volume = 500 ml
minute volume = 12 × 500 ml = 6000 ml
Tachypneic patient: f = 24, tidal volume = 250 ml
minute volume = 24 × 250 ml = 6,000 ml
Bradypneic patient: f = 6, tidal volume = 1000 ml
minute volume = 6 × 1000 ml = 6000 ml

4. Calculate and interpret the patient's alveolar ventilation at the bedside. (IC1k) [R, Ap]

Alveolar ventilation (V_A) is the amount of tidal volume that reaches the alveoli. It is calculated by subtracting the physiologic dead space (anatomic plus alveolar dead space) from the measured exhaled tidal volume. For a bedside test, it only possible to subtract the estimated anatomic dead space. It is estimated at 1 ml/pound or 2.2 ml/kg of lean body weight. The alveolar dead space measurement requires sophisticated equipment, which is usually only available in the pulmonary function testing laboratory. Clinically normal people have very little alveolar dead space.

Example:

A 154-lb/70-kg person would have an estimated anatomic dead space of about 154 ml. The measured tidal volume is 500 ml.
Calculated alveolar ventilation = 500 ml − 154 ml = 346 ml.

The following examples show how the patient's alveolar ventilation can vary considerably because of changes in the respiratory rate and tidal volume even though the minute volume remains unchanged. These examples are included to show the importance of alveolar ventilation on the patient's Pa_{CO_2} and Pa_{CO_2} values.

Examples:

a. Normal patient: f = 12, tidal volume = 500 ml, anatomic dead space = 154 ml

$$\begin{aligned} \text{minute volume} = 12 \times 500 \text{ ml} &= 6000 \text{ ml} \\ \text{minute alveolar ventilation } (\dot{V}_A) &= 12 \times (500 \text{ ml} - 154 \text{ ml}) \\ &= 12 \times 346 \text{ ml} \\ &= 4152 \text{ ml} \end{aligned}$$

This patient should have a normal carbon dioxide level.

b. Tachypneic patient: $f = 24$, tidal volume = 250 ml, anatomic dead space = 154 ml

$$\begin{aligned} \text{minute volume} = 24 \times 250 \text{ ml} &= 6000 \text{ ml} \\ \text{minute alveolar ventilation } (\dot{V}_A) &= 24 \times (250 \text{ ml} - 154 \text{ ml}) \\ &= 24 \times 96 \text{ ml} \\ &= 2304 \text{ ml} \end{aligned}$$

This patient should have a high carbon dioxide level.

c. Bradypneic patient: $f = 6$, tidal volume = 1000 mL, anatomic dead space = 154 ml

$$\begin{aligned} \text{minute volume} = 6 \times 1000 \text{ ml} &= 6000 \text{ ml} \\ \text{minute alveolar ventilation } (\dot{V}_A) &= 6 \times (1000 \text{ ml} - 154 \text{ ml}) \\ &= 6 \times 846 \text{ ml} \\ &= 5076 \text{ ml} \end{aligned}$$

This patient should have a low carbon dioxide level.

5. Measure and interpret the patient's forced vital capacity at the bedside. (IC1g and IIIE8) [R, Ap]

The forced vital capacity (FVC) is the greatest volume of gas that the patient can exhale as rapidly as possible after the lungs have been completely filled. Normally, it is the same volume as that found in a slow or nonforced vital capacity. Careful instructions, demonstrations, and coaching are needed to ensure that the patient's efforts are the best possible. At least *three* proper efforts must be obtained.

If the measurement instrument does not give a printout, simply record the patient's efforts in the chart. If the measurement instrument does give a printout, include copies of the efforts. See Figure 4-2 for the tracing of a properly performed forced vital capacity. Notice that the start of the effort is smooth and without interruption. The initial fast flow of gas from the upper airway is seen as the nearly vertical part of the tracing. The rest of the tracing is smooth without any coughing or other interruptions in the patient's effort. The tracing becomes progressively more horizontal as the end of the effort is reached. Encourage the patient to try to push out as much air as possible as the end approaches. Current guidelines require that the patient keep pushing so that the total effort lasts at least 6 seconds.

Fig. 4-2 was made on a chain-compensated, water-seal sprirometry system made by Warren E. Collins, Inc. Notice how the tracing progresses from the right to the left. This company also makes the Stead-Wells, water-seal spirometer system. The Stead-Wells system shows the same tracing "upside down" compared with the chain-compensated system. The tracing starts on the left and moves to the right. See Fig. 4-5 to 4-7. Other company's systems could show either the chain-compensated or Stead-Wells tracings in a mirror image or opposite shape. This is an important point since the NBRC can show a FVC tracing from any system and expect it to be interpreted. It is recommended that a mirror be held to this figure to create Stead-Wells or opposite tracings. The start of the effort can be determined by the near vertical portion of the tracing and the relatively small expiratory reserve volume (ERV) compared with the inspiratory reserve volume (IRV).

Now is a good time to review the normal values and relationships of the various lung volumes and capacities as shown in Table 4-1. See Fig. 4-3 for a normal spirometry tracing that is subdivided into the four volumes and four capacities. Carefully note the relationships of the volumes and capacities and how capacities are made up of two or more volumes. Note that all volumes and capacities can be directly measured by spirometry at the bedside except residual volume and functional residual capacity. The residual volume must be found by indirect methods in the pulmonary function laboratory.

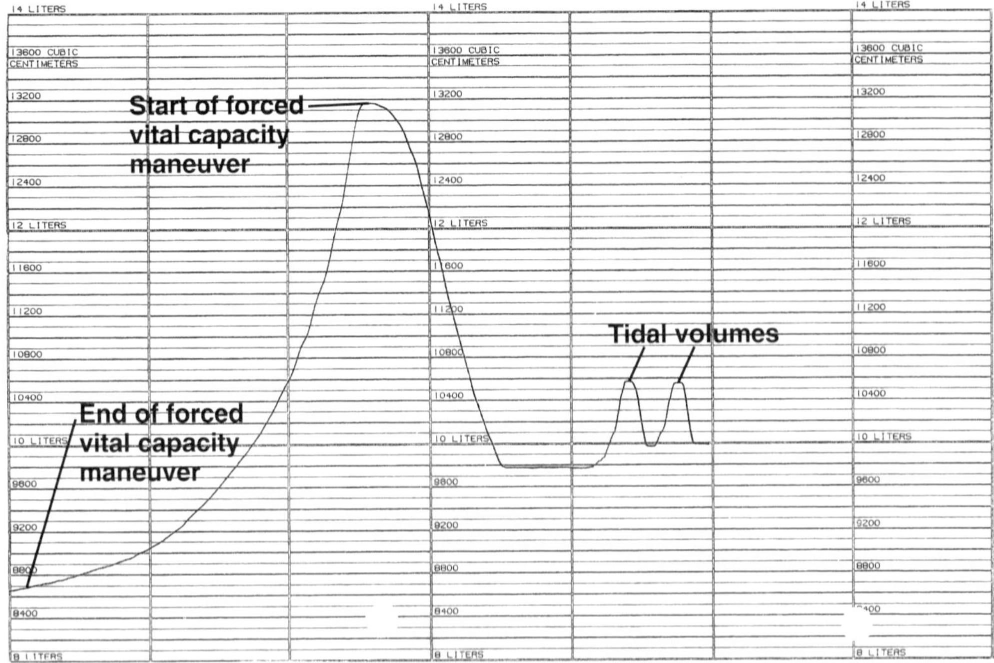

Fig. 4-2 Tracing of tidal volumes and forced vital capacity.

The predicted normal values in liters for the forced vital capacity have been reported by Morris and colleagues as follows:

- Males: [(0.148 × height in inches) − (0.025 × age)] − 4.24
- Females: [(0.115 × height in inches) − (0.024 × age)] − 2.85

Example:

Calculate the predicted forced vital capacity of a 50-year-old male who is 6 ft (72 in.) tall.

$$\begin{aligned}\text{Male FVC} &= [(0.148 \times 72) - (0.025 \times 50)] - 4.24 \\ &= [10.656 - 1.25] - 4.24 \\ &= 9.406 - 4.24 \\ &= 5.166\ \text{L}\end{aligned}$$

Table 4-1. Lung Volumes and Capacities in a Clinically Normal Young Man

Tidal volume (V_T) = 500 ml
Inspiratory reserve volume (IRV) = 3100 ml
Expiratory reserve volume (ERV) = 1200 ml
Residual volume (RV) = 1200 ml
Inspiratory capacity (IC) = 8,600 ml (made up of the V_T and IRV)
Functional residual capacity (FRC) = 2400 ml (made up of the ERV and RV)
Vital capacity (VC) = 4,800 mL (made up of the V_T, IRV, and ERV)
Total lung capacity (TLC) = 6000 mL (made up of the V_T, IRV, ERV, and RV)

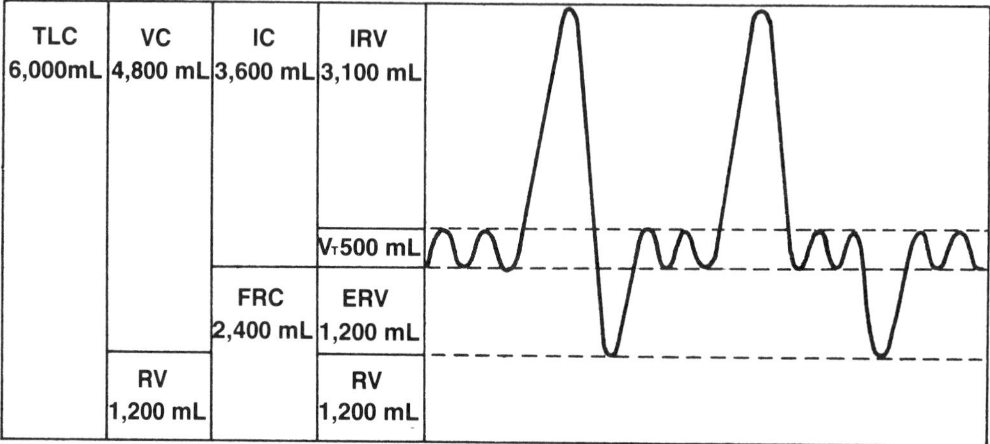

Volumes: Four primary

A. Tidal volume: The volume of gas inspired or expired during normal respiration (V_T).
B. Inspiratory reserve volume: The maximum volume of gas that can be inspired beyond a normal inspiration (IRV).
C. Expiratory reserve volume: The maximum volume of gas that can be exhaled after a normal expiration (ERV).
D. Residual volume: The volume of gas remaining in the lungs after a maximum expiration (RV).

Capacities: Four, which include two or more primary volumes

A. Total lung capacity: The total amount of gas contained in the lungs after maximum inspiration (TLC). Includes all four primary volumes –TLC = V_T + IRV + ERV + RV.
B. Vital capacity: The maximum amount of gas that can be exhaled after a maximum inspiration (VC). Includes three primary volumes–VC = V_T + IRV + ERV.
C. Inspiratory capacity: The maximum amount of gas that can be inspired after a normal expiration(IC). Includes two primary volumes – IC = V_T + IRV.
D. Functional residual capacity: The total amount of gas remaining in the lungs after normal expiration (FRC). Includes two primary volumes – FRC = ERV + RV.

Fig. 4-3 Lung volumes and capacities for a clinically normal young man.

A measured FVC that is at least 80% of that predicted is considered to be within normal limits. It is normal to see a decline in the FVC with age. Restrictive problems such as advanced pregnancy, obesity, ascites, neuromuscular disease, sarcoidosis, and chest wall or spinal deformity can also result in a small FVC. Patients with chronic obstructive lung diseases such as emphysema, bronchitis, asthma, cystic fibrosis, and bronchiectasis commonly have a small FVC. See Fig. 4-4 for a comparison of the spirometry tracings of a normal, obstructed, and restricted patient.

6. Measure and interpret the patient's timed, forced expiratory volumes at the bedside. (IC1h) [R, Ap]

The timed, forced expiratory volumes ($FEV_{0.5,\ 1,\ 2,\ \text{and}\ 3\ \text{seconds}}$) effectively "cut" the FVC into sections based on how much volume the patient forcibly exhales in 0.5, 1, 2, and 3 seconds. Some patients with severe obstructive lung disease will require several more seconds to completely exhale. In these cases, simply keep measuring the volume exhaled in each additional second.

Some bedside units will give a numerical value for some or all of the timed intervals. However, it is best to have a spirometer that produces a printout of the patient's FVC effort. See Fig. 4-5 (from a Stead-Wells system) for a FVC tracing that has been subdivided into 0.5-, 1-, 2-, and 3-second intervals.

It must be obvious that every person will exhale different volumes for these time intervals because their FVCs are all different. The way to standardize this test is to divide the timed volumes by the FVC volume and convert the fraction into a percentage. These values can then be standardized for all individuals despite each having different FVCs.

The following are predicted values for normal patients:

- $FEV_{0.5}$ = 50% to 60% of the FVC.
- FEV_1 = 75% to 85% of the FVC.
- FEV_2 = 94% of the FVC.
- FEV_3 = 97% of the FVC.

These values will normally decrease slightly in the elderly patient. Most patients with normal lungs and airways will still be able to completely exhale their FVC within 4 seconds.

Patients with restrictive lung diseases will likely exhale their FVC more quickly than expected. This abnormal finding is caused by these patients having a smaller-than-normal FVC and stiff lungs that recoil more quickly than expected to their resting volume. See Fig. 4-6 to compare the FVC curves of a patient with restrictive lung disease and one with obstructive lung disease.

Patients with obstructive lung disease will take longer than expected to exhale their FVC (see Fig. 4-6). As a result, the percentages of the FVC exhaled in the above-timed intervals will be lower than normal. A FEV_1 of less than 65% to 70% of the FVC would

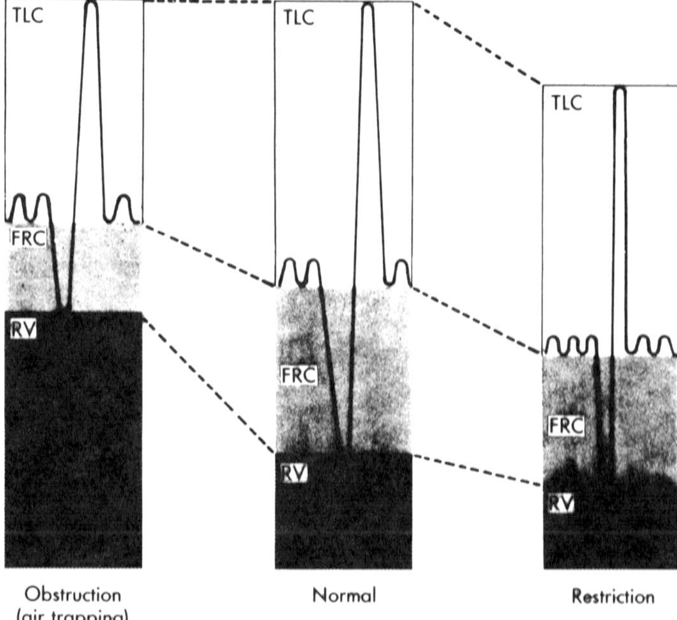

Fig. 4-4 Tracings for an obstructed, normal and restricted patient. (From Ruppel G: *Manual of Pulmonary Function Testing,* ed 4. St. Louis, Mosby, 1986. Used by permission.)

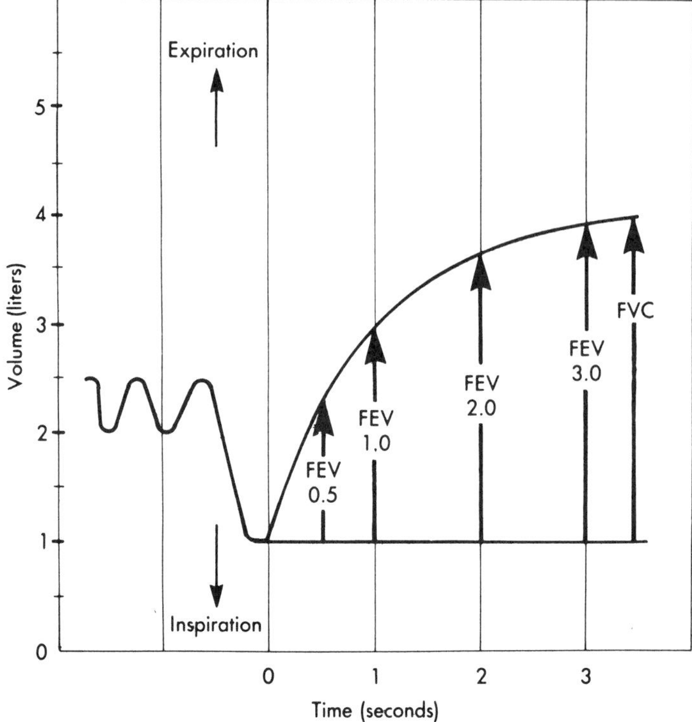

Fig. 4-5 Tracing of a forced vital capacity divided into $FEV_{0.5}$, $FEV_{1.0}$, $FEV_{2.0}$, and $FEV_{3.0}$. (From Ruppel G: *Manual of Pulmonary Function Testing,* ed 4. St. Louis, Mosby, 1986. Used by permission.)

confirm obstructive lung disease. Obviously, the lower the percentage exhaled for any timed interval, the worse the obstruction to exhalation.

7. Measure and interpret the patient's peak flow at the bedside (IC1f) [R, Ap]

The peak flow (PF) is the greatest flow rate seen in a patient's forced expiratory effort. Some authors refer to the peak flow as the peak expiratory flow rate (PEFR). It is usually seen at the beginning of the FVC effort. The instructions for the test must be simple and clear with a good demonstration. It is most important to emphasize that the patient must "blast" the air out as hard and fast as possible. It is not necessary to encourage the patient to completely empty the lungs to residual volume.

The patient's effort is easily directly measured from a hand-held peak flowmeter. If the instrument gives a printout, it will be necessary to hand draw the peak flow line and calculate the results. Fig. 4-7 shows an example. Note that the peak flow is drawn in as a tangent to the steepest (most vertical) part of the tracing. Ideally, this tangent line crosses two time lines (for 1 second) so that the answer can be read directly from the printout. The example in Fig. 4-7 shows that the answer can be found by setting up this proportional problem:

1. $\frac{4\text{ L}}{0.67\text{ sec}} = \frac{\text{unknown liters}}{1.0\text{ sec}}$ (Cross multiply.)
2. 0.67 unknown liters = 4 L

3. $\frac{0.67 \text{ unknown liters}}{0.67} = \frac{4 \text{ L}}{0.67}$ (Divide each fraction by 0.67.)
4. Unknown liters = 6 (rounded off). Peak flow is 6 L/sec.

Cherniack and Raber[1] have published the following formula for predicting peal flow in liters per second:

- Males: [(0.144 × height in inches) − (0.024 × age)] + 2.225
- Females [(0.090 × height in inches) − (0.018 × age)] + 1.130

As can be seen, the peak flow is directly related to height and indirectly related to age. Therefore, it would be expected that the taller the patient is, the greater the peak flow would be. Peak flow would be expected to decrease with age.

It is reasonable to record the patient's effort in liters per second because the effort takes place in about that much time. However, do not be confused by some measurement instruments and other prediction equations giving the value in liters per minute. Simply multiply or divide by 60 to convert your patient's effort from one time frame to the other. For example, a young man's peak flow could be recorded as 10 L/sec or 600 L/min.

The peak flow is a rather nonspecific measurement of airway obstruction. It measures flow through the upper airways and would be reduced in patients with an upper airway problem like a tumor, vocal cord paralysis, or laryngeal edema. However, the test is often given to patients having an asthma attack as a quick and easy measurement of small-airways obstruction. The following covers this topic in more detail.

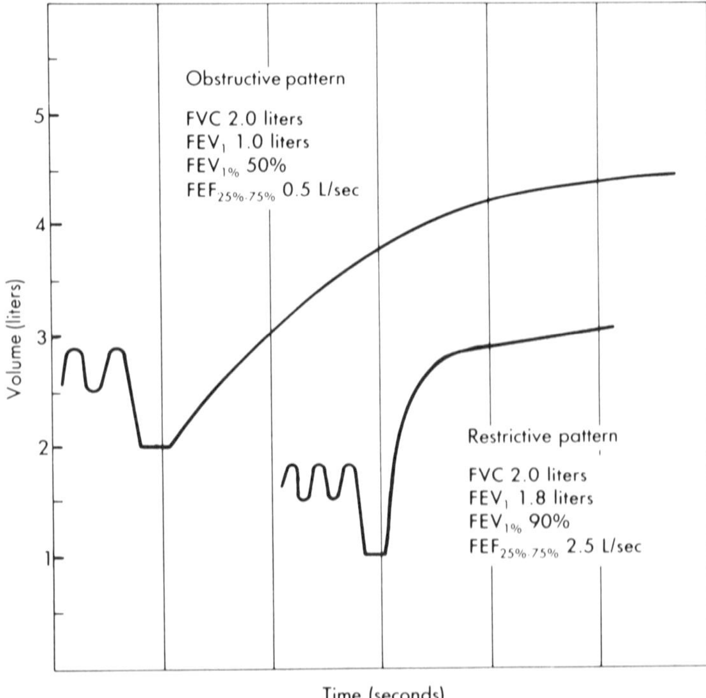

Fig. 4-6 Forced vital capacity tracings showing an obstructive flow pattern and a restrictive flow pattern. (From Ruppel G: *Manual of Pulmonary Function Testing,* ed 4. St. Louis, Mosby, 1986.)

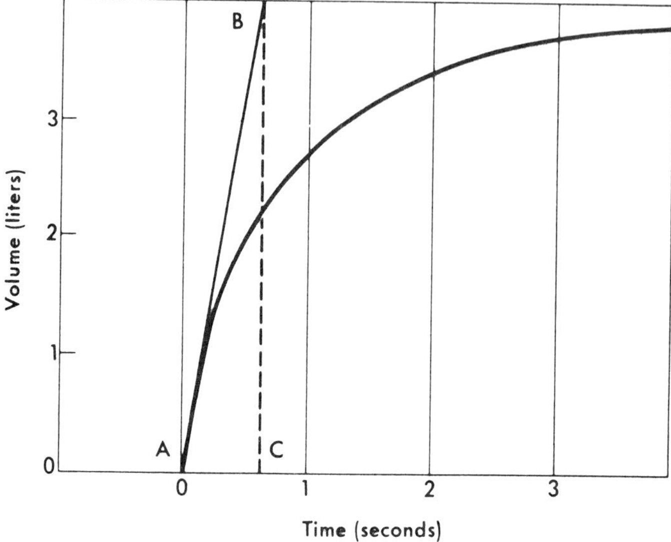

Fig. 4-7 Tracing of a forced vital capacity with the peak flow tangent line added. (From Ruppel G: *Manual of Pulmonary Function Testing,* ed 4. St. Louis, Mosby, 1986.)

8. Perform and interpret spirometry at the bedside before and/or after an aerosolized bronchodilator is given. (IC2b) [R, Ap]

The following are common indications:

1. The patient is known to have asthma or another type of chronic obstructive lung disease.
2. The patient has an $FEV_{1\%}$ of less than 70% (unless elderly).
3. To evaluate the effectiveness of a new bronchodilator.

The most commonly administered tests are the peak flow and $FEV_{1\%}$ from a forced vital capacity. Either one or both should be measured before the medication is given to determine the patient's initial airway condition. The medication can be given by intermittent positive-pressure breathing (IPPB), hand-held nebulizer, or metered dose inhaler as long as the method is done properly. Wait about 10 to 15 minutes for the medication to take effect and the patient's blood gas values to return to normal. Then, repeat the peak flow and/or $FEV_{1\%}$ test.

The percentage of improvement is calculated by using the following formula:

$$\text{Percent change} = \frac{\text{after drug air flow} - \text{before drug air flow}}{\text{before drug air flow}} \times 100$$

The medication is shown to be effective if the patient has a 15% to 20% improvement in peak flow and/or $FEV_{1\%}$. It is not uncommon to see patients with asthma improve much more than this. Other patients may not have this much improvement but do show increases in airflow and FVC and say that they feel better. In these cases, the physician may decide to continue the medication.

Remember that the raw data that have been obtained for the lung volumes and flows should be body, temperature, pressure, and water vapor saturated (BTPS) corrected. This is because as the warm exhaled gas cools on entering the measuring device it contracts in volume. The BTPS correction is needed to restore the measured volume to its original volume in the patient's lungs. The mathematical procedure involves multiplying the raw data (measured volume or flow) by the given BTPS factor. BTPS correction is usually limited to the pulmonary function laboratory and not done at the bedside. To date, the NBRC has not had these calculations on the entry level examination. However, the principle is important to be aware of.

9. Measure and interpret the patient's maximum inspiratory pressure at the bedside. (IC1e and IIIE13) [R, Ap]

The maximum inspiratory pressure (MIP) is the greatest amount of negative pressure that the patient can create when inspiring against an occluded airway. The literature includes the following names for this test: negative inspiratory force (NIF), inspiratory force, negative inspiratory pressure, maximal inspiratory force, peak negative pressure, and maximal static inspiratory pressure. The following factors affect the test results: strength of the respiratory (mainly diaphragm) muscles, lung volume when the airway is occluded, ventilatory drive, and the length of time the airway is occluded. It is most commonly used to determine the weanability of mechanically ventilated patients.

A study of the literature reveals that a number of measurement devices have been assembled and that different bedside techniques have been used to determine the effort of a patient breathing naturally, one who is intubated, and one who is breathing by way of a mechanical ventilator. There is no consensus on what is the best equipment configuration or measurement technique.

Branson et al. and Kacmarek et al. make a strong case for the use of a double one-way valve to connect the intubated patient to the manometer (Fig. 4-8). Use of the one-way valve lets the patient exhale but prevents an inhalation when the practitioner occludes the opening. This forces the patient to inhale from closer to residual volume with each breathing effort. They also recommend that the patient make inspiratory efforts for 15 to 20 seconds.

Clausen recommends that the device used for measuring the NIF of a patient with a normal airway have a small leak so that the effects of the cheek and neck muscles will not be measured (Fig. 4-9).

Steps in the NIF procedure for a normally breathing patient include the following:

1. Obtain a pressure gauge capable of measuring at least −60-cm water pressure.
2. Have the patient sit upright. Place a note in the chart if the patient is lying down.
3. Instruct the patient.
4. Simulate a demonstration of the procedure.
5. Place nose clips over the patient's nose. Have the patient seal his or her lips and teeth around the mouthpiece and breathe through the open port.
6. Tell the patient to exhale completely. Seal the port when residual volume has been reached.
7. Tell the patient to breathe in as hard as possible and hold it for 1 to 3 seconds.
8. Reteach if necessary.
9. Repeat until at least three good efforts have been performed. Record the greatest stable value seen after the first second of effort. This eliminates any artifact created by the cheeks or by chest wall movement.

It is important to monitor any patient for signs of undue stress and hypoxemia such as tachycardia, bradycardia, ventricular dysrhythmias, hypertension, hypotension, and/or decreasing saturation on pulse oximetry. If any of these are seen, the procedure should be stopped and the patient reoxygenated and ventilated. Some patients will have their best effort be the first or second inspiration and will have decreasing effort as they continue trying. This is probably because of fatigue. Stop the procedure and record the best effort.

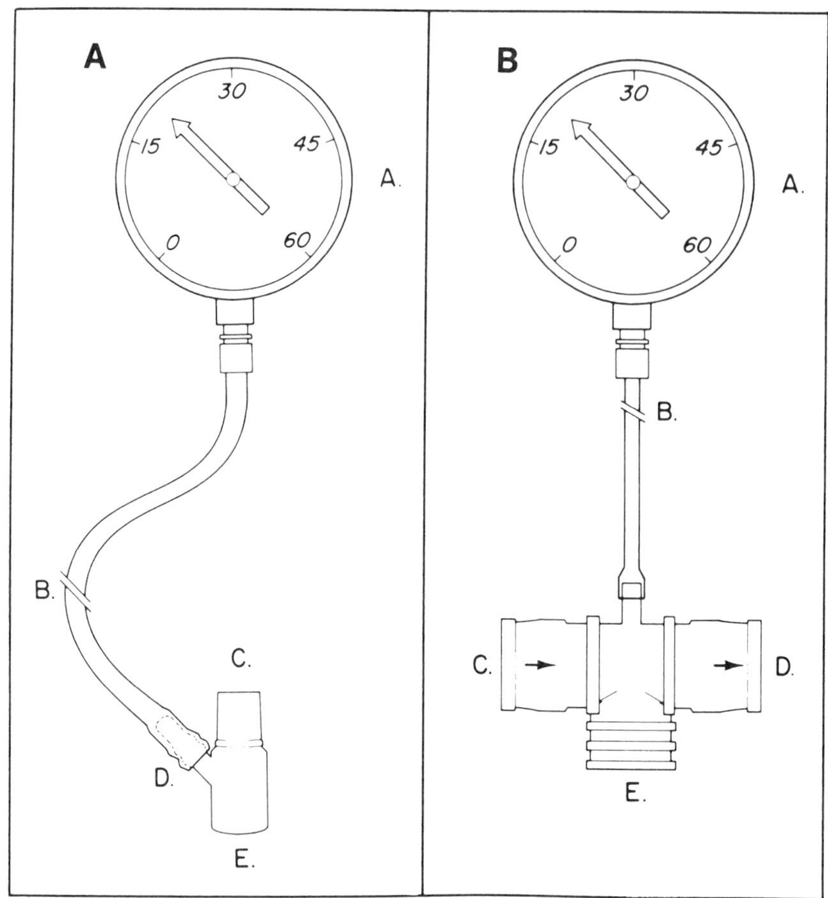

Fig. 4-8 Two systems for measuring negative inspiratory force (NIF) on a patient with an artificial airway. System **A,** Simple occlusion. *A,* Pressure manometer; *B,* Connecting tubing; *C,* Port to be occluded during the NIF effort; *D,* Connection of the adapter to the manometer; *E,* Port to connect to the patient's artificial airway. System **B,** One-way valve. *A,* Pressure manometer; *B,* connecting tubing; *C,* Inspiratory port to be occluded during the NIF effort; *D,* Expiratory port; *E,* Port to connect to the patient's artificial airway. (From Kacmarek RM, Cycyk-Chapman MC, Young-Palazzo PJ, et al: Determination of maximal inspiratory pressure: a clinical study and literature review. *Respir Care* 1989; 34:868-878.)

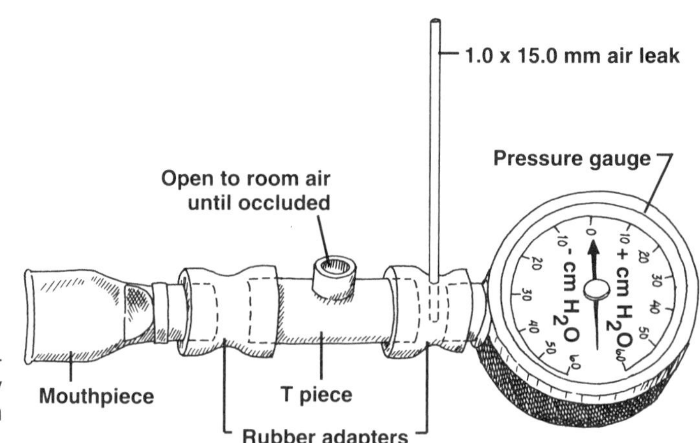

Fig. 4-9 A system for measuring negative inspiratory force (NIF) on a patient with a natural airway.

Patients of either sex and any age should be able to generate at least −60-cm H_2O. This is enough to offer assurance that the patient has enough strength and coordination to protect the airway, take a deep breath, and cough effectively. Patients with neuromuscular diseases, diseases of the respiratory muscles, thoracic injury or abnormality, and chronic obstructive lung diseases will tend to have decreased strength. The patient who cannot generate at least −20-cm H_2O is at risk. This patient probably does not have the strength to cough effectively. Depending on the blood gas values and other physical parameters, the patient may need to be endotracheally intubated and maintained on a mechanical ventilator.

Black and Hyatt have published the following MIP prediction formulas for spontaneously breathing in nonintubated subjects breathing from residual volume. The values are in centimeters of water pressure (cm H_2O).

- Males: 143 − (0.55 × age)
- Females: 104 − (0.51 × age)

These would be predictive for patients aged 20 to 86 years. As can be seen, the older the patient is, the lower the predicted negative inspiratory force would be.

Some advocate having the procedure done from the functional residual capacity instead of the residual volume. This is how the procedure should be performed if the patient is unconscious and uncooperative. In these cases, it is probably necessary to occlude the airway for several breathing efforts to obtain a realistic negative inspiratory force. The prediction formulas by Black and Hyatt would not be useful. Branson et al. found that this method of MIP measurement underestimates the MIP value when compared with the situation when a one-way valve system is used. This is because a patient breathing through the one-way valve system tended to exhale and then inspire from nearer the residual volume. In either case, a MIP of at least −20-cm H_2O would be predictive of successful weaning from the ventilator.

10. Perform and interpret the maximum expiratory pressure at the bedside. (IC1m) [R, Ap]

The maximum expiratory force (MEF) is the greatest amount of positive pressure that the patient can create when expiring from total lung capacity against an occluded airway. It is also known as a maximal expiratory pressure (MEP). The following factors affect the test results: patient cooperation and effort, strength of the accessory muscles of respiration and the abdominal muscles, lung volume when the airway is occluded, ventilatory drive, and the length of time the airway is occluded.

As with the negative inspiratory force test, a study of the literature reveals that a number of measurement devices have been assembled and that different bedside techniques have been used to determine the effort of a patient breathing naturally and one who is intubated breathing by way of a mechanical ventilator. There is no consensus on what is the best equipment configuration or measurement technique.

A strong case can be made for the use of a double one-way valve to connect the intubated patient to the manometer (see Fig. 4-8). Use of the one-way valves lets the patient inhale but prevents an exhalation when the practitioner occludes the expiratory opening. This forces the patient to exhale from closer to total lung capacity with each breathing effort. However, the expiratory efforts should not be held for more than 3 seconds. This test is similar to Valsalva's maneuver and can cause a reduction in the cardiac output because of the high intrathoracic pressure.

Steps in the MEF procedure for a normally breathing patient:

1. Obtain a pressure gauge capable of measuring at least ±60 cm water pressure.
2. Have the patient sit upright. Place a note in the chart if the patient is lying down.

3. Instruct the patient to breathe in to total lung capacity.
4. Simulate a demonstration of the procedure.
5. Place nose clips over the patient's nose. Have the patient seal his/her lips and teeth around the mouthpiece and breathe through the open port.
6. Tell the patient to inhale completely. Seal the port when total lung capacity has been reached.
7. Tell the patient to breathe out as hard as possible. Hold it for 1 to 3 seconds.
8. Reteach if necessary.
9. Repeat until at least three good efforts have been performed. Record the greatest stable value seen after the first second of effort. This eliminates any artifact created by the cheeks or chest wall movement.

It is important to monitor any patient for signs of undue stress and hypoxemia such as tachycardia, bradycardia, ventricular dysrhythmias, hypotension, and/or decreasing saturation on pulse oximetry. If any of these are seen, the procedure should be stopped and the patient reoxygenated and ventilated.

Clinically normal people of either sex and any age should be able to generate at least +80 cm water pressure. Patients with neuromuscular diseases, thoracic injury or abnormality, and COPD will tend to have decreased strength. A MEF value of $^{+}40$ cm water is probably enough to offer assurance that the patient has enough strength and coordination to cough effectively to clear secretions. However, depending on the blood gas values and other physical parameters, the patient may need to be endotracheally intubated and maintained on a mechanical ventilator.

Black and Hyatt have published the following MEF prediction formulas for spontaneously breathing nonintubated subjects breathing from total lung capacity. The values are in cm water pressure.

- Males: $268 - (1.03 \times \text{age})$
- Females: $170 - (0.53 \times \text{age})$

The lower limit of normal for men is 140 and 95 for women. These would be predictive for patients aged 20 to 86. As can be see, the the older the patient is, the lower the predicted maximal expiratory force would be.

Module B. Pulmonary function equipment.

1. Water, mercury, and anaeroid-type manometers (pressure gauges).
a. Get the necessary equipment for the procedure. (IIA8a)[R, Ap]

There are many manufacturers of manometers (pressure gauges). Work with as many of them as possible. Mercury or water-type manometers have a vertical column of the liquid as in a sphygmomanometer for measuring blood pressure. An anaeroid (spring loaded) unit is most commonly used. This is because they do not have to be kept upright to measure accurately. Anaeroid manometers can be calibrated in either mm of mercury (mm Hg) or cm of water (cm H_2O) pressure and look like a Bourdon gauge. Be able to mathematically convert cm of water to mm of mercury and vice versa by using the following formulas:

- $\text{mm Hg} = \dfrac{\text{cm } H_2O}{1.36}$
- $\text{cm } H_2O = \text{mm Hg} \times 1.36$

b. Put the equipment together, make sure that is works properly, and identify any problems with it. (IIB14a)[R, Ap]

These pressure gauges come preassembled by the manufacturer. It is only necessary to attach the pressure source to the inlet port on the unit to measure a pressure change. This connection must be air-tight or a leak will occur and the measured pressure will be wrong. Accuracy of the unit can be checked by opening the inlet port to room air and reading the pressure. A reading of zero should be seen (indicating no pressure change from atmospheric). Next, a known pressure is applied to the gauge. Often this is done by attaching it to a sphygmomanometer and pumping up the pressure to a known level such as 50 mm Hg. The pressure gauge should show the same. If not, there may be a leak in the system or the pressure gauge is miscalibrated. Do not use a pressure gauge that cannot be calibrated.

2. Inspiratory and/or expiratory force meters (pressure gauges).
a. Get the necessary equipment for the procedure. ((A8b)[R, Ap]

The maximum inspiratory pressure and maximum expiratory pressure tests are usually recorded in centimeters of water pressure. However, millimeters of mercury could be used. As shown, be able to convert between the two pressures. If a centimeters of water pressure gauge is used it should be able to record a negative and/or positive pressure of at least 100 cm H_2O). However, a unit that can record ±60 cm H_2O would probably be adequate.

b. Put the equipment together, make sure that is works properly, and identify any problems with it. (IIB14b)[R, Ap]

There is no standard setup for these devices. See Figs. 4-8 and 4-9 for two possible assemblies. The system can be sealed and pressure checked with a known force to make sure that the pressure manometer is accurate and all the connections are air-tight. Do not use a pressure gauge that cannot be calibrated. The one-way valves must function so that the patient can only exhale or inhale as needed for the test.

Module C. Patient assessment.

Review Section 1 as needed for general information on patient assessment. In general, the work and stress of the performing these procedures might cause some patients to become tachycardic or have an abnormal rhythm. This should only be a temporary condition. Seek help if the problem persists.

It is is especially important to auscultate a patient who is undergoing a before and/or after bronchodilator study. Hopefully, the bronchodilator will relieve the bronchospasm, and wheezing will decrease.

When doing any test, note in the chart if a particular medication, breathing treatment, or procedure had any benefit to the patient or caused any difficulty. Be especially careful to check your math work for accuracy.

BIBLIOGRAPHY

Beauchamp RK: Pulmonary function testing procedures, in Barnes TA (ed): *Respiratory Care Practice*. Chicago, Mosby, 1988.

Black LF, Hyatt RE: Maximal respiratory pressures: Normal values and relationship to age and sex. *Am Rev Respir Dis* 1969; 99:696-702.

Branson RD, Hurst JM, Davis K Jr, et al: Measurement of maximal inspiratory pressure: A comparison of three methods. *Respir Care* 1989; 34:789-794.

Cherniak RM: *Pulmonary Function Testing,* ed 2. Philadelphia, WB Saunders, 1993.

Cherniack RM, Rader MD: Normal standards for ventilatory function using an automated wedge spirometer. *Am Rev Respir Dis* 1972; 106:38.

Clausen JL (ed): *Pulmonary Function Testing Guidelines and Controversies.* Orlando, Fla, Grune & Stratton, 1984.

Hess D: Measurement of maximal inspiratory pressure: A call for standardization. *Respir Care* 1989; 34:857-859.

Kacmarek RM, Cycyk-Chapman MC, Young-Palazzo PJ, et al: Determination of maximal inspiratory pressure: A clinical study and literature review. *Respir Care* 1989; 34:868-878.

Madama VC: *Pulmonary Function Testing and Cardiopulmonary Stress Testing.* Albany, Delmar Publishers, Inc, 1993.

Morris JF, Koski A, Johnson LC: Spirometric standards for healthy nonsmoking adults. *Am Rev Respir Dis* 1971; 103:57.

Ruppel G: *Manual of Pulmonary Function Testing,* ed 6. St Louis, Mosby, 1994.

SELF-STUDY QUESTIONS

1. Calculate your patient's inspiratory time and expiratory time when he has an I/E ratio of 2:1 and a respiratory rate of 15/min.
   A. 2.7 seconds for inspiration and 1.3 seconds for expiration
   B. 3.3 seconds for inspiration and 1.7 seconds for expiration
   C. 1.3 seconds for inspiration and 2.7 seconds for expiration
   D. 1.7 seconds for inspiration and 3.3 seconds for expiration
   E. 13.3 seconds for inspiration and 6.7 seconds for expiration

2. When having a patient perform a maximum expiratory force test it is important that he or she:
   A. Blow out all air before starting the effort.
   B. Breathe in a tidal volume and blow out hard.
   C. Inhale to total lung capacity and blow out hard.
   D. Exhale a tidal volume breath and inhale as hard as possible.

3. Your patient weighs 100 lb/45 kg. Her predicted tidal volume would be:
   A. 600 ml
   B. 500 ml
   C. 400 ml
   D. 300 ml
   E. 200 ml

4. You receive an order to calculate your patient's alveolar ventilation. His respiratory rate is 16, and his average tidal volume is 580 mL. He weighs 170 lb. His alveolar ventilation would be:
   A. 2720 ml
   B. 410 ml
   C. 750 ml

D. 510 ml
E. 564 ml

5. Your patient has an $FEV_{1\%}$ that calculates out to be 80% of his forced vital capacity. On the basis of this finding, the patient probably:
   A. Is having an asthma attack.
   B. Has asthma but is in remission.
   C. Has a fibrotic lung disease.
   D. Has a thoracic deformity.
   E. Is clinically normal.

Note: Refer to the figure below for questions 6 and 7.

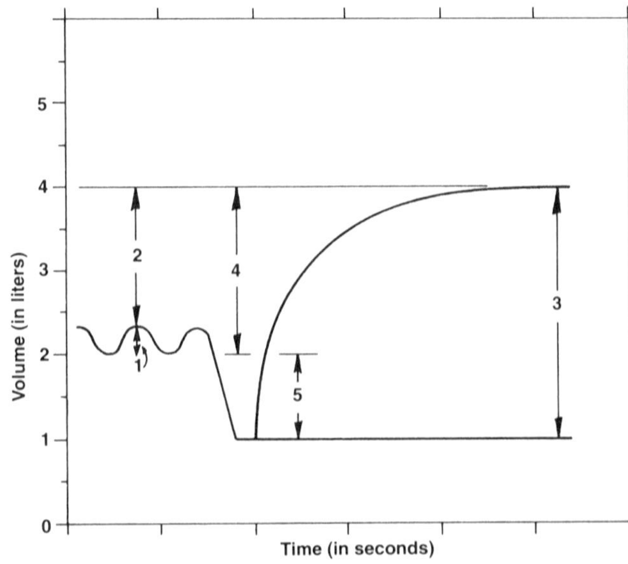

6. Which section of the spirometry tracing represents the forced vital capacity?
   A. 1
   B. 2
   C. 3
   D. 4
   E. 5

7. Which section of the spirometry tracing represents the tidal volume?
   A. 1
   B. 2
   C. 3
   D. 4
   E. 5

8. Your pediatric patient has a respiratory rate of 50, a tidal volume of 40 ml, inspiratory time of 0.3 seconds, and expiratory time of 0.9 seconds. Calculate her I/R ratio.
   A. 3:1
   B. 1:1
   C. 1:3
   D. 2:3
   E. None of the above

9. The vital capacity is made up of:
   I. Residual volume
   II. Functional residual capacity
   III. Expiratory reserve volume
   IV. Tidal volume
   V. Inspiratory reserve volume
   A. IV, V
   B. II, IV
   C. III, IV
   D. I, II, III
   E. III, IV, V

10. Bedside spirometry reveals the following patient data that have been BTPS corrected: FVC, 3600 mL; FEV_1, 2000 ml; FEV_2, 2400 mL; FEV_3, 3200 ml; FEV_4, 3400 mL; FEV_5, 3500 ml; and FEV_6, 3600 ml. Calculate her $FEV_{3\%}$.
   A. 89%
   B. 56%
   C. 67%
   D. 100%
   E. 97%

11. Which of the following are true of the peak flow measurement?
   I. It is usually seen at the end of the patient's forced vital capacity effort.
   II. It increases with height.
   III. It increases with age.
   IV. It decreases with age.
   V. It is usually seen at the beginning of the patient's forced vital capacity effort.
   A. I, II, III
   B. II, IV, V
   C. I, II, IV
   D. IV, V
   E. I, II, IV

12. The minimum safe maximum inspiratory pressure that a patient should be able to generate is:
   A. −10 cm H_2O
   B. −20 cm H_2O
   C. −30 cm H_2O
   D. −40 cm H_2O
   E. −50 cm H_2O

13. You are having your patient perform the negative inspiratory force test. His three attempts produce these results: −15 cm H_2O, −45 cm H_2O, and −20 cm H_2O. The best explanation for these values is:
   A. Confusing instructions and demonstration.
   B. The patient is starting from functional residual capacity.
   C. The equipment has a large leak.
   D. The patient is starting from residual volume.
   E. The patient is not trying his best every time.

14. The physician wants to know whether a new bronchodilator would be helpful to his asthmatic patient. He orders a before- and after-bronchodilator study. The patient has the following peak flow values: 7.5 L/min before the medication and 9.4 L/min after the medication. Calculate her percent change.

A. 80%
B. 1.25%
C. −25%
D. 25%
E. None of the above

Answer Key:

1. A; 2. C; 3. D; 4. B; 5. E; 6. C; 7. A; 8. C; 9. E; 10. A; 11. B; 12. B; 13. E; 14. D

5 Oxygen Therapy

Module A. Perform the following procedures to ensure that the patient is adequately oxygenated:

1. Oxygen administration:

a. Minimize hypoxemia by positioning the patient properly. (IIID1 and IIIF9h) [R, Ap, An]

A patient who is short of breath when lying supine in bed should be repositioned to breathe easier. Usually this means sitting more upright in a Fowler's or semi-Fowler's position. This seems to work best in patients with bilateral pulmonary problems such as congestive heart failure or pneumonia.

Sometimes the patient cannot sit up. If this is the case and the lung problem is one sided, roll the patient so that the more functional lung is down. The following are exceptions when the good lung should be positioned up:

1. Undrained pulmonary abscess that you would not want to drain into the good lung.
2. Neonatal congenital diaphragmatic hernia where you would not want the good lung to be compressed by the bowel in the chest cavity.
3. Pulmonary interstitial emphysema where, by lying on the bad lung, its air leak and functional residual capacity can be reduced.

In either case, always ask the patient whether the new position helps to make breathing easier. If not, reposition the patient again until breathing is more comfortable with less shortness of breath.

b. Administer oxygen, as needed, and make a recommendation to change the fractional inspired oxygen concentration (F_{IO_2}) or oxygen flow to spontaneously breathing patients. (IIID2, IIIF9g1 and 2) [R, Ap, An]

Oxygen is a drug that must be administered in doses that are adequate to treat hypoxemia, decrease the patient's work of breathing, or decrease the work of the heart. This means up to 100% oxygen. Because it is a drug, there must be a physician's order to give it to a patient or make a change in the percentage. The only exceptions are when there are recognized protocols in your institution to give oxygen under certain limited conditions. For example, all patients with a diagnosed heart attack are given a nasal cannula at 2 L/min, or all patients undergoing cardiopulmonary resuscitation receive 100% oxygen.

See Section 3, Module A, for a listing of indications for drawing blood for an arterial blood gas measurement. This list should be fairly complete for conditions that justify the need for supplemental oxygen. In general, the goal of giving supplemental oxygen is to keep the patient's Pao_2 level between 60 and 100 mm Hg. Exceptions include carbon monoxide poisoning, severe anemia, and cardiopulmonary resuscitation, where the hope is to fully saturate the hemoglobin and increase the plasma oxygen content as much as possible. Oxygen should not be given without proof of hypoxemia or another clinical justification. When those conditions have been corrected, the oxygen percentage should be adjusted accordingly.

Giving supplemental oxygen is not without risk. The following is a list of oxygen-related problems that may be clinically seen:

A. Oxygen-induced hypoventilation. This is something to watch for in patients who have an elevated carbon dioxide level because of severe emphysema, chronic bronchitis, or both. The clinical goal is to keep their Pao_2 level between 50 and 60 mm Hg. Check the blood gases frequently for the oxygen and carbon dioxide level.
B. Retrolental fibroplasia (RLF)/retinitis of prematurity (ROP). This type of blindness is found in some premature neonates who were given high levels of supplemental oxygen. This is commonly seen in premature neonates born with infant respiratory distress syndrome (IRDS). The exact cause is not completely understood but is related primarily to the degree of prematurity. Keeping the Pao_2 in the range of 50 to 60 mm Hg the first week and 50 to 70 mm Hg after that should help to prevent the problem.
C. Denitrogenation absorption atelectasis. Giving greater than 80% oxygen can result in atelectasis of underventilated alveoli. This is because there is not enough nitrogen in the alveoli to keep them open after the oxygen has been taken up by the hemoglobin. As a result, the patient will have an increase in shunting.
D. Central nervous system abnormalities. A patient who is breathing 100% oxygen in a hyperbaric chamber can have muscle tremors and seizures. Watch for this if your patient is receiving this treatment for carbon monoxide poisoning.
E. Pulmonary oxygen toxicity. In general, it appears that patients can breathe up to 50% oxygen for prolonged periods without significant damage. If clinically possible, many practitioners try to limit their patients to no more than 48 to 72 hours of breathing more than 50% oxygen. Breathing higher percentages for prolonged periods can result in one or more of the following problems:
    1. Redistribution of surfactant within the alveoli so that atelectasis is likely to occur.
    2. Death of alveolar type I pneumocytes.
    3. Edema of the alveolar wall with an intra-alveolar exudate giving the chest x-ray appearance of pneumonia.
    4. Swelling and possible obliteration of the pulmonary capillary bed.
    5. Formation of hyaline membranes.
    6. Pulmonary fibrosis.
    7. Bronchopulmonary dysplasia (BPD) in infants who survive the initial problem of IRDS. Vitamin E is given to these children in the hope of delaying or preventing further damage.

Note: The National Board for Respiratory Care (NBRC) is known to ask questions that relate to the proper use of oxygen and the hazards associated with its use.

c. Measure the patient's oxygen percentage, oxygen liter flow, or both. (IIIG7) [R, Ap]

Always measure the patient's oxygen percentage (F_{IO_2}) if possible. The gas sample should be taken as close as possible to the patient to minimize the chance of dilution from room air. Record the oxygen percentage on the arterial blood gas order slip, in the department records, and in the patient's chart if needed. As discussed in Section 2, the oxygen percentage must be known to interpret the patient's Pa_{O_2} level.

The oxygen liter flow is all that can be recorded with these devices: nasal cannula, nasal catheter, simple mask, partial rebreather mask, and non-rebreather mask. There is a direct relationship between the liter flow and the oxygen percentage, but it is not predictably accurate.

d. Prevent the patient from becoming hypoxemic by using proper technique. (IIID3) [R, Ap]

Use caution and plan ahead to minimize any time that the oxygen supply to the patient will be cut off or reduced. When changing equipment of any kind, have the replacement set up and tested for proper function before replacing the current setup. Quickly make sure that the new equipment is truly working properly. Only then is it safe to disassemble or discard the old equipment.

It is well known that suctioning the airway reduces the patient's oxygen level. This can result in dangerous dysrhythmias. Remember to increase the patient's inspired oxygen percentage about 1 minute before, during, and for at least 1 minute after suctioning. It is acceptable and safe to give 100% oxygen for short periods like this. Remember to reduce the oxygen percentage or liter flow to the previous level once the patient is stable after the procedure. Reanalyze the percentage if possible.

2. Oxygen analyzers:

a. Get the necessary equipment for the procedure. (IIA7e) [R, Ap]
b. Put the equipment together, make sure that it works properly, and identify and fix any problems with it. (IIB7d) [R, Ap]

Because there are so many different models available, it is not practical to discuss all of them here. Consult an equipment book or the manufacturer's literature for details of the various analyzers. All portable, hand-held analyzers fall into one of the following categories: electric, physical/paramagnetic, electrochemical, polarographic, or galvanic fuel cell.

Electric Analyzers

These are battery powered and employ a Wheatstone bridge to compare the cooling effects of the oxygen-enriched gas with a known reference gas. The oxygen-enriched gas will cool faster than the reference. This is known as the principle of thermal conductivity. Each sample must be drawn into the analyzer through a capillary line. These analyzers are designed to work only in oxygen and nitrogen gas mixes. Do *not* use them around flammable gases such as found in anesthesia. Mira and OEM are manufacturers of this type.

Calibration is done on this and all analyzers by sampling room air, adjusting a calibration control to 21% if necessary, sampling 100% oxygen, and adjusting a calibration control to 100% if necessary. In general, always follow the manufacturer's guidelines for setup and calibration. Failure to calibrate could be caused by a weak battery, a plugged capillary line, or a defect in an electrical component.

Physical/Paramagnetic Analyzers

These analyzers make use of the fact that oxygen is attracted toward a magnetic field (paramagnetic property). The more oxygen there is in a sample gas, the more the magnetic field is altered. This is called the Pauling principle after its discoverer. As mentioned earlier, each gas sample must be drawn into the analyzer by a capillary tube. These units can be used with all types of gases and are safe in the operating room with flammable and explosive anesthetics. Beckman is a manufacturer of this type.

A silica gel–filled container is in line with the capillary tube to dry out the sample gas before it gets to the analyzing chamber. Failure to calibrate could be caused by water or a defect in the analyzing chamber, a weak battery, or a plugged capillary line.

Electrochemical Analyzers

Both of these types make use of the fact that each oxygen molecule will accept up to two electrons and become chemically reduced. The more oxygen there is in the gas sample, the more electrons are released from an oxidizing electrolyte solution. This is measured as an electrical current that is proportional to the oxygen percentage. These analyzers can continuously monitor and display the oxygen percentage. Both types are safe by themselves in the presence of flammable gases, but the added alarm systems are electrically powered and may make the units unsafe.

Calibration is done as described earlier. Failure to calibrate could be caused by a weak battery, an exhausted supply of chemical reactant in the gas sampling probe, or an electronic failure. The galvanic units must have their probes kept dry to read accurately. Both types are pressure sensitive. High altitude will cause them to display a lower-than-true oxygen percentage, and high pressure as seen in a ventilator circuit with positive end-expiratory pressure (PEEP) will cause the units to display a higher-than-true oxygen percentage.

Polarographic Analyzers

These units use a battery to polarize the gas sampling probe. Because of this, they have a faster response time than do the galvanic fuel cell types. Ohio Medical Products, IMI, and Instrumentation Laboratories, Inc., are manufacturers of this type.

Galvanic Fuel Cell Analyzers

These units do not need a battery for power. However, they usually include alarms that are battery powered. The electrolyte solution will last longer in these units than in the polarographic types. Teledyne Analytic Instruments, Hudson Oxygen, and BioMarine Industries are manufacturers of this type.

Module B. Storage, hardware, and distribution of medical gases.

1. Oxygen and other gas cylinders, bulk storage systems, and manifolds.

Table 5-1. Color Codes for Gas Cylinders

Gas	Color
Oxygen	Green (white for international)
Air	Yellow
Helium	Brown
Helium and oxygen	Brown and green (check the label for the percentages of each gas)
Carbon dioxide	Gray
Carbon dioxide and oxygen	Gray and green (check the label for the percentages of each gas)
Nitrous oxide	Light blue
Cyclopropane	Orange
Ethylene	Red

a. Get the necessary equipment for the procedure. (IIA7d)[R, Ap]
b. Put the equipment together, make sure that it works properly, and identify and fix any problems with it. (IIB7c)[R, Ap]

Oxygen and Other Gas Cylinders

The different types of gases in cylinders are identified by the color code of the cylinder and the cylinder's label. Note that only E cylinders have mandatory color coding. The color codings on the other cylinders are voluntary but usually followed by the manufacturers. However, always read the label to be sure of the contents of the cylinder. The most important cylinder colors to remember are those of oxygen and air, but all are included in Table 5-1 for the sake of completeness.

The NBRC is known to ask the examinee to calculate how long a certain cylinder will last at a given gas flow. To date, only the durations of E-, H-, and K-sized oxygen cylinders have been asked. Remember that the duration of only gas-filled cylinders can be predicted. Liquid- and gas-filled cylinders such as nitrous oxide and carbon dioxide must be weighed to determine how full they are. See Table 5-2 and the following examples.

The duration of flow of a cylinder is calculated by the following formula:

$$\text{Minutes of flow (divide by 60 to calculate hours)} = \frac{\text{gauge pressure in psig} \times \text{cylinder factor}}{\text{liter flow}}$$

Table 5-2. Oxygen Cylinder Duration of Flow Factors

Cylinder Size	Factor (L/psig*)
E	0.28
H	3.14
K	3.14
D	0.16
M	1.36
G	2.41

**psig*, pounds per square inch gauge.

Example 1.

a. Calculate the duration of flow of an E cylinder with 1500 psig that is running at 6 L/min.

$$\text{Minutes of flow (divide by 60 to calculate hours)} = \frac{1500 \text{ psig} \times 0.28}{6 \text{ L}}$$

$$= \frac{420}{6}$$

Minutes of flow = 70 (this also works out to 1.16 hours, or 1 hour and 10 minutes)

Example 2.

Calculate the duration of flow of an H cylinder with 1950 psig that is running at 9 L/min.

$$\text{Minutes of flow (divide by 60 to calculate hours)} = \frac{1950 \text{ psig} \times 3.14}{9 \text{ L}}$$

$$= \frac{6{,}123}{9}$$

Minutes of flow = 680.33 (this works out to 11.34 hours, or 11 hours and 20 minutes)

Bulk Storage Systems

The bulk liquid oxygen storage system is the main source of a hospital's oxygen. A reducing valve is used to decrease the gas pressure to 50 psig before it is piped throughout the hospital for easy access. Alarms will sound if the pressure falls low or goes too high. Pressure relief valves will open if the pressure is greater than 75 psig. Zone valves are located throughout the hospital to turn off the gas if a leak develops or there is a fire.

Manifolds

A manifold is a piping system that connects the bulk storage system and hospital gas piping system with a bank of H- or K-sized cylinders. These free-standing cylinders are a backup source of oxygen in case the bulk system fails. A 24-hour supply of gas must be available.

The manifold system includes a reducing valve to decrease the gas pressure to 50 psig. Check valves are built into the manifold so that a leak in one cylinder connection will not result in all of the gas cylinders leaking out.

2. Adjunct hardware: reducing valves, flowmeters, regulators, and high-pressure hose connectors.

a. Get the necessary equipment for the procedure. (IIA7a) [R, Ap]

b. Put the equipment together, make sure that it works properly, and identify and fix any problems with it. (IIB7a) [R, Ap]

Reducing Valves

Reducing valves are used to reduce the high pressure seen in a bulk oxygen storage system, manifold, or gas cylinder. One or more stages (pressure-reducing steps) can be used to reach the working pressure of 50 psig. Adjustable or Bourdon reducing valves allow the working pressure to be adjusted from 50 to 100 psig. Single-stage reducing valves reach the pressure in a single step. Multiple-stage reducing valves give finer control over pressure and flow by dropping pressure in the first stage to about 200 psig and to 50 psig in the second stage. Occasionally three stages are seen.

All reducing valves (and regulators) have the following safety features built into them:

a. A frangible disk that breaks to release gas pressure in the event of a mechanical failure or breakage.

b. A fusible plug that melts to release gas pressure in the event of a fire.

c. American Standard Compressed Gas Cylinder Valve Outlet and Index Connections (usually called the American Standard system), which prevent the accidental connection of the wrong reducing valve (or regulator) onto a large gas cylinder. Respiratory care practitioners usually work only with air and oxygen but should familiarize themselves with the other gases and corresponding reducing valves.

d. The Pin Index Safely System (PISS) is a special section of the American Standard system that applies to E-sized gas cylinders and smaller. It is designed to prevent an accidental connection of the wrong gas with a reducing valve or regulator. These reducing valves and regulators are designed with a specifically pinned yoke to wrap around the valve stem of a gas cylinder. A soft plastic O-ring washer is included to help ensure a tight seal. Fig. 5-1 shows the location of the pinholes in the cylinder valve face. Table 5-3 shows the gases and pinhole positions. It is important to know the positions for oxygen and air; the others are included for the sake of completeness.

It is necessary to "crack" or blow some gas out of a cylinder before putting any reducing valve or regulator onto it to prevent any dust or debris from being forced into the reducing valve or regulator, which might cause a fire.

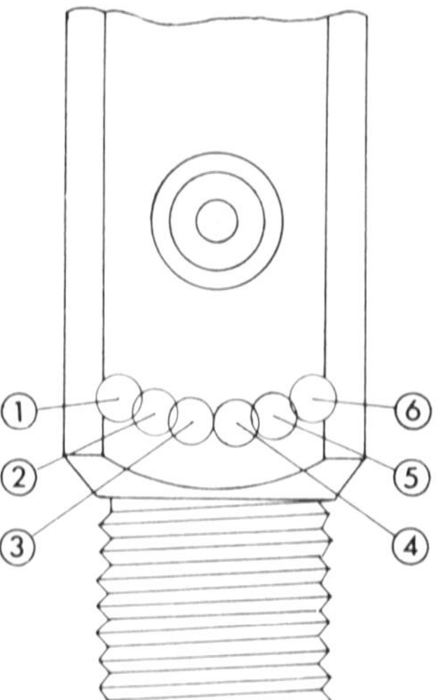

Fig. 5-1 Locations of the Pin Index Safety System holes in the cylinder valve face. (From Scanlan CL, Spearman CB, Sheldon RL [eds]: *Egan's Fundamentals of Respiratory Care,* ed 5. St Louis, Mosby, 1990. Used by permission.)

Table 5-3. Pin Index Safety System Gases and Pinhole Locations

Gas	Pinhole Locations
Oxygen	2-5
Air	1-5
Oxygen/carbon dioxide ($\leq$ 7%)	2-6
Oxygen/carbon dioxide (>7%)	1-6
Oxygen/helium (not >80% helium)	2-4
Oxygen/helium (helium >80%)	4-6
Nitrous oxide	3-5
Ethylene	1-3
Cyclopropane	3-6

Flowmeters

Flowmeters are designed to regulate and indicate flow. They also come with the following safety features so that they cannot be attached to the wrong reducing valve, regulator, high-pressure hose, or appliance:

a. Diameter-Index Safety System (DISS) inlets and outlets that are specific to the various gases so that a mix-up cannot be made. For example, the DISS inlet and outlet to an oxygen flowmeter allow it to be connected to only an oxygen reducing valve and oxygen high-pressure hose or appliance. The DISS system applies to flowmeters that attach to all American Standard and DISS reduction valves.

b. Flowmeters with quick-connect inlet adapters instead of DISS inlets. These quick-connects are designed specifically for the hospital's piped-in oxygen and air outlets.

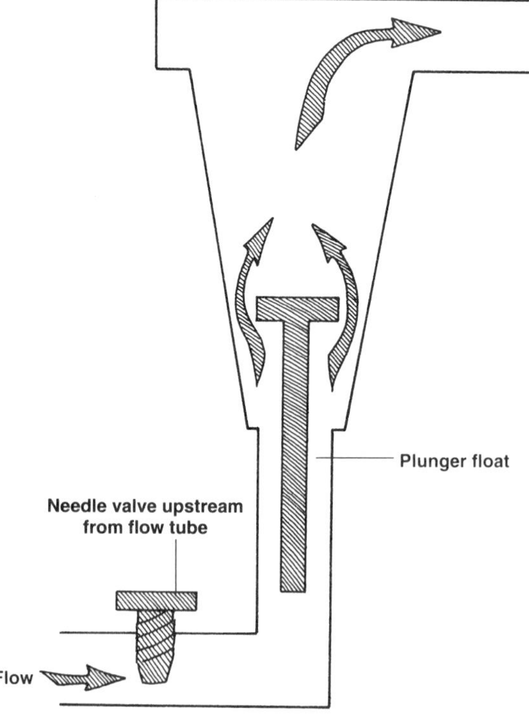

Fig. 5-2 Kinetic-type non-backpressure–compensated (pressure-uncompensated) flowmeter. (Modified from McPherson SP: *Respiratory Therapy Equipment,* ed 4. St Louis, Mosby, 1990.)

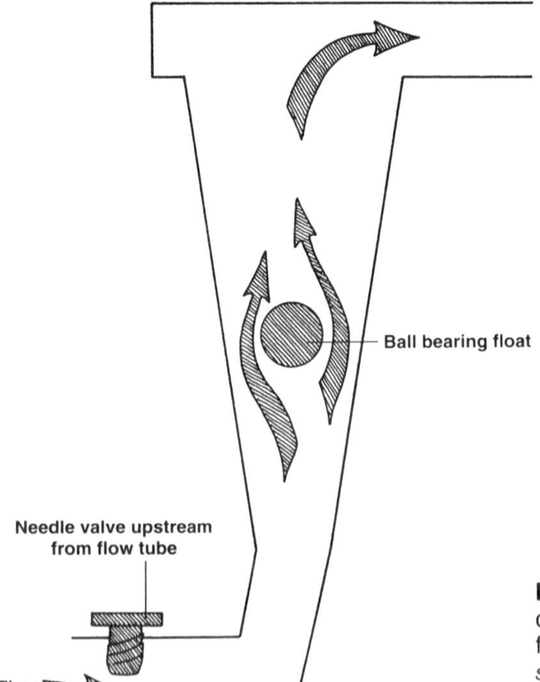

Fig. 5-3 Thorpe-type non-backpressure–compensated (pressure-uncompensated) flowmeter. (Modified from McPherson SP: *Respiratory Therapy Equipment,* ed 4. St Louis, Mosby, 1990.)

They are not interchangeable between gases or between manufacturers. Occasionally a piped oxygen outlet will jam open and let gas rapidly escape. Insert the proper flowmeter into the outlet and turn the flowmeter off. This will stop the leak until the defective wall outlet can be repaired.

Flowmeters are usually categorized by how they react to backpressure. To complicate matters further, we must remember that there are three different manufactured types of flowmeters that may or may not be backpressure compensated.

A. Non-backpressure–compensated (pressure-uncompensated) flowmeters will *inaccurately* indicate the flow through them in the face of backpressure. Figs. 5-2 to 5-4 show non-backpressure–compensated kinetic, Thorpe, and Bourdon types of flowmeters, respectively.

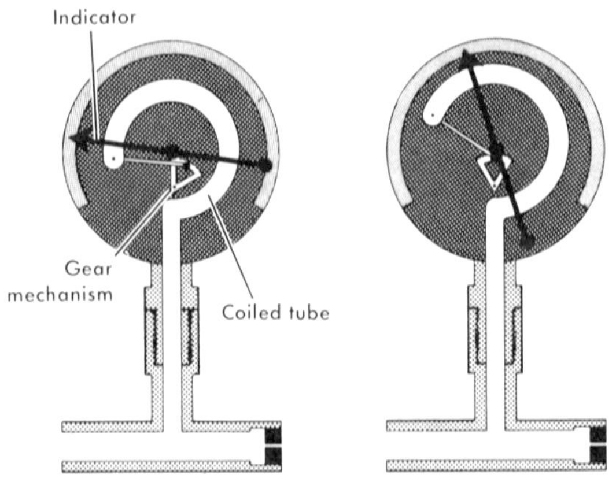

Fig. 5-4 Bourdon-type non-backpressure–compensated (pressure-uncompensated) flowmeter. (From McPherson SP: *Respiratory Therapy Equipment,* ed 4. St Louis, Mosby, 1990. Used by permission.)

Note that the Thorpe and kinetic flowmeters have the flow control valve upstream from the meter. They will read accurately if they are kept upright and do not have to "push" against any backpressure. If laid on their sides, the plunger and ball bearing will not indicate the set flow. They will both read a *lower* flow than what is actually delivered when faced with a backpressure.

The Bourdon flowmeter is designed like the Bourdon gauge in the reducing valve. The facepiece is marked in just liters of flow rather than pressure. It is the flowmeter of choice in a transport situation because it may be laid flat without affecting its flow if there is no backpressure. These flowmeters will display a *higher* flow than what is actually delivered when faced with a backpressure.

B. Backpressure-compensated (pressure-compensated) flowmeters will *accurately* indicate the flow through them in the face of backpressure. For this reason they should be used whenever possible. Figs. 5-5 and 5-6 show backpressure-compensated kinetic and Thorpe types of flowmeters, respectively.

Note that both of these flowmeters have the flow-control valve downstream from the meter. Because of this, they will read accurately in the face of backpressure as long as they are kept upright. Besides reading the label, this simple test will enable the practitioner to tell whether a flowmeter is backpressure compensated:

1. Make sure the flowmeter is turned off.
2. Plug the flowmeter into a gas outlet.
3. If the float or ball bearing bounces, the flowmeter is backpressure compensated.

These are the flowmeters of choice in all situations except during patient transport when the oxygen tank and flowmeter might be laid flat.

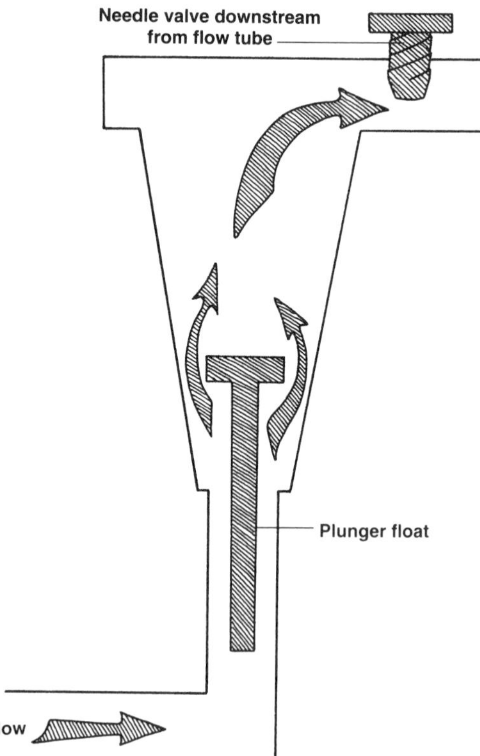

Fig. 5-5 Kinetic-type backpressure–compensated (pressure-compensated) flowmeter. (Modified from McPherson SP: *Respiratory Therapy Equipment,* ed 4. St Louis, Mosby, 1990.)

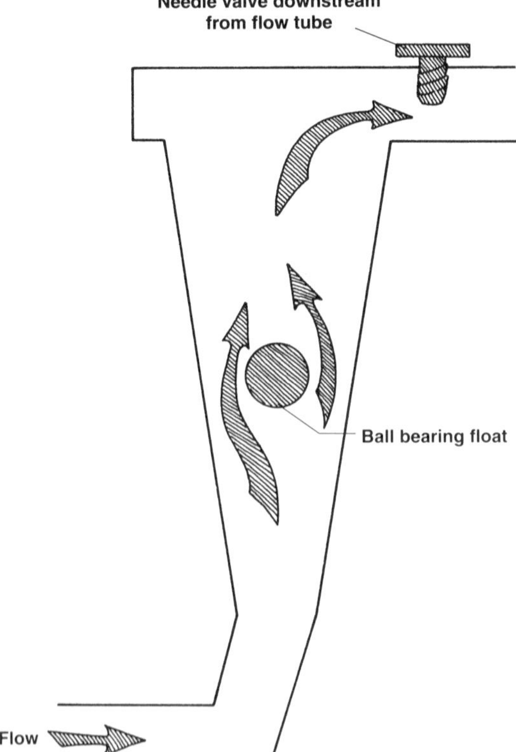

Fig. 5-6 Thorpe-type backpressure–compensated (pressure-compensated) flowmeter. (Modified from McPherson SP: *Respiratory Therapy Equipment,* ed 4. St Louis, Mosby, 1990.)

Regulators

Regulators combine a reducing valve and a flowmeter. Everything that has been discussed so far relates to regulators. Bourdon gauge reducing valves are usually seen and can have either a second Bourdon gauge added as a flowmeter or a Thorpe or kinetic flowmeter. As mentioned earlier, use a backpressure-compensated flowmeter in all situations except for patient transport.

High-Pressure Hose Connectors

These connectors and other adapters connect high-pressure hoses, flowmeters, and oxygen appliances. They have DISS inlets and outlets so that the gases cannot be cross-fitted onto the wrong equipment.

3. Air compressors.
a. Get the necessary equipment for the procedure. (IIA7b) [R, Ap]
b. Put the equipment together, make sure that it works properly, and identify and fix any problems with it. (IIB7e) [R, Ap]

Air compressors are used whenever a high-pressure gas source is needed besides oxygen. All three different types of systems are alike in that they employ an electrically powered motor, filter the room air as it enters and exists the compressor, and have a condenser to remove water vapor as it leaves the compressor.

Rotary-Type Compressor

These units generate pressure with a rotating fan. They are commonly used in volume ventilators and in the home to power hand-held medication nebulizers and intermittent positive-pressure breathing (IPPB) units.

Diaphragm-Type Compressor

These units generate pressure with a diaphragm that moves up and down within a cylinder like a piston. They also are commonly used in the home to power hand-held medication nebulizers and IPPB units.

Piston-Type Compressor

These units generate pressure by piston action within a cylinder. They are much more powerful than the previous two types of compressors. Because they are designed to generate pressures of 50 psig or greater, they are used in the hospital for its piped air system. They are also used in the home setting in oxygen concentrators.

Make sure that all of these units are operational by checking that the inlet and outlet filters are cleaned. Dirty filters will prevent proper airflow. Check the unit's pressure gauge to make sure that it is able to meet its manufacturer's specified pressure. Keep the water trap empty on the condensing unit.

4. Air/oxygen proportioners (blenders).
   a. Get the necessary equipment for the procedure. (IIA7c and IIIF6d) [R, Ap]
   b. Put the equipment together, make sure that it works properly, and identify and fix any problems with it. (IIB7b) [R, Ap]

These units are designed to change the ratio of oxygen and air so as to blend the specific percentage of oxygen from 21% to 100%. To do that, both source gases must be pressurized to 50 psig. The oxygen percentage will remain close to that desired even if there is a small drop in either one or both line pressures. Always analyze the oxygen percentage to confirm that the blend is proper. The blended gas can be sent directly to a ventilator or other device that uses 50 psig or through an added flowmeter.

Keep the gas inlets and outlets clear of any debris. All current units give an audible whistle if either one or both of the line pressures drop to an unsafe level (often about 30 psig). If the unit has a water trap at the compressed air inlet, keep it emptied of any condensate.

Module C. Administration of oxygen therapy.

1. Oxygen hoods and oxygen tents.
   a. Get the necessary equipment for the procedure. (IIA1e) [R, Ap]
   b. Put the equipment together, make sure that it works properly, and identify and fix any problems with it. (IIB1d) [R, Ap]

Oxygen Hoods

Oxygen hoods are used to provide a warmed aerosol, humidity, and a controlled oxygen percentage to pediatric patients who weigh no more than 18 lb (8.2 kg) (Fig. 5-7). In addition, the following procedures should be observed:

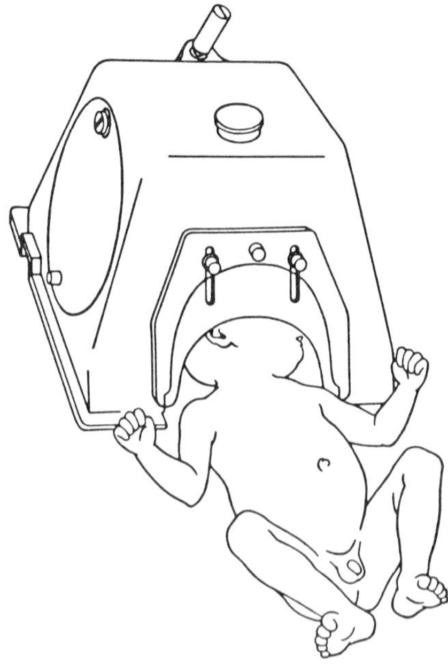

Fig. 5-7 Infant in an oxygen hood. (From Gaebler G, Blodgett D: Gas administration, in Blodgett D [ed]: *Manual of Pediatric Respiratory Care Procedures.* Philadelphia, Lippincott, 1982. Used by permission.)

a. Use an air/oxygen proportioner with a flowmeter to control the oxygen percentage and flow to the hood. The flow should be at least 7 L/min to prevent the buildup of exhaled carbon dioxide. A flow of 10 to 15 L/min is needed to keep a stable oxygen percentage. Keeping the hood sealed as much as possible and minimizing the gap between the infant's neck and the opening to the hood will also help to stabilize the oxygen percentage.

b. A warmed humidifier is needed to provide a high humidity level and to warm the oxygen to the infant's body temperature. Care must be taken with infants to ensure that they are neither heated nor cooled by the gas blowing over their heads. A thermometer should be kept in the hood to note the temperature.

c. An oxygen analyzer should be continuously monitoring how much oxygen is inside the hood. The analyzer probe should be placed at the same level as the infant's nose. This is because oxygen is heavier than air and will tend to settle toward the bottom of the hood.

The advantages of the hood over the tent are that the patient's body is accessible and the head can be reached by lifting the top off of the hood. Be aware of the noise level inside the hood to minimize damaging the infant's hearing. The sound level should be monitored and kept well below 65 dB.

Oxygen Tents

Oxygen tents were formerly used for adults but are now used only for children who are too large and active for a hood. The tent is used to control the environment by providing a cooled aerosol, humidity, and controlled oxygen percentage (Fig. 5-8). In addition, the following procedures should be observed:

a. Set an oxygen flowmeter to deliver 8 to 10 L/min to small tents and 12 to 15 L/min to large tents to keep the carbon dioxide level less than 1%. Flows of 30 L/min or greater will be needed to keep the oxygen percentage close to the 50% maximum that can be reliably maintained. (Commonly between 35% and 50% oxygen can be kept in a tent.)

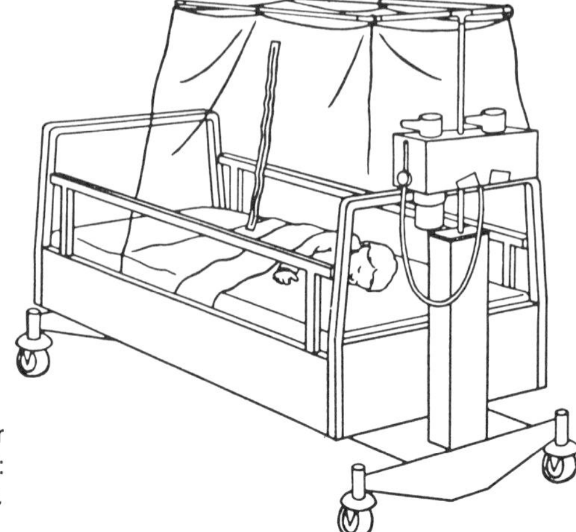

Fig. 5-8 Child in an oxygen tent. (From Gaebler G, Blodgett D: Gas administration, in Blodgett D [ed]: *Manual of Pediatric Respiratory Care Procedures.* Philadelphia, Lippincott, 1982. Used by permission.)

b. The oxygen should flow through a nebulizer or ultrasonic unit to provide the needed humidity. Try to keep the relative humidity at 60% or greater to minimize any risk of a spark causing a fire inside the tent.

c. The tent must be cooled to prevent the patient from overheating the enclosed space. Also, if the infant put into a tent has croup, the cooled air is therapeutic. The smaller, simpler units run the oxygen flow through an ice water solution. This will cool the inside about 6 to 8° F below the room's temperature. Larger, more complex units use an electrically powered refrigeration system. This more powerful system will cool the inside about 12 to 21° F below the room's temperature. Be careful not to chill the infant.

d. As with hoods, an oxygen analyzer should be continuously monitoring how much oxygen is inside the tent. The analyzer probe should be placed at the same level as the infant's nose. This is because oxygen is heavier than air and will tend to settle toward the bottom of the tent. Keep the tent sealed and the bottom edges tucked under the mattress to try to keep the oxygen percentage as high and stable as possible. The child should not be allowed to have any electrically powered toys inside the tent to minimize the risk of a spark and fire.

2. Air entrainment devices and masks.

a. Get the necessary equipment for the procedure. (IIA1c) [R, Ap]

b. Put the equipment together, make sure that it works properly, and identify and fix any problems with it. (IIB1c) [R, Ap]

Air entrainment masks are designed to provide the patient with a controlled oxygen percentage at a flow rate high enough to ensure that all of the patient's needs are met (Fig. 5-9). (The interested learner is encouraged to read about the Bernoulli principle that regulates the mixing of fluids as a result of a drop in pressure caused by a jet.) These masks are sometimes called Venturi masks, Venti masks, and high airflow with oxygen enrichment (HAFOE) systems. See Table 5-4 for specific information on available air entrainment masks.

These masks are recommended in any clinical situation where a known, certain oxygen percentage must be given to the patient. For example, even though the patient may have a variable respiratory rate, inspiratory/expiratory (I/E) ratio, tidal volume, and minute volume, the inspired oxygen percentage will remain constant. This will be true provided that the total flow through the mask meets or exceeds the patient's peak in-

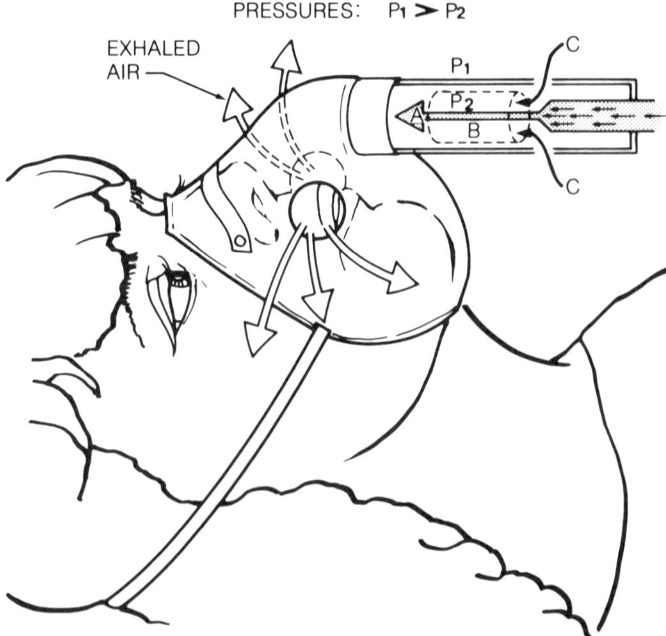

Fig. 5-9 Adult wearing an air entrainment mask. (From White GC: *Basic Clinical Lab Competencies for Respiratory Care, an Integrated Approach.* Albany, NY, Delmar, 1988. Used by permission.)

spiratory flow rate. Because this is difficult to measure clinically, the following guidelines are recommended to ensure that the patient's flow needs are met:

a. Make sure that the total flow through the mask is at least 40 L/min in a resting patient. More will be needed if the patient is breathing rapidly.
b. Provide the patient with a total flow that is four to six times his or her measured minute volume.

The total flow through the mask can be raised by increasing the oxygen flow. This should not significantly change the oxygen percentage because more room air is en-

Table 5-4. Specifications for Air Entrainment Devices and Masks

Oxygen (%)	Approximate Air/O_2 Ratio	Total Ratio Parts	O_2 Flow Rate (L/min)*	Total Flow (L/min)
24	25:1	26	4	104
28	10:1	11	4	44
30	8:1	9	6	54
35	5:1	6	8	48
40	3:1	4	10	40
45	2:1	3	15	45
50	1.7:1	2.7	15	40.5

*These flow rates were selected to ensure that the minimum total flow through the system would be at least 40 L/min. The manufacturers may recommend other minimal oxygen flow rates.

trained to keep the same ratio. However, to be certain, one should analyze the oxygen percentage inside the mask to ensure that it is as prescribed. The total flow through the mask can be calculated by adding the total of the ratio parts and multiplying by the oxygen flow rate.

Example 1.

Your patient has on a 28% air entrainment mask with an oxygen flow of 4 L/min. His condition worsens, and he increases his minute volume to 15 L/min. To ensure that he still receives his prescribed oxygen percentage, someone makes a recommendation to you to increase the oxygen liter flow to 6 L/min. The new total flow through the mask can be calculated as follows:

A 28% air entrainment mask has an air/oxygen ratio of 10:1.

a. The sum of the ratio parts is 10 + 1 = 11.
b. Total flow = 11 × 6 L/min oxygen flow = 66 L/min.
c. This flow is more than four times the patient's current minute volume. He should have all of his flow needs met.
d. Reanalyze the delivered oxygen percentage to make certain that it is as prescribed.

Example 2.

Your patient is wearing a 40% air entrainment mask that has the manufacturer's suggested 8 L/min of oxygen running into it. Her peak inspiratory flow is about 48 L/min (0.75 L/sec). To what should her oxygen flow be changed to ensure that the total gas flow is greater than her peak inspirator flow? The new oxygen flow to the mask can be calculated as follows:

A 40% air entrainment mask has an air/oxygen ratio of 3:1.

a. The sum of the ratio parts is 3 + 1 = 4.
b. Divide the sum of the ratio parts into the peak inspiratory flow: $\frac{48}{4} = 12$
c. Increase the oxygen flow from 8 to 12 L/min.

Some patients may complain that the gas coming through the mask is dry. To resolve this problem, some manufacturers have designed an aerosol adapter to add at the jet. A separate bland aerosol is then added to the room air that enters the jet stream. Make sure that the adapter fits properly and does not interfere with or block the jet or room air entrainment ports.

There are two different types of air entrainment devices based on the physical principles seen in the Bernoulli effect. It is important to know about the two different types so that you understand what can go wrong with them and how they can be fixed.

Variable Jet Diameter

Manufacturers include Vickers, OEM Medical Inc., Inspiron, and U-Mid. Notice that the jets have different diameters, but the room air entrainment ports are the same size. You will see that the *smaller* the jet diameter is, the *lower* the oxygen percentage is. This is because as the jet becomes smaller, the lateral pressure is lower. This results in more room air being brought into the entrainment ports to dilute the oxygen and raise the total flow.

Make sure that the jets are not obstructed by mucus or anything else, or the oxygen percentage will be decreased. An obstruction downstream from the jet will prevent as much room air as is normal from being brought into the mask. This will result in the oxygen percentage increasing and the total flow decreasing.

Variable Air Entrainment Ports

Manufacturers include Hudson Oxygen and Salter Labs. Notice that the jet size is fixed, but the room air entrainment ports have different sizes. It will be apparent that the *smaller* the entrainment ports, the *higher* the oxygen percentage. This is because less room air can be entrained to dilute the oxygen. The total flow is also reduced when the entrainment ports are smaller.

Make sure that the entrainment ports are not obstructed by the patient's sheet or anything else, or the oxygen percentage will increase. An obstruction downstream from the jet will also prevent as much room air as is normal from being brought into the mask. This will result in the oxygen percentage increasing and the total flow decreasing.

3. Nasal cannula.
- **a. Get the necessary equipment for the procedure. (IIA1a) [R, Ap]**
- **b. Put the equipment together, make sure that it works properly, and identify and fix any problems with it. (IIB1a) [R, Ap]**

The nasal cannula is an oxygen delivery tube that has been modified with two short prongs to deliver oxygen to the nostrils (Fig. 5-10). Care must be taken to make sure that

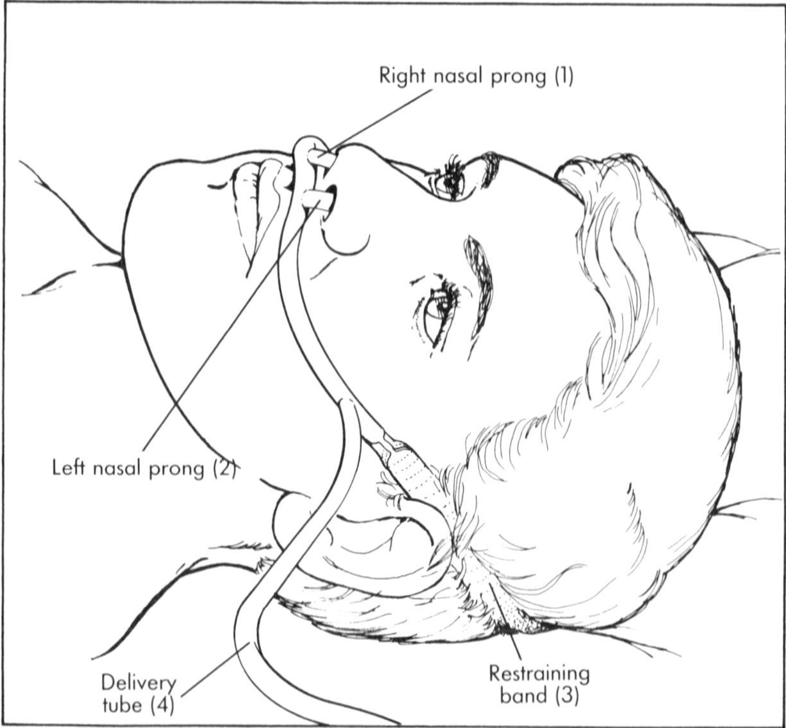

Fig. 5-10 Adult wearing a nasal cannula. (From Thalken FR: Medical gas therapy, in Scanlan CL, Spearman CB, Sheldon RL [eds]: *Egan's Fundamentals of Respiratory Care,* ed 5, St Louis, Mosby, 1990. Used by permission.)

the nares are patent and not plugged by a common cold, deviated septum, or other unseen problem. This low-flow oxygen delivery device is very widely used because it is more comfortable for many patients than an air entrainment or other type of face mask.

If a humidifier is to be used, make sure that it is properly filled with sterile water and that the oxygen bubbles through it. Check the high-pressure pop-off valve for pressure release and a whistling sound. Before placing the cannula on the patient, check to see that the oxygen is flowing through the tubing. If available, use a cannula with curved prongs. They direct the gas flow toward the back of the nasal passages for better natural humidification, as well as better patient comfort. Take care not to pull the elastic restraining band too tightly around the head. Some brands loop the oxygen tubing over the ears to be drawn up snuggly under the chin. Often this is more comfortable than the types that have the elastic band.

The problem with a nasal cannula is that the delivered oxygen percentage is unreliable. Variations in the patient's respiratory rate, I/E ratio, tidal volume, and minute volume result in different inhaled oxygen percentages. This is clearly unacceptable in an unstable patient in whom the Pa_{O_2} values are being used to help judge the changing cardiopulmonary status. Because of this clinical limitation, this device and the other low-flow oxygen delivery systems in the discussions that follow should be used only with stable patients. In the adult, the delivered oxygen percentage can be *estimated* at approximately 4% for each liter of oxygen per minute (Table 5-5). Flows are usually limited to 6 L/min to avoid excessive irritation to the nasal passages.

Flows are usually limited to 1 L/min or less in infants and 4 L/min in older children. These flows will achieve an inspired oxygen percentage in the range of 24% to 35%. The Pa_{O_2} level should be checked in patients of any age whenever a flow change is made or the patient's condition changes significantly.

The traditional cannulas are commonly used in hospitals for short-term patient use. However, in the home setting for long-term use, it is more economical to use one of the newer cannulas with a built-in oxygen reservoir because less oxygen is used. Oxymizer is a manufacturer of this type. These reservoir cannulas may be able to deliver a slightly higher oxygen percentage than the traditional types.

4. Oxygen masks: simple oxygen mask, partial rebreathing mask, nonrebreathing mask, and face tent.

a. Get the necessary equipment for the procedure. (IIA1a) [R, Ap]

b. Put the equipment together, make sure that it works properly, and identify and fix any problems with it. (IIB1a) [R, Ap]

Simple Oxygen Mask

This mask is designed to fit over the patient's nose and mouth and act as an oxygen reservoir for the next breath (Figs. 5-11 and 5-12). A bubble humidifier is often added so that the gas is not dry. Make sure that it works properly and that oxygen is flowing through the tubing before putting it on the patient. This and all other masks use an adjustable elastic strap that goes behind the head to hold it in place. Make sure that the mask fits snugly but not so tight as to cut off circulation. Various adult and pediatric sizes are available, and the patient should wear one that best fits the facial contours and size of the face. This is for comfort, as well as to try to increase the inspired oxygen percentage by decreasing the amount of room air that is inspired. Exhaled breath escapes through the exhalation ports. The patient's breathing pattern will affect the amount of room air that is breathed in through the same exhalation ports. These ports are also important in case the oxygen flow to the mask is cut off.

There is no way to make these masks provide an oxygen reservoir large enough to

Table 5-5. Estimated Delivered Oxygen Percentage in Adults Based on the Oxygen Liter Flow Through a Nasal Cannula

L/min of Oxygen	Estimated Delivered Oxygen (%)
1	24
2	28
3	32
4	36
5	40
6	44

meet the patient's tidal volume, so the inspired oxygen percentage is unpredictable. Oxygen flows between 5 and 10 L/min should provide *approximately* 35% to 60% inspired oxygen. The Pao_2 level should be checked whenever a flow change is made or the patient's condition changes significantly.

Partial Rebreathing Mask

The partial rebreathing mask is designed to fit over the patient's nose and mouth as the simple oxygen mask does. A 500- to 1000-mL plastic bag is added to the mask to act as an oxygen reservoir for the next breath (Figs. 5-13 to 5-15). When properly applied, the first third of the patient's exhaled gas from the anatomic dead space is exhaled back into this bag. This gas is close to pure oxygen and has no carbon dioxide. A bubble humidifier is often added so that the gas is not dry. Make sure that it works properly, that the oxygen is flowing through the tubing, and that the reservoir bag has been filled before putting it on the patient. Child and adult sizes are commonly available, and the mask should be conformed to fit the patient's facial contours and size as much as possible.

This is for comfort, as well as to try to increase the inspired oxygen percentage by decreasing the amount of room air that is inspired. Exhaled breath escapes through the exhalation ports. The patient's breathing pattern will affect the amount of room air that is

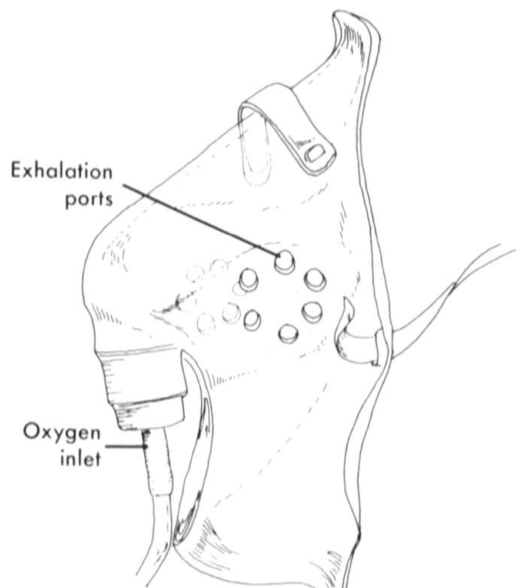

Fig. 5-11 Close up view of a simple oxygen mask. (From McPherson SP: *Respiratory Therapy Equipment,* ed 4. St Louis, Mosby, 1990. Used by permission.)

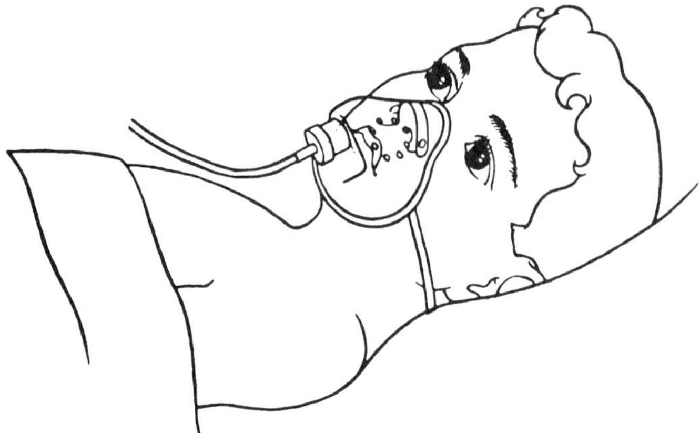

Fig. 5-12 Child wearing a simple oxygen mask. (From Gaebler G, Blodgett D: Gas administration, in Blodgett D [ed]: *Manual of Pediatric Respiratory Care Procedures.* Philadelphia, Lippincott, 1982. Used by permission.)

breathed in through the same exhalation ports. These ports are also important in case the oxygen flow to the mask is cut off. There is no way to make these masks provide an oxygen reservoir large enough to meet the patient's tidal volume, although it is much better than the simple oxygen mask. Again, the inspired oxygen percentage is unpredictable. Oxygen flows between 6 and 10 L/min should provide *approximately* 35% to 80% inspired oxygen. Adjust the flow as needed to ensure that the reservoir does not collapse by more than one third on inspiration. This will ensure that the mask and reservoir are filled with as much oxygen as possible. A Pa_{O_2} level should be checked whenever a flow change is made or the patient's condition changes significantly.

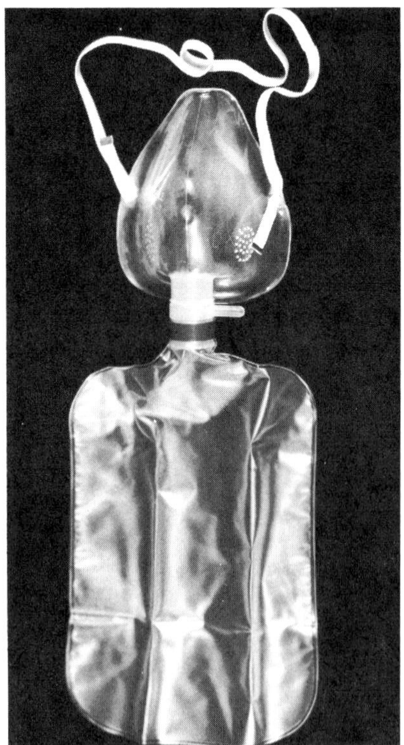

Fig. 5-13 Outside view of a partial rebreathing mask. (From McPherson SP: *Respiratory Therapy Equipment,* ed 4. St Louis, Mosby, 1990. Used by permission.)

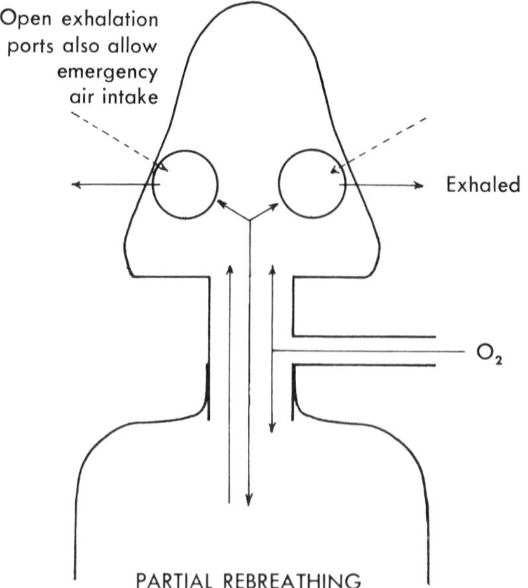

Fig. 5-14 Cutaway view of a partial rebreathing mask showing gas flow. (From Thalken FR: Medical gas therapy, in Scanlan CL, Spearman CB, Sheldon RL [eds]: *Egan's Fundamentals of Respiratory Care,* ed 5. St Louis, Mosby, 1990. Used by permission.)

Non-rebreathing Mask

The non-rebreathing mask looks initially like the partial rebreathing mask with its plastic bag added as an oxygen reservoir for the next breath (Figs. 5-16 and 5-17). However, notice that a one-way valve has been added between the mask and the reservoir bag. This allows the bag to be filled with pure oxygen that is available for the next breath. No exhaled gas can enter the reservoir. Two (sometimes one) one-way valves are added to the exhalation ports on the mask. These ensure that the patient breathes in only oxygen and not room air. Exhaled breath escapes through the exhalation ports as with the partial rebreathing mask. Not shown is an emergency pop-in valve that allows room air to be drawn into the mask if the oxygen supply should be cut off. A bubble humidifier is often added so that the gas is not dry. Make sure that it works properly, that the oxygen is flowing through the tubing, and that the reservoir bag has been filled before putting it on the patient. Adult and pediatric sizes are available. The mask should be conformed to fit the patient's facial contours and size as much as possible.

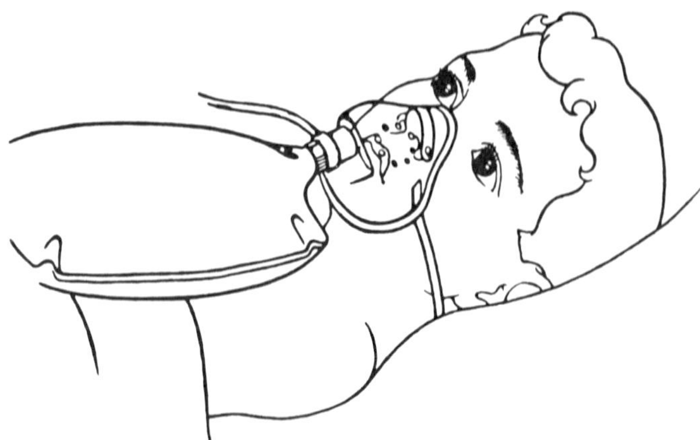

Fig. 5-15 Child wearing a partial rebreathing mask. (From Gaebler G, Blodgett D: Gas administration, in Blodgett D [ed]: *Manual of Pediatric Respiratory Care Procedures.* Philadelphia, Lippincott, 1982. Used by permission.)

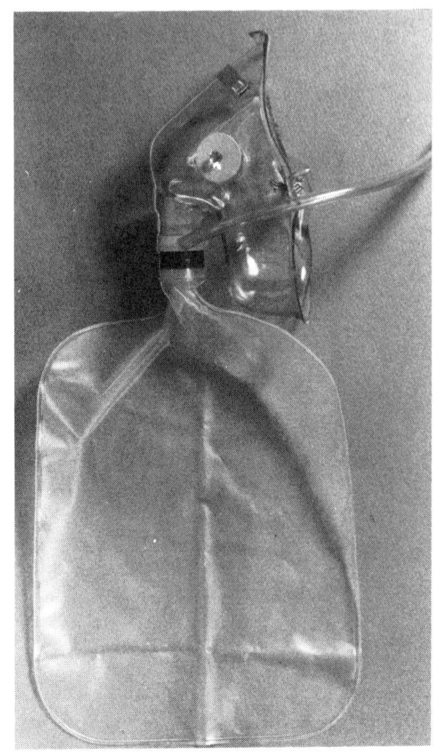

Fig. 5-16 Outside view of a non-rebreathing mask. (From McPherson SP: *Respiratory Therapy Equipment,* ed 4. St Louis, Mosby, 1990. Used by permission.)

As mentioned earlier, this is for comfort and to try to increase the inspired oxygen percentage by decreasing the amount of room air that is inspired. It is, in theory, possible to deliver 100% oxygen with this mask if the oxygen flow is high enough and the mask is airtight over the face. However, experience has shown that the disposable masks that are usually available in the hospital will not prevent room air from being drawn in. Oxygen flows between 8 and 10 L/min should provide *approximately* 60% to 80% (or

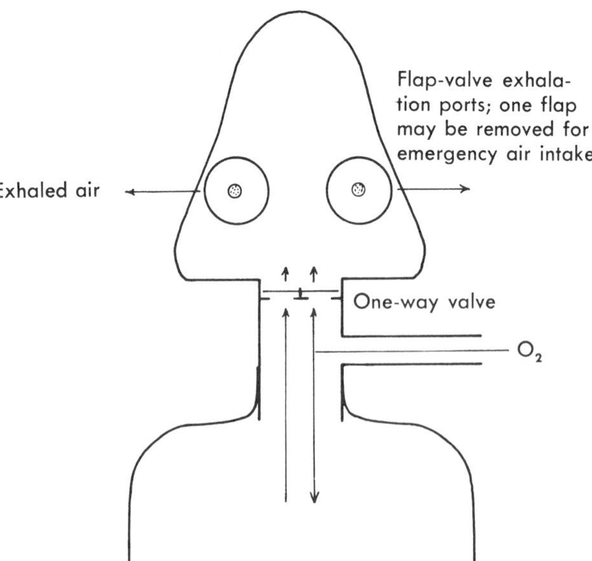

Fig. 5-17 Cutaway view of a non-rebreathing mask showing gas flow. (From Thalken FR: Medical gas therapy, in Scanlan CL, Spearman CB, Sheldon RL [eds]: *Egan's Fundamentals of Respiratory Care,* ed 5. St Louis, Mosby, 1990. Used by permission.)

more) inspired oxygen. Adjust the flow as needed to ensure that the reservoir does not collapse by more than one third on inspiration. This will ensure that the mask and reservoir are filled with oxygen and that the patient's tidal volume comes completely from the reservoir bag. The Pao_2 level should be checked whenever a flow change is made or the patient's condition changes significantly.

Face Tent

These masks are designed to fit around the patient's neck, under the jaw, and around the cheeks in front of the ears. The front edge should be higher than the level of the patient's nostrils (Fig. 5-18). These are sometimes used to provide oxygen to a patient who cannot wear a mask, cannula, or catheter because of oral and nasal trauma, burns, or surgery. These are usually ordered with the oxygen run through a humidifier or nebulizer so that the gas is not dry. Make sure that the humidifier or nebulizer is filled with sterile water, that the high pressure pop-off works, and that gas is flowing through the tubing before it is put on the patient.

The patient should be sitting as upright as possible for these masks to deliver their oxygen because oxygen is heavier than air and will tend to settle in the mask around the patient's nose and mouth if the fit is tight. If the patient is lying flat or if the mask fits loosely, the oxygen will simply "pour" down out of it. This makes it difficult to know with any certainty what inspired oxygen percentage is available to the patient. Flows of 5 to 10 of oxygen L/min are commonly used with adults. Try to analyze the oxygen percentage close to the patient's nose and mouth with as much accuracy as possible. A Pao_2 level should be checked whenever a flow change is made or the patient's condition changes significantly.

5. Tracheostomy appliances: mask/collar and Brigg's adapter/ T-adapter.

a. Get the necessary equipment for the procedure. (IIA1b) [R, Ap]

b. Put the equipment together, make sure that it works properly, and identify and fix any problems with it. (IIB1b) [R, Ap]

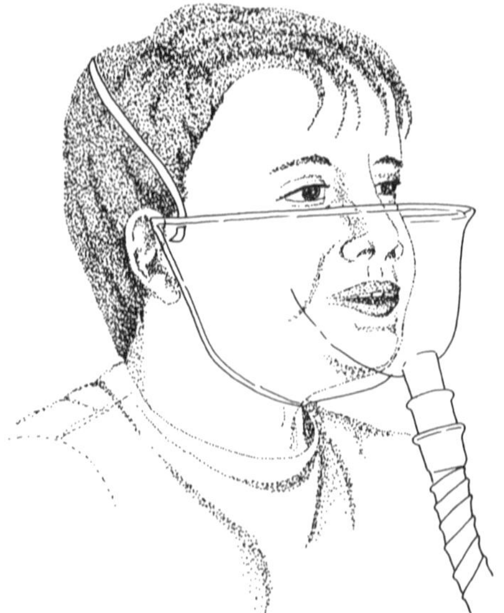

Fig. 5-18 Young adult wearing a face tent.

Tracheostomy Mask/Collar

The adult or pediatric tracheostomy mask or collar is shaped to fit over a tracheostomy tube or stoma to provide oxygen and aerosol (Fig. 5-19). A nebulizer is always used because the patient's upper airway is bypassed. Make sure that the nebulizer is filled with sterile water, that the high-pressure pop-off valve is working, and that adequate mist is flowing through to the mask before putting it on the patient.

Because this is a low-flow system with no reservoir, it is not possible to guarantee the patient's inspired oxygen percentage. Gas flows are usually set high enough to make sure that there is a good flow of aerosol and oxygen to meet as much of the patient's needs as possible. Analyze the oxygen percentage from inside the mask to try for as much accuracy as possible. A Pa_{O_2} level should be checked whenever a flow change is made or the patient's condition changes significantly.

Brigg's Adapter/T-Adapter

The Brigg's adapter or T-adapter is designed to provide air or supplemental oxygen and aerosol. It has one 15-mm–inner diameter (ID) opening that fits over any endotracheal or tracheostomy tube adapter. The other two openings are 22 mm outer diameter (OD) so that aerosol tubing can be added (Fig. 5-20). A nebulizer is commonly used because the patient's upper airway is bypassed. Make sure that the nebulizer is filled with sterile water, that the high-pressure pop-off valve is working, and that adequate mist is flowing through to the adapter before putting it on the patient.

The nebulizer is usually an air entrainment type, so the oxygen percentage can be adjusted. The addition of a length of aerosol tubing downstream from the adapter acts as a reservoir so that the inspired oxygen percentage is ensured. A reservoir of 50 to 100 mL of aerosol tubing is commonly needed for the adult. Care must be taken to adjust the gas flow so that it is high enough to meet the patient's peak inspiratory flow rate. This can be determined by watching the aerosol flow past the adapter and reservoir. Make sure that during inspiration the aerosol is still flowing past the tracheostomy/endotracheal

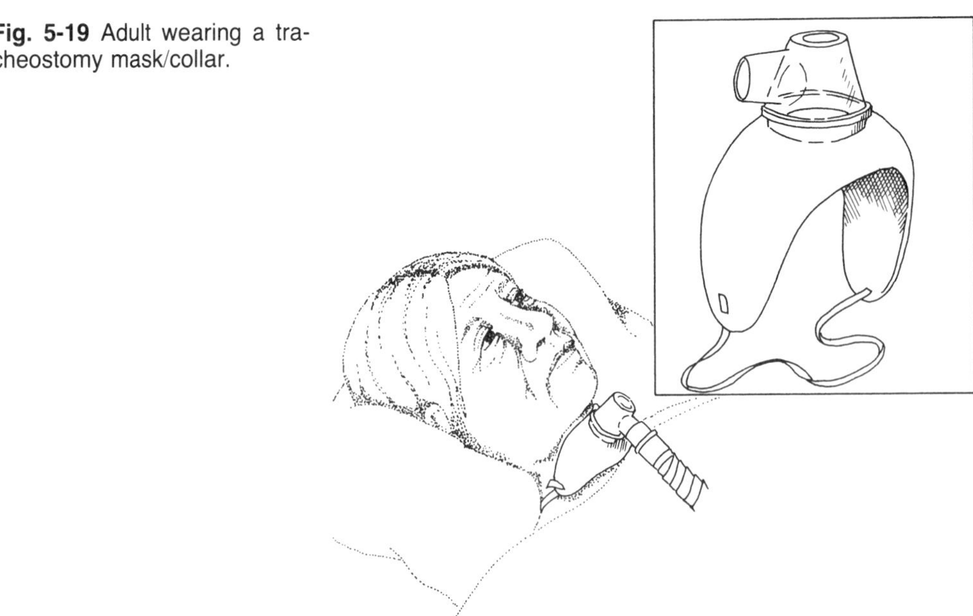

Fig. 5-19 Adult wearing a tracheostomy mask/collar.

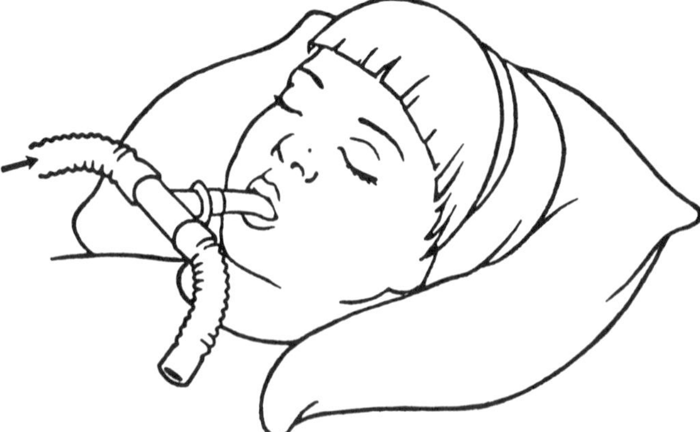

Fig. 5-20 Child with intubated airway with a Brigg's adapter/T-adapter and aerosol tubing added to the endotracheal tube. (From Gaebler G, Blodgett D: Gas administration, in Blodgett D [ed]: *Manual of Pediatric Respiratory Care Procedures.* Philadelphia, Lippincott, 1982. Used by permission.)

tube and into the reservoir. Inadequate flow could result in the patient rebreathing gas from the reservoir. This gas has just been exhaled and is high in carbon dioxide and low in oxygen.

This ends the general discussion on oxygen therapy. The entry level examination will include *direct* questions over this material. In general, Section I and the provisions discussion cover Module D. A few additional comments will be added as necessary.

Module D. Patient assessment.

1. Evaluate the patient's respiratory care plan and make any recommendations for changes, as needed. (IIIF9)[R, Ap, An]

Tachycardia and tachypnea are common findings in hypoxemic patients. Proper oxygen therapy should relieve the problem so that the patient's vital signs return toward normal. An abnormal heart rhythm as a result of hypoxemia should return to normal with the relief of the problem. Check the patient's pulse oximetry value (abbreviated Spo_2 or Sao_2) whenever there is a change in the inspired oxygen percentage or a significant change in his or her clinical condition. As discussed in Section 3, the previously healthy patient who develops cardiopulmonary failure should have the Spo_2 value kept at 90% or greater to ensure adequate oxygenation. This corresponds with a Pao_2 level of 60 mm Hg or more. The patient with chronic obstructive pulmonary disease can probably tolerate a Spo_2 value as low as 85%. This corresponds with a Pao_2 level of 55 mm Hg or more. The neonate can also tolerate a Spo_2 value of as low as 85%. Most hypoxemic patients will report that their shortness of breath is better after their Spo_2 value is greater than 90% and Pao_2 level is greater than 60 mm Hg. Watch for signs of oxygen-induced hypoventilation or other complications of the use of oxygen. This is sometimes seen in patients with end-stage emphysema who have their hypoxic drive blunted by the excessive use of oxygen and tend to become drowsy, breathe shallowly, and retain carbon dioxide. This dangerous situation must be prevented.

a. Change the oxygen percentage. (IIIF6c) [R, Ap]
b. Change the flow of oxygen. (IIIF6b) [R, Ap]
c. Change the method of administering the oxygen. (IIIF6a) [R, Ap]

Every patient's oxygen percentage or flow must be tailored to meet the patient's clinical goals. Usually this means keeping the Pao_2 level between 60 and 100 mm Hg and Spo_2 value between 90% and 97% in patients who are acutely hypoxemic. Exceptions, when the blood oxygen level is kept as high as possible, include cardiopulmonary resuscitation and the treatment of carbon monoxide poisoning.

Another exception is the chronic obstructive lung disease patient who is hypoxemic and hypercarbic. Usually these patients' conditions are maintained with a moderate hypoxemia. The Pa_{O_2} level should be between 50 and 60 mm Hg and SpO_2 value between 85% and 90%. It is imperative to keep the oxygen in this relatively narrow range. Further hypoxemia will result in pulmonary hypertension and cor pulmonale. Cardiac dysrhythmias or arrest and death can occur if the hypoxemia is severe (< 40 mm Hg). Oxygen levels in the normal range (>60 mm Hg) may result in blunting of the hypoxic drive. This could result in bradypnea and even greater carbon dioxide retention with corresponding acidemia. When the carbon dioxide pressure (Pa_{CO_2}) level exceeds 80 to 90 mm Hg, many patients become drowsy or somnolent. The treatment is to decrease the F_{IO_2} to lower the Pa_{O_2} level to 50 to 60 mm Hg. This, in turn, stimulates the hypoxic drive so that the patient increases his or her ventilation.

The advantages, disadvantages, and possible oxygen ranges for the various oxygen appliances were discussed earlier with each of them. Be prepared to make recommendations to change from one appliance to another.

BIBLIOGRAPHY

AARC clinical practice guideline: oxygen therapy in the acute care hospital. *Respir Care* 1991; 36:1410-1413.

Bageant RA: Oxygen analyzers. *Respir Care* 1976; 21:410-416.

Bakken E, Desautels DA: Oxygen therapy, in Aloan CA (ed). *Respiratory Care of the Newborn, a Clinical Manual.* Philadelphia, Lippincott, 1987.

Bohn DJ: Ask the expert, *Respir Tract* February 1988, p 9.

Cleveland DV: Oxygen therapy, in Koff PB, Eitzman DV, Neu J, (eds): *Neonatal and Pediatric Respiratory Care.* St Louis, Mosby, 1988.

Eubanks DH, Bone RC: *Comprehensive Respiratory Care,* ed 2. St Louis, Mosby, 1990.

Gaebler G, Blodgett D: Gas administration, in Blodgett D (ed): *Manual of Pediatric Respiratory Care Procedures.* Philadelphia, Lippincott, 1982.

Krider TM, Meyer R, Syvertsen WA: *Master Guide for Passing the Respiratory Care Credentialing Exams,* ed 2. Clairmont, Calif, Education Resource Consortium, 1989.

McPherson SP: *Respiratory Therapy Equipment,* ed 4. St Louis, Mosby, 1986.

Mohler JG, Collier CR, Brandt W, et al: Blood gases, in Clausen JL, (ed): *Pulmonary Function Testing Guidelines and Controversies, Equipment, Methods, and Normal Values.* Orlando, Grune & Stratton, 1984.

Moran RF: Assessment of quality control of blood gas/pH analyzer performance, *Respir Care* 1981; 26:538-546.

Product literature on Oxisensors. Nellcor Hayward, Calif.

Product literature on the model 4701A ear oximeter. Hewlett-Packard, Medical Products Group, Waltham, Mass.

Scanlan CL, Spearman CB, Sheldon RL (eds): *Egan's Fundamentals of Respiratory Care,* ed 5. St Louis, Mosby, 1990.

Shapiro BA, Harrison RA, Cane RD, et al: *Clinical Application of Blood Gases,* ed 4. Chicago, Mosby, 1989.

Shapiro BA, Harrison RA, Kacmarek RM, et al: *Clinical Application of Respiratory Care,* ed 3. Chicago, Mosby, 1985.

Ward JJ: Equipment for mixed gas and oxygen therapy, in Barnes TA (ed): *Respiratory Care Practice.* Chicago, Mosby, 1988.

White GC: *Basic Clinical Lab Competencies for Respiratory Care, an Integrated Approach.* Albany, NY, Delmar, 1988.

SELF-STUDY QUESTIONS

1. You are making general rounds in the hospital when you find a patient whose reservoir tubing has fallen off his 40% Brigg's adapter. This would result in which of the following?
   A. Decreased tidal volume
   B. Increased inspired oxygen
   C. Increased inspired carbon dioxide
   D. Decreased inspired carbon dioxide
   E. Decreased inspired oxygen

2. The risks of oxygen therapy include all of the following *except:*
   A. Pulmonary oxygen toxicity
   B. Denitrogen absorption atelectasis
   C. Oxygen-induced hyperventilation
   D. Retrolental fibroplasia in premature newborns
   E. Seizure activity

3. Your patient is wearing a face tent because of recent facial surgery. It is set at 35% oxygen. The nurse moves her from an upright to a flat position in bed. What effect will this have on her respiratory status?
   A. Decreased tidal volume
   B. Increased inspired oxygen
   C. Increased inspired carbon dioxide
   D. Decreased inspired carbon dioxide
   E. Decreased inspired oxygen

4. To minimize the risk of hypoxemia during a treatment or procedure, you would do which of the following?
   I. Increase the oxygen percentage by 20% above the normal setting before suctioning or changing equipment.
   II. Keep the oxygen percentage the same as normal if the patient is not hypoxemic at this time.
   III. Minimize the time that the patient would be breathing room air.
   IV. Increase the oxygen percentage to 100% before suctioning.
   V. Make sure the replacement equipment is working properly before placing it on the patient.
   A. I, III
   B. III, IV, V
   C. II, V
   D. III, IV
   E. II, III

5. You are working with a patient whose airway is mechanically ventilated. The oxygen analyzer is a galvanic fuel cell type. Every time that the patient's airway pressure fluctuates during a mechanical breath, the oxygen percentage goes up and then down. This could be caused by:
   A. Plugged capillary line
   B. Dry analyzing chamber
   C. Variable pressure against the analyzer probe
   D. Weak battery
   E. Exhausted supply of chemical reactant

6. Your patient is wearing a partial rebreathing mask. The reservoir bag almost totally collapses during her inspiration. You would do which of the following?
   A. Decrease the oxygen flow
   B. Put a nasal cannula on her

C. Tell her to breathe more rapidly
D. Increase the oxygen flow
E. Remove the reservoir bag because it is not functional

7. Your patient is a 36-year-old woman who suddenly developed a pulmonary embolism. The minimally safe Spo_2 value for her would be:
A. 100%
B. 95%
C. 90%
D. 85%
E. 80%

8. What oxygen delivery device would you recommend for a patient who has a variable respiratory rate, I/E ratio, and tidal volume?
A. Nasal cannula
B. Air entrainment mask
C. Simple oxygen mask
D. Face tent
E. Non-rebreathing mask

9. The physician asks you which oxygen delivery device would be best for a patient who needs about 75% oxygen. You would recommend which of the following?
A. Nasal cannula
B. Air entrainment mask
C. Simple oxygen mask
D. Face tent
E. Non-rebreathing mask

10. A patient has a nasal cannula and needs to be transported with an E oxygen cylinder while lying flat on the stretcher. You would recommend using which of the following flowmeters?
A. Backpressure-compensated Thorpe
B. Non-backpressure–compensated Thorpe
C. Bourdon
D. Backpressure-compensated kinetic
E. Non-backpressure–compensated kinetic

11. An E cylinder oxygen regulator would have which pinhole locations?
A. 1-5
B. 2-6
C. 3-5
D. 2-5
E. 3-6

12. Calculate the duration of flow of an E cylinder with 1700 psig that is running at 5 L/min.
A. 17.8 hours
B. 0.9 hour
C. 7.7 hours
D. 13.7 hours
E. 1.6 hours

13. You are called to draw an arterial blood sample from a patient who is wearing a 35% air entrainment mask. When you enter the room, you notice that his covers are drawn up over the air entrainment ports of the mask. How would this affect the function of the mask?
A. The total flow will be increased.
B. There will be no effect.

C. The oxygen percentage will be increased.
D. The oxygen percentage will be decreased.
E. The device will function normally if the reservoir bag is inflated at least one third on inspiration.

Answer Key:

1. E; 2. C; 3. E; 4. B; 5. C; 6. D; 7. C; 8. B; 9. E; 10. C; 11. D; 12. E; 13. C.

6 Hyperinflation Therapy

Module A. Coughing and deep breathing.

1. Perform the following procedures with the patient to help make breathing more effective.

a. Teach the patient the best techniques for breathing efficiently. (IIIC1) [R, Ap]

Teach the following steps to patients with obstructive airways diseases:

a. Have the patient lie in a comfortable supine position; knees can be flexed.
b. Instruct the patient to relax physically as much as possible, especially the shoulders.
c. Use soothing music, meditation, or other techniques for mental relaxation.
d. Instruct the patient to concentrate on breathing more slowly.
e. Emphasize pursed lip breathing where the patient breathes slowly in through the nose with the abdominal muscles relaxed and slowly out through pursed (slightly opened) lips. Breathing with pursed lips keeps some backpressure on the airways so that they stay open longer. The technique will help to improve gas exchange so that the patient feels less dyspnea.

b. Reinforce to the patient the need to breathe deeply. (IIIC2) [R, Ap]

Explain to the patient that by taking in deep breaths, the lungs will be kept healthy and have less chance of developing pneumonia. Hopefully the patient will be able to go home sooner.

Deep breathing and coughing are indicated in patients with atelectasis, pulmonary infiltrates, or pneumonia. These exercises should help to raise secretions. It may be possible to prevent or limit atelectasis and pneumonia by deep breathing and coughing. This is especially important for patients who have just had a cholecystectomy or splenectomy.

c. Teach the patient proper coughing techniques and coach him or her to cough productively (IIIB2a) [R, Ap]

Ideally the patient is taught these techniques before surgery. If not, teach the postoperative patient the following cough techniques:

a. Minimize traction or tension on the incision to decrease the pain. This can be done by placing your or the patient's hands on both sides of the incision, or a pillow can be held against the incision by the practitioner or patient.

b. Instruct the patient to breathe two or three times in through the nose and out through the mouth.

c. Instruct the patient to take in as deep a breath as possible and perform a normal cough.

d. If the patient cannot cough normally because of pain, a serial or huff cough can be performed.

Teach the patient with obstructive airways disease the following cough techniques:

a. Avoid an ineffective, shallow, hacking cough.
b. Position the patient in a sitting position, bent slightly forward, with feet on the floor or supported. The patient who must lie in bed can be positioned on the preferred side with the legs flexed at the knees and hips.
c. Instruct the patient to perform a midinspiratory cough:
    1. Breathe two or three times in through the nose and out through the mouth.
    2. Breathe in to a comfortable volume larger than the tidal volume but not as deeply as possible.
    3. Briefly hold the breath.
    4. Cough hard or perform a serial cough at relatively low flows. This should help to raise secretions without causing airway collapse.
d. Squeezing the knees and thighs together at the instant of coughing helps to increase the air flow and volume.

Coaching is important because patients in pain or suffering from chronic lung disease tend to be uncooperative and not try hard. Give positive reinforcement when the patient does well. Correct any problems the patient is having with following the instructions. Demonstrations are often useful so that the patient can copy a good example.

Module B. Incentive spirometry.

Incentive spirometry (IS) is a technique whereby a patient is encouraged to breathe deeply by seeing his or her inhaled volume on the spirometry device. The patient receives positive feedback by seeing that the volume gradually increases as his or her condition improves. It is also known as incentive breathing and sustained maximal inspiration (SMI). It is indicated in any patient who has or is likely to develop atelectasis. Examples of conditions where atelectasis is likely to be seen include postoperative thoracic or upper abdominal surgery cases, the aged, the obese, airway obstruction, inadequate sigh, and cardiopulmonary disease.

The goal of IS is to prevent or treat atelectasis. This is done by having the patient inhale a near-normal inspiratory capacity (IC). It is even more beneficial if the patient can hold the IC for several seconds, also referred to as SMI. The cooperative surgical patient should have the IC measured before the operation. It can be measured at the bedside or calculated from a pulmonary function test where vital capacity is measured. (Review Section 4 for IC information.) the IC is then measured again postoperatively.

1. Teach the patient the proper techniques for IS, and evaluate the patient's ability to perform it. (IIIC3) [R, Ap]

Before starting the instruction, make sure that the patient is alert and cooperative enough to follow instructions. The patient's respiratory rate should be less than 25 breaths/min to perform the procedure properly.

Use the following steps in teaching IS:

a. Have the patient in semi-Fowler's position, on the edge of the bed, or up to a chair.

b. Set an initial goal of twice the patient's tidal volume.

c. Tell the patient what the purpose of the treatment is and how to perform it properly.

d. Simulate the procedure for the patient.

e. Put the unit within easy reach. It must be kept sitting upright.

f. Have the patient exhale normally (to functional residual capacity), seal the lips around the mouthpiece, and inspire maximally through the unit. It is important that the patient inspire in a slow, controlled effort.

g. Hold the inspiratory capacity for *at least* 3 seconds before exhaling. This is the sustained maximal inspiration. Do not hold the breath for longer than 15 seconds.

h. Proceed to increase the patient's goal as tolerated and indicated earlier.

i. The patient should perform the deep breath at least 10 times each hour while awake. A rest period with normal breathing should take place between each large breath.

Monitor your patient's progress in these ways:

a. If the patient cannot meet the initial goal, reconsider whether this is the best form of treatment. Intermittent positive-pressure breathing (IPPB) might be a better choice to provide a deep breath.

b. Stop the treatment temporarily if the patient has signs of hyperventilation such as dizziness or tingling of the fingertips. A few minutes of normal breathing should result in a normal feeling again. Have the patient take longer rest periods between maximal breaths.

c. Stop the treatment if the patient complains of acute chest pain. It is possible to cause pulmonary barotrauma by breathing in as deeply as possible. Evaluate the patient's pulmonary condition, and call the physician if indicated.

2. Increase or decrease the patient's IS goal. (IIIF4b) [R, Ap]

See Table 6-1 for IS guidelines. In addition, the following guidelines are suggested:

a. Set the initial IC goal at twice the tidal volume.

b. Increase the goal in 200-ml increments as the patient tolerates.

c. Have a final IC goal of greater than 12 ml/kg of ideal body weight.

d. Or, have a forced vital capacity (FVC) goal of greater than 15 ml/kg of ideal body weight.

e. A normal person should have an IC of about 75% of his or her FVC. For example, a predicted FVC of 5.166 L was calculated for a male patient in Section 4. His predicted IC would be calculated as 5.166 L × 0.75 = 3.875 L. However, because of natural variations in people, he could inhale only 80% of this (3.1 L) and still be considered within normal limits. Use this as a guideline for anticipating a patient's maximum IC. Do not expect your patient to inhale a greater IC than is physically possible.

Consider increasing the IS goal if (1) the patient is easily able to reach the set goal, or (2) the patient's breath sounds are diminished in the bases. Consider decreasing the IS goal if (1) the patient cannot reach the set goal because it is too large, (2) the patient is frustrated and discouraged at his or her inability to reach the set goal, or (3) excessive surgical site pain prevents the patient from reaching the set goal.

Table 6-1. Guidelines for the Use of Incentive Spirometry

Postoperative Bedside Spirometry	Treatment Modality
IC* > 80% of the preoperative value	No treatment needed unless there is radiographic or clinical evidence of atelectasis
IC at least 33% of the preoperative value; or, FVC* of at least 10 ml/kg	IS* is indicated
IC < 33% of the preoperative value; or FVC < 10 ml/kg	IPPB* is indicated

**IC,* Inspiratory capacity; *FVC,* forced vital capacity; *IS,* incentive spirometry; *IPPB,* intermittent positive-pressure breathing.

Module C. IS equipment.

1. Get the necessary equipment for the procedure. (IIA10) [R, Ap]
2. Put the equipment together, make sure that it works properly, and identify and fix any problems with it. (IIB10) [R, Ap]

There are two basic types of IS equipment.

Flow Displacement

Flow displacement units work by having the patient breathe in a flow great enough to raise one or more plastic balls in calibrated cylinders (Fig. 6-1). The patient is encouraged to try to keep the ball (or balls) suspended by breathing in more deeply.

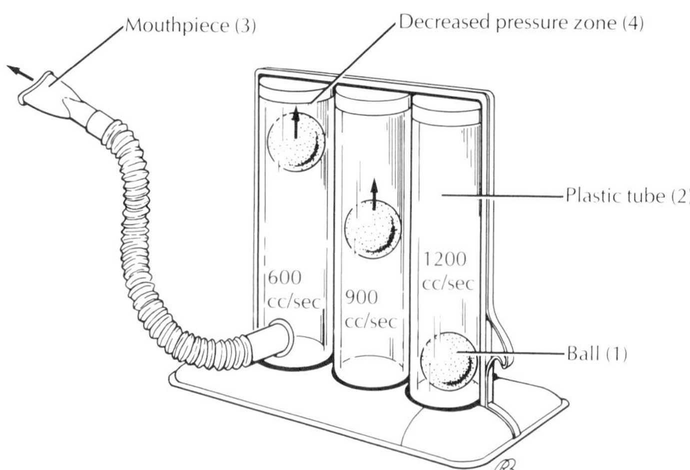

Fig. 6-1 TriFlo II incentive deep breathing exerciser. (From Eubanks DH, Bone RC: *Comprehensive Respiratory Care,* ed 2. St Louis, Mosby, 1990. Used by permission.)

Encourage the patient to breathe in *slowly* to suspend the balls for as long as possible. Have the patient watch as the balls are held up by the inspired breath as positive reinforcement for doing a good job. It is not helpful to breathe in a fast, short breath and have the balls pop up and down. Volume is calculated by multiplying the flow per second needed to suspend the balls by the number of seconds that the balls are suspended. For example:

$$600 \text{ cc/sec} \times 2 \text{ seconds} = 1200 \text{ cc IC}.$$

Assembly is performed by attaching the flow tube to the unit and the mouthpiece to the flow tube. An obstruction to the flow tube or mouthpiece or a built-in leak in the calibrated cylinders will stop airflow. No balls will rise despite the patient's inspiratory effort.

Manufacturers include Sherwood Medical with Triflo and Triflo II, Dart Respiratory with Expand-A-Lung, and Spirocare Incentive Breathing Exerciser, among others.

Volume Displacement

Volume displacement units work by having the patient breathe in a preset volume goal from the reservoir bellows (Fig. 6-2). Many of these units have a whistle built into them to warn if the breath is too fast. Some also have a small built-in leak so that the patient must continue inspiring to keep the bellows suspended. Have the patient watch as the bellows is suspended as positive reinforcement for doing a good job. Volume is marked on the bellows container. If the unit has a built-in leak, multiply the volume inspired by the time the bellows is suspended. For example:

$$800 \text{ ml} \times 3 \text{ seconds} = 2400 \text{ ml IC}.$$

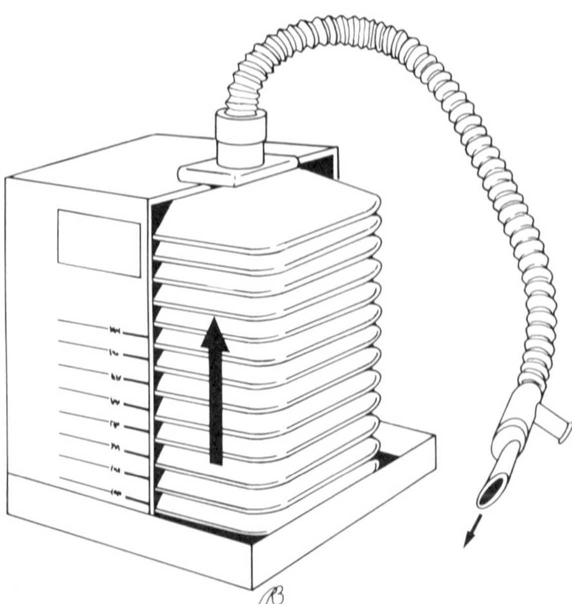

Fig. 6-2 Volume incentive breathing exerciser. (From Eubanks DH, Bone RC: *Comprehensive Respiratory Care,* ed 2. St Louis, Mosby, 1990. Used by permission.)

Assembly is performed by attaching the flow tube to the unit and the mouthpiece to the flow tube. An obstruction to the flow tube, mouthpiece, or built-in leak will stop air flow. The bellows will not rise despite the patient's inspiratory effort.

Manufacturers include Sherwood Medical with its Voldyne volumetric exerciser, Argyle with its Tru-vol, and DHD Medical Products with its Volurex.

3. Make a change in the type of IS. (IIIF4a) [R, Ap]

Although there are a number of manufacturers, there are just two different styles: flow displacement and volume displacement. Be prepared to make a recommentation to make a change if the patient seems unable to operate or benefit from the type that he is she is currently using. It has been presented that patients at risk of developing inspiratory muscle fatigue should use an incentive spirometer that has the lowest imposed work of breathing by its design. These types of patients include those that are using their auxiliary respiratory muscles, have abdominal distention, or are hyperinflated. The same study ranked the following brands of incentive spirometer from least to most imposed work of breathing: Air_x (flow displacement), Voldyne 5000 (volume displacement), Coach (volume displacement), Triflow II (flow displacement), Lung Volume Exerciser (flow displacement), and Coach Jr (volume displacement).

This ends the general discussion on hyperinflation therapy. The entry level examination will include *direct* questions over this material. Review sections 1 and 4 and the previous discussion when considering Module D.

Module D. Patient assessment.

1. Determine and continue to monitor how the patient responds to the treatment or procedure.

The following should be considered to evaluate the patient's response:

- The opening of atelectatic areas would be signaled by the return of normal rather than diminished or absent breath sounds.
- Acute chest pain could be the result of a pneumothorax from barotrauma. A chest x-ray film would be needed to confirm or deny the presence of a pneumothorax. Stop the treatment if a pneumothorax is suspected.
- Be prepared to measure tidal volume, vital capacity, and IC to determine the patient's goals and evaluate his or her progress.
- The patient may have an increase in sputum production if the deep breathing exercises and IS open up atelectatic areas. The patient may have a more productive cough because of a greater vital capacity.

BIBLIOGRAPHY

AARC clinical practice guidelines: incentive spirometry. *Respiratory Care*, December 1991, Vol. 36, No. 12, pp. 1402-1405.

Douce FH: Incentive spirometry and other aids to lung inflation, in Barnes TA (ed): *Respiratory Care Practice*. Chicago, Mosby, 1988.

Eubanks DH Bone RC: *Comprehensive Respiratory Care, a Learning System*, ed 2. St Louis, Mosby, 1990.

Johnson NT and Pierson DJ: The spectrum of pulmonary atelectasis: pathophysiology, diagnosis, and therapy. *Respir Care* 1986; 31:1107-1120.

Mang H, Obermayer A: Imposed work of breathing during sustained maximal inspiration: comparison of six incentive spirometers. *Respir Care* 1989; 34:1122-1128.

Scuderi J, Olsen GN: Respiratory therapy in the management of postoperative complications. *Respir Care* 1989; 34:281-291.

Scanlan CL, Spearman CB, Sheldon RL (eds): *Egan's Fundamentals of Respiratory Care*, ed 5. St Louis, Mosby, 1990.

Shapiro BA, Harrison RA, Kacmarek RM, et al: *Clinical Application of Respiratory Care*, ed 3. Chicago, Mosby, 1985.

Wojciechowski WV: Incentive spirometers and secretion evacuation devices, in Barnes TA (ed): *Respiratory Care Practice*. Chicago, Mosby, 1988.

SELF-STUDY QUESTIONS

1. A patient with obstructive airways disease should be taught all of the following cough techniques *except:*
   A. Hold the breath in briefly before coughing.
   B. Take two to three breaths in and out before coughing.
   C. Breathe in a volume larger than the tidal volume but less than than the vital capacity.
   D. Perform a normal cough.
   E. Perform a midinspiratory cough.

2. Incentive spirometry is indicated when a patient's postoperative inspiratory capacity is what percentage of the preoperative inspiratory capacity?
   A. Less than 30%
   B. Between 30% and 50%
   C. Between 50% and 80%
   D. Between 80% and 90%
   E. Greater than 90%

3. Incentive spirometry can be started on a patient who meets the following condition(s):
   I. The patient is alert and cooperative.
   II. His respiratory rate is less than 25 breaths/min.
   III. The patient is semicomatose.
   IV. His respiratory rate is 25 to 30 breaths/min.
   V. His respiratory rate is greater than 30 breaths/min.
   A. I
   B. I, II
   C. III, V
   D. V
   E. III, IV

4. If pulmonary function results are not available, where should the initial incentive spirometry goal be set?
   A. The inspiratory capacity that is measured at the bedside
   B. Half of the vital capacity measured at the bedside
   C. The vital capacity measured at the bedside
   D. Three times the tidal volume measured at the bedside
   E. Twice the tidal volume measured at the bedside

5. Your patient has an ideal body weight of 200 lb (90 kg). What would be his initial inspiratory capacity goal?
   A. His vital capacity
   B. At least half of his vital capacity
   C. At least 1080 ml
   D. At least 540 ml
   E. At least 1620 ml

6. It is recommended that incentive spirometry be performed how often?
   A. At least 10 times/hour while awake.
   B. At least 5 times/hour while awake.
   C. At least 20 times/hour while awake.
   D. At least 10 times/day while awake.
   E. Frequency does not relate to the opening of atelectatic areas.

7. Your patient has just performed several excellent incentive spirometry efforts. She complains of tingling fingers and dizziness. Your response would be to:
   A. Have her continue with more incentive spirometry maneuvers.
   B. Call her physician immediately to warn him of her condition.
   C. Check her fingers and forehead for cyanosis.
   D. Call her physician to cancel the treatment order.
   E. Tell her to relax and breathe quietly until she feels normal again.

8. Your patient has a flow displacement type of incentive spirometry device. She is attempting to inhale forcibly through it but is unable to. What is the most likely problem?
   A. The airflow is obstructed.
   B. She is not really trying.
   C. The flow resistance is set too high.
   D. The bellows is in the locked-down position.
   E. The flow resistance is set too low.

9. If incentive spirometry has been successful, you will hear the following breath sounds in the areas where atelectasis was noted before the treatment:
   A. Bronchial
   B. Absent
   C. Normal vesicular
   D. Tracheal
   E. Fibrotic

10. Your patient's incentive spirometry device is a flow displacement type. With good coaching, he is able to raise a ball requiring 900 cc/sec of flow. He can keep it elevated for 1.5 seconds. What is his inspiratory capacity?
   A. 450 cc
   B. 900 cc
   C. 1350 cc
   D. 1800 cc
   E. 2700 cc

Answer Key:

1. D; 2. C; 3. B; 4. E; 5. C; 6. A; 7. E; 8. A; 9. C; 10. C.

7 Humidity and Aerosol Therapy

Module A. Humidity and aerosol therapy.

1. Provide humidity and aerosol therapy to aid in the clearance of bronchopulmonary secretions. (IIIB2f) [R, Ap]

A study of the content of the available entry level examinations shows that the examinee will need to understand the following terms and concepts, as well as additional material presented here, to be as prepared as possible for the examinations. The National Board for Respiratory Care (NBRC) incorporates this material into its question and possible answers.

The majority of patients receiving respiratory care will have either supplemental humidity or aerosol delivered to their airways and lungs. This is for either or both of two reasons. First, patients with excessive pulmonary secretions are benefited by the inhalation of extra humidity or an aerosol to reduce the viscosity of their secretions. This makes it easier for them to cough or to be suctioned out. Second, supplemental oxygen from either the central delivery system or cylinders is absolutely dry. Adding humidity or aerosol to the oxygen makes it easily breathable. The following material will elaborate on these basic concepts.

a. Terms and concepts relating to humidity and aerosol therapy

i. Humidity and water vapor.

Humidity is moisture in the air (or any gas) in the form of water vapor. Water vapor is molecular water (H_2O molecules).

ii. Absolute humidity.

Absolute humidity is the water content in vapor form present in a given volume of gas. It is expressed in units of grams per cubic meter or, more commonly for our purposes, as milligrams per liter. This amount varies directly with the gas temperature, that is, warmer gas can hold more moisture than cooler gas can. Rarely does the gas hold as much moisture as it possibly can. When the gas, at a given temperature, is holding as much water vapor as it can, it is said to be saturated. Absolute humidity is sometimes referred to as vapor density. See Fig. 7-1 for how absolute humidity is related to temperature.

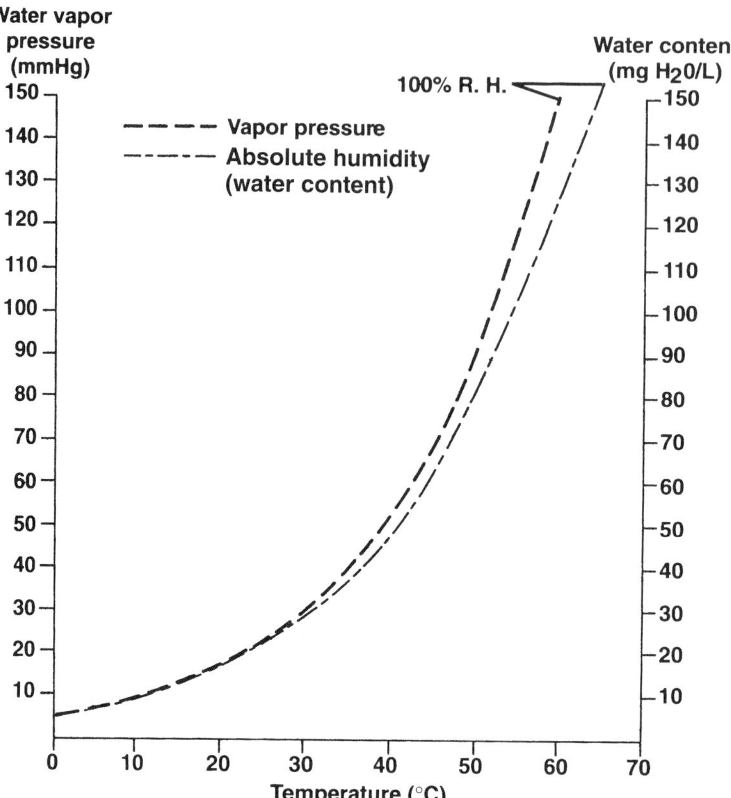

Fig. 7-1 Absolute humidity/water content and vapor pressure curves showing 100% relative humidity (RH). (Adapted from Sykes MK, McNichol MW, Campbell EJM: *Respiratory Failure,* ed 2. Boston, 1976, Blackwell Scientific Publications. Used by permission.)

iii. Vapor pressure (P_{H_2O}).

Vapor pressure is the amount of atmospheric pressure caused by water vapor. It is expressed in units of millimeters of mercury. The amount of available water vapor, as well as the gas temperature, will influence the vapor pressure. Saturated air has a vapor pressure range from 4.58 mm Hg (at the freezing point) to 760 mm Hg (at the boiling point when the air is saturated). See Fig. 7-1 for how vapor pressure is related to temperature.

iv. Relative humidity.

Relative humidity (RH) is the ratio between the amount of water in the air and the capacity of the air for water at a given temperature. This is an important concept to understand because any gas must be saturated with water by the time it reaches the alveoli. It is for this reason that many respiratory care devices add humidity to the relatively dry room air or medical gases. Hospitals usually have temperatures in the range of 21° to 23° C (70°-73° F) and have about 40% RH. Gas released from cylinders is cooler than room temperature and absolutely dry.

RH is usually listed as a percentage as seen in this formula:

$$RH = \frac{\text{actual water content}}{\text{water capacity}} \times 100$$

The answer can be calculated in two ways: (1) absolute humidity (mg/L), or (2) vapor pressure (mm Hg). See Fig. 7-1 for how the temperature influences absolute humidity and vapor pressure. See Table 7-1 for the more important absolute humidity and vapor pressure values.

Example:

Calculate the RH of a hospital room at 21° C (70° F). Refer to Table 7-1 for saturated gas values. The actual water content values were measured with a hygrometer.

$$RH = \frac{7.34 \text{ mg/L}}{18.35 \text{ mg/L}} \times 100 = 40\%$$

$$RH = \frac{7.45 \text{ mm Hg}}{18.62 \text{ mm Hg}} \times 100 = 40\%$$

As can be seen, the RH can be calculated by either method.

v. Dew point and dew point line.

The dew point is the temperature of the air at which dew begins to form. Dew is moisture that condenses from the air and collects in small drops on any cooler surface. Another way to think of the dew point is to realize that it shows 100% RH (saturated air) at a given temperature.

The dew point line is a series of dew points plotted at various temperature (Fig. 7-2). Note that the line is the same as the 100% RH line in Fig. 7-1. As the temperature of the gas cools, its capacity to hold water decreases. The water vapor condenses as liquid water (dew) on any cool surface. The air remains 100% saturated with water vapor, but the content of the water decreases.

Pure oxygen, air-oxygen mixes, and other gas mixes will have dew point lines that vary from that of room air. However, in general, all of this discussion applies to any other gas mixes.

vi. Body humidity.

Body humidity is the water saturation condition of the gas in the lungs. Under normal conditions with air, it is 43.8 (44) mg/L absolute humidity and 46.90 (47) mm Hg at a

Table 7-1. Saturated Air Values for Absolute Humidity and Vapor Pressure Under Room and Body Temperature Ranges*

Temperature			
° C	° F	Absolute Humidity (mg/L)	Vapor Pressure (mm Hg)
21	70	18.35 (18)	18.62 (19)
22	71.6	19.42 (19)	19.79 (20)
23	73	20.58 (21)	21.02 (21)
33	92	35.61 (36)	37.59 (38)
34	93	37.57 (38)	39.75 (40)
35	95	39.60 (40)	42.02 (42)
36	97	41.70 (42)	44.40 (44)
37†	98.6	43.90 (44)	46.90 (47)
38	100	46.19 (46)	49.51 (50)
39	102	48.59 (49)	52.26 (52)
40	104	51.10 (51)	55.13 (55)
41	106	53.70 (54)	58.14 (58)

*As can be seen, the warmer the air is, the more water it can hold.
†So-called normal body temperature. Body temperature normally varies under different conditions.

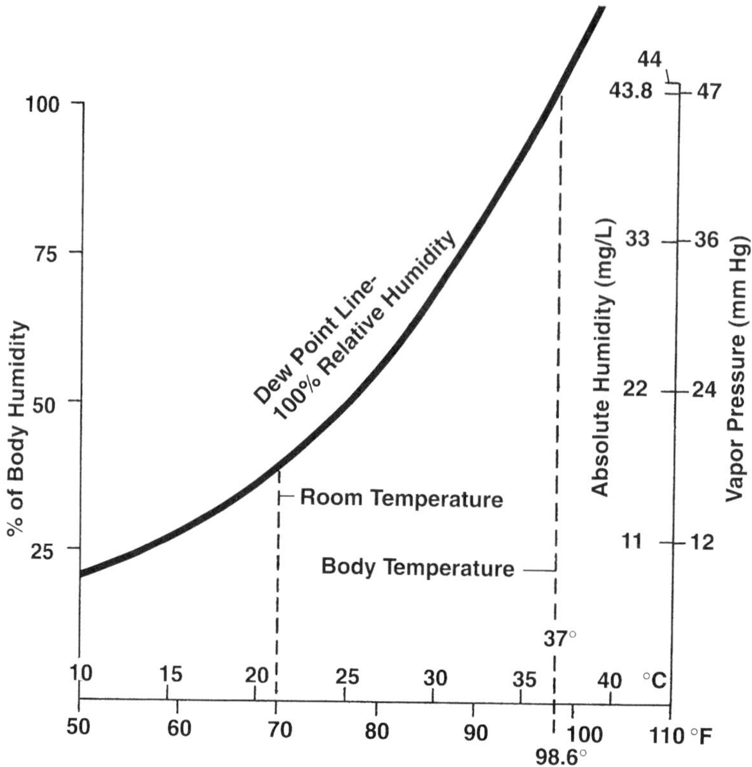

Fig. 7-2 Dew point line, 100% RH.

temperature of 37° C (98.6° F). In other words, air is always warmed to body temperature and saturated with water by the time it reaches the lungs. As seen in Table 7-1, the water content and vapor pressure in the lungs varies with the patient's temperature.

vii. Humidity deficit.

Humidity deficit is the difference between the body humidity conditions and the room air (or other gas) conditions. Because the air must be warmed to body temperature and saturated by the time it reaches the lungs and room conditions are rarely like those in the lung, it is normal to have a humidity deficit. The humidity deficit is eliminated by the respiratory passages warming and humidifying the inhaled air. See Fig. 7-3 for humidity deficit in terms of absolute humidity. The humidity deficit can also be calculated in terms of vapor pressure.

Example:

Calculate the humidity deficit under normal body conditions and room air conditions of 40% RH at 21° C (70° F):

a. Deficit = 44 mg/L − 7.34 mg/L = 36.66 mg/L that must be made up by the body.
b. Deficit = 47 mm Hg − 7.45 mm Hg = 39.55 mm Hg that must be made up by the body.

Remember that a clinically normal person can eliminate the humidity deficit without difficulty. This is done by evaporation from the mucous membranes of the nose and first few airway generations. This water lost by evaporation is called insensible loss and amounts to about 250 to 500 ml/day in an adult. However, a patient with an endotracheal

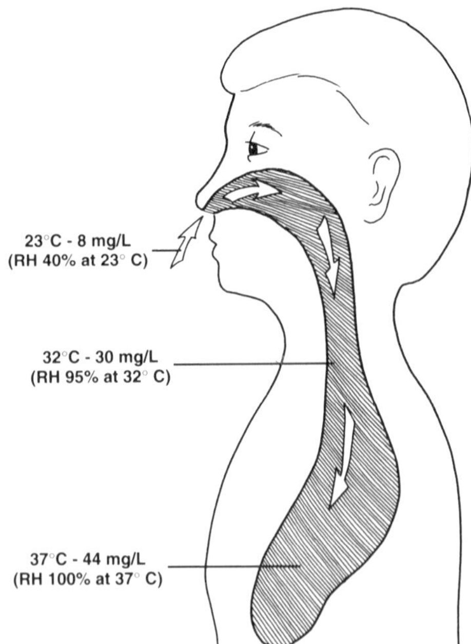

Fig. 7-3 Humidity deficit in terms of absolute humidity.

or tracheostomy tube or one who has a fever, is dehydrated, or is breathing in very cold and dry gas will have difficulty warming and saturating the inhaled gas. This can lead to drying and irritation of the mucosa, drying of secretions, chest discomfort, and even bronchospasm in susceptible patients. Under these conditions, the humidity deficit must be reduced or eliminated by warming and humidifying the inspired gas before it reaches the patient.

viii. Aerosol.

Aerosol is a suspension of liquid or solid particles in a gas. The use of therapeutic aerosols in respiratory care includes medications, saline solutions, or sterile water. Dust, pollen, and fumes can also form an aerosol. These are often very irritating to the airways and can induce a cough or even bronchospasm in a person with asthma.

ix. Aerosol characteristics and factors that influence deposition in the airways and lungs.

(1) Particle size and mass median aerodynamic diameter

There is some controversy over what sized particles deposit in the airways and lungs. Table 7-2 lists what seems to be a majority opinion. Aerosol particle diameter sizes are listed in units of micrometers. A micrometer is one thousandth of a millimeter. (As a point of clarification, some references list the symbol for a micron as μ (mu); others use the International System unit of micrometer, which is symbolized as μm.)

Mass median aerodynamic diameter (MMAD) is where the *mass* of the aerosol is centered. An equal amount of mass of aerosol will be found on both sides of the MMAD in larger and smaller particles. The MMAD is important therapeutically because it shows the size of the particle where most of the medication will be delivered to the airways. For example, if the clinical goal is to deliver an aerosol to the upper airway, an MMAD of 10 μm or greater would be best. However, if the clinical goal is to deposit the aerosol in the small airways and alveoli, a MMAD of 2 to 5 μm would be best.

Check the manufacturer's literature to determine the MMAD of an aerosol generator

Table 7-2. Aerosol Particle Sizes and Their Likely Deposition Point in the Airways and Lungs

Location	Particle Size (μm)
Nose or mouth to larynx	≥10
Trachea to terminal bronchioles	5-9
Respiratory bronchioles to alveoli	2-5
Likely to be exhaled	≤1

so that the correct one can be found to produce the desired aerosol particle size. Some manufacturers will list the mass median diameter (MMD) instead of the MMAD. It has the same meaning as far as aerosol deposition is concerned. (The MMAD is also listed as the aerodynamic mass median diameter, or AMMD, in some references.)

(2) Gravity

Larger, more massive particles are more likely to be affected by gravity than are smaller, less massive particles. Because of this, larger particles are likely to settle out and impact on an airway faster than smaller particles are. This results in larger, more massive particles impacting on larger airways and smaller, less massive particles impacting on smaller airways or the alveoli.

(3) Inertia

One of the principles of inertia is the fact that an object in motion tends to stay in motion until acted on. An aerosol particle being carried by a gas will tend to travel in a straight line even if the gas changes course at a pulmonary bifurcation. This is an important consideration when the patient is inhaling relatively large particles at relatively fast flows. Under these conditions, the particles will impact in the upper airway. Smaller particles traveling at slower speeds will tend to impact more deeply in the smaller airways.

(4) Nature of the particle

The composition of the particles may cause them to either add water vapor and enlarge or lose water vapor and shrink. As discussed earlier, this will have a major influence on their point of impaction. The following terms relate to the nature of the particles:

(a) Hygroscopic—tends to absorb water vapor and enlarge
(b) Hygrophobic—tends to lose water vapor and shrink
(c) Isotonic solution (0.9%) saline)—is a fairly stable particle because it has the same osmotic (chemical) concentration as the body
(d) Hypertonic solution (greater than 0.9% saline)—tends to absorb water vapor and enlarge
(e) Hypotonic solution (<0.9% saline)—tends to lose water vapor and shrink

(5) Temperature and humidity

If an aerosol is added to a warmed and humidified carrier gas, the aerosol particles will tend to enlarge because of water vapor coalescence on the particles. This will aid in upper airway impaction. If an aerosol is added to a cool and dry carrier gas, the aerosol particles will tend to shrink because of evaporation. This will aid in lower airway impaction.

(6) Patient's breathing pattern

Patients will breathe with whatever pattern and rate is easiest for them. Although this will have some benefits to a patient because of the minimized work of breathing and fewest calories being burned, it may not be best for the pulmonary condition. Frequently sick patients breathe in a rapid and shallow pattern. Any therapeutic aerosol particles will tend to be deposited in the first few airway generations and not reach their intended target in the smaller airways. Encouraging the patient to breathe more deeply and slowly will help to deposit the aerosol in the smaller airways. This topic will be covered in more detail later in Module C.

(7) Kinetic activity

Kinetic activity is the constant, random movement of aerosol droplets and carrier gases. Particles smaller than 1 μm are most affected by kinetic activity. Because aerosols this small are not used in respiratory care, this factor is of minor concern.

b. Indications for humidity therapy.

i. Rehumidification of dry therapeutic medical gases in patients with normal upper airways.

There is some controversy over whether it is necessary to humidify dry oxygen delivered by low-flow oxygen masks, nasal cannulas, and nasal catheters. The guidelines set at the National Conference on Oxygen Therapy of the American College of Chest Physicians state that supplemental humidity is not needed for oxygen at flows of 4 L/min or less. This would include nasal cannulas, nasal catheters, and some air entrainment mask settings. As long as the patient has a normal upper airway and the hospital has a RH of about 40%, the patient should be able to fully saturate the gas without any adverse effects.

Some clinicians believe that *any* oxygen flow through a nasal cannula or nasal catheter should be humidified. This is to prevent the local mucosa from drying out. Usually an unheated bubble-type humidifier is used to deliver about 40% RH at room temperature. The patient is able to then fully saturate the gas. All agree that dry oxygen at flows of greater than 4 L/min by any device must be humidified. Humidifier options are discussed in Module B.

ii. Elimination of humidity deficit in patients with bypassed upper airways.

There is no doubt that patients with bypassed upper airways must have their humidity deficit eliminated. Failure to do so will result in drying and crusting of the mucosa and mucus plugging. It is recommended that a heated humidifier be used. It should be set to deliver gas at 32° to 37° C (90°-99° F) to the patient and able to provide 80% to 100% RH in those temperature ranges.

iii. Reduction of airway resistance.

There is strong evidence that patients with exercise-induced asthma and cold air–induced asthma will be less likely to experience bronchospasm if they inhale warmed, humidified gas while exercising. The clinical goal in this case would be to prevent an increase in airway resistance.

c. Indications for aerosol therapy.

i. Rehumidification of dry therapeutic medical gases.

Aerosol particles heated to body temperature can fully saturate the inhaled carrier gas through evaporation of some of the particles. This would be indicated in patients who need the humidity *and* a medicinal aerosol. This is not the preferred way to deliver just humidity to a patient. It is possible to overhydrate the airway, especially in neonates, by long-term aerosol therapy. It must be remembered that aerosol particles can carry bacteria and other pathogens while humidity (water vapor) alone cannot.

ii. Soothe an irritated upper airway.

There are two generally accepted indications for delivering a bland aerosol (sterile water or normal saline solution) to soothe an irritated upper airway: following extubation or laryngotracheobronchitis (LTB, or pediatric croup). Generally a cool (room temperature) aerosol is delivered to reduce airway edema.

iii. Deliver medications to the airways and lungs.

All nebulized medications with the exception of the bland aerosols just discussed are included. This subject is covered in more detail in Module B, and the medications is discussed in Section 8.)

iv. Increased clearance of secretions.

Traditionally many patients with a mild case of bronchitis or those who recently had surgery were given breathing treatments with a bland aerosol as a way to help them mobilize secretions. These often consisted of breathing in about 5 ml of normal saline solution three or four times daily while awake for several days. Intermittent positive-pressure breathing (IPPB) or a hand-held nebulizer was used to deliver the aerosol.

It was thought that the aerosol added enough liquid to the secretions to enable the patient to cough them out. It is now understood that the patient could cough more effectively because the aerosol irritated the airway enough that the patient's own bronchial/submucosal glands poured out more mucus. This reflex is mediated by the vagus nerve.

This form of therapy is probably not indicated in most situations. It is more clinically effective to have the patient increase fluid intake so that the bronchial/submucosal glands can produce less viscous secretions. It may also be necessary to start the patient on a regimen of continuous aerosol therapy or other respiratory care treatment modalities such as incentive spirometry and chest physical therapy with postural drainage.

v. Induce sputum production for a sputum specimen.

Patients who have few, if any, secretions but in whom a sputum specimen is needed can have sputum production induced. Examples include patients with suspected tuberculosis or lung cancer. The mechanism of action is as described earlier. Typically the patient inhales an aerosol of sterile water or hypertonic saline solution for about 5 to 10 minutes. Ultrasonic nebulizers are often used because they produce a dense mist of small particles.

2. Observe the patient for changes in sputum quantity and consistency. (IIIE5) [R, Ap]

It is important to follow the patient's sputum quantity and consistency to know if the humidity or aerosol therapy is effective. Review Section 1, Module C, 6 and Module D, 14 for the discussion and see Fig. 1-25 and Table 1-7 for more information.

Module B. Humidity and aerosol generators and administrative devices.

1. Humidity delivered through small-bore tubing.

These patients have normal upper airways and can add humidity to the inhaled gas in the usual way.

a. Bubble-type humidifiers.

i. Get the necessary equipment for the procedure. (IIA2a) [R, Ap]

ii. Put the equipment together, make sure that it works properly, and identify and fix any problems with it. (IIB2a) [R, Ap]

The bubble-type humidifiers are used on patients with normal upper airways who need some supplemental humidity because of the dryness of medical oxygen. These devices are not usually heated and, in fact, deliver gas cooled to less than room temperature. They provide around 40% RH at the delivered gas temperature. The balance has to be made up by the patient (Figs. 7-4 and 7-5). It is possible to add a wrap-around type of heater if it is clinically indicated to raise the temperature of the delivered gas and reduce the patient's humidity deficit.

There are three different types of these humidifiers designed to add some humidity

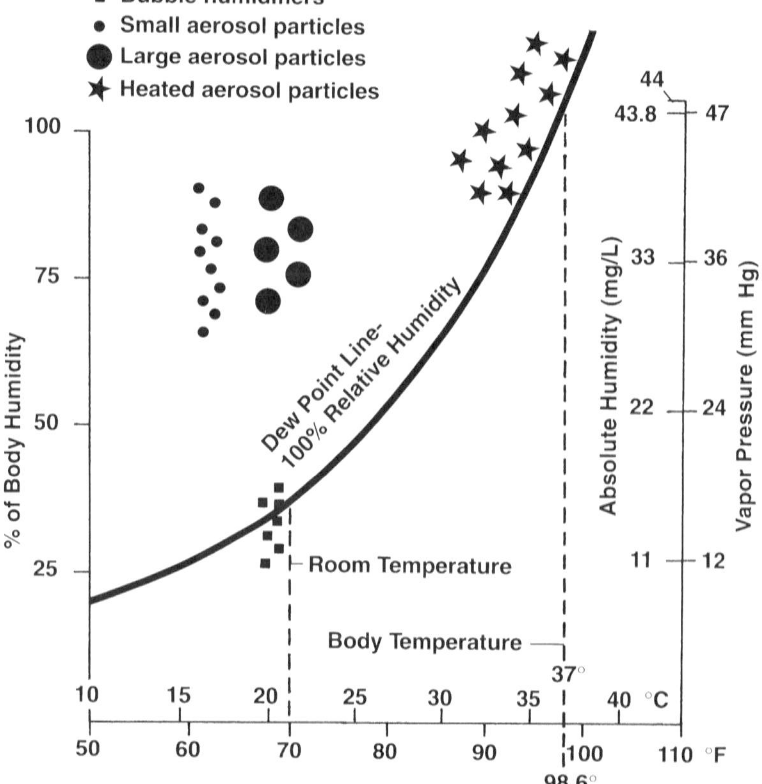

Fig. 7-4 Comparison of humidity content provided by bubble-type humidifiers and various nebulizers.

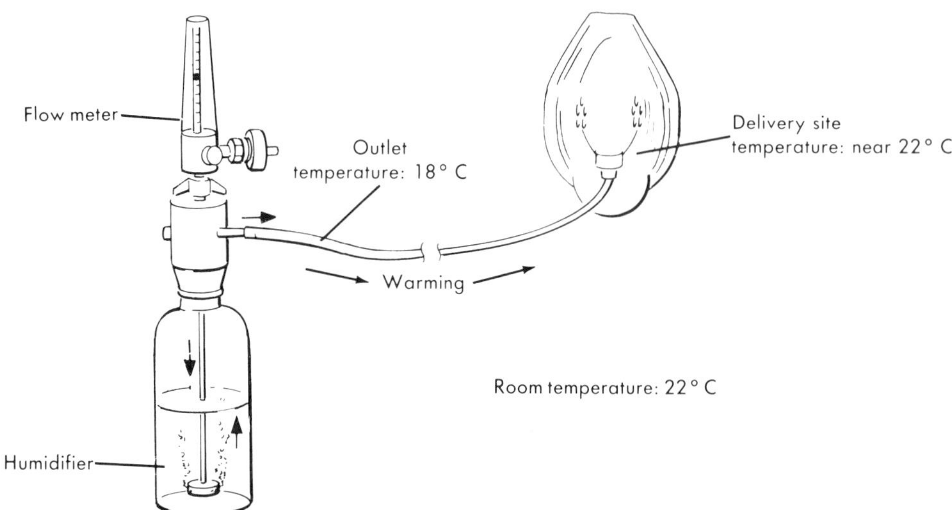

Fig. 7-5 Gases leaving outlet of the simple humidifier are cooler than room temperature because of evaporation. Warming toward room temperature occurs en route to the patient delivery site. (From Scanlan CL: Humidity and aerosol therapy, in Scanlan CL, Spearman CB, Sheldon RL [eds]: *Egan's Fundamentals of Respiratory Care,* ed 5. St Louis, Mosby, 1990. Used by permission.)

to dry oxygen delivered through small-bore tubing: tradition bubble humidifiers, jet humidifiers, and underwater jet humidifiers.

Traditional Bubble Humidifiers

Traditional bubble humidifiers use a perforated capillary tube or porous diffusion head to break the oxygen into small bubbles (Fig. 7-6). This allows for more surface area contact of the oxygen with the water and raises the RH by evaporation. It is important to keep the water level in the reservoir within the manufacturers' specifications and, if possible, as full as possible. The lower the water level is, the lower the RH will be because there is less time for evaporation. The faster the oxygen flow, the lower the RH.

Jet Humidifiers

Jet humidifiers create an aerosol that is baffled out of the delivered gas flow. The RH is increased by evaporation of some of the aerosol droplets. These units deliver a higher RH than do the bubble types just described. They have the additional advantages of delivering the same RH at higher flow levels and as the water level drops.

Underwater Jet Humidifiers

Underwater jet humidifiers create water vapor and an aerosol. The aerosol is not baffled out as it is in the jet humidifiers. Because of this, these units deliver the highest RH. They can deliver the same humidity level at high gas flows and as the water level drops. The aerosol particles can carry pathogens, so stricter infection control standards must be met to protect the patient. The water and humidifier must be changed at least every 24 hours. The Ohmeda Ohio Jet humidifier is an example of a reusable unit. If the patient

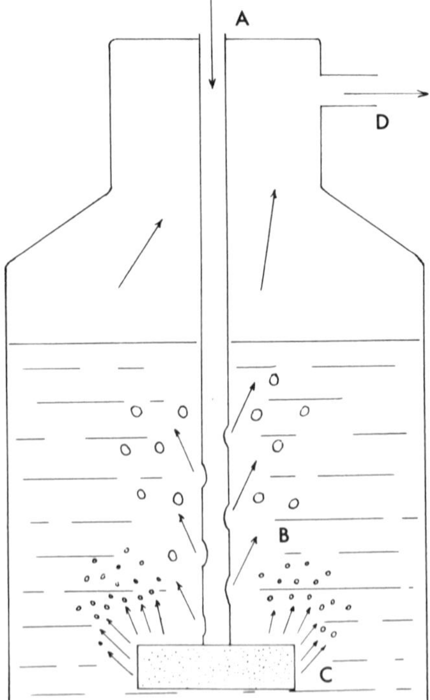

Fig. 7-6 The bubble-diffusion humidifier bubbles therapeutic gas. *A,* through a perforated tube, *B,* or a porous diffusion head, *C.* The larger the number of small bubbles, the greater the evaporation area to humidity the gas leaving outflow port, *D.* (From Scanlan CL: Humidity and aerosol therapy, in Scanlan CL, Spearman CB, Sheldon RL [eds]: *Egan's Fundamentals of Respiratory Care,* ed 5, St Louis, Mosby, 1990. Used by permission.)

needs a higher delivered RH, a jet humidifier or underwater jet humidifier would be a better choice than a bubble type.

Many of the simple bubble humidifiers come prepackaged with sterile water. They can be used for many short-term patients (e.g., those in the recovery room) or for a single long-term patient. When the water runs low, they are discarded.

The bubble and other types of humidifiers consist of a reservoir jar for the water and a Diameter-Index Safety System (DISS) oxygen connector lid that screws on. Turn on the flowmeter, and make sure that oxygen flows through the delivery tube and bubbles into the water. Failure to bubble usually indicates that the lid and jar are not screwed together tightly or the delivery tube is plugged. If the tube cannot be cleared, it must be replaced.

Most of the newer bubble-type units have a pop-off type of high-pressure relief valve that is released if the pressure builds up to either 40 mm Hg or 2 psi. Pinch closed the small-bore tubing to build up pressure and test the pop-off valve. Feel for the gas to escape from the valve. Many will whistle to signal a gas leak. Do not use a unit whose pop-off valve will not open under pressure.

b. Nasal cannulas.

As discussed earlier, the guidelines set at the National Conference on Oxygen Therapy of the American College of Chest Physicians state that humidity does not need to be added to these devices if the flow is 4 L/min or less. It is clear that adding a humidifier to every low-flow system will increase the cost to the patient. However, some patients will complain of nasal dryness and discomfort if the cannula's oxygen is not humidified. The physician and practitioner may believe that the patient's discomfort warrants the addition of a bubble-type humidifier. There is agreement that humidity should be added to flows of greater than 4 L/min. See Fig. 7-7 for a humidified nasal cannula setup.

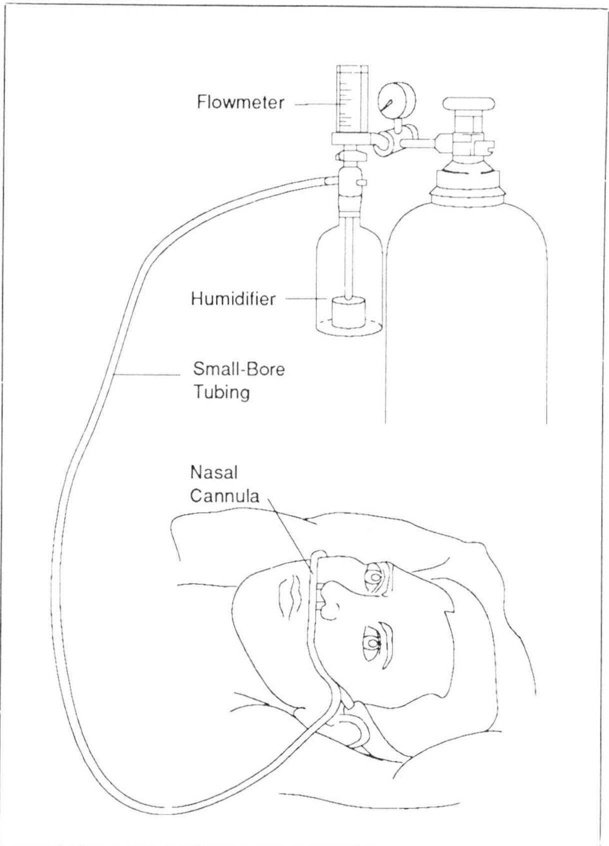

Fig. 7-7 Adult wearing a nasal cannula delivering oxygen humidified by a bubble-type humidifier. (From Guidelines for disinfection of home equipment. *Respir Care* 1988; 33:801-808. Used by permission.)

c. Oxygen masks.

As stated earlier, it is not believed to be necessary to add humidity to any oxygen mask that has an oxygen flow of 4 L/min or less. This probably includes only low–oxygen percentage air entrainment masks. A significant amount of humidified room air is entrained into these masks.

Humidity should be added to any mask that has more than 4 L/min of oxygen added. This would include simple oxygen masks at higher flows, higher–oxygen percentage air entrainment masks, partial rebreathing masks, and non-rebreathing masks.

2. Humidity delivered through large-bore tubing.

Most of these patient's have had their upper airway bypassed by an endotracheal or tracheostomy tube. Because of this, they cannot humidify inspired gas in the normal manner. In some other cases, the patient is receiving oxygen, and humidity is added so that the gas is not dry.

As stated earlier, it is recommended that a heated humidifier be used with these patients. It should be set to deliver gas at 32° to 37° C (90°-99° F) to the patient and able to provide 80% to 100% RH in those temperature ranges.

Note: All of the following humidity- and aerosol-generating devices deliver the conditioned gas to the patient through large-bore (also known as aerosol or corrugated) tubing. This tubing is discussed in more detail later.

a. Cascade-type humidifiers.
i. Get the necessary equipment for the procedure. (IIA2a) [R, Ap]
ii. Put the equipment together, make sure it works properly, and identify and fix any problems with it. (IIB2a) [R, Ap]

Note: It is beyond the scope of this book to go into detail on all of the different models of humidifiers that use large-bore tubing. Rather, some common features are briefly described. All of these humidifiers have an adjustable heater so that the water in the reservoir is at or greater than body temperature. This enables them to provide up to 100% of the patient's body humidity. It is necessary with all of these units to measure the temperature of the inspired gas near the patient. The gas temperature is usually kept the same as the patient's or a few degrees cooler (Fig. 7-8).

As the heated gas passes through the large-bore tubing, there will be some cooling. This will result in condensation that must be drained out. Water traps placed in the lowest loops in the tubing will help in this and keep the tubing clear. Remember to look periodically for water puffing or sloshing back and forth in the lower points of the tubing. Even though some of the water vapor condenses out, the RH remains 100% as the gas cools along the dew point line. The absolute humidity, however, will drop (see Fig. 7-2).

The Bennett Cascade is the most well know of these types of humidifiers (Fig. 7-9). It is most commonly used with a mechanical ventilator but can be used with other types of systems for delivering humidity with or without oxygen. Its basic principle of operation is an efficient bubble-type humidifier. The inspiratory gas must flow through the water for evaporation to occur. A variety of similar devices are now on the market and include the Bourns humidifier, Ohio Heated humidifier, Monaghan Model 610, Chemetron HR-1 Humidity Center, and Bennett's Cascade II. It is important with the Cascade humidifier and the others discussed later on that they be properly assembled. This is es-

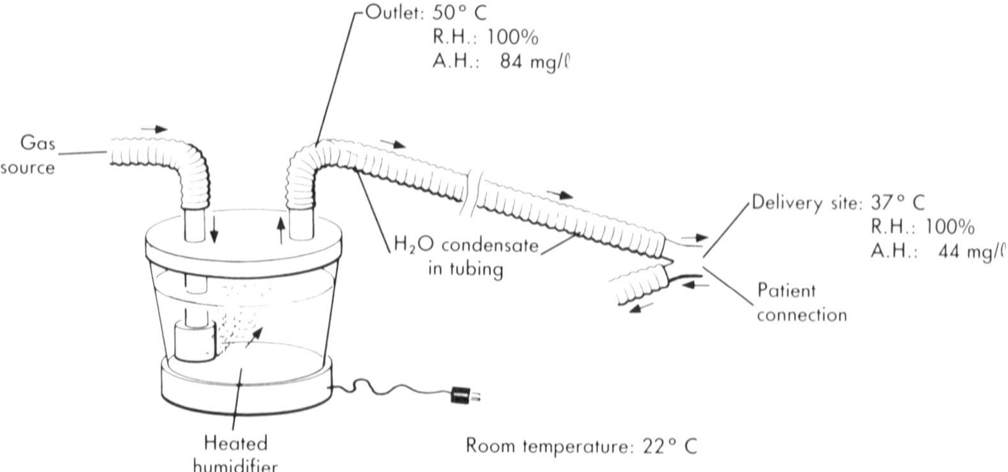

Fig. 7-8 Gases leaving outlet of heated humidifier are hot and saturated with water vapor. As cooling occurs in tubing, vapor condenses and absolute humidity *(A.H.)* decreases while relative humidity *(R.H.)* remains 100% (saturated). Note that almost half the original water vapor is "lost" to condensate in this example. (From Scanlan CL: Humidity and aerosol therapy, in Scanlan CL, Spearman CB, Sheldon RL [eds]: *Egan's Fundamentals of Respiratory Care,* ed 5. St Louis, Mosby, 1990. Used by permission.)

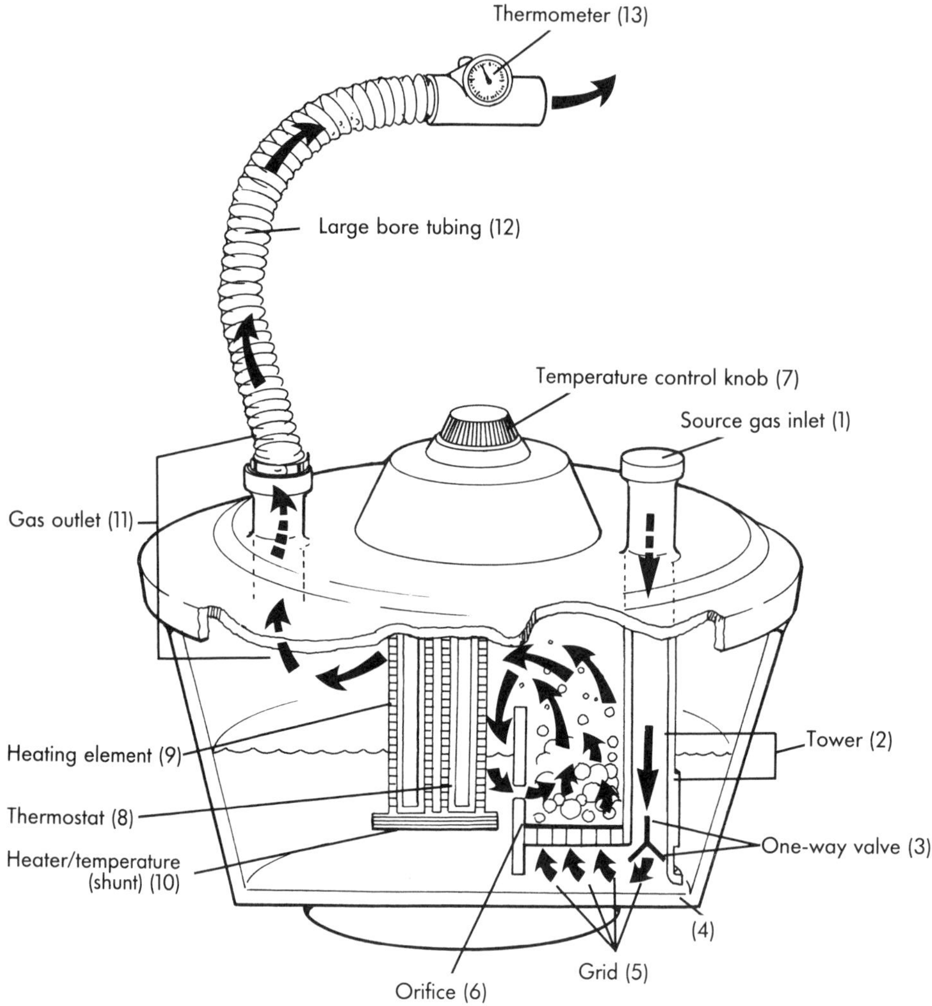

Fig. 7-9 Cascade humidifier. (From Scanlan CL: Humidity and aerosol therapy, in Scanlan CL, Spearman CB, Sheldon RL [eds]: *Egan's Fundamentals of Respiratory Care,* ed 5. St Louis, Mosby, 1990. Used by permission.)

pecially important when they are used to humidify a mechanical ventilator. Any loose connections will result in an air leak and loss of tidal volume.

b. Wick-type humidifiers.

i. Get the necessary equipment for the procedure. (IIA2a) [R, Ap]

ii. Put the equipment together, make sure that it works properly, and identify and fix any problems with it. (IIB2a) [R, Ap]

This second type of heated humidifier employs a wick, often made of sponge or paper, to soak up water for evaporation. The water, wick, or both are heated so that 100% RH can be delivered. These units are also used with mechanical ventilators or other systems, including air entrainment devices. This is because they have very little resistance to the gas flowing through them as evaporation occurs. Examples include the HLC 37 by

Travenol Laboratories, Inc., Dual Servo MR500 by Fisher and Paykel Medical, Inc., Conchapak by Respiratory Care, Inc., and the Bird Humidifier Model 3000.

c. Passover-type humidifiers.

i. Get the necessary equipment for the procedure. (IIA2a) [R, Ap]

ii. Put the equipment together, make sure that it works properly, and identify and fix any problems with it. (IIB2a) [R, Ap]

This third type of unit simply has the patient gas passing over the surface of a reservoir of hot water. They are sometimes called "hot pots" and have been used in Emerson ventilators. By themselves, these units are probably the least effective at humidifying gas. When they are used on ventilators, other features such as copper mesh in a heated inspiratory tube are used to increase the surface area for evaporation.

d. Infant hoods.

Infant hoods were first discussed in Section 5 on oxygen therapy as an oxygen delivery system. A decision must also be made on which humidification system to use. The oxygen must be heated to body temperature to eliminate the humidity deficit and keep the infant from chilling or overheating. The temperature should be measured inside the hood. Aerosols are not recommended for long-term use because of the risk of overhydration. Infants are also sound sensitive, so a quiet system is preferred. For all of these reasons, a heated cascade or wick type of humidifier is recommended.

e. Mechanical ventilator systems.

Any of the aforementioned heated humidification systems can be used with a mechanical ventilator to provide 100% body humidity. This subject is covered in more detail in Section 14.

3. Nebulizers and related delivery systems.

a. Ultrasonic nebulizers.

i. Get the necessary equipment for the procedure. (IIA3b) [R, Ap]

ii. Put the equipment together, make sure that it works properly, and identify and fix any problems with it. (IIB3b) [R, Ap]

Ultrasonic nebulizers work by converting electrical energy into sound energy that creates aerosol particles. The heart of the system is a ceramic piezoelectric crystal that changes its shape and vibrates (piezoelectric quality) at the same rate as the electrical current that is sent through it. The frequency is usually set at 1,350,000 cycles/sec (1.35 Mc or MHz) but may vary among manufacturers. The frequency is vital because it results in a stable aerosol with a mean particle size that is about 3 μm in diameter. This is an ideal size to penetrate deeply into the lungs. The only control on these units is for amplitude (power) to control the aerosol output. The range is usually up to 3 to 6 ml/min depending on the model. This output is greater than most pneumatic nebulizers can produce. The aerosol can be carried to the patient by a built-in fan or by an outside oxygen source (Fig. 7-10). The patient's humidity deficit will be minimized by the warm aerosol that is created.

Ultrasonic units are often chosen for delivering bland solutions to the lower airways because of the small particle size and the high output. The ultrasonic should not be cho-

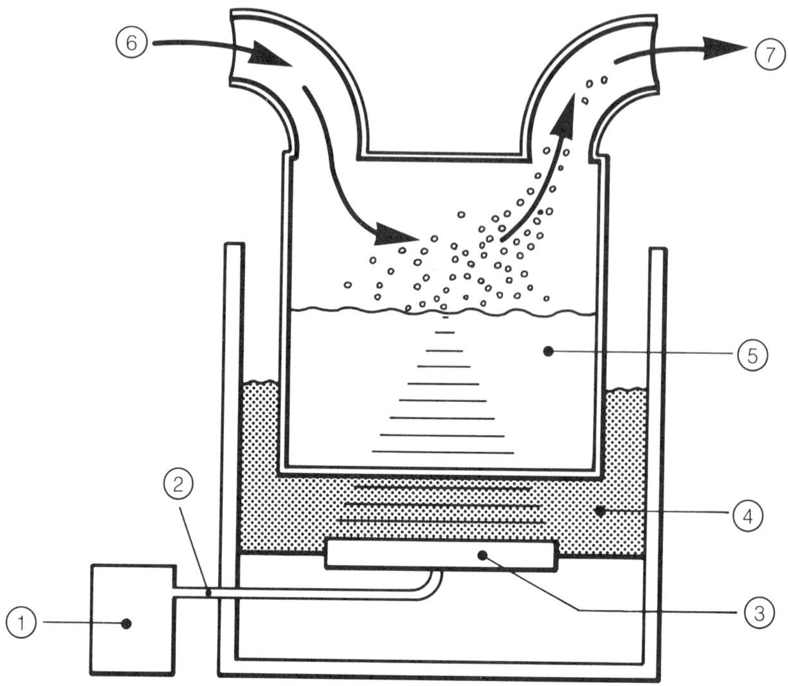

Fig. 7-10 Functional diagram of the ultrasonic nebulizer: *(1)* electric current generator, *(2)* cable, *(3)* piezoelectric crystal, *(4)* couplant chamber, *(5)* solution cup, *(6)* carrier gas inlet, and *(7)* aerosol outlet. (From Op't Holt T: Aerosol generators and humidifiers, in Barnes TA [ed]: *Respiratory Care Practice,* Chicago, Mosby, 1988. Used by permission.)

sen for upper airway aerosol deposition or for administering pharmacologically active medications such as bronchodilators, mucolytics, and antibiotics. These active medications may not nebulize at the same rate as the diluent, which creates the risk of delivering a very concentrated dose at the end of the treatment. Some of the medications may also be mechanically broken down by the high-frequency vibration and made useless.

Always follow the manufacturer's instructions when setting the system up. There are too many brands and models to discuss here. Fig. 7-10 shows the common features and Table 7-3 describes how to troubleshoot many common problems. It seems that many of the clinical difficulties have to do with keeping the proper fluid levels in the couplant chamber and the solution cup. If the sterile water in the couplant chamber is too low, the vibration cannot reach the solution cup, and no aerosol will be produced. If the saline level in the solution cup is either too low or too high, the vibrational energy will not focus properly on the surface of the saline solution, and no aerosol will be produced. Water should not be allowed to condense out and fill any low points in the large-bore tubing. If this were to occur, the ultrasonic particles would liquify as the carrier gas is forced to pass through the condensate. The exiting gas would be humidified through evaporation but carry no aerosol particles. If the carrier gas is oxygen enriched through a high airflow with oxygen enrichment (HAFOE) system, the backpressure could result in an increase in the oxygen percentage and a decrease in the total flow. Remember to always measure the oxygen percentage near the patient.

b. Large-volume nebulizers.

i. Get the necessary equipment for the procedure. (IIA3a) [R, Ap]

Table 7-3. Ultrasonic Nebulizer Troubleshooting

Symptom	Possible Problem	Suggested Check
1. Unit installed and connected as specified, but pilot light does not turn on when switch is turned to the "on" position	Electrical outlet defective Circuit breaker tripped Fuse blown	Check outlet with lamp or other appliance Reset the circuit breaker, or change fuse on the power switch; if the circuit breaker continues to trip or the fuse blows again, service is needed
2. Unit installed and connected as specified. Power pilot light turns on, normal ultrasonic activity visible in nebulizer chamber, but no aerosol output	Nebulizer chamber contaminated	Wash nebulizer chamber, decontaminate
3. Unit installed and connected as specified. Power pilot light turns on, but there is little ultrasonic activity visible in the nebulizer chamber, and aerosol output is low (even when on the no. 10 power setting)	Couplant water excessively aerated Nebulizer module and couplant water too cold Diaphragm distorted, permitting air bubbles to interfere with proper transmission of vibrational energy into the nebulizer chamber Couplant contaminated	Wait for deaeration Use warmer couplant water Check to see that diaphragm is properly shaped and installed; be sure the concave (recessed) side faces the interior of the chamber Clean couplant compartment and replace couplant water
4. Same as symptom no. 3 but at a lower power setting	Power setting too low to start and establish nebulization	Turn output control knob to maximum power setting, then reduce to desired setting
5. Unit installed and connected as specified. Power pilot light turns on. "Add couplant" light is on, and there is no ultrasonic activity visible in the nebulizer chamber	Insufficient couplant water	Add water to the couplant compartment
6. Unit installed and connected as specified. Power pilot light turns on, "Add couplant" light is off, but there is no ultrasonic activity visible in the nebulizer chamber.	Power supply overheated and its thermostatic control opened	The cooling air has been restricted, or cooling fins need cleaning; the switch will reset when the equipment returns to room temperature
7. Liquid reservoir filled and properly connected to nebulizer chamber, but chamber does not fill (for *continuous-feed system only*)	Foreign material or air bubbles in feed tubes Liquid level control in nebulizer chamber plugged with foreign material Air leaks at tube connections or reservoir cap	Flush the system Clean or flush the system Tighten all connections by pushing tubes into fittings

From Op't Holt T: Aerosol generators and humidifiers, in Barnes TA (ed): *Respiratory Care Practice*. Chicago, Mosby, 1988. Used by permission.

ii. Put the equipment together, make sure that it works properly, and identify and fix any problems with it. (IIB3a) [R, Ap]

Large-volume nebulizers all share the common feature of having a water reservoir of at least 250 ml, hence the name large-volume nebulizer. Commonly they also will entrain room air to increase the total gas flow. It is beyond the scope of this book to cover all of the different brands of large-volume and air entrainment nebulizers in detail. Rather, the discussion covers some common features, the three main groupings, and how the water reservoir is warmed in the first large group.

Pneumatic nebulizers share these common features:

1. All are powered by air or oxygen delivered through a flowmeter. As the gas flow drops, the aerosol output decreases.
2. All make use of Bernoulli's principle with a jet that is used to entrain liquid, room air, or both into the main gas flow.
3. All have a reservoir jar that can be filled with 250 to 2500 ml of liquid.
4. All have a capillary tube that allows the liquid to flow *up* to the jet for nebulization. (Remember that with the bubble-type humidifiers, the oxygen flows *down* the capillary tube.)
5. All have a baffle that the aerosol is sprayed against to create a more uniform particle size.

Many, but not all, of the pneumatic nebulizers allow for a changeable inspired oxygen percentage. Provided that the jet is powered by oxygen, the air entrainment ports can be opened up more to increase air entrainment (lowering the inspired oxygen percentage), or closed down to decrease air entrainment (raising the inspired oxygen percentage). The reusable units have several fixed oxygen percentages (usually 35% to 40%, 60% to 70%, and 100%). The disposable units are more flexible and usually allow for continuous dialing from 35% to 100% oxygen. Remember to always analyze the inspired oxygen percentage near the patient because water in the aerosol tubing and backpressure will decrease the entrained air and raise the oxygen percentage.

A. The largest and oldest group of pneumatic nebulizers look similar to the bubble-type humidifiers. The key components include a large reservoir jar and a top with a DISS oxygen connector and capillary tube to the jet. Examples include the reusable Puritan All Purpose and Ohio Deluxe units and many disposable types. These allow for variable oxygen percentages. Keep the capillary tube and jet clear of debris, or the aerosol output will drop. Keep the air entrainment ports open so that proper gas mixing will occur and the desired oxygen percentage will be provided (Fig. 7-11).

   Heating of the water or aerosol or both is accomplished in one of the following ways:

   1. A heated metal rod is immersed in the reservoir water through a port in the top of the nebulizer. Examples include the Puritan All Purpose and Ohio Deluxe units. A dial is used to control how hot the rod gets, but it has no automatic shutoff feature. The water temperature varies depending on how deep it is, so as the water level drops, the remaining water gets hotter. It is very important to measure the gas temperature near the patient and keep the water level stable to prevent burning the airway. The heated rod presents a risk of burns to a practitioner who accidentally touches it while it is still hot. It must be disinfected between patients and changed as often as the nebulizer is.

      There are two other systems that are variations on the previously mentioned idea of directly heating the water in the reservoir jar. The first

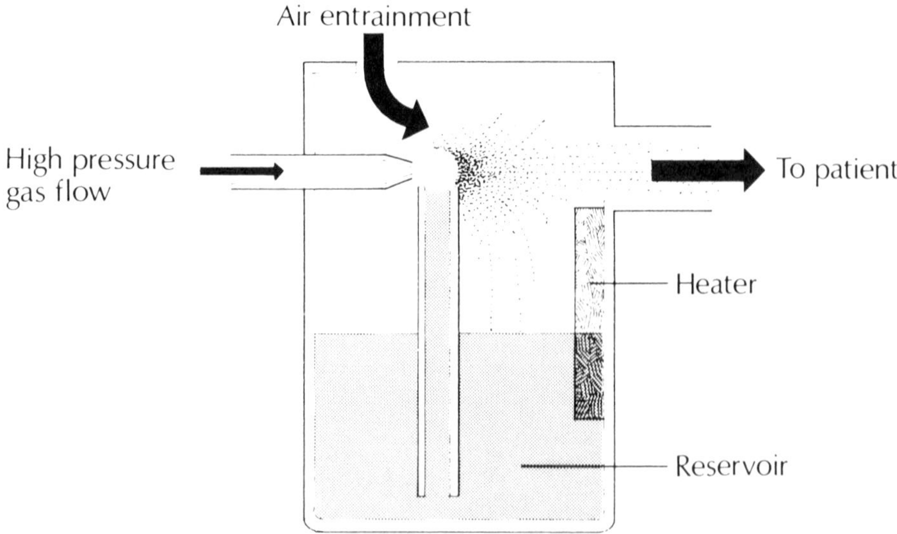

Fig. 7-11 Large-reservoir, air entrainment nebulizer. (From Shapiro BA, Harrison RA, Kacmarek, RM, et al: *Clinical Application of Respiratory Care,* ed 3, Chicago, Mosby, 1989. Used by permission.)

heats the water as it passes through the capillary tube. Examples include the Chemtron Heated Nebulizer, Aquatherm I, II, and III by Respiratory Care, Inc.; and Corpak company's nebulizer. All have the advantage of a short warm-up time when compared with all of the other systems. The Chemetron and Aquatherm units have an external temperature probe to place in the aerosol tubing. It acts as a servocontroller of the heating unit for better temperature regulation.

The second nebulizer, called the NEBULO 28 by the Inspiron Respiratory Division of C.R. Bard, Inc., directly heats only a small amount of the reservoir water just before it is aerosolized.

2. A flexible heater is wrapped around the outside of the reservoir. A dial is used to control how hot the heater gets, but it has no automatic shutoff feature. The water temperature will increase as the water level drops. Monitor the gas temperature near the patient for safety purposes.
3. A clip-on heating base plate can be added to special reservoir jars with a metal plate. These are preferable to the previously mentioned types because they are thermostatically controlled. High- and low-temperature limits can be set, and the unit will shut itself off if the limits are reached. They also ensure a constant temperature to the aerosol as the water level drops. Examples include the Ohio Deluxe nebulizer top and the Puritan All Purpose nebulizer top.

Heating the water or aerosol reduces the patient's humidity deficit and is usually done if the secretions are thick. See Fig. 7-12 for a comparison of an unheated and a heated system. See Fig. 7-4 for the location of the aerosol particles and their relationship with the dew point and the patient's body humidity.

B. The Babington principle is a variation on the previously mentioned types of pneumatic nebulizers. Its main difference is in how the jet is constructed. These units have a more controlled particle size than those other types. Examples include the Solo-Sphere, Hydro-Sphere, and Maxi-Cool by Airlife/American Pharmaseal Company (Fig. 7-13). These units are quite complex and have many parts compared with the other types of nebulizers.

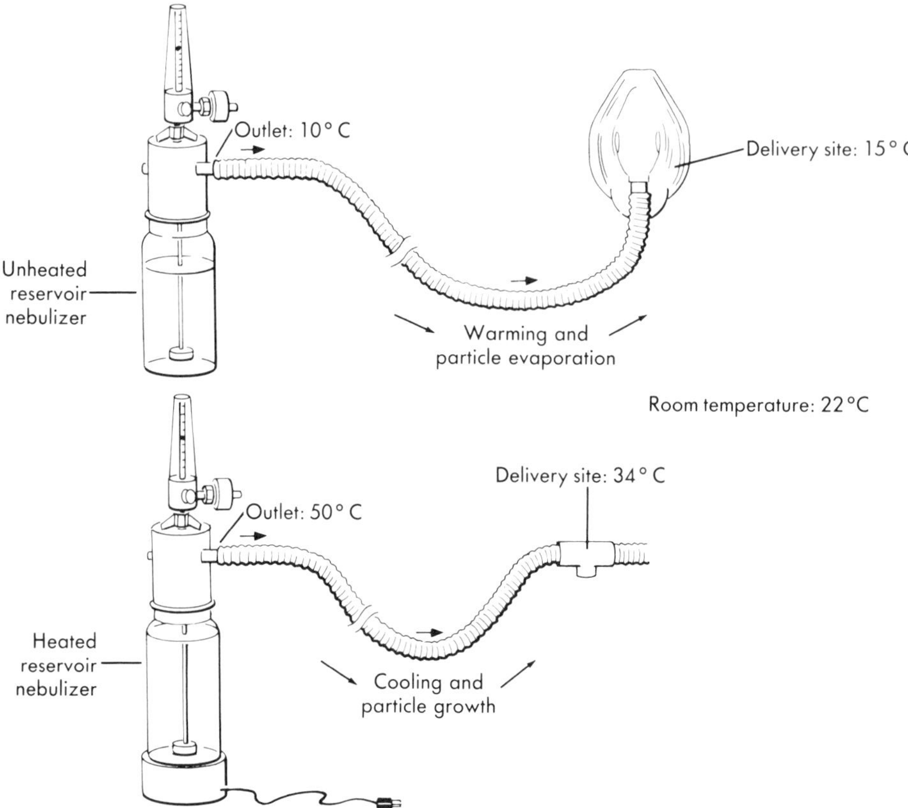

Fig. 7-12 Comparison of unheated vs. heated reservoir nebulizers. Output from the unheated (cool) nebulizer is cooler than room temperature because of evaporation of aerosol in the nebulizer. As the aerosol warms on the way to the patient delivery site, further evaporation of particles occurs. Output from the heated nebulizer is hot and humid. Cooling occurs as the aerosol travels through tubing exposed to cooler room and water vapor condenses on aerosol particles, causing them to "grow" larger. (From Scanlan CL: Humidity and aerosol therpay, in Scanlan CL, Spearman CB, Sheldon RL [eds]: *Egan's Fundamentals of Respiratory Care,* ed 5. St Louis, Mosby, 1990. Used by permission.)

C. Another variation is called the floating island nebulizer. Models are made by Win-Liz and Air Shields.

c. Aerosol delivery systems.

i. Large-bore tubing.

Large-bore tubing (also known as aerosol tubing or corrugated tubing) is needed to connect the aerosol generator with the patient. This tubing is 22 mm in internal diameter (ID). It is very flexible because of the corrugations and comes in two different types. One type has the corrugations going through to the inside of the tubing whereas the other is smooth internally. The internally smooth tubing is preferable for mechanical ventilators or other systems where it is desirable to minimize the airflow resistance. It also may allow more aerosol to pass through because there is a smaller surface area for impaction. There are flat areas spaced out periodically through both types of tubing for easy cutting. This is so that the tube length can be tailored to the patient's needs; and temperature probes and water traps can be added as necessary. The smooth areas fit over all of the 22-mm–outer diameter (OD) ports of the various aerosol generators that were just presented, as well as the heated humidifiers presented earlier and the various masks and adapters presented later on.

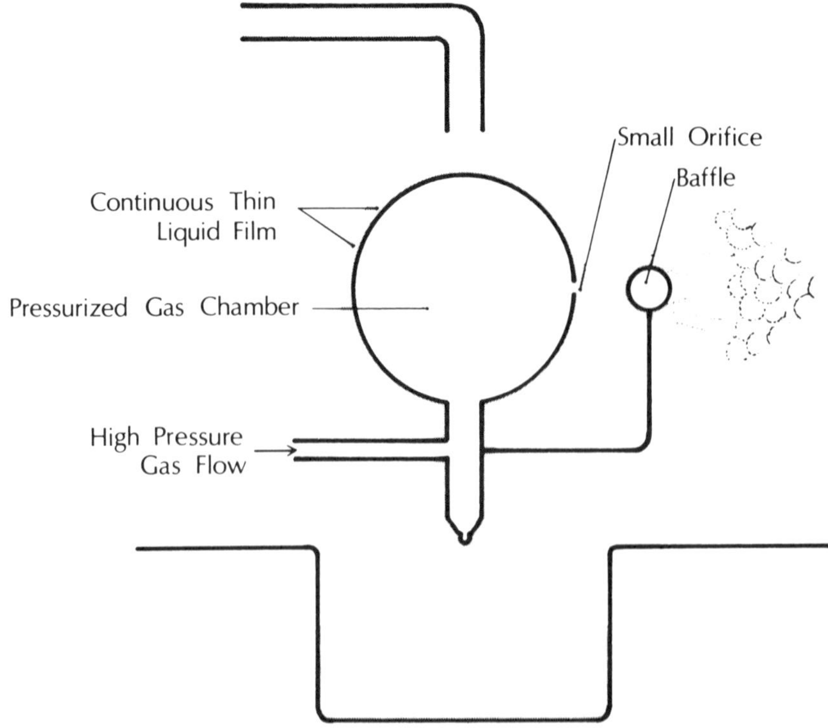

Fig. 7-13 Babington principle/hydronamic nebulizer. (From Shapiro BA, Harrison RA, Kacmarek, RM, et al: *Clinical Application of Respiratory Care,* ed 3. Chicago, Mosby, 1988. Used by permission.)

ii. Aerosol masks.

The aerosol mask looks similar to the simple oxygen mask except that it has larger side ports for exhalation and has a 22-mm-OD adapter for the large-bore tubing to attach to (Fig. 7-14). This is often considered to be a low-flow oxygen mask because the ports are open to room air. Because of this, it is difficult to ensure that the patient will receive the oxygen percentage that has been set. If the flow is high enough that aerosol mist can

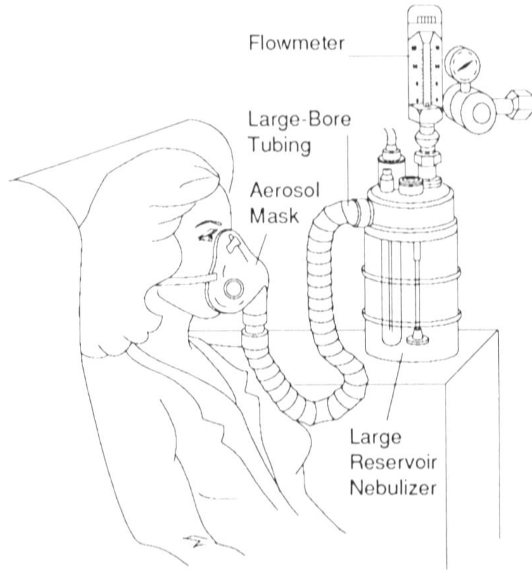

Fig. 7-14 Adult wearing an aerosol mask. (From Guidelines for disinfection of home equipment. *Respir Care* 1988; 33:801-808. Used by permission.)

be seen flowing out of the side ports during an inspiration, little room air is being inspired. It is best to analyze the oxygen percentage inside the mask to be sure. Any of the previously mentioned humidity or aerosol devices can be used and powered by compressed air or oxygen.

iii. Face tents.

The face tent is discussed in Section 5, Module C, 4. Any of the humidity or aerosol devices just discussed can be used with it and powered by compressed air or oxygen.

iv. Tracheostomy masks/collars.

The tracheostomy masks/collars are discussed in Section 5, Module C, 5. Any of the previously mentioned humidity or aerosol devices can be used with it and powered by compressed air or oxygen (Fig. 7-15).

v. Brigg's adapter/T-adapters.

The Brigg's adapter/T-adapter was discussed in Section 5, Module C, 5. Any of the previously mentioned humidity or aerosol devices can be used with it and powered by compressed air or oxygen.

vi. Aerosol (mist) tents.

(1) Get the necessary equipment for the procedure. (IIIA13) [R, Ap]

(2) Put the equipment together, make sure that it works properly, and identify and fix any problems with it. (IIB11) [R, Ap]

Oxygen tents are discussed in Section 5, Module C, 1. The aerosol or mist tents are essentially like the oxygen tents. The main difference is that no supplemental oxygen is used because the patient does not need it. The top of the canopy can be now be left open for better flow-through ventilation. At least 10 L/min of compressed air should still be run through the nebulizer to make sure that there is no carbon dioxide buildup. The

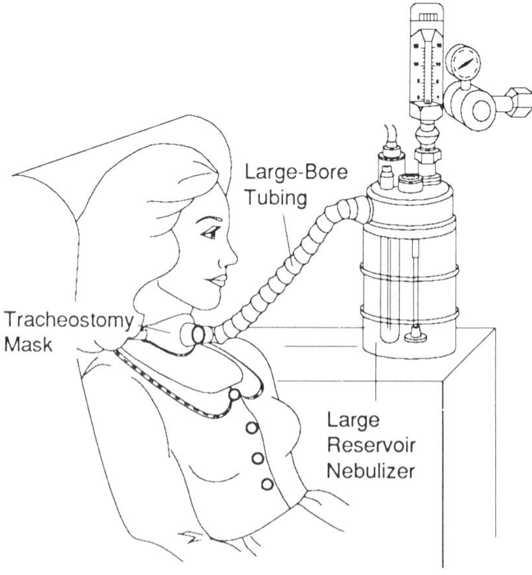

Fig. 7-15 Adult wearing a tracheostomy mask/collar. (From Guidelines for disinfection of home equipment. *Respir Care* 1988; 33:801-808. Used by permission.)

nebulizer or ultrasonic system should be cared for as described earlier to ensure that there is enough aerosol to treat the condition.

Aerosol tents are sometimes used to treat upper respiratory tract problems such as laryngotracheobronchitis (LTB or pediatric croup). A cool aerosol seems to be clinically preferred because it reduces airway edema. Never use so much aerosol that the child cannot be seen in side the tent. Also, be wary of fluid overloading the young patient who is in the tent for a prolonged period.

d. Medication delivery systems.

i. Gas-powered systems.

(1) Small-volume nebulizers

Small-volume nebulizers are designed to hold a relatively small volume of fluid, typically 10 ml or less. They are designed to nebulize liquid medications such as bronchodilators and mucolytics for inhalation. Either compressed air or oxygen can be used to generate the mist. These units operate under the same physical principles as the large-volume nebulizers described earlier. There are two different types: mainstream and sidestream.

Mainstream nebulizers are designed so that the main flow of gas to the patient flows through the aerosol as it is produced. A second high-pressure gas flow is used to power the jet to create the aerosol (Fig. 7-16). The Bird Corporation makes a reusable type called the Micronebulizer for its IBBP (intermittent positive-pressure breathing) circuit. *Sidestream nebulizers* are designed so that the aerosol is produced out of the main flow of gas and added to it by the jet's gas flow (Fig. 7-17). The Puritan-Bennett Corporation makes a reusable type called the Slipstream for its IPPB circuits.

Many manufacturers produce disposable medication nebulizers for IPPB circuits or hand-held circuits. Most of these are sidestream nebulizers. Select the nebulizer that produces a particle size that matches the therapeutic target. Table 7-2 lists the particle sizes with their likely locations for impaction.

See Fig. 7-18 for a typical hand-held nebulizer circuit. The nebulizer can be powered by either air or oxygen. Typically, flows of 4 to 6 L/min are use to nebulize 3 to 5 ml of medication in about 10 minutes. The nebulizer finger control allows the patient to power the nebulizer by covering the open hole in the "T." Uncovering the hold permits the gas to exit and the medication is not nebulized and wasted. The reservoir tube serves to hold oxygen and medication for the next inspiration.

A concern has been raised recently about two risks to practitioners related to using

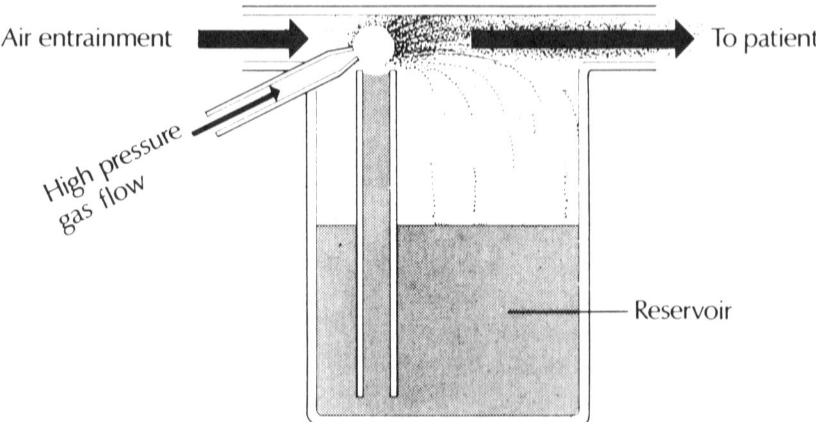

Fig. 7-16 Mainstream medication nebulizer. (From Shapiro BA, Harrison RA, Kacmarek, RM, et al: *Clinical Application of Respiratory Care,* ed 3. Chicago, Mosby, 1985. Used by permission.)

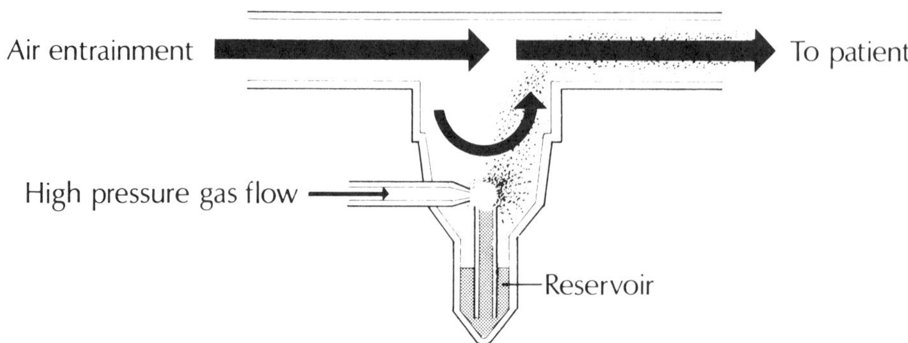

Fig. 7-17 Sidestream medication nebulizer. (From Shapiro BA, Harrison RA, Kacmarek, RM, et al: *Clinical Application of Respiratory Care,* ed 3. Chicago, Mosby, 1989. Used by permission.)

small-volume nebulizers. First, any aerosolized medications that escape into the room air may be inhaled. It is possible that the practitioner, or anyone else who happens be near, may have an allergic or other adverse reaction. Second, nebulized secretions from the patient's airway and lungs may be inhaled. This may place the practitioner or others at risk of acquiring a pulmonary infection from the patient. Although it is unlikely that many actual problems like this occur, it is a possibility. If either of these situations is a

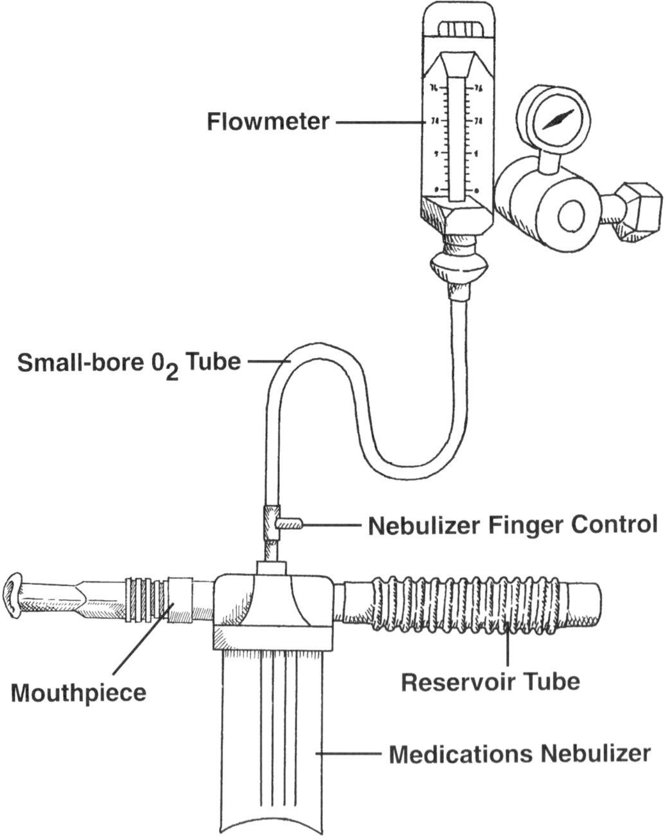

Fig. 7-18 Hand-held medication nebulizer circuit. (Adapted from Guidelines for disinfection of home equipment. *Respir Care* 1988; 33:801-808.)

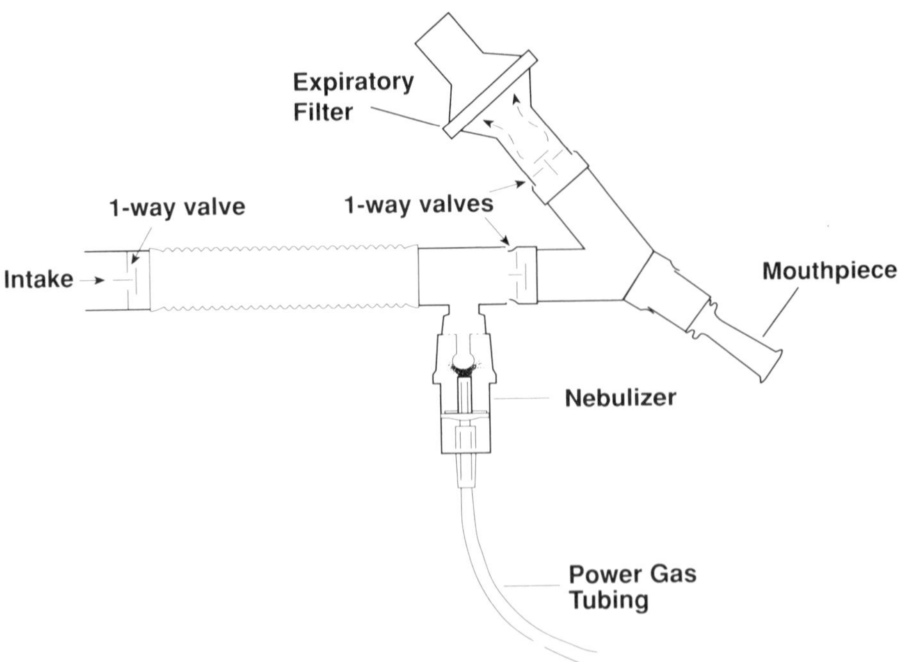

Fig. 7-19 Diagram of the Respirgard II nebulizer system shows one way valves and expiratory filter to scavenge exhaust aerosol. (From Rau Jr JL: *Respiratory Care Pharmacology,* ed 4. Chicago, Mosby, 1994. Used by permission.)

concern, a small small-volume nebulizer with a downstream particle filter should be used. This filter will trap any exhaled aerosol droplets.

Marquest Medical Products, Inc., manufactures the original Respirgard and newer Respirgard II Nebulizer System (Fig. 7-19). They have been recommended for use when nebulizing pentamidine isethionate (Pentam). Flows of 5 to 7 L/min are used, and the particle size is small enough to reach the alveolar level. The system is different from traditional small-volume nebulizers in that it has three one-way valves and an exhalation side filter. This ensures that the patient breathes in the medication and that none escapes to the room air. Although designed for nebulizing pentamidine, it could be used for any other antibiotic or medication that should not contaminate the room air. More recently Cadema has manufactured the AeroTech II. Although it differs in basic design from the Respirgard II, it also features one-way valves and an exhalation side filter to prevent any aerosolized particles from reaching room air. Either could be used to ensure that room air contamination is prevented.

If any small-volume nebulizer fails to generate an aerosol, make sure that the jet and capillary tube are not plugged with debris. Sometimes they can be cleared by running them under water or pushing a needle through the channel. Do not use a nebulizer that does not generate an aerosol.

(2) SPAG II (Small-Particle Aerosol Generator

The original SPAG and newer SPAG II are produced by ICN Pharmaceuticals (Fig. 7-20). It generates a particle with a mass median aerodynamic diameter of 1.2 to 1.3 μm for deep deposition. They are used to nebulize ribavirin (Virazol). The medication is used to treat the respiratory syncytial virus that can cause a serious pneumonia in neonates. The usual treatment time is about 6 hours. The nebulizer is designed to be used with an

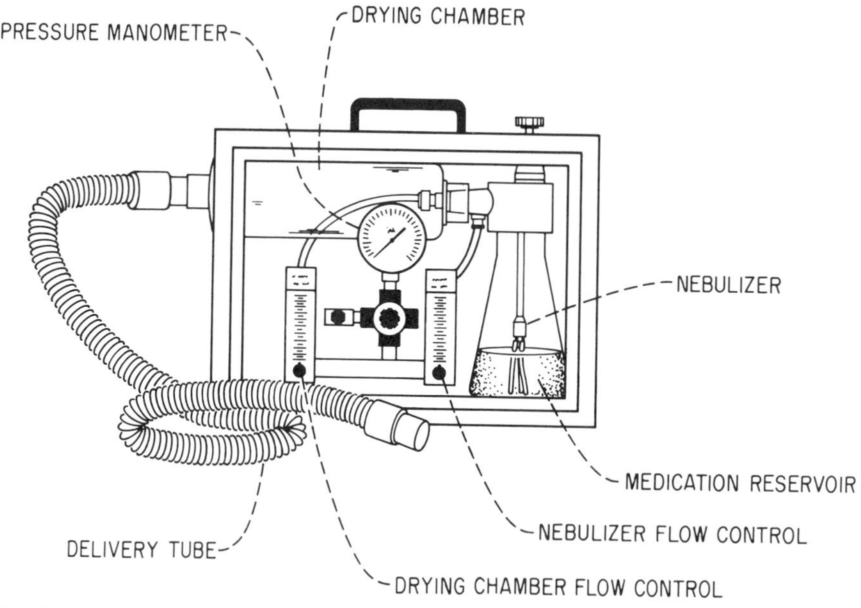

Fig. 7-20 SPAG (small-particle aerosol generator) unit. (From Scanlan CL: Humidity and aerosol therapy, in Scanlan Cl, Spearman CB, Sheldon RL [eds]: *Egan's Fundamentals of Respiratory Care,* ed 5. St Louis, Mosby, 1990. Used by permission.)

infant hood or other open system. Some practitioners have adapted the SPAG II so that the medication can be delivered to infants on mechanical ventilators.

(3) Metered Dose Inhalers (MDIs)

MDIs are designed to dispense a premeasured amount of medication. Each activation increases the amount of medication that is taken by the patient. There are two main types of MDIs: dry powder and Freon powered.

(a) Dry powder inhalers (DPIs)

(i) Get the necessary equipment for the procedure (IIA14) [R, Ap]

(ii) Put the equipment together, make sure that it works properly, and identify and fix any problems with it. (IIB13) [R, Ap]

These inhalers dispense a dry medicinal powder into the patient's airways and lungs when he or she inhales deeply. The medicine is held in a plastic capsule until released. The device is designed to open the capsule and allow it to be inhaled by the patient. The drug manufacturer sells both the medication and the dispenser to the patient. At this writing only three medications and their DPI units can be obtained, as discussed later on. However, it is likely that others will become available in the future.

The Spinhaler is used to pierce the gelatin capsule holding cromolyn sodium (Intal and Aarane) and dispense it into the patient's airway. As the patient inhales rapidly (flow rates of 40-100 L/min are needed), the plastic rotor blades spray the powder into the inhaled stream of air. The patient should inhale as deeply as possible and hold the breath for at least 10 seconds for maximum deposition in the small airways and alveoli. Care must be taken to hold the unit upright when the capsule is pierced and the powder is inhaled or it will spill (Fig. 7-21). Cromolyn sodium is used to prevent the onset of an asthma attack and is useless after an attack has begun.

The Rotahaler is designed to break in half a capsule containing a powdered form of either albuterol (Proventil or Ventolin) or beclomethasone dipropionate (Vanceril). Albuterol is a sympathomimetic bronchodilator, and beclomethasone is a corticosteroid. Care must be taken with the Rotahaler to hold it horizontally after the capsule has been broken, or the medication will spill out. A fast inhalation with a breath hold is recommended to deliver the medication to the airways and lungs.

Some practice is needed is using both units. The two main pieces must be unscrewed so that the capsule can be placed in the holding chamber. With the Spinhaler the plastic slide must be moved up and down once to pierce the capsule. With the Rotahaler the mouthpiece is twisted around to break open the capsule. The medication is then forcefully inhaled. Unscrew both units to remove the empty capsule.

(b) Freon-powered inhalers and spacers

(i) Get the necessary equipment for the procedure. (IIA14) [R, Ap]

(ii) Put the equipment together, make sure that it works properly, and identify and fix any problems with it. (IIB13) [R, Ap]

Many pharmaceutical companies have developed a Freon gas–powered metered dose inhaler device to dispense the medication to the patient. All of the devices operate in the same way. They have several milliliters of medication and Freon (or another compressed inert gas) contained inside of a metal container with a built-in jet nozzle. A plastic actuator opens the jet when pressed into the container (Fig. 7-22). The patient can inhale the medication through the built-in mouthpiece. Also, there are adapters so that the medication can be sprayed into a mechanical ventilator circuit or through a bronchoscopy adapter to an endotracheal tube. A specific amount of medication is nebulized with each actuation of the device. The metering chamber is filled with medicine by tipping it over and back upright. Patients should be instructed to wash the actuator out daily to keep the aerosol channel open and the unit clean.

THE SPINHALER TURBO-INHALER

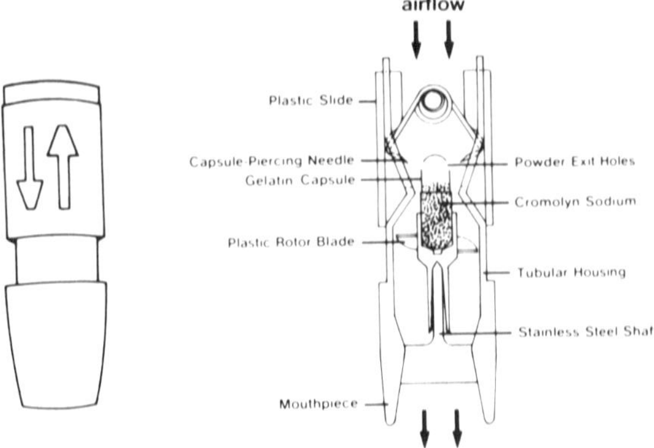

Fig. 7-21 Sketch of the Spinhaler device used for inhalation of the dry powder form of cromolyn sodium. (From Rau Jr JL: *Respiratory Care Pharmacology,* ed 3. Chicago, Mosby, 1989. Used by permission.)

MDI AUXILIARY DEVICES

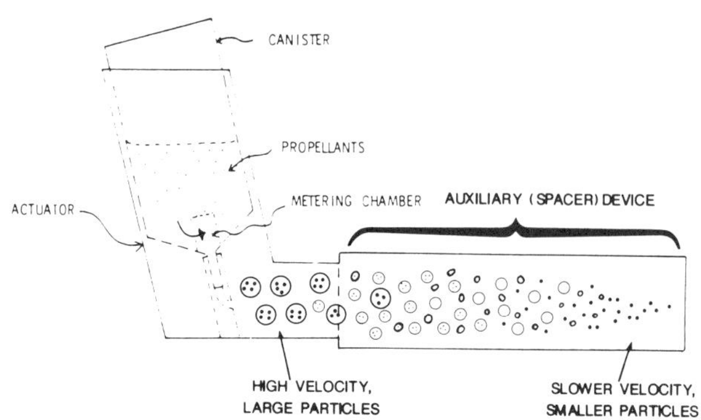

Fig. 7-22 The effect of an extension device on aerosol particle size and velocity from a Freon-powered metered dose inhaler. (From Rau Jr JL: *Respiratory Care Pharmacology,* ed 3. Chicago, Mosby, 1989. Used by permission.)

It has been shown that the addition to some sort of spacer between the actuator and the patient's mouth increases the amount of medication that is inhaled. These devices slow the aerosol down so that less impacts on the back of the throat. Also, the patient is better able to coordinate the breath with the actuator spraying the medication. Some of the spacers have a built-in whistle that sounds if the patient is inhaling too quickly (see Fig. 7-22 and 7-23). Some spacers are designed to fit with only one actuator. Others will adapt to fit to any actuator.

Patients must be instructed to wash out any of these medication dispensers on a daily basis. Warm, soapy water and a thorough rinsing are usually adequate for home use. However, a disinfecting liquid such as Cidex is preferable if the patient can afford it.

Module C. Coached patient breathing patterns. (IIIF5d) [R, Ap]

1. Upper airway deposition.

Particles 10 μm or larger are more likely to impact on the upper airway when the patient is coached to:

a. Inhale at a normal or faster speed. The flow should be greater than 30 L/min.
b. Inhale a normal tidal volume.
c. Breathe in a normal pattern.

2. Lower airway and alveolar deposition.

Particles 2 to 5 μ are more likely to deposit on the smaller airways and in the alveoli when the patient is coached to:

a. Inhale at a slow speed. The flow should be less than 30 L/min.
b. Inhale an inspiratory capacity.
c. Hold the full breath in for 10 seconds if possible before exhaling.

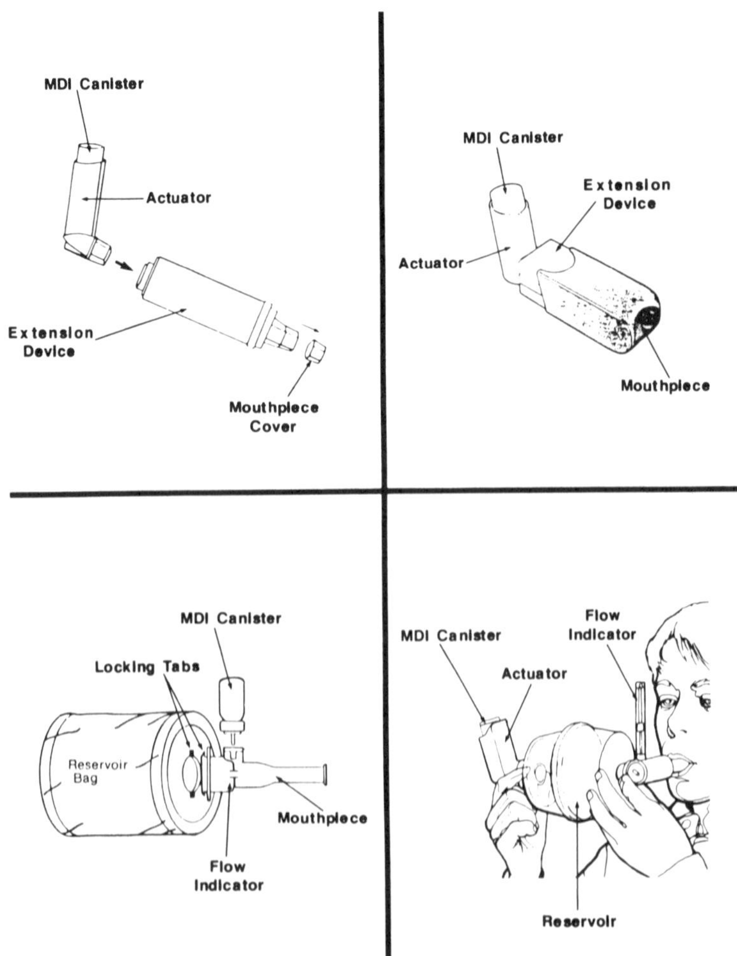

Fig. 7-23 Representative spacer devices. Clockwise, from upper left: Monaghan Aero-chamber, Giegy Breathancer, InspirEase and Inhal-Aid (both from Key Pharmaceuticals). (From Rau Jr JL: *Respiratory Care Pharmacology,* ed 3. Chicago, Mosby, 1989. Used by permission.)

Obviously, all patients will not be able to perform these techniques perfectly, but to the extent that they can, the medication will be deposited where it is needed and the treatment will be more effective.

This ends the general discussion on humidity and aerosol therapy. The entry level examination will include *direct* questions over this material and include it in other questions that relate to gas therapy and mechanical ventilation. In general, Section 1 and the previous discussion cover Module D.

Module D. Patient assessment.

1. Determine and continue to monitor how the patient responds to the treatment or procedure.

The patient with a secretion problem should be helped by the addition of an aerosol or medication and better able to clear them out effectively. This should result in the patient feeling better, as well as having improved vital signs, oxygenation, breath sounds, and spirometry values.

The use of aerosol therapy can cause bronchospasm in some asthmatic patients. Patients with thick, dry secretions can have their airways occluded if aerosol therapy causes the secretions to take in water and swell. The patient must be able to cough out the thinned secretions, or suctioning equipment must be available to remove them.

2. Modify the treatment or procedure and recommend any changes in the patient's respiratory care plan, depending on the response.

a. Change the type of equipment being used. (IIIF5a) [R, Ap]

Be prepared to change the type of humidity and aerosol delivery system from among those discussed in this section based on the patient's condition. Review the indications, contraindications, uses, and limitations of the various systems.

b. Adjust the temperature of the liquid being used in the equipment. (IIIF5c) [R, Ap]

In general, a cool humidity or aerosol system is used with patients with the following conditions:

a. Pediatric croup
b. Upper airway irritation such as after extubation or a bronchoscopy procedure

In general, a body temperature humidity or aerosol system is used with patients with the following conditions:

a. Bypassed upper airway
b. Viscous secretions
c. Hypothermia
d. Neonate to maintain a neutral thermal environment

c. Change the output of aerosol by the equipment. (IIIF5e) [R, Ap]

Neonates are sensitive to overhydration. Long-term aerosol therapy for them should be avoided or minimized. Adult patients with heart failure or pulmonary edema should also not be given long-term aerosol therapy. Instead, a Cascade-type humidifier can be used.

The adult patient who has viscous secretions may be aided by long-term aerosol therapy of a dense mist at body temperature. The secretions will often be liquified and made easier to cough or suction out. An ultrasonic nebulizer is often used for this purpose. The child with croup is usually given a dense mist of a cool bland aerosol in a mist tent. This therapy is usually needed for only a few days. Be wary of fluid overload if the mist is needed for a longer period.

BIBLIOGRAPHY

AARC Aerosol Consensus Statement—1991. *Respir Care* 1991; 36:916-921.

AARC Clinical Practice Guideline: Selection of aerosol delivery device. *Respir Care* 1992; 37:891-897.

ARRC Clinical Practice Guideline: Bland aerosol administration. *Respir Care* 1993; 38:1196-1200.

Dolovich M: Clinical aspects of aerosol physics. *Respir Care* 1991; 36:931-938.

Eubanks DH, Bone RC: *Comprehensive Respiratory Care*, ed 2, St Louis, Mosby, 1990.

Fuller HD, Dolovich MB, Posmituck G, et al: Pressurized aerosol versus jet aerosol delivery to mechanically ventilated patients: comparison of dose to the lungs. *Am Rev Respir Dis* 1990; 141:440-444.

Helmholz Jr HF, Burton GG: Applied humidity and aerosol therapy, in Burton GG, Hodgkin JE (eds): *Respiratory Care—a Guide to Clinical Practice*, ed 2. Philadelphia, Lippincott, 1984.

Hess D: The delivery of aersolized bronchodilator to mechanically ventilated intubated adult patients. *Respir Care* 1990; 35:399-404.

Kacmarek RM, Hess D: The interface between patient and aerosol generator. *Respir Care* 1991; 36:952-976.

Krider TM, Meyer R, Syvertsen WA: *Master Guide for Passing the Respiratory Care Credentialing Exams*, ed 2. Clairmont, Calif, Education Resource Consortium, 1989.

Manufacturer's literature on the AeroVent, Monaghan Medical Corporation, Plattsburg, NY.

Manufacturer's literature on the Respirgard II. Marquest Medical Products, Englewood, Colo.

McPherson SP: *Respiratory Therapy Equipment*, ed 4. St Louis, Mosby, 1990.

Op't Holt T: Aerosol generators and humidifiers, in Barnes TA (ed): *Respiratory Care Practice*, Chicago, Mosby, 1988.

Rau Jr RL: Humidity and aerosol therapy, in Barnes TA: (ed): *Respiratory Care Practice*, Chicago, Mosby, 1988.

Rau JR JL: *Respiratory Care Pharmacology*, ed 3. Chicago, Mosby, 1989.

Scanlan CL: Humidity and aerosol therapy, in Scanlan CL, Spearman CB, Sheldon RL (eds): *Egan's Fundamentals of Respiratory Care*, ed 5. St Louis, Mosby, 1990.

Shapiro BA, Harrison RA, Kacmarek RM, et al: *Clinical Application of Respiratory Care*, ed 3. Chicago, Mosby, 1989.

Vinciguerra C, Smaldone G: Treatment time and patient tolerance for pentamidine delivery by Respirgard II and AeroTech II. *Respir Care* 1990; 35:1037-1041.

SELF-STUDY QUESTIONS

1. A patient's humidity deficit is going to be the *smallest* under which the following conditions:
   A. Breathing in regular hospital room air at 72° F and 40% relative humidity.
   B. Breathing in outside air at −10° F
   C. Breathing in outside air at 80° F and 50% relative humidity
   D. Breathing in 6 L/min of oxygen through a nasal cannula running through an unheated bubble humidifier
   E. Breathing in 5 L/min of oxygen through a cascade-type humidifier at 95° F to an aerosol mask

2. An ultrasonic nebulizer works by which of the following principles or actions?
   A. Vibration
   B. Bernoulli's
   C. Venturi's
   D. Hydronamic
   E. Air entrainment

3. Your patient has an endotracheal tube. Which of the following devices would be the *least* effective in reducing this patient's humidity deficit?
   A. Wick-type humidifier set at 35° C
   B. Cascade-type humidifier set at 35° C

C. Unheated bubble-type humidifier
D. Ultrasonic nebulizer
E. Heated air entrainment nebulizer

4. Your patient has a temperature of 98.6° F. To saturate the inhaled air, how much absolute humidity must be provided?
   A. 37° C
   B. 47 mm Hg
   C. 760 mm Hg
   D. 44 mg/L
   E. 1034 cm H_2O

5. Your heated humidifier unit has a water reservoir temperature of 40° C. The humidified gas is traveling through large-bore tubing to the patient. Which of the following statements are true?
   I. Condensation will occur.
   II. The gas will warm and expand as it travels to the patient.
   III. The gas will remain saturated.
   IV. The relative humidity will decrease.
   V. The relative humidity will increase.
   A. II
   B. I, III
   C. IV
   D. V
   E. I, IV

6. The pop-off valve is whistling on your patient's bubble humidifier to a 28% oxygen, air entrainment mask. What could be the problem?
   A. The reservoir jar is not screwed tightly into the top.
   B. The air entrainment mask should be set at 24% oxygen.
   C. The small-bore tubing is pinched.
   D. The air entrainment mask should be set at 35% oxygen.
   E. The water level is too low.

7. Complications of aerosol therapy include all of the following *except:*
   A. Decreased humidity deficit
   B. Aerosol-induced bronchospasm
   C. Fluid overload in the infant
   D. Swollen secretions causing an increase in the work of breathing
   E. Possible patient contamination if the reservoir water is infected

8. Your patient's air entrainment nebulizer is not putting out as much aerosol as it was a short time ago. To correct the problem, you would check which of the following:
   I. Make sure that the water level is correct.
   II. Make sure the hydronamic valve is patent.
   III. Make sure the jet is patent.
   IV. Make sure the oxygen can flow *down* the capillary tube.
   V. Make sure the water can flow *up* the capillary tube.
   A. I, II
   B. I, III, IV
   C. II, IV
   D. I, III, V
   E. III, IV, V

9. Which of the following would you recommend to add moisture to your infant patient's oxygen hood?
   A. Unheated bubble humidifier
   B. Heated large-reservoir nebulizer
   C. Cascade- or wick-type heated humidifier
   D. Unheated large-reservoir nebulizer
   E. Hydrosphere nebulizer

10. Your patient's airway has just been extubated and shows signs of laryngeal edema. What size particle generator would you recommend to treat the problem?
    A. 20 to 50 μm
    B. 10 to 20 μm
    C. 4 to 6 μm
    D. 1 to 3 μm
    E. Smaller than 1 μm

11. Your DeVilbiss ultrasonic nebulizer has a flashing couplant indicator light. You notice that the output has decreased from what it was earlier. The most likely problem is:
    A. Too much water in the solution cup
    B. Too much water in the couplant chamber
    C. Not enough water in the solution cup
    D. Not enough water in the couplant chamber
    E. Loose electrical cable

12. You notice that water has collected at the low point of the large-bore tubing of your patient's heated aerosol system. The aerosol is "puffing" out of the end of the tubing. Your reaction should be to:
    A. Keep it as it is because it is operating normally.
    B. Add water to the reservoir jar.
    C. Empty water from the reservoir jar.
    D. Empty the water from the large-bore tubing into a waste water jar.
    E. Empty the water from the large-bore tubing into the reservoir jar so that it is not wasted.

13. Saturated air at body temperature would have which of the following characteristics?
    I. 40% relative humidity
    II. 100% relative humidity
    III. 47 mm Hg vapor pressure
    IV. 44 mm Hg vapor pressure
    V. 44 mg/L absolute humidity
    A. II, IV
    B. II, III, V
    C. I, III, V
    D. I, IV
    E. II, III, V

14. It is best to coach your patient to breathe in the following pattern for particle deposition in lower airways and alveoli:
    I. Inhale a tidal volume.
    II. Inhale rapidly.
    III. Inhale an inspiratory capacity.
    IV. Hold the breath in for 10 to 15 seconds before exhaling.
    V. Inhale at a slow speed

A. I, II
B. III, IV, V
C. I, V
D. II, III
E. I, II, IV

Answer Key:

1. E; 2. A; 3. C; 4. D; 5. B; 6. C; 7. A; 8. D; 9. C; 10. B; 11. D; 12. D; 13. E; 14. B.

8 Pharmacology

Module A. Recommend or administer the following types of aerosolized medications.

The wording in the National Board of Respiratory Care's (NBRC's) examination content outline is vague as to what specific categories of medications will be tested on the entry level examination. Only a few classes of medications are specified. The aerosolized bronchodilators, saline solutions, mucolytics, and cromolyn sodium are the only exclusively inhaled medications tested on the entry level self-assessment examination versions II, III, and IV. They are discussed in some detail in this text. Note that the entry level self-assessment examination version IV has three questions that together include the following medications: cortisone, ampicillin, atropine, furosemide (Lasix), phenobarbitol, theophylline (Aminophylline), succinylcholine (Anectine), and pancuronium (Pavulon). It seems apparent that the NBRC expects examinees to have a general understanding of the effects of a wide variety of medications that may be used in the patient population. However, it has not tested over such detailed information as dosages, indications, and contraindications on these or other medications. The wise learner will attempt to gain a broader understanding of medications beyond those that are directly administered by respiratory care practitioners.

A study of the NBRC's examination content outline for the written registry examination shows the following medications are tested at that level: vasoconstrictors, vasodilators, inotropic agents, antibiotics, sedatives, analgesics, respiratory stimulants, diuretics, artificial surfactants, and nicotine therapy agents.

1. Bronchodilators.

a. Recommend their use. (IIIF9d) [R, Ap, An]

b. Administer the prescribed medication. (IIIB2g and IIIC4) [R, Ap]

The aerosolized bronchodilators are medications designed to relax the bronchial muscles so that the airways dilate, airway resistance is reduced, and breathing is easier. This group of medications is often called sympathomimetic amines or sympathomimetic bronchodilators. They have the effect of stimulating the body's sympathetic nerves, which results in bronchodilation and other effects.

A brief review of the autonomic nervous system will help in understanding how these medications work and some side effects to look out for. The autonomic nervous system is not under voluntary control. It is an automatic system designed to regulate metabolism and the vital signs. It is made up of two branches: the sympathetic nervous system and the parasympathetic nervous system. The lungs, heart, and most other organs are innervated by both branches. The blood vessels in the mucous membranes are innervated only by the sympathetic branch. The parasympathetic nervous system is usually dominant and keeps the body functioning normally. The sympathetic nervous system is an "emergency" system that is dominant in times of great stress. It is sometimes called the "fight or flight" system. Adrenaline (or epinephrine) is released by the adrenal glands in these emergencies. Adrenaline causes a number of effects, including the one that many of our patient's need: bronchodilation. The sympathetic nervous system has the following three different types of receptors that are located in different organs and are affected by adrenaline:

1. The α_1-receptors (alpha$_1$) are located in the blood vessels of the mucous membranes (and other tissues not of interest to us in this discussion). Vasoconstriction results when these are stimulated.
2. The β_1-receptors (beta$_1$) are located in the heart. Tachycardia, increased stroke volume, and possibly dysrhythmias result when they are stimulated.
3. The β_2-receptors (beta$_2$) are located in the airways. Bronchodilation results when these are stimulated.

Aerosolized bronchodilators are usually recommended under one of the three following situations:

Acute Bronchospasm With Severe Shortness of Breath

This patient is in need of rapid relief. Recommend a fast-acting medication such as isoetharine (Bronkosol or Bronkometer). The other catacholamines are less desirable because of unnecessary α_1- and β_1-effects or longer onset and peak times. The resorsinols and saligenin classes also have longer onset and peak times.

Chronic But Stable Bronchospasm With Moderate Shortness of Breath

These patients are in need of a dependable medication of longer duration. This is especially true if the patient is planning to go home soon. Recommend bitolterol (Tornalate), terbutaline (Brethaire, Brethine, and Bricanyl), albuterol (Proventil and Ventolin), or metaproterenol (Alupent and Metaprel) by aerosol. Terbutaline and albuterol also come in oral preparations. All of these medications have a longer duration of action than isoetharine so that fewer treatments are needed.

The medication nebulizer and breathing pattern to treat bronchospasm are discussed in detail in Section 7. To summarize:

1. Use a nebulizer that generates particles 2 to 5 μm.
2. Use a spacer on a metered dose inhaler (MDI).
3. Have the patient inhale an inspiratory capacity.
4. Have the patient inhale slowly (<30 L/min, or 0.5 L/sec).
5. Have the patient hold his or her breath in for 10 seconds, if possible.

Treatment of the Patient With Laryngeal Edema

This type of problem requires the administration of a medication that will reduce the swelling of the mucosa of the larynx and epiglottis. Racemic epinephrine (MicroNefrin, Vaponefrin, and AsthmaNefrin) is the medication of choice because it stimulates α_1-receptors. This results in vasoconstriction of the mucosal blood vessels. Because of this the swelling is reduced, the patient's airway is enlarged, and breathing is easier.

The medication nebulizer and breathing pattern to treat laryngeal edema are discussed in detail in Section 7. To summarize:

1. Use a nebulizer that generates particles 10 μm or larger.
2. Have the patient inhale a normal tidal volume.
3. Have the patient inhale at a normal or faster speed (>30 L/min, or 0.5 L/sec).
4. Have the patient breathe in a normal pattern.

Most of the medications listed in this section are chemically derived from adrenaline. They are somewhat different in their structures so that the desired effects and side (unwanted) effects vary. See Table 8-1 for the side effects of the aerosolized bronchodilators. Clinically the most dangerous of these side effects are palpitations, tachycardia, and hypertension.

There are three different classes of aerosolized bronchodilators based on their chemical structures. The following medications are grouped by their respective classes. The information listed is not meant to be a comprehensive description of each medication. Refer to the *Physicians' Desk Reference*, the drug producer's literature, or other authoritative source for complete information.

Catecholamine

A. Epinephrine (Adrenalin)
   1. Cardiopulmonary indications: bronchospasm, mucosal congestion, and restoring the heart's rhythm in a cardiac arrest situation except when caused by cardiac failure.
   2. Contraindications/warnings/precautions: cardiovascular disease, hypertension, congestive heart failure, diabetes, and hyperthyroidism.
   3. Administration method, strength, and dosage: see Table 8-2.
   4. Receptor site, onset, peak, and duration: see Table 8-3.
   5. Miscellaneous: Broken down by exposure to light, heat, and oxygen. Do not use if pink or brown or contains a precipitate. This medication stimulates α-, β_1-, and β_2-receptors about equally. Tachycardia and other cardiac effects can be expected. Repeated use of the medication can result in β-receptor blockade from a metabolic by-product. If this happens, use of the medication must be stopped and another substituted.

Table 8-1. Clinically Observed Side Effects of Sympathomimetic Aerosolized Bronchodilators From the Most Commonly Seen to the Least Commonly Seen

1. Tremor—gentle, uncontrollable, involuntary muscle shaking
2. Palpitations and tachycardia—irregular heart beats and fast heart rate
3. Headache
4. Increased blood pressure—possibly from both the α_1-effect on blood vessels and tachycardia
5. Nervousness and irritability
6. Dizziness
7. Nausea
8. Decreased Pa_{O_2}* level from a worsening of the ventilation/perfusion ratio

*Pa_{O_2}, Arterial oxygen pressure.

Table 8-2. Dosages and Strengths Used for Various Methods of Administering Beta-Adrenergic Bronchodilators

Drug	Brand Names	Administration Method	Strength	Dosage
Epinephrine	Adrenalin	Nebulizer	1:100 (1%)	0.25-0.5 ml qid
Racemic epinephrine	MicroNefrin Vaponefrin AsthmaNefrin	Nebulizer	2.25%	0.25-0.5 ml qid
Isoproterenol	Isuprel	Nebulizer	1:200 (0.5%)	0.25-0.5 ml qid
	Isuprel Mistometer	MDI	131 μg/puff	1-2 puffs qid
Isoetharine	Bronkosol	Nebulizer	1%	0.25-0.5 ml qid
	Bronkometer	MDI	340 μg/spray	1-2 puffs qid
Metaproterenol	Alupent	Nebulizer	5%	0.3 ml tid, qid
	Metaprel	MDI	0.65 mg/puff	2-3 puffs q4h
		Tablets	10, 20 mg	20 mg tid, qid
		Syrup	10 mg/5 ml	10 mg tid, qid
Terbutaline	Brethaire	MDI	0.2 mg/puff	2 puffs q4-6h
	Brethine	Injection	1 mg/ml	0.25 mg SC
	Bricanyl	Tablets	2.5, 5 mg	2.5 or 5 mg tid
Albuterol	Proventil	Nebulizer	0.5%	0.5 ml tid, qid
	Ventolin	MDI	90 μg/puff	2 puffs tid, qid
		DPI	200 μg/caps.	1 caps. q4-6h
		Tablets	2, 4 mg	2 or 4 mg tid, qid
		Extended-release tablet	4 mg	q12h
		Syrup	2 mg/5 ml	2 or 4 mg tid, qid
Bitolterol (colterol)	Tornalate	MDI	0.37 mg/puff	2 puffs q8h
		Nebulizer	0.2%	1.25 ml tid or as ordered
Pirbuterol	Maxair	MDI	0.2 mg/puff	2 puffs q4-6h

From Rau JL: *Respiratory Care Pharmacology,* ed 4. Chicago, Mosby, 1994. Used by permission.

B. Racemic epinephrine (MicroNefrin, Vaponephrine, and AsthmaNefrin)
   1. Cardiopulmonary indications: bronchospasm, mucosal edema, laryngeal edema, laryngotracheobronchitis (LTB or pediatric croup).
   2. Contraindications/warnings/precautions: cardiovascular disease, hypertension, congestive heart failure, diabetes, and hyperthyroidism.
   3. Administration method, strength, and dosage: see Table 8-3.
   4. Receptor site, onset, peak, and duration: see Table 8-3.
   5. Miscellaneous: Broken down by exposure to light, heat, and oxygen. Do not use if pink or brown or contains a precipitate. Racemic epinephrine has about half of the effects of epinephrine in all three receptor sites. It is the drug of choice for treating laryngeal edema and croup because of its ability to shrink the mucous membrane with only a moderate increase in the heart rate.

C. Isoproterenol (Isuprel and Mistometer)
   1. Cardiopulmonary indications: bronchospasm, bradycardia.
   2. Contraindications/warnings/precautions: preexisting tachycardia, transient hypertension, palpitations, coronary insufficiency, diabetes, and hyperthyroidism.
   3. Administration method, strength, and dosage: see Table 8-2.
   4. Receptor site, onset, peak, and duration: see Table 8-2.
   5. Miscellaneous: broken down by exposure to light, heat, and oxygen. Do not use if pink or brown or contains a precipitate. This medication is the most powerful stimulator of β_1- and β_2-receptors available. It has fallen out of favor as a bronchodilator because of the problems of tachycardia and palpitations.

Table 8-3. Receptor Preference and Basic Pharmacokinetics of the β-Adrenergic Bronchodilators

Drug	Receptor	Onset (min)	Route*	Peak (min)	Duration (hr)
Noncatecholamine					
Ephedrine	α + β†	15-60	PO	2‡	3-5
Catecholamines					
Epinephrine	α + β	3-5	INH	5-20	1-3
		6-15	SC		
Isoproterenol	β	2-5	INH	5-30	½-2
Isoetharine	β_2	1-6	INH	15-60	1-3
Bitolterol	β_2	3-4	INH	30-60	5-8
Resorcinol					
Metaproterenol	β_2	1-5	INH	60	2-6
		15-30	PO		
Terbutaline	β_2	5-30	INH	30-60	3-6
		6-15	SC	30-60	1½-4
		30	PO	2-4‡	4-8
Saligenin					
Albuterol	β_2	15	INH	30-60	3-8
		30	PO	1-2‡	4-6
Other					
Pirbuterol	β_2	5	INH	30	5

From Rau JL: *Respiratory Care Pharmacology*, ed 4. Chicago, Mosby, 1994. Used by permission.
**PO,* orally; *INH,* inhalation; *SC,* subcutaneously.
†β, Beta nonspecific, β_1 and β_2 receptors.
‡Hours.

Repeated use of the medication can result in β-receptor blockade from a metabolic by-product. If this happens, use of the medication must be stopped and another substituted.

D. Isoetharine (Bronkosol and Bronkometer)
   1. Cardiopulmonary indication: bronchospasm.
   2. Contraindications/warnings/precautions: same as earlier. Problems are rare because this and the following medications are almost specifically pure β_2-receptor stimulators. The vital signs must still be monitored.
   3. Administration method, strength, and dosage: see Table 8-2.
   4. Receptor site, onset, peak, and duration: see Table 8-2.
   5. Miscellaneous: broken down by exposure to light, heat, and oxygen. Do not use if pink or brown or contains a precipitate. Its fast onset and peak make it a drug of choice for the patient suffering from acute, severe bronchospasm.

E. Bitolterol (colterol, Tornalate)
   1. Cardiopulmonary indications: bronchospasm.
   2. Contraindications/warnings/precautions: same as earlier.
   3. Administration method, strength, and dosage: see Table 8-2.
   4. Receptor site, onset, peak, and duration: see Table 8-3.
   5. Miscellaneous: This medication must be metabolically altered to its active state. The peak effect is delayed because of this. It is one of the aerosol drugs of choice for the stable patient because it has the longest duration of any sympathomimetic bronchodilator.

Resorcinol

A. Metaproterenol (Alupent and Metaprel)
   1. Cardiopulmonary indication: bronchospasm.

2. Contraindications/warnings/precautions: same as earlier.
3. Administration method, strength, and dosage: see Table 8-2.
4. Receptor site, onset, peak, and duration: see Table 8-3.
5. Miscellaneous: This medication can be taken orally in prepared forms.

B. Terbutaline (Brethaire, Brethine, and Bricanyl)
1. Cardiopulmonary indication: bronchospasm.
2. Contraindications/warnings/precautions: Same as earlier.
3. Administration method, strength, and dosage: see Table 8-2.
4. Receptor site, onset, peak, and duration: see Table 8-3.
5. Miscellaneous: It is twice as potent a bronchodilator as metaproterenol. It can be taken orally in prepared forms. This is one of two drugs of choice when a long duration of action is needed and the options of an aerosol or oral preparation are clinically desirable.

Saligenin

A. Albuterol (Proventil and Ventolin)
1. Cardiopulmonary indication: bronchospasm.
2. Contraindications/warnings/precautions: Same as earlier.
3. Administration method, strength, and dosage: see Table 8-2.
4. Receptor site, onset, peak, and duration: see Table 8-3.
5. Miscellaneous: It can be taken orally in prepared forms. This is one of two drugs of choice when a long duration of action is needed and the options of an aerosol or oral preparation are clinically desirable.

2. Corticosteroids.
a. Recommend their use. (IIIF9d) [R, Ap, An]
b. Administer the prescribed medication. (IIIB2g and IIIC4) [R, Ap]

Corticosteroids are a class of hormone that are produced by the cortex of the adrenal gland. They have a wide variety of effects. Corticosteroids affect the respiratory system in two ways. First, they potentiate the effects of the sympathomimetic agents. The patient who is diagnosed with status asthmaticus should have systemic corticosteroids promptly given by the intravenous route. Second, they stop the inflammatory response seen in the airways of asthmatics after exposure to an allergen. This prevents mucosal edema from developing. The patient with chronic airflow obstruction such as mild asthma or asthmatic bronchitis should be given inhaled corticosteroids. When they are used as directed, there is little systemic (bodily) absorption.

These drugs can be lifesavers if use properly. However, chronic use of large oral or intravenous doses can lead to serious systemic complications such as immunosuppression and adrenal gland insufficiency. The patient who is using inhaled corticosteroids must gargle and rinse out his or her mouth after each use of the MDI. If not, the patient runs the risk of developing a fungal infection of the mouth and throat. Fungal species include *Candida albicans*, which causes oral candidiasis (oral thrush), and *Aspergillus niger*. Commonly used inhaled corticosteroids include beclomethasone dipropionate (Beclovent and Vanceril), triamcinolone acetonide (Azmacort), flunisolide (Aerobid), and dexamethasone sodium (Decadron Respihaler).

All of these medications have similar beneficial affects, as discussed earlier. They all are given by a Freon-powered metered dose inhaler. See Table 8-4 for specific strength and dosage information. The best patient breathing pattern for this type of MDI was discussed earlier. An advantage of giving these medications by the inhalation route is that there are fewer systemic side effects than by the oral or intravenous route because there is little absorption into the general circulation. However, if a patient has been taking sys-

Table 8-4. Corticosteroids Available by Aerosol for Inhalation Administration

Drug	Strength	Dosage
Dexamethasone sodium phosphate (Decadron Respihaler)	84 μg/puff	Adults: 3 puffs tid or qid Children: 2 puffs tid or qid
Beclomethasone dipropionate (Beclovent, Vanceril)	42 μg/puff	Adults: 2 puffs tid or qid Children: 1-2 puffs tid or qid
Triamcinolone acetonide (Azmacort)	100 μg/puff	Adults: 2 puffs tid or qid Children: 1-2 puffs tid or qid
Flunisolide (Aerobid)	250 μg/puff	Adults: 2 puffs bid Children: 2 puffs bid

From Rau JL: *Respiratory Care Pharmacology,* ed 3. St Louis, Mosby, 1989. Used by permission.

temic corticosteroids for an extended time, they should be gradually weaned off of them after the inhaled corticosteroids have been started. It is dangerous to just stop an oral or intravenous corticosteroid that has been used for a prolonged time.

Examples of commonly used systemic corticosteroids include methylprednisolone (Medrol and Solu-Medrol), prednisone (Deltasone), prednisolone (Meticortelone and Delta-Cortef), cortisone (Cortone), and hydrocortisone (Cortef and Solu-Cortef). Generally these are used only if the patient is suffering from status asthmaticus or is not responding to inhaled corticosteroids.

3. Mucolytics.
a. Recommend their use. (IIIF9d) [R, Ap, An]
b. Administer the prescribed medication. (IIIB2g) [R, Ap]

The information listed is not meant to be a comprehensive description of each medication. Refer to the *Physicians' Desk Reference*, the drug producer's literature, or other authoritative source for complete information.

A. Acetylcysteine (Mucomyst)
   1. Cardiopulmonary indications: viscous mucus, mucus plugs.
   2. Contraindications/warnings/precautions: bronchospasm in asthmatic patients, nausea and vomiting from the bad odor (rotten eggs).
   3. Administration method, strength, and dosage:
      a. Hand-held nebulizer or intermittent positive-pressure breathing (IPPB): 3 to 5 ml of the 20% solution or 6 to 10 ml of the 10% solution. The 20% solution is often diluted with an equal volume of normal saline solution or 2% to 7.5% sodium bicarbonate. After three fourths of the original solution has been nebulized, add an equal volume of sterile water or the original diluent so that the medication is not too concentrated.
      b. Direct instillation into the trachea: 1 to 2 ml of either strength as often as hourly.
      c. Oxygen/mist tent: as much as needed of either strength to produce a heavy mist for the desired time period. As much as 300 ml in a single treatment period is reported.
   4. Site of effect: The disulfide bonds in mucus are chemically broken. This results in the mucus becoming less viscous. The bronchial/submucosal glands may also be stimulated to secrete more sol.
   5. Miscellaneous: It is often wise to either pretreat the patient with an aerosolized bronchodilator or mix one with the acetylcysteine before it is nebulized for the patient. Any bronchodilator can be used in the usual dose. The manufacturer recommends that all of the medication in a vial be used within 96 hours or discarded. It should be stored in the refrigerator. A slightly pur-

ple color is commonly seen after the vial has been opened; it can still be used safely.

B. Dornase alfa (Pulmozyme)

Pulmozyme has been approved for use in the treatment of patients with cystic fibrosis. It works by breaking up strands of DNA found in the secretions of patients with a pulmonary infection. Usually a single daily dose of 2.5 ml of solution (containing 2.5 mg of dornase alfa) is inhaled by small-volume nebulizer. Store the drug in a refrigerator and protect it from strong light. It has no serious side effects.

4. Saline solutions and water.
a. Recommend their use. (IIIF9d) [R, Ap, An]
b. Administer the prescribed medication. (IIIB2g and IIIC4) [R, Ap]

The various saline solutions and sterile water are known collectively as "bland" aerosols because they have no direct pharmacologic effect on the lungs and airways.

A. Saline solutions: normal saline, 0.9%; hypotonic saline, 0.45%; and hypertonic saline, 1.8% to 20%.
   1. Cardiopulmonary indications: irritated upper airway, liquifying secretions, and sputum induction.
   2. Contraindications/warnings/precautions: bronchospasm in asthmatic patients, irritated cough; avoid use in patients on a low-salt diet. Prolonged use of these solutions in aerosol form can lead to fluid overload in pediatric patients.
   3. Administration method, strength, and dosage: see Table 8-5.
   4. Site of effect: a vagally mediated reflex causes the bronchial/submucosal glands to secrete more sol when irritated by these aerosols.
   5. Miscellaneous: see Table 8-5. Many saline solutions come with a bacteriostatic agent added. These solutions should not be used for any sputum inductions because the bacteria will not grow.

Table 8-5. Saline Solutions Used as Mucolytics

Normal saline solution, 0.9% saline
- Direct instillation into the airway:
  - Infants may be given about 1 mL several times daily before suctioning.
  - Adults may be given about 3-5 ml several times daily before suctioning.
- Aerosol: Most medication nebulizers hold 3-5 ml that is nebulized several times daily.
- Miscellaneous:
  - Usually is well tolerated because it is isotonic to the body.
  - Particle size is fairly stable as nebulized.

Hypotonic saline solution, 0.45% saline
- Direct instillation into the airway: same as earlier.
- Aerosol: Same as earlier. Many practitioners use this concentration in ultrasonic nebulizers.
- Miscellaneous: Particles tend to shrink because of evaporation. This results in smaller particles than nebulized that are closer to isotonic. Impaction is more likely in the smaller airways.

Hypertonic saline solution, 1.8%-20% saline
- Aerosol: Some practitioners use a large-reservoir nebulizer with a heater to generate the aerosol.
  - Hypertonic saline solution is most commonly used to induce a cough and sputum sample for cytology (lung cancer) or fungal or mycobacteria (tuberculosis) culture. It should not be used for a general bacteria culture because the high salt concentration inhibits the growth of most bacteria.
- Miscellaneous:
  - Particles tend to enlarge because of the absorption of water vapor. This results in larger particles than nebulized that are closer to isotonic. Impaction is more likely in the upper airway.
  - This concentration is the most likely to cause bronchospasm in asthmatic patients because it is the farthest from isotonic and, therefore, the most irritating.

B. Sterile water
   1. Cardiopulmonary indications: humidification, irritated upper airway, liquifying secretions, and sputum induction.
   2. Contraindications/warnings/precautions: bronchospasm in asthmatic patients, irritated cough. Prolonged use in aerosol form can lead to fluid overload in pediatric patients.
   3. Administration method, strength, and dosage: most commonly used in large-reservoir humidifiers and air entraiment nebulizers to humidify dry medical gases. Sterile water is used as it comes from the manufacturer. Distilled, sterile water is not commonly used because it is very irritating.
   4. Site of effect: same as earlier.
   5. Miscellaneous: Water is the best overall mucolytic agent when given orally or intravenously. The surface goblet cells and bronchial/submucosal glands will maintain the proper consistency of mucus when the body and lungs are properly hydrated.

5. Cromolyn sodium (Intal and Aarane).
a. Recommend their use. (IIIF9d) [R, Ap, An]
b. Administer the prescribed medication. (IIIB2g and IIIC4) [R, Ap]

A. Cardiopulmonary indications: bronchial asthma. Exercise-induced asthma can be prevented in some patients if the medication is taken between 10 and 60 minutes before exercising.

B. Contraindications/warnings/precautions: status asthmaticus, coronary artery disease, or cardiac arrhythmias due to the propellant used in the inhaler; bronchospasm from inhaling the powder; throat irritation or dryness, bad taste, cough, and nausea.

C. Administration method, strength, and dosage:
   1. Spinhaler: 20-mg gelatin capsule. The usual dose for prevention of asthma is one capsule four times daily. The usual dose for prevention of exercise-induced asthma is one capsule 10 to 60 minutes before exercise. The Spinhaler device and the proper inhalation technique for deep deposition are described in Section 7.
   2. Medication nebulizer: 20 mg in 2 ml of water. Nebulizer particle sizes should be between 2 and 5 μm. The patient should use the same breathing pattern as with an inhaled sympathomimetic bronchodilator, as discussed earlier.
   3. MDI: 800 μg per actuation. The usual dose for prevention of asthma is two actuations four times daily. The usual dose for prevention of exercise-induced asthma is two actuations 10 to 60 minutes before exercise. The patient breathing is the same as with an inhaled sympathomimetic bronchodilator.

D. Site of effect: Mast cells in the airway are stabilized so that contact with an allergen will not cause an asthma attack.

E. Miscellaneous: The medication may have to be used for several weeks before it is proved to have any effect. If an asthma attack is in progress, cromolyn sodium is not effective. In fact, the powdered form should not be taken because it can be an airway irritant. Instead, rely on the sympathomimetic amines to treat the bronchospasm.

Note: A contraindication to these medications, or any medication, is a hypersensitivity or allergic reaction to it or any preservative or other included component of the medication.

Module B. Drug dosage calculations.

The NBRCs Examination Content Outline does not specifically list drug dosage calculations, and none has been tested on previous Entry Level Examinations. They are included here for the sake of completeness and understanding.

The problems will be easier to solve if the following are remembered:

a. One milliter = 1 cc = 1 g.

b. Most drug doses are listed in milligrams instead of grams. Convert grams to milligrams by moving the decimal point three places to the right (the same as multiplying by 1000). For example, 0.5 g equals 500 mg.

c. Know how to interconvert fractions, decimal fractions, and percentages. For example: 1:100 = 1/100 = 0.01 = 1%.

One common way to solve any drug dosage calculation is by the creation of a proportional problem. To do this the drug concentration must be converted into a fractional form. The proportional problem can then be set up to solve for the unknown. For example:

1. How much active ingredient would be in 0.5 ml of 1:100 Isuprel?

A 1:100 drug concentration means that there is 1 part of active ingredient in 100 parts of the solution. Or, there would be 1 ml or g of active ingredient in 100 ml or g of the solution. This can be set up in the following proportion:

$$\frac{\text{1 ml active ingredient}}{\text{100 ml total solution}} = \frac{\text{unknown active ingredient or } x}{\text{0.5 ml solution}} \quad \text{(Cross multiply.)}$$

$$100x = 0.5 \text{ ml (Divide both sides of the equation by 100.)}$$
$$x = 0.005 \text{ ml} = 0.005 \text{ g} = 5 \text{ mg active ingredient}$$

2. How much active ingredient would be in 0.25 mL of Alupent? Alupent is 5.0% active ingredient.

A 5.0% drug concentration means that there are 5 parts of active ingredient in 100 parts of the solution. So, there would be 5 ml or g of active ingredient in 100 ml or g of the solution. This can be set up in the following proportion:

$$\frac{\text{5 ml active ingredient}}{\text{100 ml total solution}} = \frac{\text{unknown active ingredient or } x}{\text{0.25 ml solution}} \quad \text{(Cross multiply.)}$$

$$100x = 1.25 \text{ ml (Divide both sides of the equation by 100.)}$$
$$x = 0.0125 \text{ ml} = 0.0125 \text{ g} = 12.5 \text{ mg active ingredient}$$

Thus, it can be seen that the amount of active ingredient can be calculated if the drug concentration is given in either a fractional or percentage form.

The next two examples deal with calculating the volume of medication needed to deliver a desired amount of active ingredient. With these types it is necessary to convert to consistent units, usually converting grams to milligrams. For example:

3. How much 1:100-strength Isuprel would be needed to give a patient 2.5 mg of active ingredient by IPPB?

A 1:100 drug concentration means that there is 1 part of active ingredient in 100 parts of the solution. Or, there would be 1 ml or g of active ingredient in 100 ml or g of the solution. This converts to 1000 mg/100 ml. Set up the following proportion:

$$\frac{1000 \text{ mg active ingredient}}{100 \text{ ml total solution}} = \frac{2.5 \text{ mg}}{X \text{ ml needed}} \text{ (Cross multiply.)}$$

$$250 \text{ ml} = 1000X \text{ (Divide both sides of the equation by 1000.)}$$
$$X = 0.25 \text{ ml of Isuprel should be given.}$$

4. How much 4% Xylocaine would be needed to give a patient 100 mg of active ingredient by hand-held nebulizer before a bronchoscopy?

A 4.0% drug concentration means that there are 4 parts of active ingredient in 100 parts of the solution. So, there would be 4 ml or g of active ingredient in 100 ml or g of the solution. This converts to 4000 mg/100 ml. Set up the following proportion:

$$\frac{4000 \text{ mg active ingredient}}{100 \text{ ml total solution}} = \frac{100 \text{ mg}}{X \text{ ml needed}} \text{ (Cross multiply.)}$$

$$10{,}000 \text{ ml} = 4000X \text{ (Divide both sides of the equation by 4000.)}$$
$$X = 2.5 \text{ ml of Xylocaine should be given.}$$

So, it can be seen that the volume of medication needed to deliver a given amount of active ingredient can be calculated if the drug concentration is given in either a fractional or percentage form.

This ends the general discussion on pharmacology and the delivery of aerosolized medication. The entry level examination will include *direct* questions over these topics. In general, Sections 1 and 7 and the previous discussion will cover Module C that follows. A few comments are added as needed.

Module C. Patient assessment.

1. Determine and continue to monitor how the patient responds to the treatment or procedure.

Many treatment protocols require the practitioner to count the patient's heart rate before, at least one time during, and after an aerosolized bronchodilator is given. This is because of the risk of tachycardia. It is generally acceptable to count for 30 seconds and multiply by 2 for 1 minute's count. Record the various heart rates. The heart rhythm can be determined as the pulse is measured. A stethoscope can be used to be more sure of an abnormality.

Listen for a reduction in wheezing after the administration of an aerosolized bronchodilator as proof that it has been effective at reducing bronchospasm. Listen for a reduction in airway secretions after a productive cough. The mucolytics should be helpful in making the secretions less viscous.

If the patient's condition does not improve after the administration of the prescribed medication, there may be another problem. A chest x-ray film might help to clarify the situation.

See Section 4 for details on spirometry. If the patient is being given an aerosolized bronchodilator for bronchospasm, it would be expected that the patient's spirometry results would move toward more normal values as the bronchospasm is reduced. The two most important bedside spirometry values to follow are the peak flow and forced expiratory volume in 1 second (FEV_1). A 15% to 20% improvement in either one or both after the inhalation of an aerosolized bronchodilator proves (1) the medication works, and (2) the patient has reversible bronchospasm.

Most patients will gladly tell you if their breathing is easier after the delivery of the proper medication. It is just as important to know when the patient does *not* feel any better. Possibly the medication does not work, or the dose is insufficient.

2. Modify the treatment or procedure and recommend any changes in the patient's respiratory care plan depending on the response.

Watch for tachycardia and palpitations with an aerosolized bronchodilator. A common policy is to stop the treatment if the patient's pulse increases by more than 20% from the initial level. For example, the patient's initial pulse was 100 and is now 120 beats/min. The treatment should be stopped.

Watch for bronchospasm from the the bland aerosols (expecially hypertonic saline solution) or Mucomyst. Compare the patient's initial breath sounds with the breath sounds during the treatment. Ask if the patient's breathing is all right or if the chest fells "tight." Stop the treatment if the patient develops or has worsening bronchospasm during the treatment.

If these problems persist despite changes in the medication doses or addition of a bronchodilator to Mucomyst, the treatment should probably be discontinued. Stop a breathing treatment any time the patient appears to have had an allergic reaction to a medication. Tell the patient's physician and ask for further orders.

3. Make a recommendation to change the dosage or concentration of an aerosolized medication. (IIIF9c) [R, Ap, An]

Bronchodilators

Make a recommendation to increase the amount of medication if the patient's bronchospasm is not reversed and there are no adverse side effects. Make a recommendation to decrease the amount of medication if the patient is having serious side effects such as tachycardia or palpitations.

Mucomyst or Saline Solutions

Make a recommendation to increase the amount of medication if the patient's secretions are still too thick to cough out or suction and there are no adverse side effects. Make a recommendation to decrease the amount of medication if the patient's secretions are thin enough for expectoration or suctioning or if there are side effects like bronchospasm.

4. Change the dilution of a medication used in aerosol therapy. (IIIF5b) [R, Ap]

The various saline solutions and sterile water are known collectively as "bland" aerosols because they have no direct pharmacologic effect on the lungs and airways. They are used to increase the volume of liquid in a small-volume nebulizer after the medication has been added. Most of these nebulizers work most efficiently when they hold about 3 to 5 ml of liquid. Usually normal saline solution (0.9% sodium chloride) is added.

Adding little or no saline to the medication will result in the patient inhaling a very concentrated solution. The nebulizer will aerosolize the medication within a few minutes. The patient should quickly feel the beneficial effects of the treatment. However, depending on the nature of the medication, the patient might find it to be quite irritating to the airway. Coughing or bronchospasm could result. Side effects, such as tachycardia, should be watched for with sympathomimetic agents because the medication will enter the blood stream so quickly.

The more saline that is added, the less concentrated the solution will be. The nebulizer will take longer to aerosolize the medication because of the added volume. Relief of symptoms will take longer. However, it will be less likely to irritate the airway. Side effects with sympathomimetic agents could be less severe because the drug is given over a longer period. But, remember that increasing the amount of saline makes no difference on the total amount of medication that is given to the patient. Tachycardia or other side effects may still be seen if the total amount of medication is given.

Saline-only aerosol treatments, as for an induced sputum, will be more effective at higher concentrations of saline. See Table 8-5 for complete information on the saline solutions.

BIBLIOGRAPHY

Au JP, Ziment I: Drug therapy and dosage adjustment in asthma. *Respir Care* 1986; 31:415-418.

Barnes TA (ed): *Respiratory Care Practice*. Chicago, Mosby, 1988.

Barnhart ER (ed): *Physicians' Desk Reference*, ed 46. Oradell, NJ, Medical Economics, 1992.

Eubanks DH, Bone RC: *Comprehensive Respiratory Care*, ed 2. St Louis, Mosby, 1990.

Howder CL: *Cardiopulmonary pharmacology: a Handbook for Respiratory Practitioners and Other Allied Health Personnel*. Baltimore, Williams & Wilkens, 1992.

Kacmarek RM, Mack CW, Dimas S: *The Essentials of Respiratory Care*, ed 3. St Louis, Mosby, 1990.

Lehnert BE, Schachter EN: *The Pharmacology of Respiratory Care*. St Louis, Mosby, 1980.

Peters JA, Peters BA: Pharmacology for respiratory care, in Scanlan CL, Spearman CB, Sheldon RL (eds): *Egan's Fundamentals of Respiratory Care*, ed 5. St Louis, Mosby, 1990.

Rau JL: *Respiratory Care Pharmacology*, ed 2. Chicago, Mosby, 1984.

Rau JL: *Respiratory Care Pharmacology*, ed 3. Chicago, Mosby, 1989.

Tashkin DP: Dosing strategies for bronchodilator aerosol delivery. *Respir Care* 1991; 36:977-988.

Ziment I: *Respiratory Pharmacology and Therapeutics*. Philadelphia, Saunders, 1978.

Ziment I: Drugs used in respiratory therapy, in Burton GG, Hodgkin JE, Ward JJ (eds): *Respiratory Care: a Guide to Clinical Practice*, ed 3. Philadelphia, Lippincott, 1991.

SELF-STUDY QUESTIONS

1. Your patient's airway was extubated 30 minutes ago. She is complaining of hoarseness and "tightness in my throat." The drug of choice to treat this problem is:
   A. Racemic epinephrine
   B. Acetylcysteine
   C. Isoproterenol
   D. Isoetharine
   E. Cromolyn sodium

2. Your patient is coughing very hard to bring up thick mucus with plugs. The drug of choice to treat this problem is:
   A. Racemic epinephrine
   B. Acetylcysteine
   C. Isoproterenol
   D. Isoetharine
   E. Cromolyn sodium

3. What is the minimum amount of time that a pulse rate should be checked when an aerosolized bronchodilator medication is given?
   A. 15 seconds
   B. 20 seconds
   C. 30 seconds
   D. 45 seconds
   E. 60 seconds

4. You receive an order to administer 5 ml of isoetharine (Bronkosol) by hand-held nebulizer. You would proceed to:
   A. Give the treatment.
   B. Call the physician about changing the order to an IPPB treatment.
   C. Have the shift supervisor give the treatment.
   D. Call the physician to check on the medication dose.
   E. Give 0.5 ml of medication because that is probably what the physician meant to write.

5. The best aerosol medication to treat a patient with bronchitis and viscous secretions is:
   A. 0.9% (normal) saline solution
   B. Acetylcystine (Mucomyst)
   C. Sterile water
   D. 0.45% (hypotonic) saline solution
   E. 10% (hypertonic) saline solution

6. When the medication cromolyn sodium (Intal) is administered, it is important to monitor the patient for:
   A. Tachycardia
   B. Bradycardia
   C. Watery secretions
   D. Oral candidiasis (oral thrush)
   E. Bronchospasm

7. Your patient is in the emergency room with severe bronchospasm from an asthma attack. The drug of choice to treat this problem is:
   A. Racemic epinephrine
   B. Acetylcysteine
   C. Isoproterenol
   D. Isoetharine
   E. Cromolyn sodium

8. How much active ingredient would be in 0.25 ml of 1:200 isoproterenol (Isuprel)?
   A. 1.25 ml
   B. 0.5 g
   C. 1.25 mg
   D. 500 mg
   E. 0.00125 mg

9. How much active ingredient would be in 0.6 ml of 2.25% racemic epinephrine (Vaponephrine)?
   A. 26.7 g
   B. 26,700 mg
   C. 0.0267 mg
   D. 13.5 g
   E. 13.5 mg

10. The aerosol bronchodilators work by stimulating which receptor(s)?
   A. β_1
   B. β_1 and β_2
   C. β_2
   D. α and β_2
   E. α

11. You are administering an aerosolized bronchodilator to your patient. Her pretreatment pulse was 85 beats/min. You would stop the treatment if her pulse reached:
   A. 90 beats/min
   B. 100 beats/min
   C. 110 beats/min
   D. 120 beats/min
   E. 130 beats/min

12. Your patient is using a metered dose inhaler. To increase the amount of medication deposited in the lower airway you would have the patient do all of the following *except:*
   A. Have the patient breathe in slowly.
   B. Have the patient inspire an inspiratory capacity.
   C. Use a spacer between the metered dose inhaler and lips.
   D. Have the patient hold the medication in for 10 to 15 seconds.
   E. Have the patient breathe in a normal pattern.

13. Side effects of the aerosolized bronchodilators include:
   I. Bradycardia
   II. Tremor
   III. Headache
   IV. Nervousness and irritability
   V. Tachycardia
   A. I, II
   B. III, IV, V
   C. II, III, IV, V
   D. II, IV
   E. I, II, III, IV

14. Your patient is being discharged and will receive aerosolized bronchodilator therapy at home. The best medication for this chronically sick but stable patient is:
   A. Metaproterenol
   B. Isoetharine
   C. Racemic epinephrine
   D. Bitolterol
   E. Epinephrine

15. Your patient has an order for an induced sputum sample to look for tuberculosis. The best medication for this is:
    A. Mucomyst
    B. 10% saline solution
    C. 0.9% saline solution
    D. Sterile water
    E. 0.45% saline solution

16. After finishing an aerosolized dose of Mucomyst, your patient's breath sounds reveal wheezing. They were not present at the start of the treatment. What medication should be added to the Mukomyst for the next treatment to prevent the bronchospasm?
    A. Bronkosol
    B. Sterile water
    C. Tornalate
    D. 0.9% saline solution
    E. 0.45% saline solution

Answer Key:

1. A; 2. B; 3. C; 4. D; 5. B; 6. E; 7. D; 8. C; 9. E; 10. C; 11. C; 12. E; 13. C; 14. D; 15. B; 16. A.

9 Postural Drainage Therapy

Module A. Perform postural drainage therapy (PDT).

PDT is also known as chest physiotherapy, chest physical therapy, bronchopulmonary drainage, postural drainage and percussion, and percussion and vibration.

1. Make a recommendation to begin PDT procedures. (IIIF9f5) [R, Ap, An]

See Table 9-1 for indications for turning, postural drainage, percussion, and vibration. Contraindications are listed in Table 9-2. Besides the indications listed in Table 9-1, the following should be evaluated to determine if PDT is needed:

a. PDT is not indicated if an optimally hydrated patient is coughing out less than 25 ml/day with the procedure.
b. A dehydrated patient should have apparently ineffective PDT continued for at least 24 hours after the patient is rehydrated. The combination of rehydration and PDT may help to mobilize previously viscous secretions.
c. PDT is not indicated in a patient who is producing greater than 30 ml of secretions daily if the treatments do not increase the sputum production. This is because the patient is already able to effectively cough out the sputum.

2. Perform the following procedures to help the patient cough out bronchopulmonary secretions.

a. Turning.

Turning involves rotating the patient's body in the longitudinal (head to toe) axis. It is done to promote unilateral or bilateral lung expansion. This should help to improve arterial oxygenation. Patients can be turned from their back (prone) to one side, side to side, or one side to back to other side, depending on the patient's need. The bed may be moved to any head-up or head-down position as the patient needs and tolerates. Patients who are critically ill or on a mechanical ventilator should be turned every 1 to 2 hours around the clock as tolerated. Other patients should be turned every 2 hours as tolerated. The patient can turn himself or herself, be turned by a caregiver, or be placed in a bed that is motorized and programmed to change its position in a set pattern. See Table 9-1 for the indications for turning, Table 9-2 for assessing the patient's need, and Tables 9-3 and 9-4 for the contraindications and hazards.

Table 9-1. Indications for Turning, Postural Drainage, and Percussion and Vibration

Turning:
1. Patient is unable to change his or her body position. For example, the patient has a cerebral injury or neuromuscular disease, is being mechanically ventilated, or has been medicated to cause sedation or paralysis.
2. Atelectasis or the potential for its development.
3. Hypoxemia associated with a particular position. Commonly, if one-sided lung disease is present, the patient is turned so that the affected lung is superior.
4. Patient has an artificial airway.

Postural Drainage:
1. Mobilize retained secretions so that they can be coughed or suctioned out. Patient has difficulty coughing out secretions but produces more than 25-30 ml/day. Evidence or indications that a patient with an artificial airway has retained secretions.
2. Atelectasis that is known or believed to be caused by mucus plugging.
3. Patient has a diagnosis of cystic fibrosis, bronchiectasis, or cavitating lung disease.
4. Foreign body in an airway.
5. Removal of aspirated foreign body or stomach contents.

Percussion and Vibration:
1. Patient receiving postural drainage who has a large volume of viscous sputum. This suggests that the external manipulation of the thorax would assist gravity in its movement toward a more central airway.

Based on information found in AARC Clinical Practice Guidelines: Postural drainage therapy. *Respir Care,* 1991; 36:1418-1426.

b. Perform postural drainage. (IIIB2b) [R, Ap]

Postural drainage (bronchopulmonary drainage) is performed to clear secretions or prevent the accumulation of secretions. See Table 9-1 for the indications for postural drainage, Table 9-2 for assessing the patient's need, and Tables 9-3 and 9-4 for the contraindications and hazards. The patient is positioned so that the bronchus of a particular segment is as vertical as possible. Gravity will then pull the secretions toward a major bronchus or the trachea. From there the secretions are either coughed or suctioned out.

Postural drainage and the external manipulation of the patient's thorax (percussion and vibration) can be very strenuous or contraindicated in some patients. See Table 9-3

Table 9-2. Assessment of the Patient's Need for PDT*†

- Excessive production of sputum
- Ineffectiveness of cough
- Patient history of PDT helpful in treating past problem (for example, bronchiectasis, cystic fibrosis, lung abscess, etc.)
- Abnormal breath sounds (for example, decreased, crackles, or rhonchi suggesting airway secretions)
- Change in the patient's vital signs
- Abnormal chest x-ray finding consistent with infiltrates, atelectasis, and/or mucus plugging

Based on information found in AARC Clinical Practice Guidelines: Postural drainage therapy. *Respir Care,* 1991; 36:1418-1426.

**PDT,* Postural drainage therapy.

†These problems should be assessed *together* to evaluate the patient's need for PDT. Not all patients will experience all of these problems. The seriousness of these problems should be used in determining which patients will benefit from PDT.

Table 9-3. Contraindications of Turning/Postural Drainage and Percussion and Vibration

Turning/Postural Drainage:*

All positions are contraindicated for patients with:

1. Unstabilized head or neck injury, or both. (Absolute)
2. Active hemorrhage and hemodynamic instability. (Absolute)
3. ICP† greater than 20 mm Hg.
4. Recent spinal surgery, such as a laminectomy, or acute spinal injury.
5. Active hemoptysis.
6. Empyema.
7. Bronchopleural fistula.
8. Pulmonary edema secondary to congestive heart failure.
9. Large pleural effusions.
10. Advanced age, anxiety, or confusion and intolerant of position changes.
11. Fractured rib(s) with or without flail chest.
12. Healing tissue or surgical wound.

Trendelenburg position is contraindicated in patients with:

1. ICP greater than 20 mm Hg.
2. Sensitivity to increased ICP (eg, neurosurgery, cerebral aneurysms, or eye surgery).
3. Uncontrolled hypertension.
4. A distended abdomen.
5. Esophageal surgery.
6. Recent gross hemoptysis. (Especially if the hemoptysis is associated with lung cancer that was recently treated surgically or by radiation therapy.)
7. An uncontrolled airway who are at risk of aspirating (recent meal or tube feeding). Many authors list less than one hour since eating as a contraindication.

Reverse Trendelenburg position is contraindicated in patients who:

1. Are hypotensive.
2. Are receiving a vasoactive medication.

Percussion and Vibrations:

1. All of the previously listed contraindications.
2. Subcutaneous emphysema. (Several authors list an untreated pneumothorax as an absolute contraindication.)
3. Spinal anesthesia or recent epidural spinal infusion for pain control.
4. Recent thoracic skin grafts or skin flaps.
5. Thoracic burns, open wounds, or skin infections.
6. Transvenous or subcutaneous pacemaker that has been recently placed. (Expecially true if a mechanical percussor/vibrator is to be used.)
7. Suspicion of pulmonary tuberculosis.
8. Lung contusion.
9. Bronchospasm.
10. Osteomyelitis of the ribs.
11. Osteoporosis.
12. Clotting disorder (coagulopathy).
13. Complaints of chest-wall pain.

Additionally, a number of authors have listed the following as contraindications to percussion and vibration:

1. Not over bare skin.
2. Not over buttons, zippers, folded clothes, seams of clothing.
3. Not over female breast tissue.
4. Not over the spine, sternum, or kidneys.
5. Not over an area with a known lung tumor.

Based on information found in AARC Clinical Practice Guideline: Postural drainage therapy. *Respir Care,* 1991; 36:1418-1426.

*These are relative contraindications except those marked as absolute

†*ICP,* Intracranial pressure.

Table 9-4. Hazards/Complications, With Recommended Actions, and Limitations of Postural Drainage and Percussion and Vibration

Hazards/Complications:

1. *Hypoxemia.* The patient known to be hypoxic or prone to hypoxemia during the procedure should be given a higher inspired oxygen percentage. Give 100% oxygen to any patient who becomes hypoxic during the procedure. Stop the treatment, return the patient to the original resting position, make sure ventilation is adequate, and consult with the physician before continuing.
2. *Increased intracranial pressure.* If this happens, stop the treatment, return the patient to the original resting position, and consult with the physician before continuing.
3. *Acute hypotension during the procedure.* If this happens, stop the treatment, return the patient to the original resting position, and consult with the physician before continuing.
4. *Pulmonary hemorrhage.* If this happens, stop the treatment, return the patient to the original resting position, and call the physician immediately. Give the patient supplemental oxygen and keep an open airway until the physician responds.
5. *Pain or injury to the patient's muscles, ribs, or spine.* Stop the therapy that seems to be causing the problem. Carefully move the patient to a more comfortable position and call the physician before continuing.
6. *Vomiting and aspiration.* Stop the treatment, apply suction as needed to clear the airway, give supplemental oxygen, maintain a patent airway, return the patient to the original resting position, and call the physician immediately.
7. *Bronchospasm.* If this happens, stop the treatment, return the patient to the original resting position, give or increase the supplemental oxygen while calling the physician. Give the patient any aerosolized bronchodilators that the physician orders.
8. *Dysrhythmias.* If this happens, stop the treatment, return the patient to the original resting position, give or increase supplemental oxygen while calling the physician.

Limitations:

1. Be careful to give PDT* only to those patients who would benefit from it. Do not rely on past experiences with other patients when judging current ones.
2. Patients with ineffective coughs may unable to clear their airways as well as desired.
3. Critically ill patients are difficult to position optimally.

Based on information found in AARC Clinical Practice Guideline: Postural drainage Therapy. *Respir Care,* 1991; 36:1418-1426.

**PDT,* Postural drainage therapy.

for the contraindications and Table 9-4 for hazards or complications and limitations to these procedures. There is some disagreement in the literature whether it is better to approach postural drainage of all lobes in one or both lungs from an apices to bases or bases to apices pattern. This is discussed in more detail later. For now, the key steps in each drainage position in a bases to apices pattern are presented because this pattern is the most commonly recommended.

It is wise to review the anatomy of the pulmonary lobes with their segments and respective bronchi. Fig. 9-1 shows them in detail. Note that each segment and its bronchus adjoins the right or left mainstem bronchus at a particular angle. This critical angle determines the positioning that must be used to drain the various segments. Obviously, putting the patient in the wrong position will do nothing to drain the desired segment.

Fig. 9-2 to 9-5 show the anterior, posterior, and lateral views of the patient's chest with the lungs and other landmarks added. Auscultation, palpation, and percussion of the chest should lead the practitioner to know where the secretions are located.

Individual segments should be drained when the physician's order specifies them or when the practitioner determines that secretions are present. Some practitioners perform postural drainage in clear segments as a preventive treatment in certain patients such as those who are aged and bedridden. Some practitioners also believe it is wise to drain the lung segment opposite the one that has been therapeutically drained to minimize the risk of secretions from the infected segment contaminating the normal segment. In general,

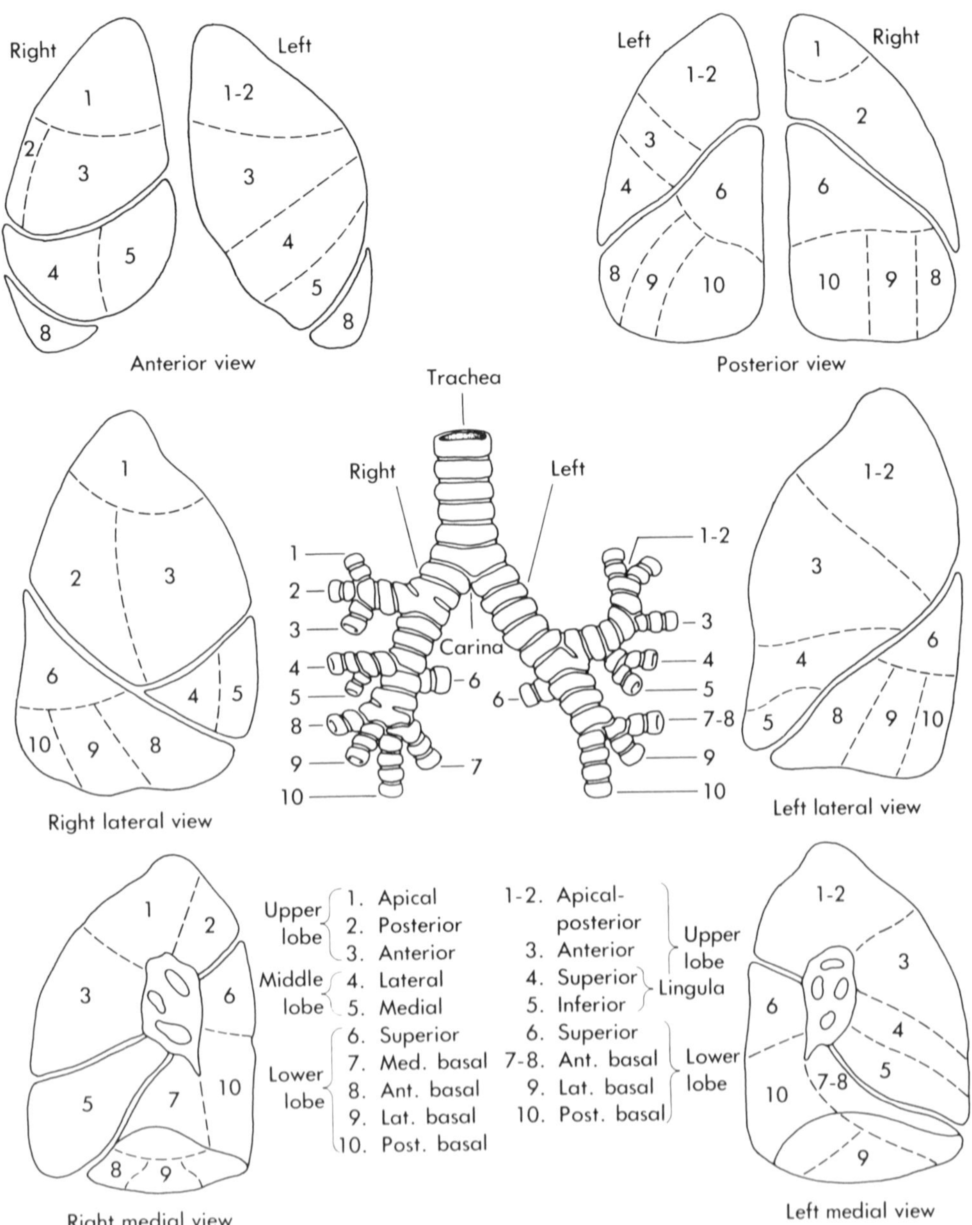

Fig. 9-1 Names and locations of the segments with their respective bronchi. (From Shibel EM, Moser KM [eds]: *Respiratory Emergencies,* St Louis, Mosby, 1977. Used by permission.)

individual segments are drained for 3 to 15 minutes. It may be necessary to provide drainage for a longer period in special situations.

Watch for hypoxemia or an increase in dyspnea in the patient. If the patient normally has supplemental oxygen, it should be kept on while in the drainage positions. Some patients need supplemental oxygen only when in certain positions. It must be made available to them.

Coughing should be encouraged after each segment is drained. However, you do *not* want the patient to cough in a head-down position. This is because of the risk of an increase in intracranial pressure. Have the patient sit up to cough vigorously.

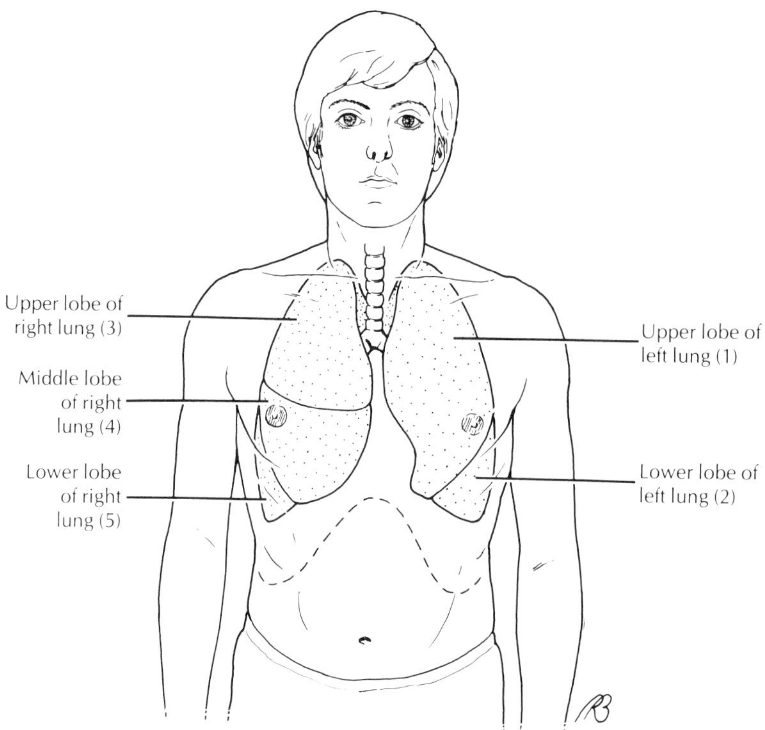

Fig. 9-2 Anterior view of the chest showing the lobes of the lungs. (From Eubanks DH, Bone RC: *Comprehensive Respiratory Care,* ed 2. St Louis, Mosby, 1990. Used by permission.)

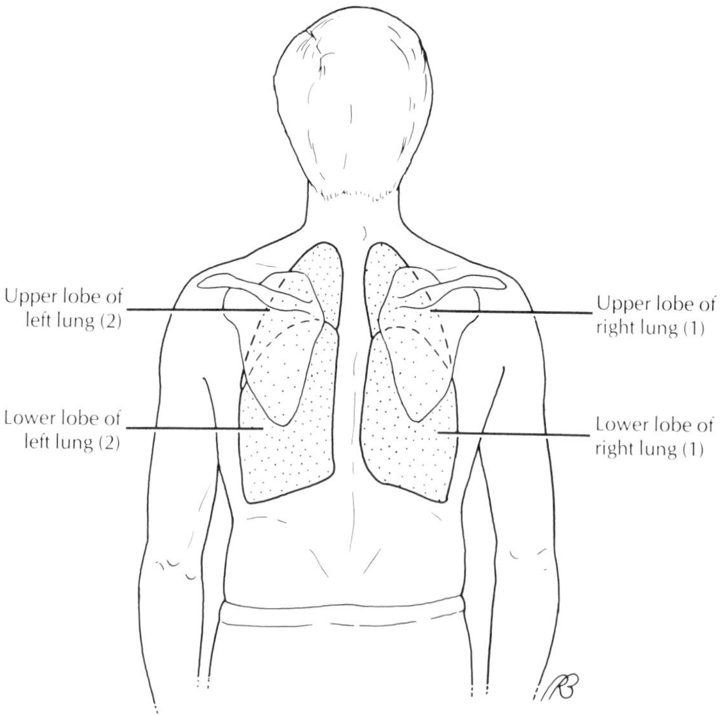

Fig. 9-3 Posterior view of the chest showing the lobes of the lungs. (From Eubanks DH, Bone RC: *Comprehensive Respiratory Care,* ed 2. St Louis, Mosby, 1990. Used by permission.)

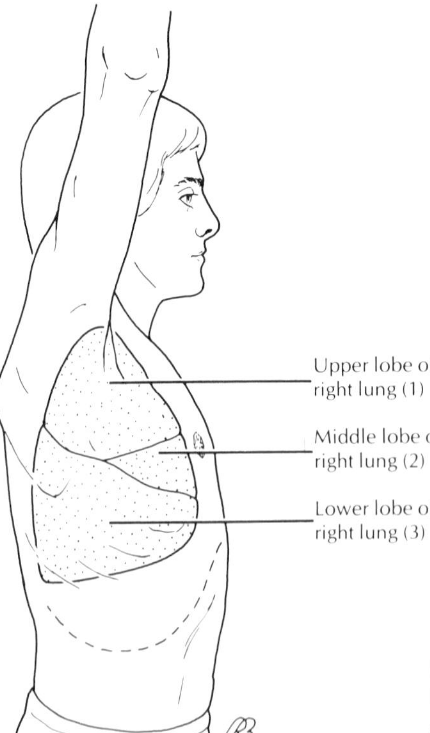

Fig. 9-4 Right lateral view of the chest showing the lobes of the lungs. (From Eubanks DH, Bone RC: *Comprehensive Respiratory Care,* ed 2. St Louis, Mosby, 1990. Used by permission.)

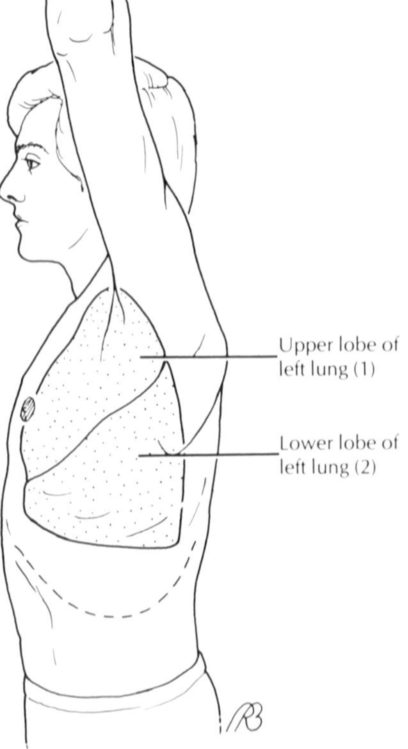

Fig. 9-5 Left lateral view of the chest showing the lobes of the lungs. (From Eubanks DH, Bone RC: *Comprehensive Respiratory Care,* ed 2. St Louis, Mosby, 1990. Used by permission.)

Pulmonary Drainage Positions

Lower Lobes

A. Posterior basal segment.
   1. See Fig. 9-6.
   2. The patient lies face down on the bed. A pillow is placed beneath the hips.
   3. The foot of the bed is elevated 18 inches or 30 degrees.
   4. If ordered, percussion or vibration would be performed over the lower ribs near the spine on either or both sides, depending on whether one or both segments are to be drained. See the shaded areas.

B. Lateral basal segment.
   1. See Fig. 9-7. The patient is shown in a position to drain the right lateral basal segment. The left lateral basal segment would be drained by placing the patient the same way on the opposite side.
   2. The patient lies one-fourth turn up from face down on the bed. A pillow may be placed in front of the patient for support or between the knees for comfort.
   3. The foot of the bed is elevated 18 inches or 30 degrees.
   4. If ordered, percussion or vibration would be performed over the posterolateral areas of the lower ribs. See the shaded areas.

C. Anterior basal segment.
   1. See Fig. 9-8. The patient is shown in a position to drain the left anterior basal segment. (**Note:** This is a combined segment that is the anatomic equivalent

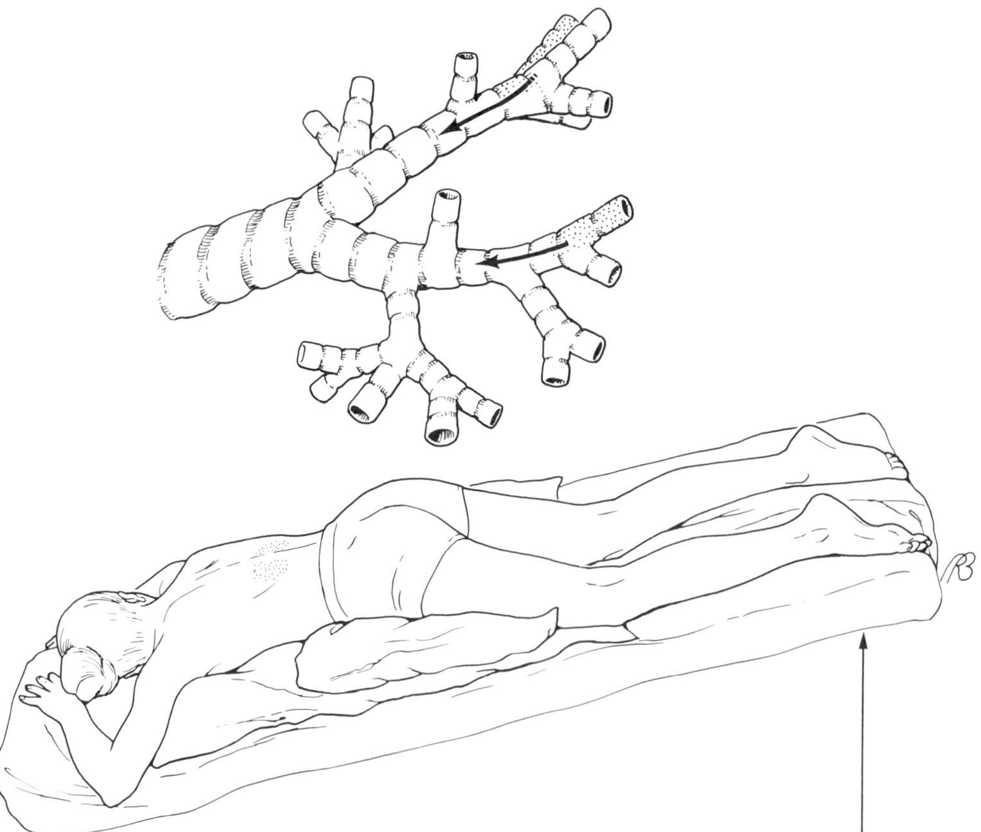

Fig. 9-6 Drainage position for the posterior basal segments of both lower lobes. (From Eubanks DH, Bone RC: *Comprehensive Respiratory Care,* ed 2. St Louis, Mosby, 1990. Used by permission.)

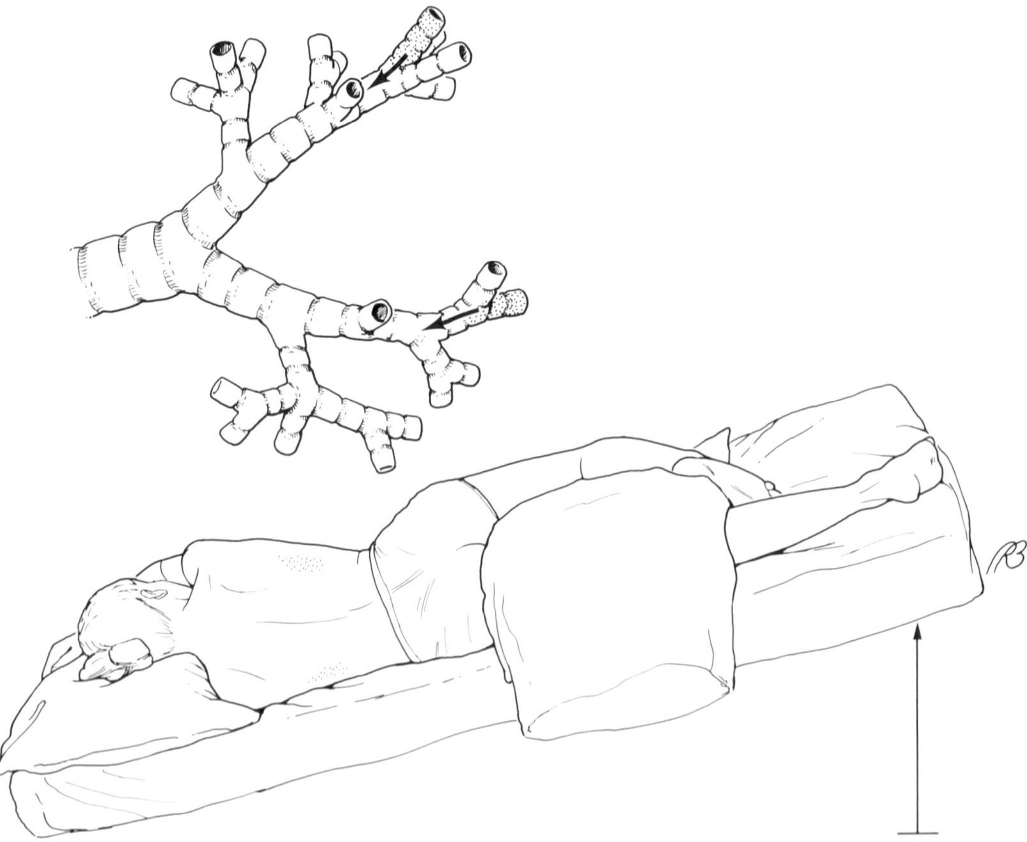

Fig. 9-7 Drainage position for the lateral basal segment of the right lower lobe. The same segment in the left lung would be drained by positioning the patient similarly on the right side. (From Eubanks DH, Bone RC: *Comprehensive Respiratory Care,* ed 2. St Louis, Mosby, 1990. Used by permission.)

of the medial basal segment and anterior basal segment of the right lung.) The right anterior basal and medial basal segments would be drained by placing the patient the same way on the opposite side.

2. The patient lies straight up on his or her side. Pillows may be used in front or behind (or both) the patient for positioning or between the knees for comfort.
3. The foot of the bed is elevated 18 inches or 30 degrees.
4. If ordered, percussion or vibration would be performed over the lower ribs below the axilla. See the shaded areas.

D. Superior segment.

1. See Fig. 9-9.
2. The patient lies face down on the bed. A pillow is placed beneath the hips.
3. The bed is flat.
4. If ordered, percussion or vibration would be performed over the middle of the back below the scapula on either or both sides of the spine depending on whether one or both segments are to be drained. See the shaded areas.

Right Middle Lobe and Left Lingula

A. Right lateral and medial segments.

1. See Fig. 9-10. The same position is used to drain both segments.
2. The patient lies one-fourth turn up from back down on the bed. A pillow may

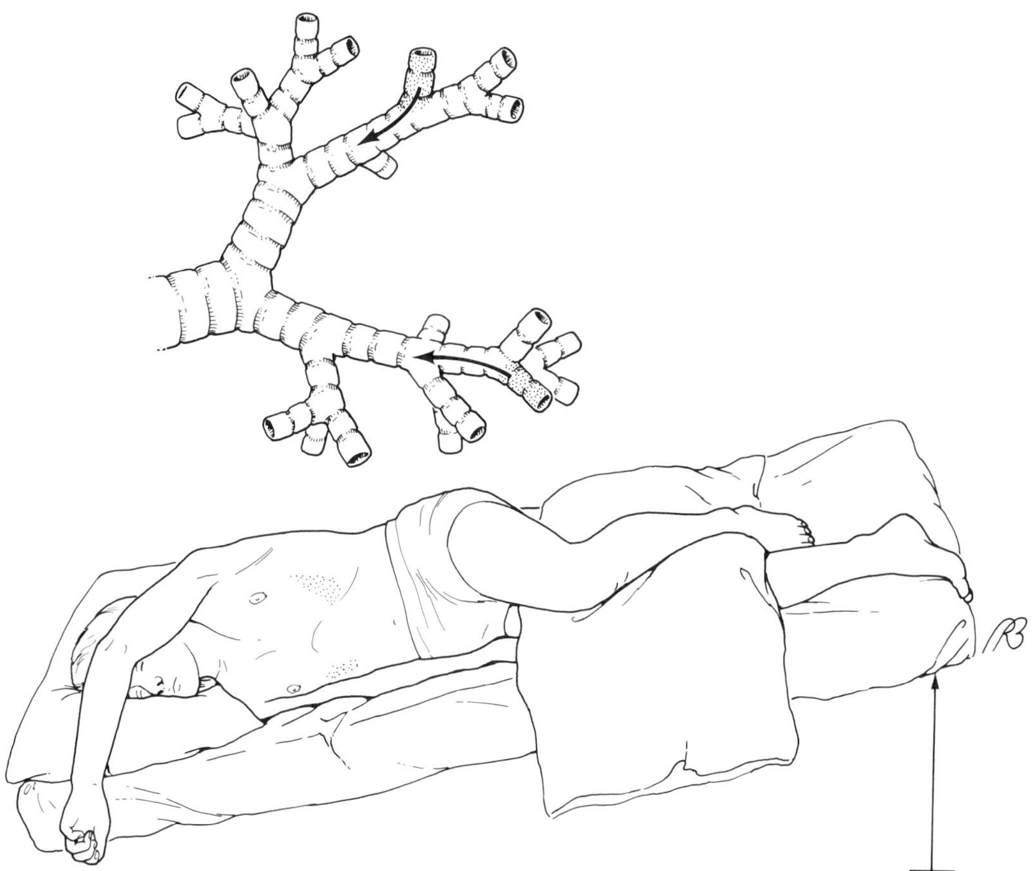

Fig. 9-8 Drainage position for the anterior basal segment of the left lower lobe. The same segment in the right lung would be drained by positioning the patient similarly on the left side. (From Eubanks DH, Bone RC: *Comprehensive Respiratory Care,* ed 2. St Louis, Mosby, 1990. Used by permission.)

be placed in back of the patient for support or between the flexed knees for comfort.

3. The foot of the bed is elevated 14 inches or 15 degrees.
4. If ordered, percussion or vibration would be performed over the right nipple area in a male patient. See the shaded area. Percussion and vibration may not be possible on a female patient.

B. Left superior and inferior lingular segments.

1. See Fig. 9-11. The same position is used to drain both segments.
2. The patient lies one-fourth turn up from back down on the bed. A pillow may be placed in back of the patient for support or between the flexed knees for comfort.
3. The foot of the bed is elevated 14 inches or 15 degrees.
4. If ordered, percussion or vibration would be performed over the left nipple area in a male patient. See the shaded area. Percussion and vibration may not be possible on a female patient.

Upper Lobes

A. Posterior segment.
   1. See Fig. 9-12.
   2. The patient leans forward 30 degrees. This can be over the back of a chair, as shown, or in bed. A pillow can be used to lean against or support the chest.
   3. If ordered, percussion or vibration would be performed over the upper portion of the back on either or both sides of spine, depending on whether one or both segments are being drained. See the shaded areas.

B. Apical segment.
   1. See Fig. 9-13.
   2. The patient leans backward 30 degrees. This can be done in bed, as shown, or in a chair. A pillow can be leaned against to support the lower portion of the back.
   3. If ordered, percussion or vibration would be performed between the clavicle and the top of the scapula on either or both sides, depending on whether one or both segments are being drained. See the shaded areas.

C. Anterior segment.
   1. See Fig. 9-14.
   2. The patient lies supine in bed. A pillow should be placed behind the knees. This enables the abdominal muscles to relax so that the patient can breathe more easily.
   3. If ordered, percussion or vibration would be performed between the clavicle

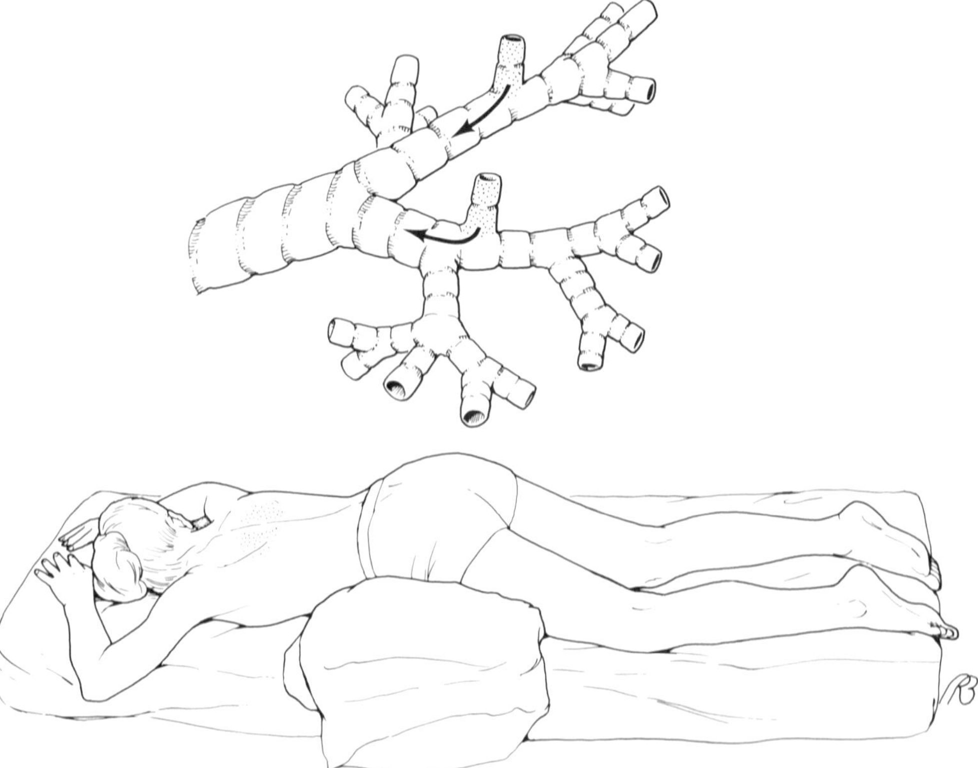

Fig. 9-9 Drainage position for the superior segments of both lower lobes. (From Eubanks DH, Bone RC: *Comprehensive Respiratory Care,* ed 2. St Louis, Mosby, 1990. Used by permission.)

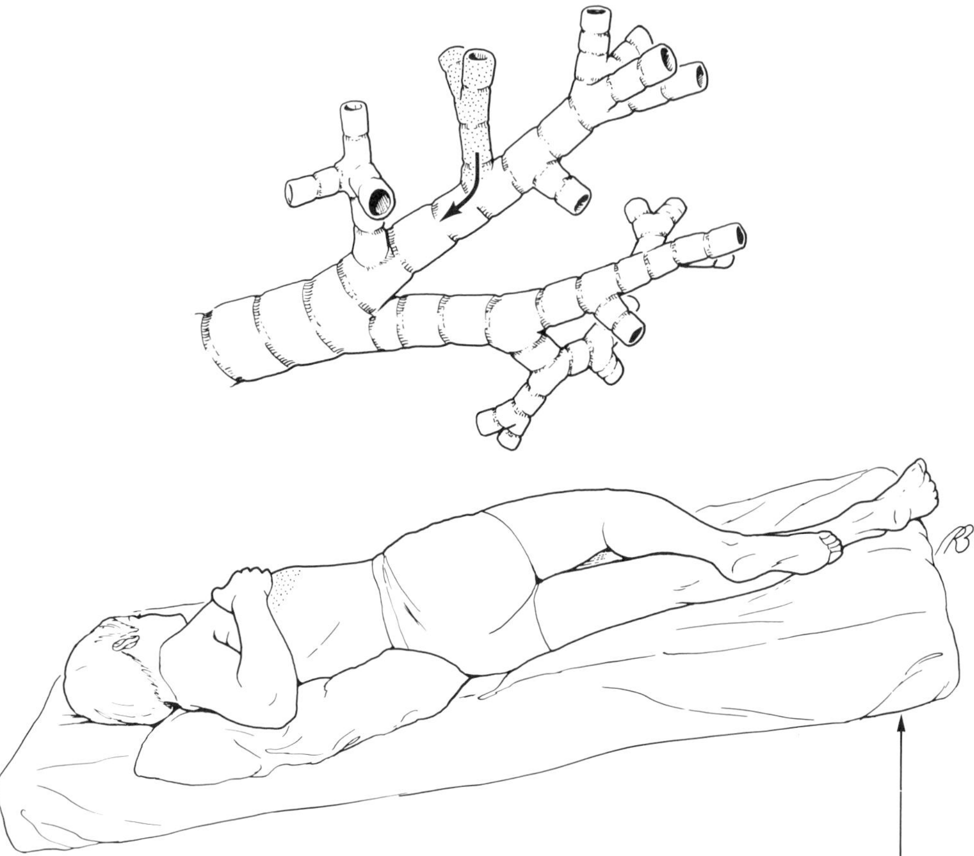

Fig. 9-10 Drainage position for the lateral and medial segments of the right middle lobe. (From Eubanks DH, Bone RC: *Comprehensive Respiratory Care,* ed 2. St Louis, Mosby, 1990. Used by permission.)

and the nipple of a male patient on either or both sides, depending on whether one or both segments are being drained. See the shaded areas. Percussion and vibration may not be possible on a female patient.

Some authors may list slightly different positions or several additional positions. The most commonly accepted postural drainage positions have been presented.

The postural drainage positions in the infant are basically the same as in the adult. Positioning can be accomplished more easily by the use of pillows. See Fig. 9-15 for the various segmental drainage positions.

c. Perform percussion. (IIIB2c) [R, Ap]

Percussion (also known as clapping, cupping, and tapotement) is the act of rhythmically striking the patient's chest with cupped hands over an area with secretions. (Note that the AARC Clinical Practice Guideline on Postural Drainage Therapy lists percussion and vibration together as External Manipulation of the Thorax. Do not be confused by varying terminology.) Its purpose is to vibrate the secretions so that they will flow more quickly down the vertical bronchus. Percussion will not work to move secretions if the patient is not in the proper postural drainage position. It is performed throughout the breathing cycle.

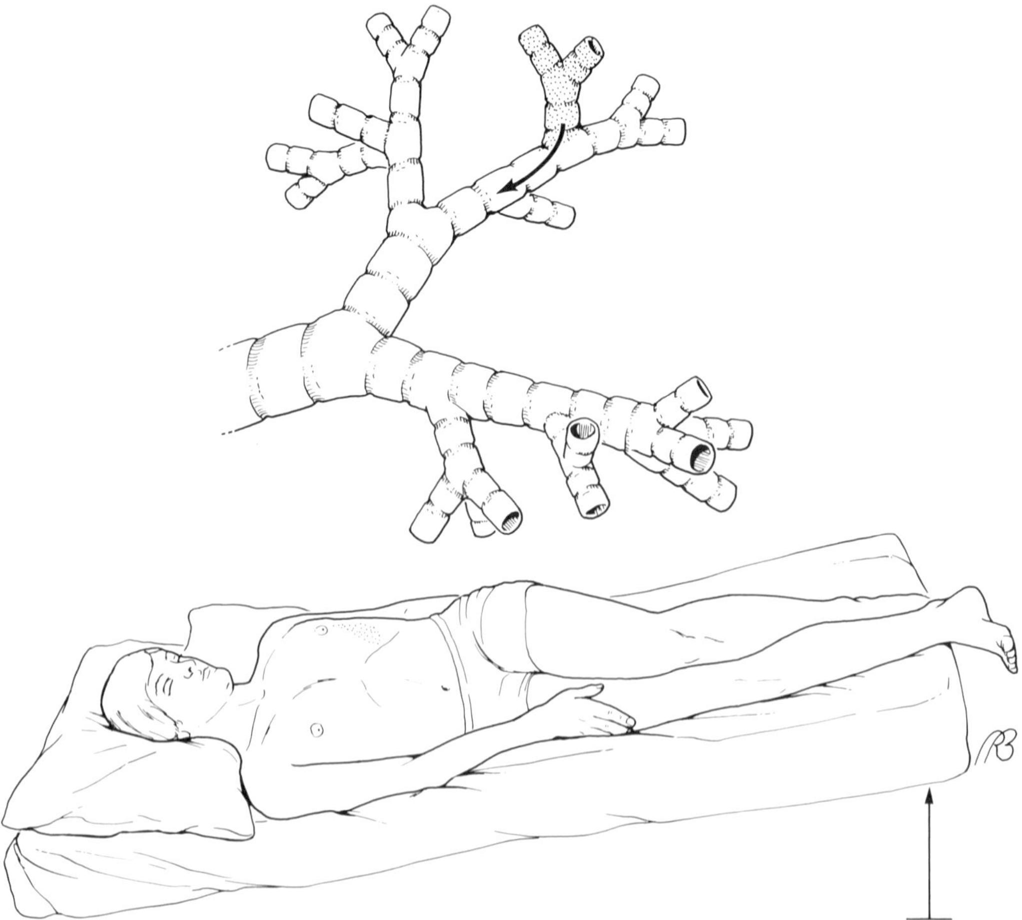

Fig. 9-11 Drainage position for the superior and inferior segments of the lingula. (From Eubanks DH, Bone RC: *Comprehensive Respiratory Care,* ed 2. St Louis, Mosby, 1990. Used by permission.)

Percussion can be done with one or both hands. A properly cupped hand will trap air against the chest and cause a popping sound. It should not be painful to the patient. If it is, the technique must be altered. As an added precaution, most authors recommend that the chest be covered lightly with the patient's gown or towel. Percussion should not be done over buttons or zippers. The wrists, elbows, and shoulders should be kept as loose as possible. This will enable the practitioner to keep the proper loose waving motion of the hand and minimize fatigue (Fig. 9-16).

It has been recommended that percussion be performed for 5 minutes or longer in each position. Some patients may not tolerate it for that long. One minute would seem to be the shortest time that would still have any therapeutic benefit. There is no agreement on the ideal rate of percussion. The practitioner must vary the rate, depending on how the patient feels and what seems to produce the best clearance of secretions. It can become exhaustive to perform manual percussion on a series of patients.

Infants can be percussed by putting the index, middle, and ring fingers together into a kind of three-sided tent. This enables the practitioner to percuss a small area of the chest wall.

Mechanical percussors/vibrators and other devices may be used to supplement manual percussion. They are discussed later on.

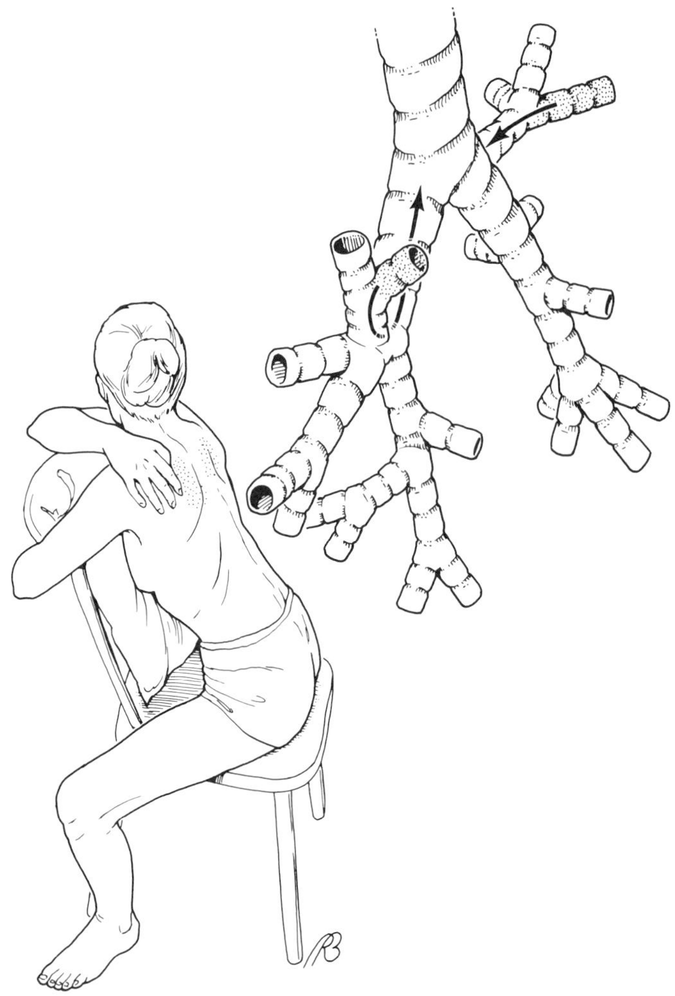

Fig. 9-12 Drainage position for the posterior segments of both upper lobes. (From Eubanks DH, Bone RC: *Comprehensive Respiratory Care,* ed 2. St Louis, Mosby, 1990. Used by permission.)

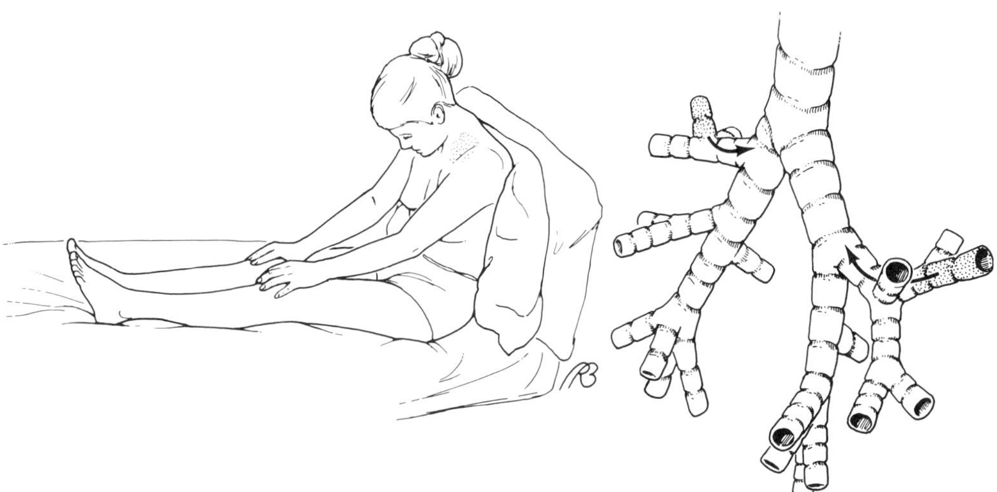

Fig. 9-13 Drainage position for the apical segments of both upper lobes. (From Eubanks DH, Bone RC: *Comprehensive Respiratory Care,* ed 2. St Louis, Mosby, 1990. Used by permission.)

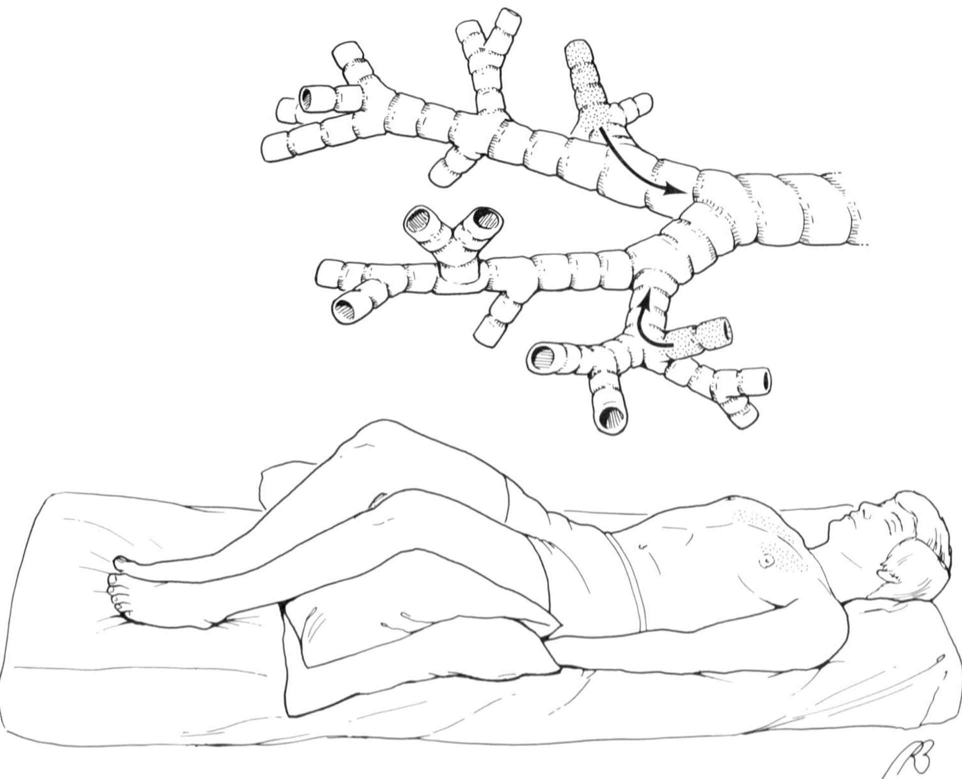

Fig. 9-14 Drainage position for the anterior segments of both upper lobes. (From Eubanks DH, Bone RC: *Comprehensive Respiratory Care,* ed 2. St Louis, Mosby, 1990. Used by permission.)

d. Perform vibration. (IIID3) [R, Ap, An]

Vibration is the gentle, rapid shaking of the chest wall directly over the lung segment that is being drained. It may be performed along with percussion or by itself. (Note that the AARC Clinical Practice Guideline on Postural Drainage Therapy lists percussion and vibration together as External Manipulation of the Thorax. Do not be confused by varying terminology.) The practitioner places his or her hands side by side if the chest area is large enough or one on the other for a smaller chest area. The elbows are locked with the arms straight (Fig. 9-17). The patient's chest is gently but effectively shaken during exhalation. The patient should exhale at least the complete tidal volume as the chest wall is vibrated. Blowing out the expiratory reserve volume should help to clear out more secretions. A vibration rate of 200/min (about 3/sec) has been recommended as ideal to help move secretions. The literature differs as to how the patient should exhale during the procedure. Both breathing out slowly through pursed lips and breathing out forcefully through an open mouth have been recommended. It seems reasonable that a pursed-lip exhalation patterns should be used if the patient has a problem with bronchospasm and air trapping. A patient without this problem should exhale forcefully because this will help to clear more secretions. Vibration should be performed for several expiratory efforts or until it is no longer effective in helping to mobilize secretions.

There is mention in the literature of some patients needing a more vigorous form of vibration called shaking. It would be indicated in patients with thick secretions that cannot be cleared by other methods. With shaking, the patient's chest is pumped in and out

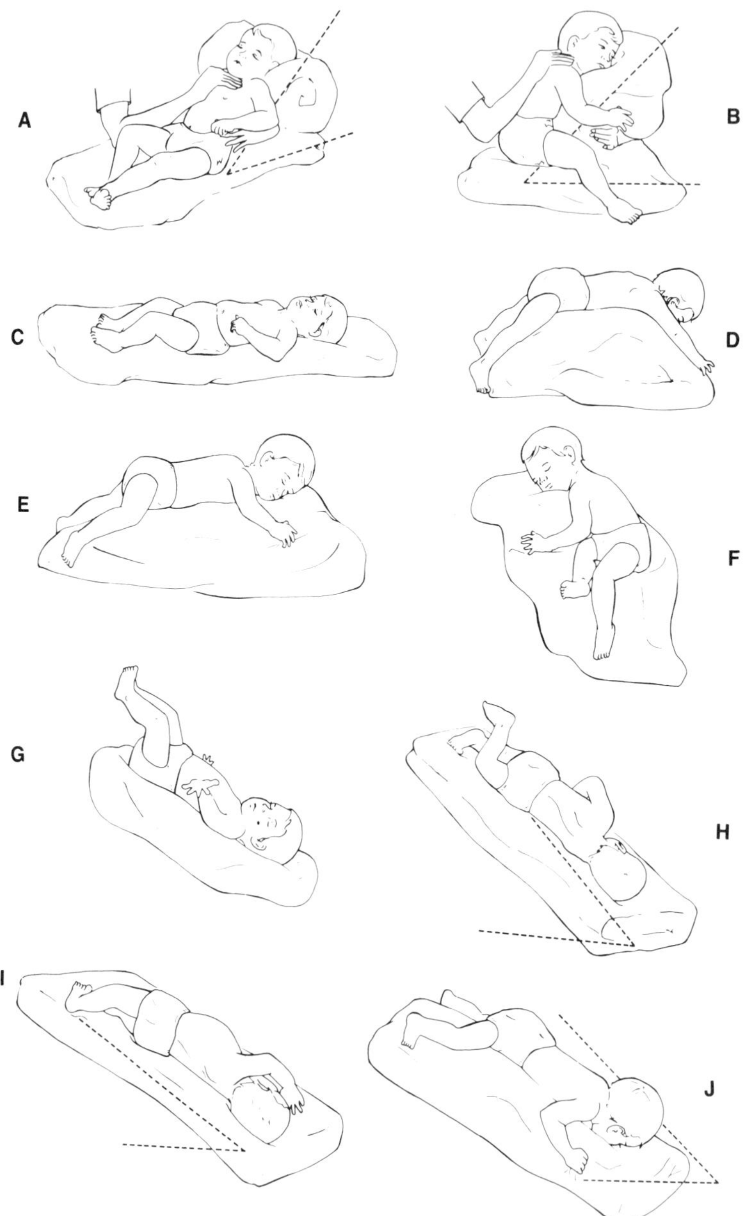

Fig. 9-15 Drainage positions in infants. **A,** apical segments of upper lobes. **B,** posterior segments of upper lobes. **C,** anterior segments of upper lobes. **D–F,** superior segments of lower lobes. **G** and **H,** anterior basal segments of both lower lobes (H on right and left sides). **I,** segments of the right middle lobe and lingula (shown). **J,** posterior basal segments of the lower lobes. (From Crane L: Physical therapy for the neonate with respiratory disease, in Irwin S, Tecklin JS [eds]: *Cardiopulmonary Physical Therapy*. St Louis, Mosby, 1985. Used by permission.)

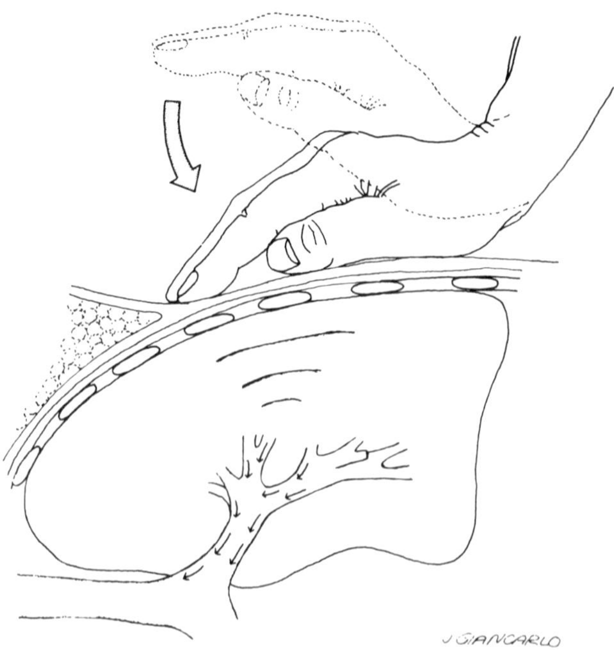

Fig. 9-16 Movement of the cupped hand at the wrist during chest percussion. (From Shapiro BA, Harrison RA, Kacmarek RM, et al: *Clinical Application of Respiratory Care,* ed 3. Chicago, Mosby, 1985. Used by permission.)

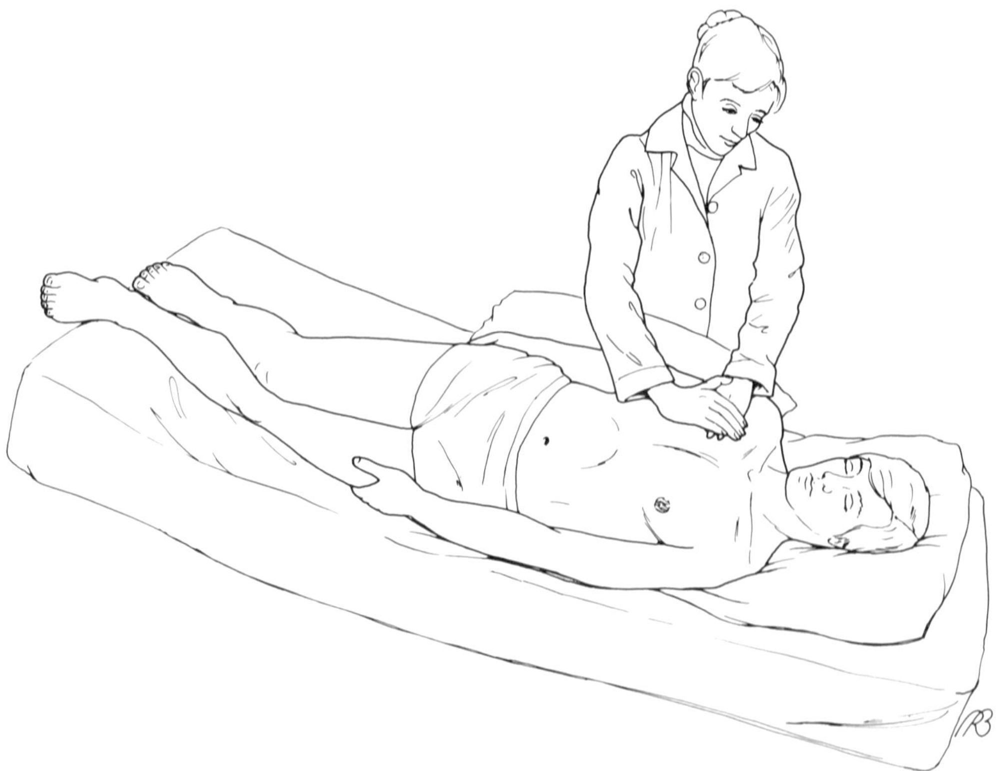

Fig. 9-17 Vibration of the chest in a postural drainage position. (From Eubanks DH, Bone RC: *Comprehensive Respiratory Care,* ed 2. St Louis, Mosby, 1990. Used by permission.)

to forcefully move air during exhalation. This technique must only be performed on patients with normally compliant chest walls.

3. Modify the postural drainage therapy in the following ways:
a. Change the length of time of the treatment. (IIIF2a) [R, Ap]

Lung segments should generally be drained for 3 to 15 minutes. If the patient is tolerating the position and secretions are still being cleared, the position can be held longer. Stop the treatment if the patient is showing any signs of intolerance as listed in Tables 9-3 and 9-4.

It is generally recommended that the total time of the procedure be no longer than 30 to 40 minutes. This is because the patient may become exhausted by the various position changes. If this is the case, the practitioner must select the worst segments to be drained first. It may take several drainage sessions to get to all of the involved segments.

b. Change the treatment techniques used. (IIIF2c) [R, Ap]

Be prepared to modify the postural drainage, percussion, and vibration procedures, depending on how the patient tolerates them. For example:

1. Some patients will not tolerate certain positions, especially head down, because of pain, shortness of breath, hypoxemia, or elevated blood pressure.
2. Percussion rate, pressure, and hand position may need to be modified, depending on the patient's tolerance, chest size, and secretion clearance.
3. It may not be possible to percuss or vibrate female patients in the right middle lobe and left ligula positions because of breast tissue.
4. Hypoxemia should be prevented with supplemental oxygen in those patients who need it. Pulse oximetry could be performed before and during the procedure to monitor the patient's oxygen saturation (Spo_2). The patient's oxygen saturation should improve as atelectatic areas open up and secretions are removed. Ventilation should then better match with perfusion. Refer to Section 5 for details on oximetry.
5. Cardiac patients should have their heart rate, heart rhythm, and blood pressure monitored. Check the heart rate before the procedure and with each position change.
6. Postoperative or trauma patients may not tolerate certain positions or percussion or vibration because of pain.
7. Patients with copious secretions that cannot be coughed out should not be put in a compromising situation. Suctioning equipment must be available. This situation may include patients who are not alert or who have a tracheostomy.
8. Very obese patients may not tolerate any head-down positions because of increased shortness of breath.

c. Organize the sequence of drainage positions and treatment techniques. (IIIF2d) [R, Ap]

There are differences of opinion as to the sequence in which the segments should be drained. Some authors state that an apices-to-bases approach is better, whereas others state that a bases-to-apices pattern is preferred.

It makes sense to take an apices-to-bases approach for a first treatment when all lobes are to be drained. This pattern gives the patient time to get used to the whole procedure. It may also be safer because the practitioner can evaluate the patient through a sequence of positions that progresses from the least to the most stressful.

If the patient is known to tolerate all positions without any difficulties and the lower lobes are the worst in terms of secretions, choose to drain the lower lobes first. If time permits, work up through the middle lobe and lingula to the upper lobes.

Careful study of the positions will show that the patient's work can be minimized by sequencing them properly. For example:

1. Drain the upper lobes in a posterior, apical, anterior sequence.
2. Drain the lateral basal and anterior basal segments of either lower lobe.
3. Drain the superior and posterior basal segments of either lower lobe.

It is also recommended that the total procedure take no longer than 30 to 40 minutes. Many patients will not tolerate a longer treatment. The practitioner may find that the worst segments need to be drained first and that less involved segments will have to be drained at a later time.

Module B. Postural drainage therapy equipment: percussors and vibrators.

1. Get the necessary equipment for the procedure. (IIA12) [R, Ap]

The terms *percussor* and *vibrator* are sometimes used interchangeably. It is not clear whether there is a difference in cycling rate or stroking distance between the two. Check the manufacturer's information for specific details. There are several manufacturers who produce either electrically or pneumatically powered percussors/vibrators. Some are large enough to be wheeled into the patient's room. See Fig. 9-18 for a drawing

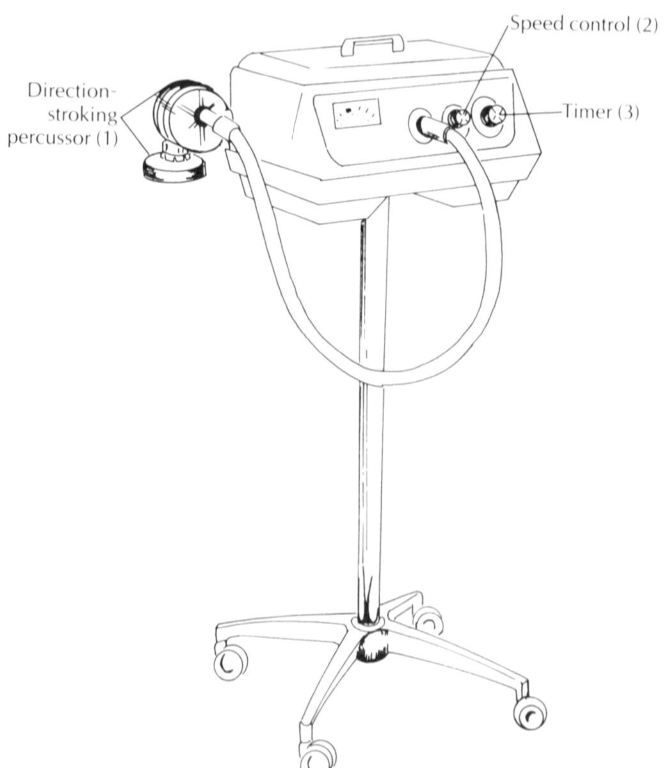

Fig. 9-18 An electrically powered mechanical percussor/vibrator. (From Eubanks DH, Bone RC: *Comprehensive Respiratory Care,* ed 2. St Louis, Mosby, 1990. Used by permission.)

of the Vibramatic produced by General Physiotherapy, Inc. (St. Louis). Obviously, electrically powered units need a standard electrical outlet for power, whereas the pneumatically powered units need to be plugged into a 50-psi oxygen or air source. Some electrical units are small enough to fit over the hand and are battery powered.

Pediatric units must be smaller to accurately focus on the much smaller target area of the infant's chest. They are battery powered. The Neocussor produced by General Physiotherapy, Inc. is an example. Some practitioners find that an electric toothbrush with padded bristles works very well. Manual percussion of infants can be aided by using soft rubber palm cups that come in several pediatric sizes. Some practitioners prefer to make their own infant percussion aids out of a pediatric resuscitation mask, an adapter, and an end cap (Fig. 9-19).

2. Put the equipment together, make sure that it works properly, and identify and fix any problems with it. (IIB12) [R, Ap]

Based on the previous discussion, it is known that the various devices are powered by wall electrical output, 50-psi source gas (±5 psi), or batteries. Check the power source if the device fails to work.

Some units have different patient applicators and connectors. These must be fastened properly so that the vibrating action will not cause them to loosen or fall off. For example, the Vibramatic has several patient applicators that must be screwed into the percussion adaptor, which is then screwed into the ring adaptor (Fig. 9-20).

3. Modify the equipment used. (IIIF2b) [R, Ap]

Some electrically powered units use a rubber belt and different-sized wheels to change gears and produce several vibration rates. Others electrically vary the motor

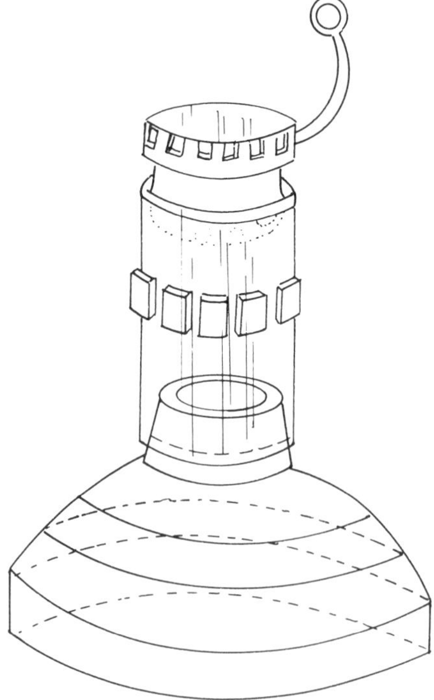

Fig. 9-19 A manual chest percussion aid for use with an infant. (From Eubanks DH, Bone RC: *Comprehensive Respiratory Care,* ed 2. St Louis, Mosby, 1990. Used by permission.)

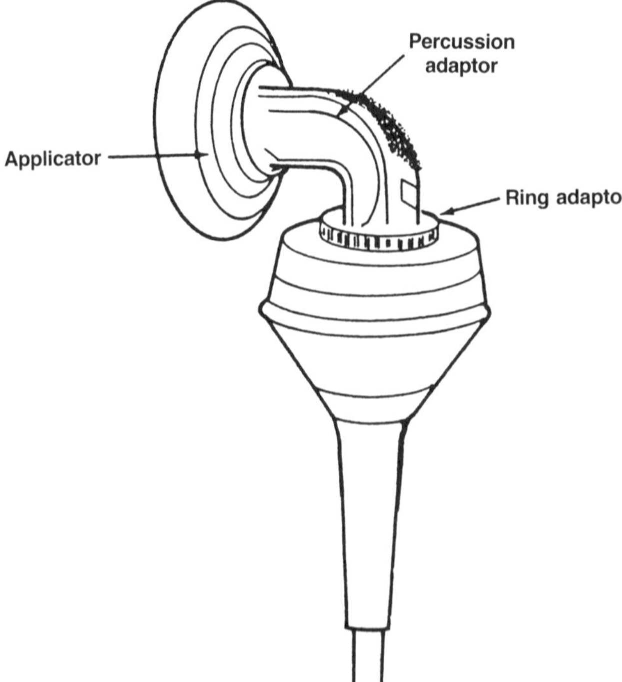

Fig. 9-20 Right-angle adaptor for percussor of Vibramatic chest percussor. Make sure that the percussion adaptor is tightly screwed into the ring adaptor and the various patient applicators are tightly screwed into the percussion adaptor. (Courtesy of General Physiotherapy, Inc, St Louis.)

speed to change the vibration rate. Some pneumatically driven units can have their percussion force and rate varied.

General Physiotherapy, Inc., recommends the following percussion rates for its Vibramatic and other models:

a. Twenty to 30 cps (or Hz) for an average-sized adult
b. Less than 20 cps for larger adults
c. Greater than 30 cps for smaller adults or children

One author lists an ideal rate of 25 to 35 cps to mobilize secretions. It seems reasonable that the practitioner should use whatever rate is tolerated by the patient and seems to best help mobilize the secretions.

Some adult percussors/vibrators come with a variety of patient contact pads. Select the one that best fits the patient's chest area that needs to be percussed. For example, a flat pad would be used over a broad area of the patient's back, whereas a U-shaped pad would be used around a patient's side.

It is important that the practitioner use the mechanical percussor/vibrator properly. General Physiotherapy, Inc., recommends that the patient applicator be held in one place for only 30 to 60 seconds. Longer may cause skin irritation. The applicator should be held loosely in the operator's hand; it is not necessary to press down on the patient. Because the patient applicator moves horizontally and vertically (Fig. 9-21), it must be used properly to help move the secretions. Fig. 9-22 shows how the patient applicator should be used to direct the loosened secretions to the draining bronchus and trachea.

• • •

This ends the general discussion on postural drainage therapy. The following information may be included in the questions offered by the NBRC. The general discussion of these topics was covered in Section 1. Some additional comments that relate directly to chest physiotherapy have been added.

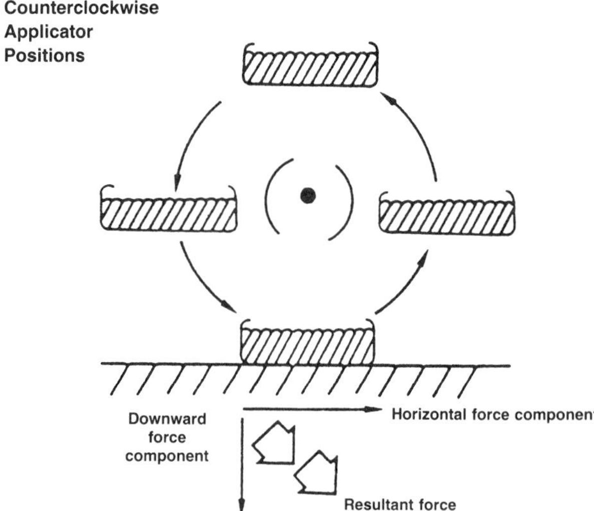

Fig. 9-21 Horizontal and perpendicular force components of the patient applicator for the Vibramatic chest percussor. Note the resultant force that propels secretions. (Courtesy of General Physiotherapy, Inc, St Louis.)

Module C. Patient assessment.

1. Determine and continue to monitor how the patient responds to the treatment or procedure.

Be prepared to measure the patient's blood pressure, heart rate, and respiratory rate before, during, and after a change in position. Minor changes (<20%) can be expected. Positional hypoxemia may result in arrhythmias. The intracranial pressure should also be monitored if available.

The patient's oxygenation should improve as secretions and mucous plugs are removed and atelectatic areas open up. This is because ventilation will better match with perfusion. Pulse oximetry should be used throughout the procedure if there is any concern for the patient having transient hypoxemia during position changes.

The patient's breath sounds should be auscultated before the treatment begins to determine which segments are silent or have secretions. Auscultate each segment after it

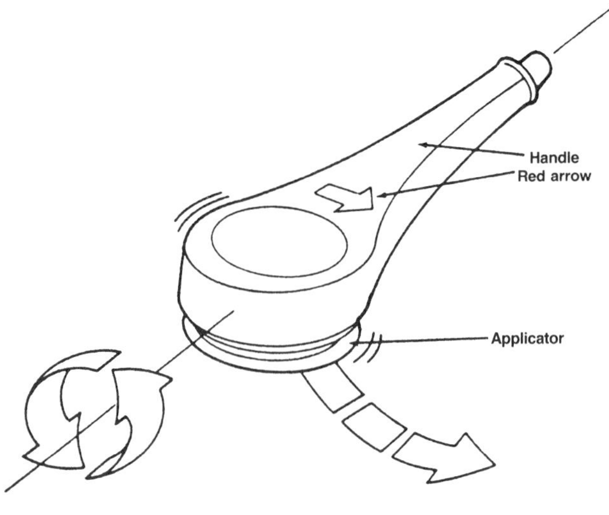

Fig. 9-22 Directional stroking percussor for the Vibramatic and Multimatic chest percussors. Note how the red arrow on the handle points the direction secretions will flow when the patient is positioned properly and the applicator is placed correctly over the desired lung segment. (Courtesy of General Physiotherapy, Inc, St Louis.)

has been drained and the patient has coughed. Listen to hear if air is moving into formerly silent areas or if secretions have been cleared.

Make a recommendation for a chest x-ray film to find specific areas for chest physiotherapy. A white shadow on a chest x-ray film over what should be normal lung may indicate areas of atelectasis or infiltrates that can be targeted for treatment. Repeat chest x-ray films should be performed to look for an improvement in the lungs. The resolution may be slow or dramatic, depending on the original problem and how it responds to the various treatments used on it.

Ask the patient how he or she feels before, during, and after the treatment. This is very important because the patient is being positioned in unnatural ways that may result in discomfort, shortness of breath, dizzyness, or nausea. Percussion and vibration rates and force should not be uncomfortable.

2. Modify the treatment or procedure and recommend any changes in the patient's respiratory care plan, depending on the response.

Postural drainage therapy should not be performed for at least 1 hour after a patient has eaten. This is to help minimize the chances of nausea and vomiting from the head-down positions. Avoid PDT immediately before a meal because the patient may be to tired to eat properly.

The practitioner may have to determine which segments need to be drained if the physician's order is nonspecific. The practitioner may have to also determine if any treatment modifications are needed or if a mechanical percussor is indicated. The practitioner may find that different segments need to be drained than originally ordered or indicated. Make note of any treatment modifications that have been started and how the patient tolerated them. These procedures should not be performed if they are not indicated or if the patient has a contraindicating condition.

As mentioned earlier, each position should be drained for 3 to 15 minutes. Cut the time short if the patient does not tolerate it. Add to the time if the patient tolerates it and secretions are still being produced. The total procedure should not exceed 40 minutes. A 20% increase or decrease in any of the vital signs should cause the treatment to be stopped. Also, stop the treatment if the patient becomes hypoxemic, complains of worsening shortness of breath, or has frank hemoptysis. Repeated difficulties may mean that the patient cannot tolerate the procedure under any circumstances or modifications and the procedure should be canceled.

BIBLIOGRAPHY

AARC Clinical Practice Guideline: Postural drainage therapy. *Respir Care* 1991:36:1418-1426.

Barrascout JR: Chest physical therapy and related procedures, in Burton GG, Hodgkin JE (eds): *Respiratory Care*, ed 2. Philadelphia, Lippincott, 1984.

Eubanks DH, Bone RC: *Comprehensive Respiratory Care*, ed 2. St Louis, Mosby, 1990.

Frownfelter DL: Chest physical therapy and airway care, in Barnes TA (ed): *Respiratory Care Practice*. Chicago, Mosby, 1988.

Meyer CL: Chest physiotherapy in infants requiring ventilatory assistance. *Respir Ther* 1984; January/February.

Rarey KP, Youtsey JW: *Respiratory Patient Care*. Englewood Cliffs, NJ, Prentice-Hall, 1981.

Scanlan CL: Chest physical therapy, in Scanlan CL, Spearman CB, Sheldon RL (eds): *Egan's Fundamentals of Respiratory Care*, ed 5. St Louis, Mosby, 1990.

Scott AA, Koff PB: Airway care and chest physiotherapy, in Koff PB, Eitzman DV, Neu J (eds): *Neonatal and Pediatric Respiratory Care*. St Louis, Mosby, 1988.

Shapiro BA, Harrison RA, Kacmarek RM, et al: *Clinical Application of Respiratory Care*, ed 3. Chicago, Mosby, 1985.

White GC: *Basic Clinical Lab Competencies for Respiratory Care*. Albany, NY, Delmar, 1988.

Wojciechowski WV: Incentive spirometers and secretion evacuation devices, in Barnes TA (ed): *Respiratory Care Practice*. Chicago, Mosby, 1988.

SELF-STUDY QUESTIONS

1. Manual percussion should be performed with:
   I. The hand cupped
   II. A tight, fixed wrist position
   III. The elbows relaxed
   IV. The hand flat
   V. The wrist relaxed
   A. III, IV, V
   B. II, III, IV
   C. II, IV
   D. I, II
   E. I, III, V

2. Vibration should be performed:
   I. On inspiration
   II. At a rate of 20 to 30 cps
   III. On expiration
   IV. At a rate of 3 cps
   V. Throughout the breathing cycle
   A. I, IV
   B. I, IV
   C. III, IV
   D. IV, V
   E. II, V

3. Contraindications for postural drainage include all of the following *except:*
   A. Increased intracranial pressure in a patient with head injury
   B. Broken ribs
   C. Stroke
   D. Small vital capacity in a bedridden patient
   E. Immediately after eating

4. You receive an order to perform postural drainage, percussion, and vibration on a patient. No segments are specified. On reviewing the chest x-ray film, you notice infiltrates in the lower right lung field. You would proceed to treat the following segments:
   I. Apical
   II. Lateral basal
   III. Superior
   IV. Medial
   V. Posterior basal
   A. II, V
   B. III, IV, V
   C. I, IV
   D. II, III, V
   E. All of the above.

5. To drain the superior and inferior lingular segments the patient should be positioned:
   I. With the foot of the bed elevated 14 inches
   II. One-fourth turn up from front down on the bed
   III. One-fourth turn up from back down on the bed
   IV. With the foot of the bed elevated 30 degrees
   V. Flat on his or her back
   A. I, III
   B. IV, V
   C. I, II
   D. I, V
   E. III, IV

6. Contraindications to percussion and vibrations include all of the following *except:*
   A. Over the kidneys
   B. To mobilize thick secretions
   C. Over bare skin
   D. Over or near a surgical site
   E. Over a known lung tumor

7. A patient is positioned on her left side with the foot of the bed raised 18 inches. She would be draining which lung segment?
   A. Anterior basal
   B. Superior
   C. Lateral and medial lingular
   D. Posterior basal
   E. Posterior

8. Before using a Vibramatic mechanical percussor on an average-sized adult patient, you would set the cycling rate at:
   A. 5/sec
   B. 15/sec
   C. 25/sec
   D. 35/sec
   E. 45/sec

9. Indications for postural drainage include all of the following *except:*
   A. Atelectasis
   B. The patient has retained secretions
   C. Cystic fibrosis
   D. To drain an empyema
   E. Removal of an aspirated foreign body

10. You receive an order to perform postural drainage, percussion, and vibration on a 23-year-old female patient. The lateral and medial segments of the right middle lobe are among those that need to be treated. You would procede to:
   A. Drain, percuss, and vibrate the segments.
   B. Drain and vibrate the segments.
   C. Drain but not percuss or vibrate those segments.
   D. Position her more straight up on her side so that the breast would shift out of the way and percussion could be performed.
   E. Drain and use a mechanical percussor.

Answer key:

1. E; 2. C; 3. D; 4. D; 5. A; 6. B; 7. A; 8. C; 9. D; 10. C.

10 Cardiopulmonary Resuscitation (Emergency Care)

Module A. Perform cardiopulmonary resuscitation (CPR) and related functions.

1. Establish that the patient is unresponsive and needs CPR. (IIIG1) [R, Ap]

Observing a patient who *appears* to be dead does not prove that the patient needs CPR. Clinical death must be proved before CPR is begun.

Adults should be tapped or gently shaken while shouting, "Are you okay?"

Infants should have the bottom of their feet gently slapped while shouting, "Wake up!" The rescuer can also clap his or her hands together loudly to wake a sleeping infant.

CPR should never be started on a person who does not need it!

2. Call out for help. (IIIG2) [R, Ap]

Call out for help if the victim does not respond to any attempts at arousal. The second rescuer should be told to call in the cardiac arrest team. Many hospitals have a cardiac arrest button in each patient's room. If this is the case, the first rescuer can push the button while calling out for help. Dial 911 on the telephone for help if the victim is found at home.

3. Open the airway. (IIIG3) [R, Ap]

The head-tilt/chin-lift maneuver is the procedure of choice for opening the airway of all victims except those with a known or suspected cervical (neck) spine injury. The victim is gently positioned on his or her back. In an adult, the head is firmly pushed back with one hand, and the jaw is pulled upward with the fingers of the other hand (Fig. 10-1). In an infant, it is not necessary to tilt the head back beyond a neutral position. Children may need to have the head pushed back slightly beyond neutral (Fig. 10-2).

The jaw-thrust maneuver is the procedure of choice for opening the airway of all victims with a known or suspected cervical spine injury. The rescuer's elbows are rested on the ground, and the hand are placed on either side of the victim's jaw. Lifting of the jaw usually opens the airway the need to tilt the head back. See Fig. 10-3 for the adult maneuver and Fig. 10-4 for the infant maneuver.

Anything that can be seen in the mouth or throat should be removed. The cross-finger technique can be used to open the mouth wide enough so that a finger or suction device can be inserted to remove a blockage (Fig. 10-5). An oral airway should be used

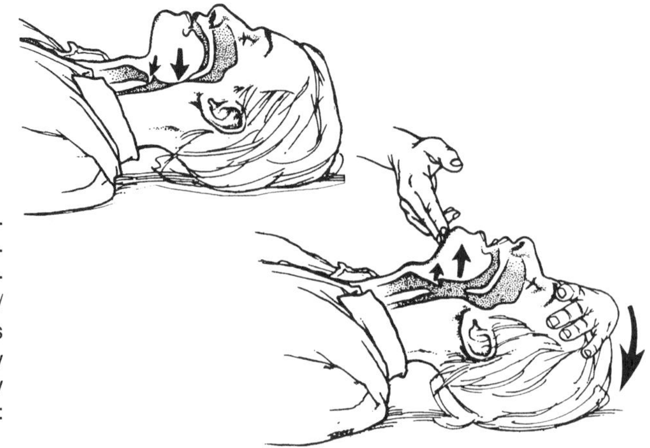

Fig. 10-1 Opening the adult's airway. *Top,* Airway obstruction produced by the tongue and epiglottis. *Bottom,* Relief by head-tilt/chin-lift method. (From Standards and guidelines for cardiopulmonary resuscitation [CPR] and emergency cardiac care [ECC]. *JAMA* 1992; 268: 2186. Used by permission.)

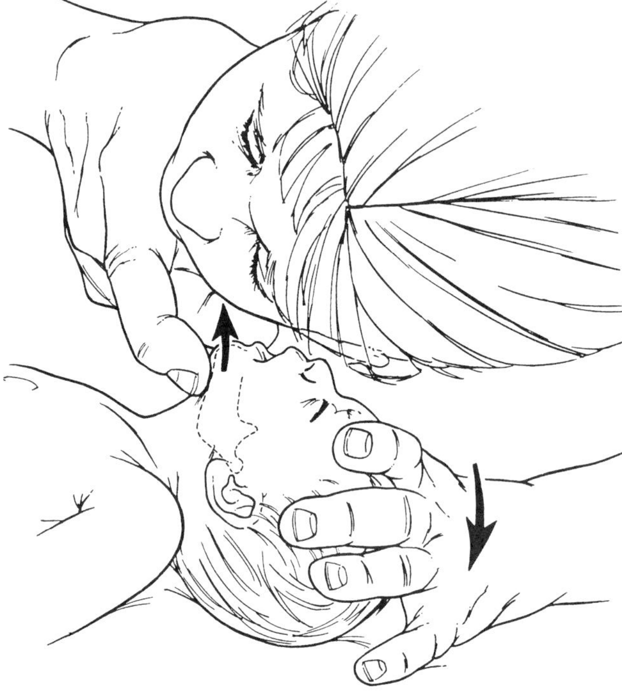

Fig. 10-2 Opening the infant's airway by the head-tilt/chin-lift method. (From Standards and guidelines for cardiopulmonary resuscitation [CPR] and emergency cardiac care [ECC]. *JAMA* 1992; 268:2253. Used by permission.)

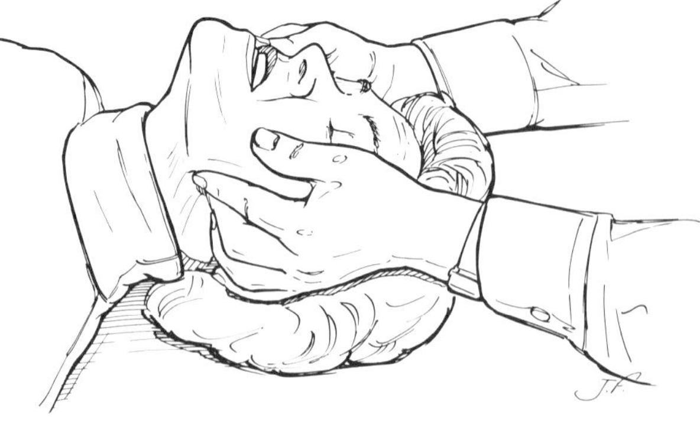

Fig. 10-3 Opening the adult's airway by the jaw thrust method. (From Watson MA: Cardiopulmonary resuscitation, in Barnes TA [ed]: *Respiratory Care Practice,* Chicago, Mosby, 1988. Used by permission.)

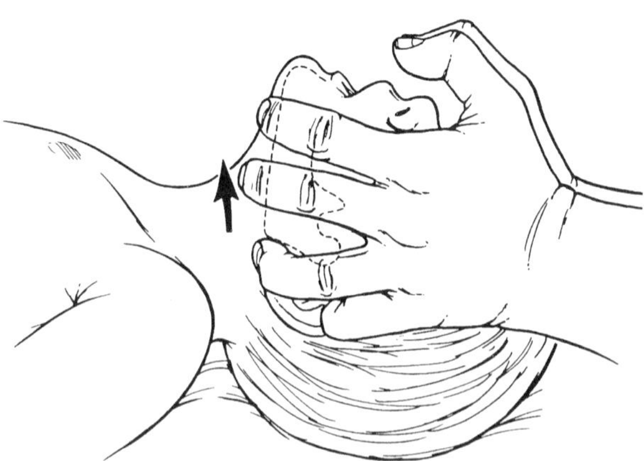

Fig. 10-4 Opening the infant's airway by the jaw thrust method. (From Standards and guidelines for cardiopulmonary resuscitation [CPR] and emergency cardiac care [ECC]. *JAMA* 1992; 268:2254. Used by permission.)

only in an unconscious patient to keep the tongue from falling back and blocking the airway.

4. Determine that the patient is not breathing. (IIIG8) [R, Ap]

The rescuer places his or her face close to the victim's so that he or she can *look* for rising and falling of the chest, *listen* for air movement, and *feel* any air movement from the victim's breathing (Fig. 10-6). This should be done for 3 to 5 seconds to be sure that the patient is really apneic and not just breathing slowly.

5. Ventilate the patient's airway. (IIIG4) [R, Ap]

a. Mouth-to-mouth breathing.

The first rescuer should begin mouth-to-mouth breathing as soon as possible if their is no spontaneous breathing by the victim once the airway is opened. No matter the age of the victim, there must be an effective seal between the rescuer and the victim. The adult victim's nose must be pinched closed; often the infant's nosed can be blocked by the cheek of the rescuer. Both the nose and mouth of an infant can be covered by the mouth of the rescuer. Alternative methods of ventilation include mouth to nose and mouth to stoma (Fig. 10-7).

In an adult, two breaths large enough to raise the victim's chest should be given. An adequate volume of 800 ml; up to 1200 ml may be given. Blow into the victim's mouth

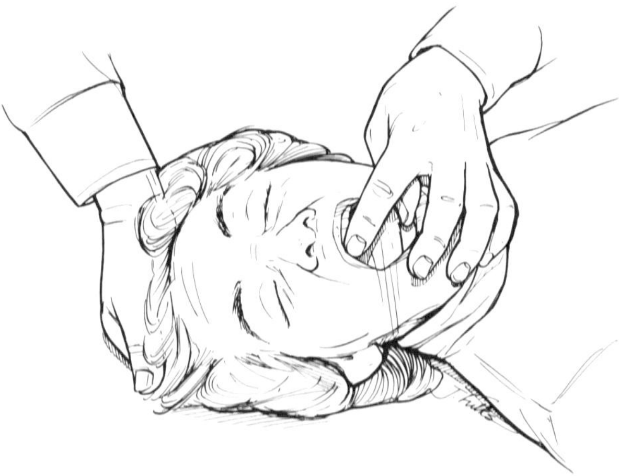

Fig. 10-5 The cross-finger method of opening the victim's mouth to look for an obstruction. (From Watson MA: Cardiopulmonary resuscitation, in Barnes TA [ed]: *Respiratory Care Practice,* Chicago, Mosby, 1988. Used by permission.)

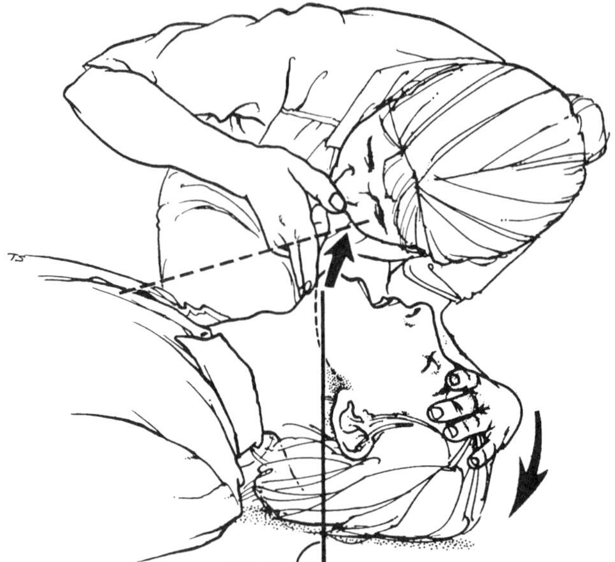

Fig. 10-6 Determine breathlessness by looking, listening, and feeling. (From Standards and guidelines for cardiopulmonary resuscitation [CPR] and emergency cardiac care [ECC]. *JAMA* 1992; 268:2187. Used by permission.)

for 1 to 1.5 seconds. This is to ensure a large enough volume without having to use much pressure. Keeping the ventilating pressure as low as possible will minimize the risk of forcing air into the stomach. Ensure that the victim exhales completely by watching the chest fall and feeling the air escape against your cheek. Rescue breathing should be performed at a rate of 10 to 12 times/min (every 6 seconds) if the victim has a pulse but is apneic.

In a child, two breaths large enough to raise the victim's chest should be given. The volume will obviously be less than that needed in an adult. All of the same considerations apply as in the adult. Rescue breathing should be performed at a rate of 20/min (every 3 seconds) in an infant and 15/min (every 4 seconds) in a child (Fig. 10-8).

If the victim's airway cannot be ventilated, reposition the head and attempt to ventilate again. Failure to ventilate a second time means that the victim has an obstructed airway. The following steps should be taken:

A. Unconscious adult obstructed airway maneuvers:
   1. Position the victim on his or her back if not already there.
   2. Perform the Heimlich maneuver several times if needed. This is done by kneeling astride the victim, placing the heel of one hand midline on the abdomen slightly above the navel but well below the xiphoid process. The other hand is placed on top, and both are quickly thrust upward toward the chest (Fig. 10-9). The markedly obese or obviously pregnant victim can have chest thrusts performed on them. The rescuer's hands should be placed on the lower half of the sternum as with cardiac compressions. Several compressions should be performed slowly but similarly to how a cardiac compression would be done.
   3. Attempt to clear out any foreign body with a finger sweep. First, grasp the victim's tongue and jaw between your thumb and fingers, and lift the jaw open. Next, insert the index finger of the other hand along the inside of the victim's cheek and down the back of the throat so as to hook and remove food, gum, dentures, and so on.

B. Unconscious child (≤1 year) obstructed airway maneuvers:
   1. Same as adult.
   2. Same as adult with up to five thrusts performed if needed. Chest thrusts are not used.

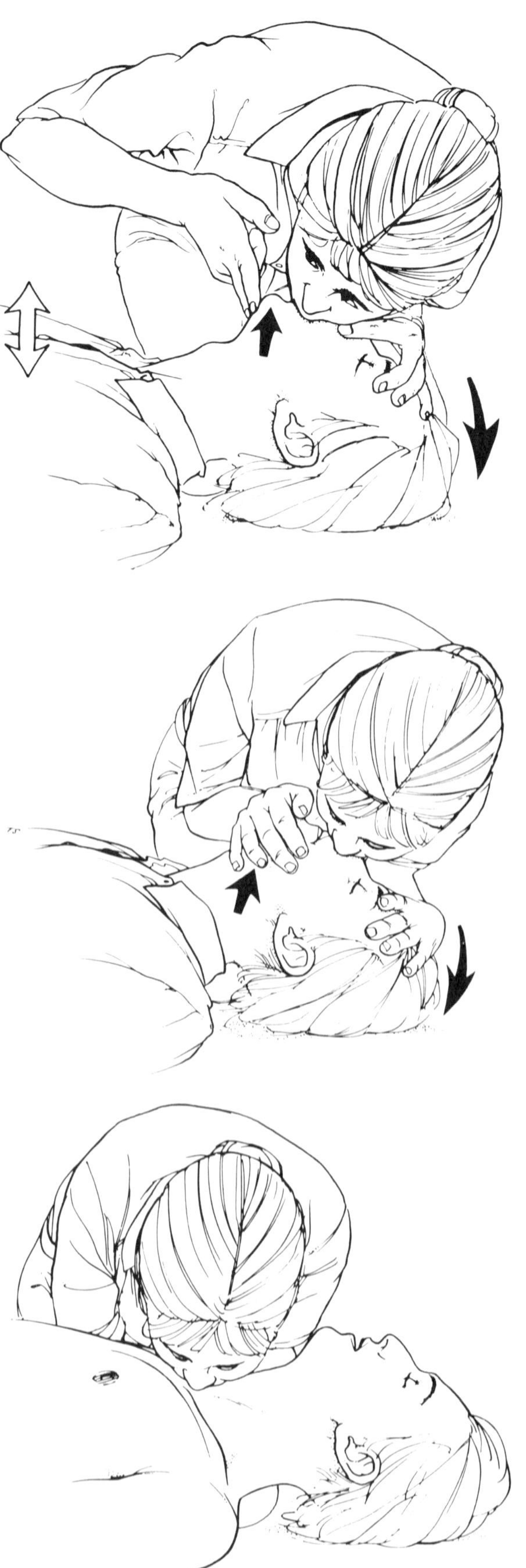

Fig. 10-7 Adult mouth-to-mouth, mouth-to-nose, and mouth-to-stoma ventilation. (From Standards and guidelines for cardiopulmonary resuscitation [CPR] and emergency cardiac care [ECC]. *JAMA* 1992; 268: 2188. Used by permission.)

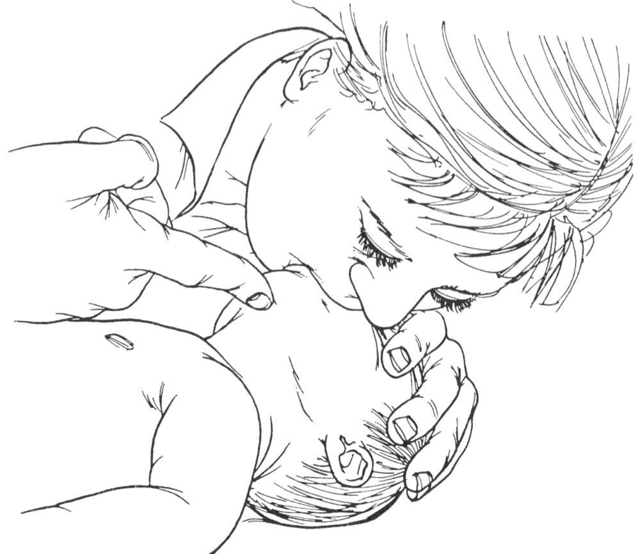

Fig. 10-8 Infant mouth-to-mouth ventilation with the cheek used as a nose seal. (From Standards and guidelines for cardiopulmonary resuscitation [CPR] and emergency cardiac care [ECC]. *JAMA* 1992; 268:2254. Used by permission.)

3. Same as the adult except that the index finger is inserted only when a foreign body has been seen. Blindly inserting the index finger may push a foreign body further down the throat.

C. Unconscious infant obstructed airway maneuver:
   1. The infant is straddled over one forearm of the rescuer. His or her jaw and head are held by the hand. The infant's head should be lower than the body. Five firm back blows are delivered between the shoulder blades with the heel of the rescuer's other hand (Fig. 10-10).
   2. The infant is sandwiched by the rescuer's other arm, and his or her body are supported head are turned to a supine position. The head should remain

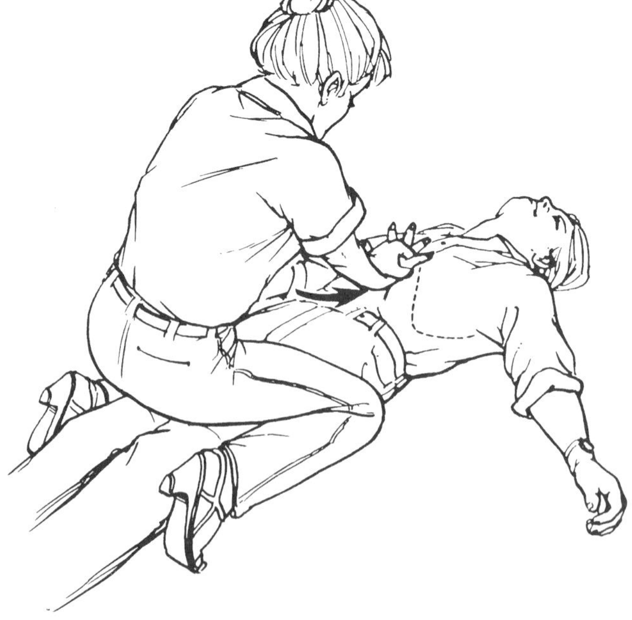

Fig. 10-9 Administering the Heimlich maneuver to an unconscious adult victim of an airway obstruction. (From Standards and guidelines for cardiopulmonary resuscitation [CPR] and emergency cardiac care [ECC]. *JAMA* 1992; 268:2193. Used by permission.)

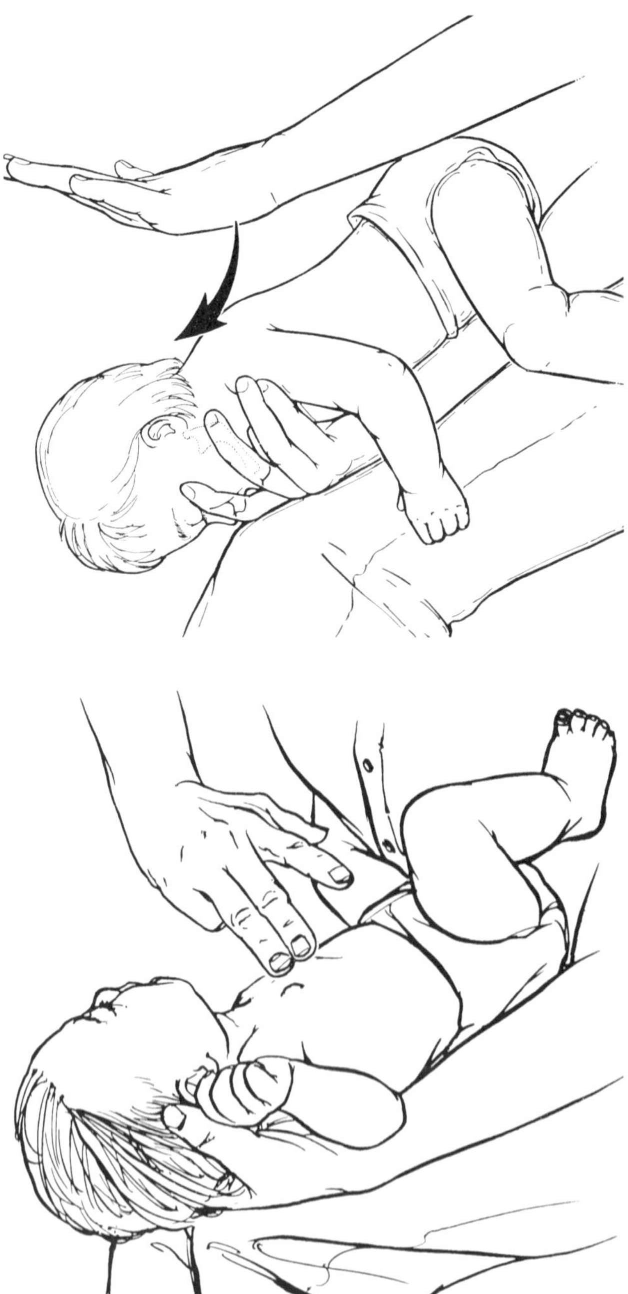

Fig. 10-10 Administering back blows and chest thrusts to an infant victim of an airway obstruction. (From Standards and guidelines for cardiopulmonary resuscitation [CPR] and emergency cardiac care [ECC]. *JAMA* 1992; 268:2258. Used by permission.)

lower than the body. Five chest thrusts are performed in the same location and manner as cardiac compressions but at a slower rate. Steps 1 and 2 can be done by placing the infant on the rescuer's lap.

3. Same as step 3 in the unconscious child mentioned earlier.

b. Manual resuscitator (bag-valve).

A manual resuscitator should be used during hospital-based CPR as soon as one is available. The resuscitation mask must be held to the face so that there is no air leak during the forced inspiration (Fig. 10-11.) An assistant can hold the mask tightly to the

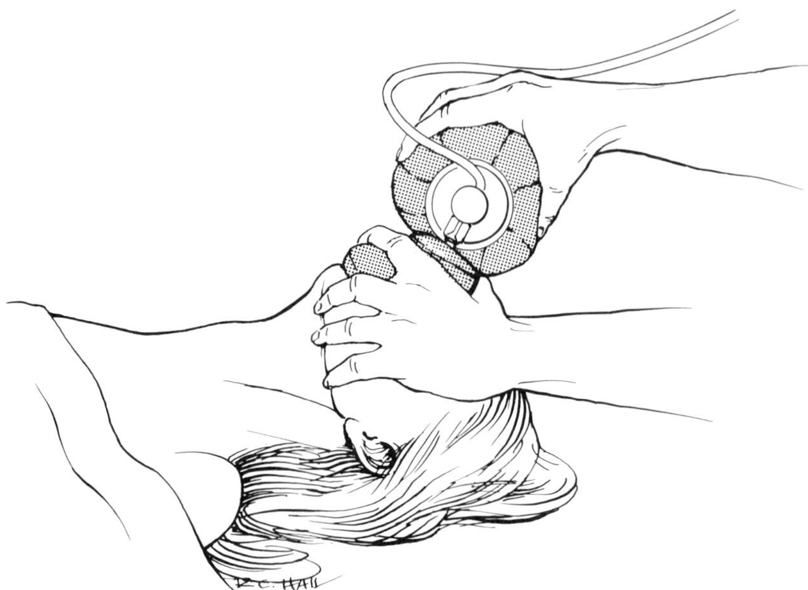

Fig. 10-11 Ventilation of an adult with a manual resuscitation bag and mask. (From Eubanks DH, Bone RC: *Comprehensive Respiratory Care,* ed 2. St Louis, Mosby, 1990. Used by permission.)

face so that the rescuer who is pumping the resuscitation bag can use both hands. This has been shown to produce a larger tidal volume. If the victim's airway contains an endotracheal or tracheostomy tube, the valve adapter fits directly over the tube adapter. Rescue breathing would continue with the previously mentioned considerations for volume and rate.

c. Mouth-to-valve mask ventilation.

A mouth-to-valve mask device (often called a pocket mask) combines a resuscitation mask with a one-way valve mouthpiece. It is used to ventilate an apneic patient rather than perform mouth-to-mouth breathing. Concerns about protecting the rescuer from patient infections such as hepatitis have lead to their widespread acceptance. As shown in Fig. 10-12, the patient's neck is hyperextended, the mask is applied over the mouth and nose to get an airtight seal, and the rescuer breathes into the mouthpiece. It is best if the rescuer is positioned at the victim's head so that the chest can be seen to rise with each delivered breath. The one-way valve is designed so that the victim's exhaled gas is vented out to the room air. Some units have a nipple adapter so that supplemental oxygen can be added to the delivered breath. Simply attach oxygen tubing between the nipple and oxygen flowmeter and turn the flowmeter on to the manufacturer's recommended flow. For example, the Laerdal pocket mask can have between 5 and 15 L of oxygen/min added to it to supplement the rescuer's breathing. It is best if these devices be replaced by a manual resuscitator as soon as possible.

6. Add supplemental oxygen. (IIIG10) [R, Ap]

The victim should be given 100% oxygen as soon as possible. There is no contraindication for giving pure oxygen during a resuscitation effort. This can be done easily only if a manual resuscitator is used to ventilate the victim. Most modern units have the capability of giving 100% oxygen if the oxygen flow is high enough and a reservoir is added. Some older units can give supplemental oxygen at some percentage less than 100%.

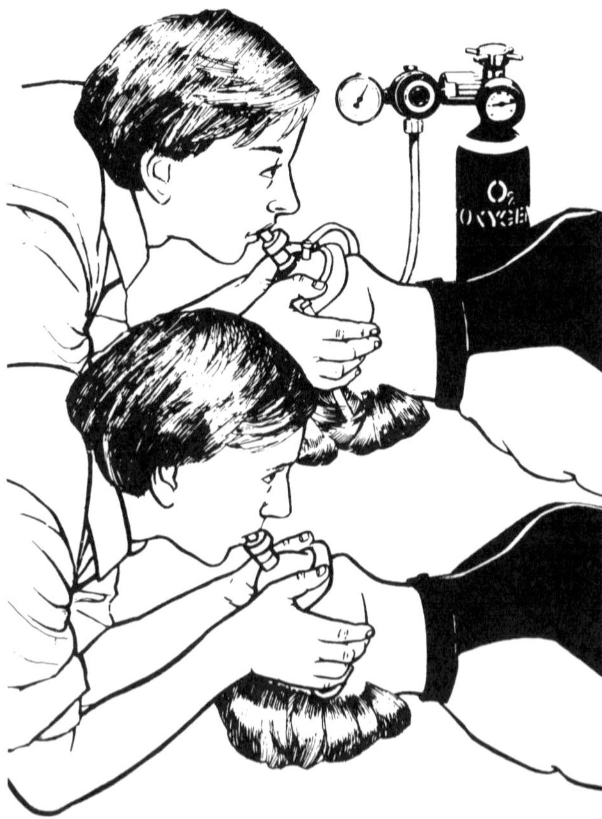

Fig. 10-12 Proper positioning to use a mouth-to-valve mask resuscitator. The top rescuer has added supplemental oxygen to the device. The bottom rescuer is ventilating without the use of added oxygen. (Courtesy of Laerdal Medical Corporation, Armonk, NY.)

These are still better than using room air but should be replaced with a unit capable of delivering 100% oxygen as soon as possible.

7. Determine pulselessness. (IIIG6) [R, Ap]

The carotid pulse is felt for in all victims except children younger than 1 year. The carotid pulse is found by gently feeling with two or three fingers in the groove between the larynx and the sternocleidomastoid muscle on either side of the neck (Fig. 10-13). Check for 5 to 10 seconds to be sure that the victim is pulseless and not just bradycardiac. An infant younger than 1 year should have the pulse felt in the brachial artery (see Fig. 10-14). This is because the carotid artery is difficult to find in such young children with short, chubby necks.

The femoral pulse can be felt for as an alternative site in all victims. This is limited to victims in the hospital who are wearing few clothes. Once the CPR team has arrived and two-person CPR is instituted, the femoral pulse may the one that is most accessible for monitoring the pulse and the effectiveness of the chest compressions.

8. Perform external chest compressions. (IIIG5) [R, Ap]

The absence of a pulse confirms a cardiac arrest. Blood must be pumped by external chest compressions of the heart. The victim must be supine on a hard surface. A CPR backboard is placed behind a victim who is in bed.

In adults and large children or those more than 8 years old, the heel of the rescuer's hand is placed over the lower half of the sternum. This is found by placing the middle finger of one hand in the notch where the ribs meet the sternum, placing the index fin-

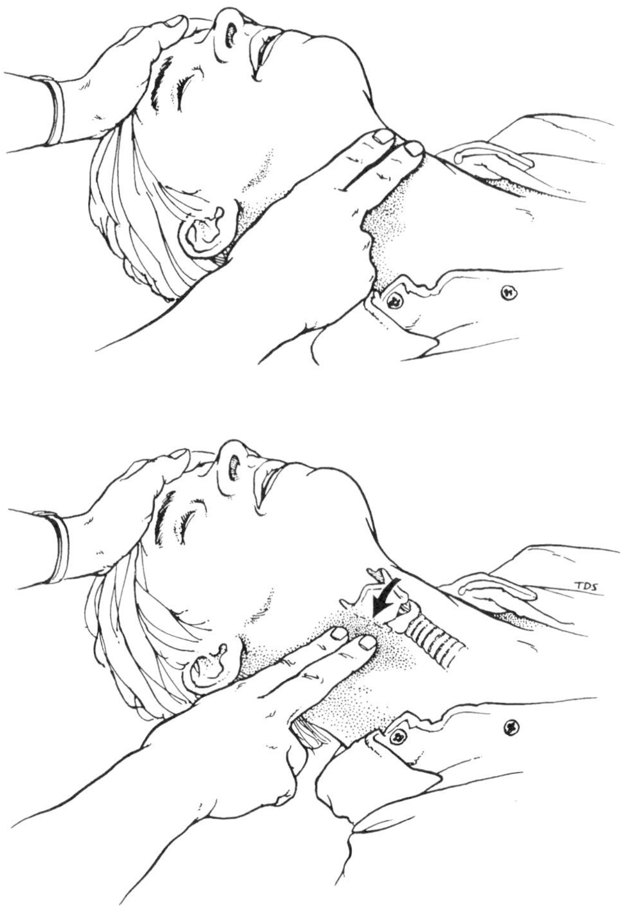

Fig. 10-13 Determining pulselessness by checking the carotid pulse of an adult. (From Standards and guidelines for cardiopulmonary resuscitation [CPR] and emergency cardiac care [ECC]. *JAMA* 1992; 268:2189. Used by permission.)

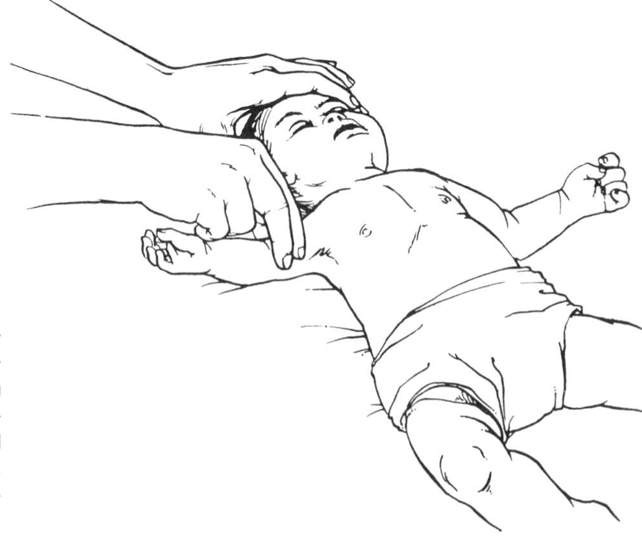

Fig. 10-14 Determining pulselessness by checking the brachial pulse of an infant. (From Standards and guidelines for cardiopulmonary resuscitation [CPR] and emergency cardiac care [ECC]. *JAMA* 1992; 268:2255. Used by permission.)

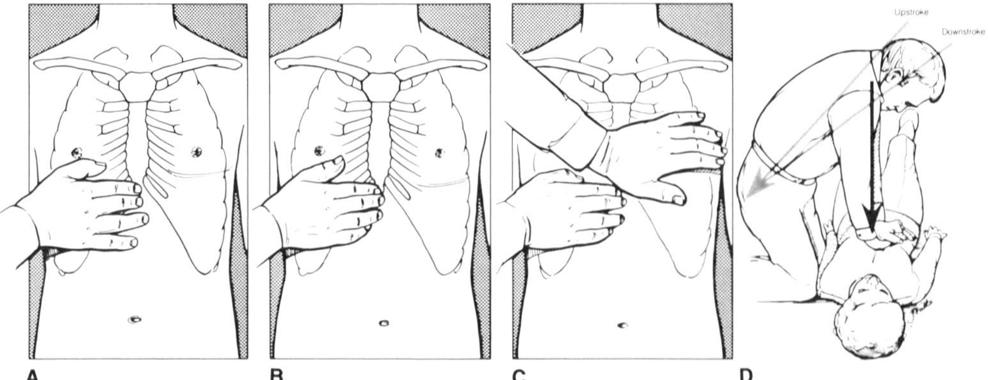

Fig. 10-15 Cardiac compression on an adult. **A,** locate tip of xiphoid process. **B,** place two fingertips at xiphoid process. **C,** place palm of other hand on sternum next to fingers. **D,** arm and body positions for cardiac compression. (From Barnes TA: *Respiratory Care Practice,* Chicago, Mosby, 1988, p 255. Used by permission.)

ger next to it, and placing the other hand next to the finger. The first hand is placed over it, the elbows are locked, and the shoulders are directly over the hands. This creates the most efficient pumping action (Fig. 10-15). The rescuer pivots from the hips, with half of the time spent pumping down and half of the time releasing pressure. The hands should always touch the victim's chest. The sternum must be compressed 1.5 to 2.0 inches (3.8-5.0 cm) in an average adult. The compression rate should be between 80 and 100/min.

In a child 8 years or younger, hand position is found as in the adult (Fig. 10-16). The child's sternum must be compressed with *one* hand to a depth of 1 to 1.5 inches (2.5-3.8 cm). Half of the time should be spent on compression and half on relaxation. The rate should be 100/min to achieve a rate of 80/min between ventilations.

In an infant, two or three fingers are placed over the middle of the sternum one finger width below an imaginary line drawn between the nipples (Fig. 10-17). The child's sternum must be compressed to a depth of 0.5 to 1 inch (1.3-2.5 cm). Half of the time should be spent on compression and half on relaxation. The rate should be at least 100/min.

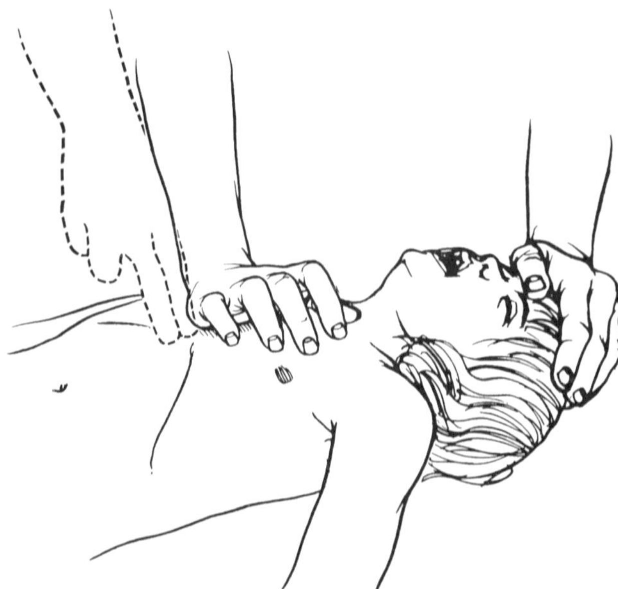

Fig. 10-16 Locating the proper hand position for chest compressions in the child. Use the other hand to keep the proper head position for ventilations. (From Standards and guidelines for cardiopulmonary resuscitation [CPR] and emergency cardiac care [ECC]. *JAMA* 1992; 268:2257. Used by permission.)

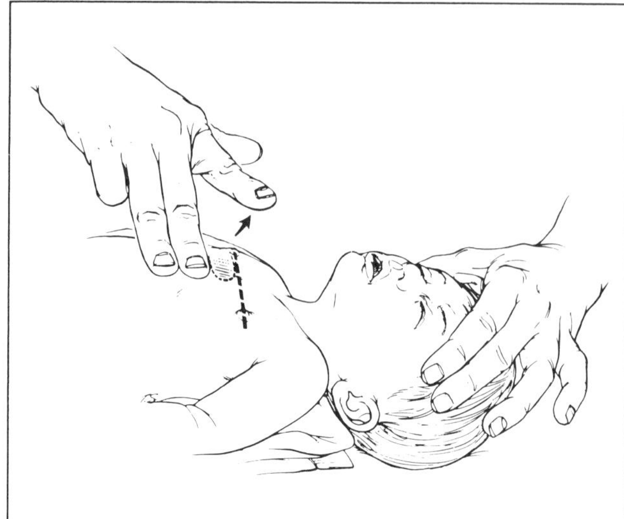

Fig. 10-17 Locating the proper finger position for chest compressions in the infant. (From Standards and guidelines for cardiopulmonary resuscitation [CPR] and emergency cardiac care [ECC]. *JAMA* 1992; 268: 2256. Used by permission.)

Even though the examination content outline of the National Board of Respiratory Care (NBRC) does not specifically list one- and two-person CPR, they are included for the sake of completeness.

A. Adult one-rescuer CPR:
   1. Assess the victim's need for CPR.
   2. Call out for help.
   3. Open the airway.
   4. Assess the victim's lack of breathing.
   5. Give two rescue breaths.
   6. Assess the victim's lack of a pulse.
   7. Perform 15 chest compressions at a rate of 80 to 100/min. Count them out as "one and, two and, three and . . ."
   8. Reopen the airway and give two breaths.
   9. Repeat this cycle (15:2 ratio) a total of four times.
   10. Check the victim's carotid pulse from 5 seconds. If it has not returned, give two breaths and continue with compressions.
   11. If the pulse has returned, check on the return of breathing. If it has not returned, give 12 breaths/min.
   12. If CPR is continued, check for the return of a heartbeat and breathing every few minutes.

B. Adult two-rescuer CPR:
   1. Perform steps 1 to 6 as earlier.
   2. The first rescuer performs five chest compressions at a rate of 80 to 100/min. Count them out as "one and, two and, three and . . . ."
   3. The second rescuer gives one breath during a 1.5- to 2-second pause between sets of compressions.
   4. Repeat this cycle (5:1 ratio) several times.
   5. The second rescuer calls for a 5-second pause after 1 minute and checks for the return of pulse or breathing.
   6. Provide breathing, circulation, or both as needed. If CPR is continued, check for the return of a heartbeat and breathing every few minutes.
   7. Switch positions whenever one rescuer becomes tired. Make the switch at the end of a cycle, check the victim for a return of pulse or breathing, and continue as needed.

C. Infant and child one and two-rescuer CPR:
   1. Perform steps 1 to 6 as earlier.
   2. In either case, a rescuer performs sets of five chest compressions. These are delivered at a rate of at least 100/min to deliver at least 80 compressions/min between ventilations. Count them out as "one and, two and, three and . . ."
   3. One breath is given during a 1- to 1.5-second pause between sets of compressions.
   4. Repeat this pattern (5:1 ratio) for about 1 minute (20 cycles).
   5. The second rescuer calls for a 5-second pause and checks for the return of pulse or breathing.
   6. Provide breathing and/or circulation as needed. If CPR is continued, check for the return of a heartbeat and breathing every few minutes.
   7. Switch positions whenever one rescuer becomes tired. Make the switch at the end of a cycle, check the victim for a return of pulse or breathing, and continue as needed.

9. Make a recommendation for an arterial blood gas measurement. (IIIG9) [R, Ap, An]

Blood for arterial blood gas determination is usually drawn in any hospital-based CPR effort. It should not be done at the expense of time that should be spent in starting effective ventilations and chest compressions or defibrillating the heart.

The blood gas values give important information on the patient's oxygenation and whether the patient is acidotic. Changes in the ventilation efforts and medications such as bicarbonate are based on information from the arterial blood gases.

The femoral site is usually the best to draw from in a CPR situation. This is because it is the largest artery and easiest to hit and because it is far enough from the chest to not interfere with the chest compression efforts.

Module B. CPR equipment.

1. Manual resuscitator (bag-valve).

a. Get the necessary equipment for the procedure. (IIA9a) [R, Ap]

The first consideration when one decides which manual resuscitator to select is the size of the patient. Although the volume of the reservoir bag and the tidal volume that will be expelled from it vary among the types of bags, there are three basic sizes. An infant or newborn unit typically has a reservoir bag volume of about 250 ml. Examples include Penlon and Laerdal Infant. A pediatric unit usually has a reservoir bag volume of about 250 to 500 ml. Examples include Hope and Hope II (pediatric), AMBU E-2 Infant, Laerdal Child, Hudson Lifesaver and Lifesaver II (pediatric), and AIRbird (pediatric). An adult unit typically has a reservoir bag volume of 1500 to 2000 ml. Examples include Hope and Hope II (adult), Air Viva, AMBU E-2 Adult Mark II, Laerdal RFB-II, PMR and High Oxygen PMR, AIRbird (adult), and Hudson Lifesaver and Lifesaver II (adult). In addition to all of these reusable units, there are a number of disposable units that are thrown away after one patient use. They also come in comparable infant, pediatric, and adult reservoir bag volumes. Only use a resuscitator that meets the following guidelines set by the American Society for Testing and Materials (ASTM) and the American Medical Association (AMA):

a. The non-rebreathing one-way valve to the patient should not stick at an oxygen flow of 15 L/min. Ideally it should not stick at a flow of 30 L/min.

b. AMA standards are that the unit should deliver 100% oxygen at the flow rate of 15 L/min; ASTM standards are that it should deliver at least 85% oxygen. An oxygen reservoir system will need to be added to the basic unit to achieve these oxygen percentages.

c. The valve to the patient must be clearable within 20 seconds if it becomes fouled by vomitus, sputum, or blood.

d. The valve to the patient must have a connector with a 15-mm–inside diameter (ID) fitting for any endotracheal tube adapter and a 22-mm—outside diameter (OD) fitting for any patient face mask. The endotracheal tube adapter should be "slip proof" to prevent any accidental disconnections. All internal one-way valves should have a fail-safe design so that they cannot be reversed or switched during assembly.

e. Neonatal and pediatric units must have a pressure-release (pop-off) valve that opens at 40 cm H_2O pressure. The pressure may be adjustable. If an adult unit has a pressure release valve, it must have an override system that is easy to operate.

f. The unit must be able to operate if dropped 1 m onto a concrete surface.

g. The unit must be able to operate under any environmental conditions that may be encountered. It should not freeze up in subzero conditions.

b. Put the equipment together, make sure that it works properly, and identify and fix any problems with it, (IIB4a) [R, Ap]

Learners and examinees should disassemble and reassemble as many different models as possible in all three sizes. See Fig. 10-18 for line drawings of a complete set of

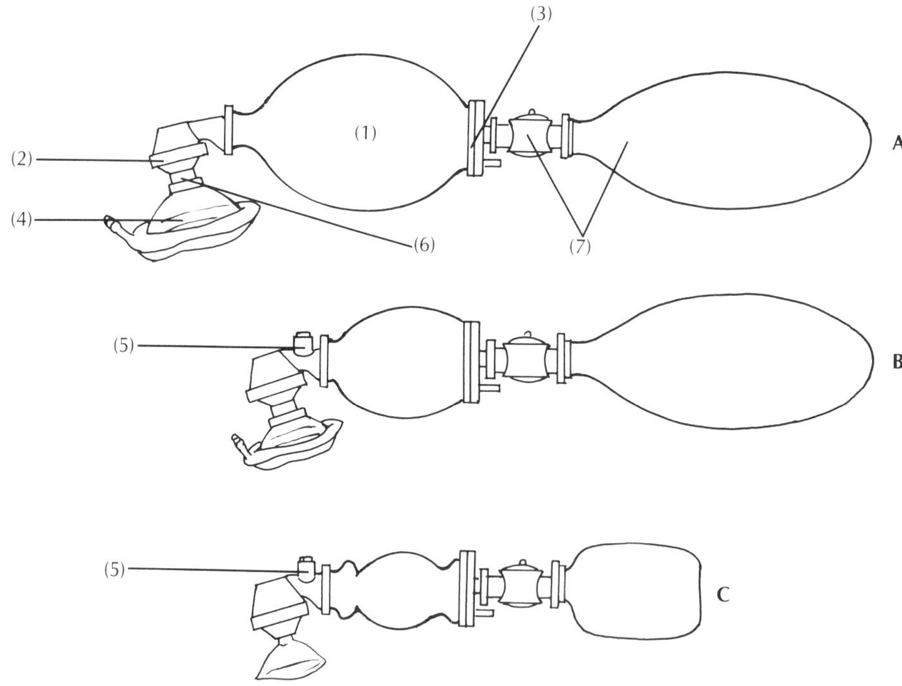

Fig. 10-18 Laerdal manual resuscitator (bag-valve) devices. **A,** Adult unit. **B,** Child unit. **C,** Infant unit. These and many other similar devices have these features: *(1)* Self-filling vinyl bag. *(2)* One-way exhalation valve. *(3)* Nipple and one-way valve to add supplemental oxygen. *(4)* Transparent plastic face mask with cushion. *(5)* Child and infant units containing a pressure-limiting (pop-off) valve. *(6)* Standard 15-mm-I.D./22-mm-O.D. connector for attaching to an endotracheal tube or face mask. *(7)* Reservoir system for delivering up to 100% oxygen. (From Eubanks DH, Bone RC: *Comprehensive Respiratory Care,* ed 2. St Louis, Mosby, 1990. Used by permission.)

Laerdal infant, pediatric, and adult manual resuscitators. Most other units have similar features. It is beyond the scope of this book to go into detail on all of the available units. However, the following steps should be taken when the function of a manual resuscitator is evaluated:

a. Squeeze and release the bag to see if the non-rebreathing valve and air/oxygen reservoir intake valve open and close properly.
b. Feel the air leave the outlet port of the non-rebreathing valve when the bag is squeezed.
c. Occlude the outlet port and squeeze the bag. No gas should leak out. If present, the pop-off valve should open at the correct pressure.
d. The face mask should fit onto the 22-mm-OD fitting and have its cushion properly inflated.

Check for a reversed or improperly seated one-way valve if the gas does not enter or exit the unit as it should. In clinical use, mucus, vomitus, and blood can foul the non-rebreathing valve system and must be cleared within 20 seconds. Do this by disconnecting the unit from the patient, aiming the adapter into a neutral area, and squeezing the bag to blow out the obstruction. Replace a unit that cannot be promptly cleared.

2. Mouth-to-valve mask resuscitator.

a. Get the necessary equipment for the procedure. (IIA9b) [R, Ap]

The following are important considerations when the best device for the victim is selected:

1. The first consideration in selection of the proper device is that the mask fits the victim's face so that there is no air leak. There should be infant, child, and adult sizes available.
2. The mouth piece should be designed so that it fits only one way into the mask. Some units include a short length of aerosol tubing between the mouthpiece and mask for greater flexibility.
3. The one-way (non-rebreathing) valve should be designed to ensure that all of the rescuer's breath is directed into the victim and the victim's exhaled breath is vented to room air rather than back at the rescuer. Some units include a bacteria filter in the one-way valve between the rescuer and victim.
4. It should be possible to add supplemental oxygen through a T-piece or nipple on the mask. This is important for hospital or ambulance use. If a T-piece is added, it must be designed to easily fit between the mouthpiece and face mask. An oxygen administration nipple should have a cap over it when not in use to prevent any leakage of the delivered breath.

There are at least 20 manufacturers of these devices. Common producers include Laerdal with its Pocket Mask, Respironics with its Seal Easy, Armstrong Medical Industries, Inc. with its Armstrong CPR mask, and CODEPAK with its CODEPAK Resuscitator.

b. Put the equipment together, make sure that it works properly, and identify and fix any problems with it. (IIB4b) [R, Ap]

As mentioned earlier, these are relatively simple devices. Most have only two or three pieces: face mask, mouthpiece with a one-way valve, and possibly an oxygen T-piece (Fig. 10-19.) The "male" and "female" connections are designed to fit together

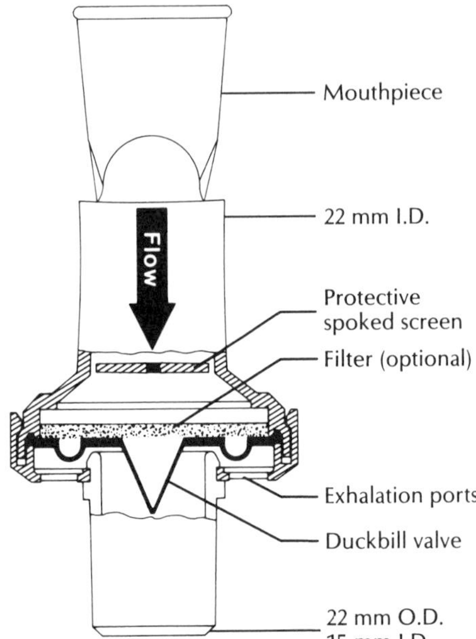

Fig. 10-19 Cut-away view of a mouthpiece and one-way valve that would attach to the mask of a mouth-to-valve mask resuscitator. (Courtesy of RCI Hudson, Temecula, Calif.)

only one way. When they are properly assembled, there should be no air leaks when the breath is delivered to the victim. If the breath cannot be delivered, check the one-way valve to make sure that it has not been put together backward. Reverse it, if necessary, and ventilate the victim's airway. Keep the oxygen nipple on the mask or T-piece capped off if it is not being used. Air will leak out during the delivered breath if the cap is left off the nipple.

This ends the general discussion on cardiopulmonary resuscitation. The entry level examination will ask *direct* questions over this material. The following topics are covered in detail in Section 1. A few additional comments are added as necessary.

Module C. Patient assessment.

1. Determine and continue to monitor how the patient responds to the procedure.

The survivor's condition and circumstances will likely be very different now than they were before the cardiac arrest. Make note of any special considerations. Evaluate any new patient care orders.

2. Modify the procedure and recommend any changes in the patient's respiratory care plan, depending on the response.

The practitioner should make a recommendation to the physician to stop a procedure being performed as an adjunct to CPR if the patient is suffering an adverse reaction to it. For example, bag and mask ventilation may force air into the stomach; recommend intubation. Always notify the physician of any change in the patient's condition or if there is a complication to any CPR-related procedure.

It is common for patients who have had a heart attack to develop pulmonary edema. Fulminating pulmonary edema is seen as pink, frothy secretions in the lungs and airway. These must be suctioned out to clear the airway.

BIBLIOGRAPHY

AARC Clinical Practice Guideline: Resuscitation in acute care hospitals. *Respir Care* 1993; 38:1197-1198.

Eubanks DH, Bone RC: *Comprehensive Respiratory Care*, ed 2. St Louis, Mosby, 1990.

Ferko JG: Airtight advice. *Emergency* January 1988, pp 31-36.

Harrison RR, Maull KI, Keenan RL, et al: Mouth-to-mask ventilation: a superior method of rescue breathing. *Ann Emerg Med* 1982; 11:39-41.

Hess D, Goff G, Johnson K: The effect of hand size, resuscitator brand, and use of two hands on volumes delivered during adult bag-valve ventilation. *Respir Care* 1989; 34:805-810.

Madama VC: Safe mouth-to-mouth resuscitation requires adjunct equipment, caution. *Occupat Health Safety* 1991:60(1); 56-64.

McPherson SP: *Respiratory Therapy Equipment*, ed 4. St Louis, Mosby, 1990.

Standards and guidelines for cardiopulmonary resuscitation (CPR) and emergency cardiac care (ECC). *JAMA* 1992; 268:2171-2295

Stephenson Jr HE: Cardiopulmonary resuscitation, in Burton GG, Hogkin JE (eds): *Respiratory care—a Guide to Clinical Practice*, ed 2. Philadelphia, Lippincott, 1984.

Watson MA: Cardiopulmonary resuscitation, in Barnes TA (ed): *Respiratory Care Practice*. Chicago, Mosby, 1988.

SELF-STUDY QUESTIONS

1. You enter a patient's room to check on her nasal cannula. You notice that she is slumped over in her chair and appears cyanotic. Your first reaction would be to:
   A. Open the airway.
   B. Determine whether the patient is responsive.
   C. Call out for help.
   D. Begin mouth-to-mouth ventilation.
   E. Check for a pulse.

2. You are working in the emergency room when an automobile accident victim is brought in. You suspect that the driver has a cervical spine injury. What is the best way to open the airway?
   A. Cricothyrotomy
   B. Tracheostomy
   C. Head-tilt/chin-life maneuver
   D. Jaw-thrust maneuver
   E. Nasal intubation

3. To determine breathlessness it is best to:
   I. Feel for air movement with your cheek by the victim's mouth.
   II. Feel the chest rise and fall with your hand.
   III. Listen for air movement with your ear by the victim's mouth.
   IV. Look at the victim's chest for a rising and falling movement.
   V. Look at the victim's face for nasal flaring.
   A. I, II
   B. III, V
   C. I, III, IV
   D. IV, V
   E. I, II, III, IV, V

4. The best way to determine pulselessness in a 10-month-old infant is by checking the:
   A. Brachial pulse for 5 to 10 seconds
   B. Carotid pulse for 3 to 5 seconds
   C. Femoral pulse for 3 to 5 seconds
   D. Brachial pulse for 3 to 5 seconds
   E. Carotid pulse for 5 to 10 seconds

5. While doing oxygen equipment rounds, you come upon a cyanotic patient who is not breathing. As you reposition the patient and hyperextend his neck, you notice that he has open lip ulcers. What would be the best way to ventilate this patient?
   A. Perform mouth-to-mouth ventilation.
   B. Use a mouth-to-valve device stored in the room for this purpose.
   C. Run to the CPR crash cart and get a manual resuscitation bag and mask.
   D. Wait for the anesthesiologist to intubate the patient's airway and then use a manual resuscitation bag.

6. During a CPR attempt you are handed a manual resuscitator. You use it to deliver a tidal volume but notice that the victim does not exhale. Looking at the flowmeter, you notice that it is running at flush (about 50 L/min). Your reaction should be to:
   I. Give another breath and see whether the victim exhales.
   II. Turn the flow up higher.
   III. Check the non-rebreathing valve for debris.
   IV. Remove the resuscitator so that the victim can exhale.
   V. Turn the flowmeter down to about 15 L/min.
   A. I
   B. II, III
   C. II, IV
   D. IV, V
   E. IV

7. Adult two-rescuer CPR should be performed at what chest compression/ventilations ratio?
   A. 15 to 2
   B. 5 to 2
   C. 5 to 1
   D. 15 to 1
   E. 1 to 5

8. To make sure that a manual ventilator is ready for use you would:
   I. Make sure that no gas escapes through the outlet port when it is closed off and the bag is squeezed.
   II. Squeeze the bag and make sure the air/oxygen reservoir intake valve closes properly.
   III. Squeeze the bag and make sure the non-rebreathing valve opens properly.
   IV. Feel air leave the outlet port when the bag is squeezed.
   V. Squeeze the bag, and make sure the air/oxygen reservoir intake valve opens properly.
   A. I, II, III, IV
   B. I, II, V
   C. IV, V
   D. II, III
   E. I, IV

9. Blood for an arterial blood gas measurement needs to be drawn during a CPR attempt. You would recommend which site be used?
   A. Carotid
   B. Radial

C. Brachial
D. Dorsalis pedis
E. Femoral

Answer Key:

1. B; 2. D; 3. C; 4. A; 5. B; 6. D; 7. C; 8. A; 9. E.

11 Airway Management

Module A. Perform the following procedures, and care for the following artificial airways and equipment to maintain a patent airway.

1. Open the patient's airway. (III B1a) [R, Ap]

a. Identify an airway obstruction problem.

Patients who suddenly experience upper airway obstruction will show some or all of the following signs or symptoms:

a. Holding onto the throat or gesturing toward their mouth
b. Panic or fear
c. Inspiratory stridor or muffled speaking if an incomplete obstruction
d. Apnea and inability to speak if a complete obstruction
e. Suprasternal, substernal, intercostal, or supraclavicular retractions or combination thereof (see Fig. 1-7)
f. Nasal flaring (see Fig. 1-7) or open mouth
g. Increased use of accessory muscles of ventilation (see Fig. 1-12)
h. Diaphoresis
i. Cyanosis

Most of these topics are discussed in Section 1. Airway obstruction is a medical emergency and must be dealt with immediately. Unconsciousness and then death will result if the airway cannot be opened so that the patient can breathe.

A foreign object in the mouth can be removed to clear the airway. Relaxation of the tongue and soft tissues of the mouth and throat are frequently a cause of obstruction in an unconscious patient who is supine (see later discussion. Various artificial devices can be used to keep an airway open and are discussed in this section. Suctioning to remove foreign matter from the airway is discussed in Section 12.

b. Properly position the patient with airway obstruction.

Positioning of the head to open the airway is discussed in Section 10 on cardiopulmonary resuscitation. Briefly, use the head-tilt/chin-lift maneuver to hyperextend the neck of an adult, and slightly extend the neck of a child to open the airway (see Figs. 10-1 and 10-2). You can place a small pad behind the neck and head to put the patient in the "sniff position." Always keep the head in line with the body.

If the patient has a known or suspected cervical spine injury, the neck cannot be hyperextended. Instead, open the airway with the jaw-thrust maneuver (see Figs. 10-3 and 10-4). Keep the head in line with the body.

The patient may be supine during the airway-opening procedures just mentioned. Frequently, however, the patient is positioned with the head and body elevated. An unconscious patient is less likely to vomit and aspirate in either of these two positions:

- Fowler's—the head and body are elevated about 45 degrees; knees are kept straight (Fig. 11-1).
- Semi-Fowler's—the head and body are elevated about 45 degrees; knees are bent to prevent slipping down in bed (Fig. 11-2).

The combination of either of these body positions and the head and neck hyperextended into the sniff position will probably keep the airway open, minimize the risk of aspiration of vomitus, and minimize the patient's work of breathing.

c. Perform the Heimlich maneuver.

The Heimlich maneuver (also known as subdiaphragmatic abdominal thrusts or abdominal thrusts) is used to clear out a foreign body from the upper portion of the airway or trachea. The residual volume of air in the lungs is used to propel the obstruction up to the mouth, where it can be coughed or pulled out.

Obstructed airway maneuvers for an unconscious victim are discussed in Section 10 on cardiopulmonary resuscitation.

The following steps would be followed for a conscious victim with an obstructed airway:

1. Assess that the patient cannot breathe. The victim will not be able to speak or cough and will be holding his or her throat or motioning toward the mouth. Ask, "Are you choking?" The victim should nod, "Yes."

2. Perform the Heimlich maneuver on the victim. Get behind the victim and wrap your arms around his or her waist. Make a fist with one hand and place its thumb side between the victim's navel and xiphoid process. Place the other hand over the first. Pull quickly and firmly up and into the victim's abdomen (Fig. 11-3). Repeat this as often as necessary until the foreign object is coughed out or the victim becomes unconscious. In-

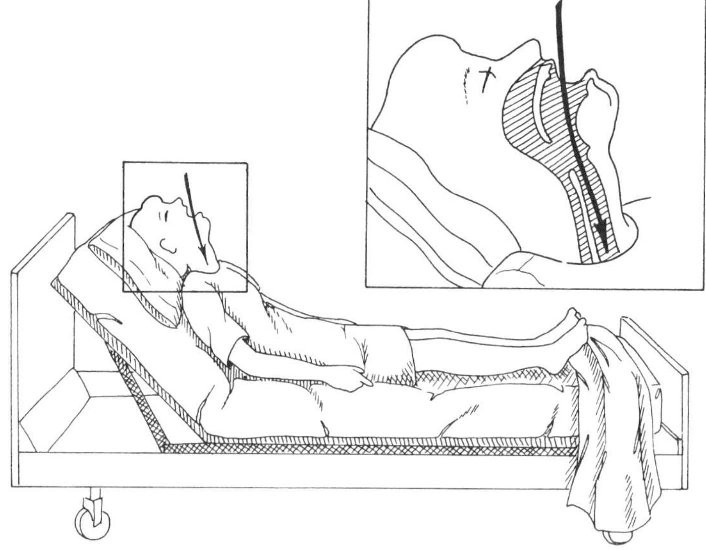

Fig. 11-1 Fowler's position with the head and neck hyperextended into the sniff position for keeping an open airway.

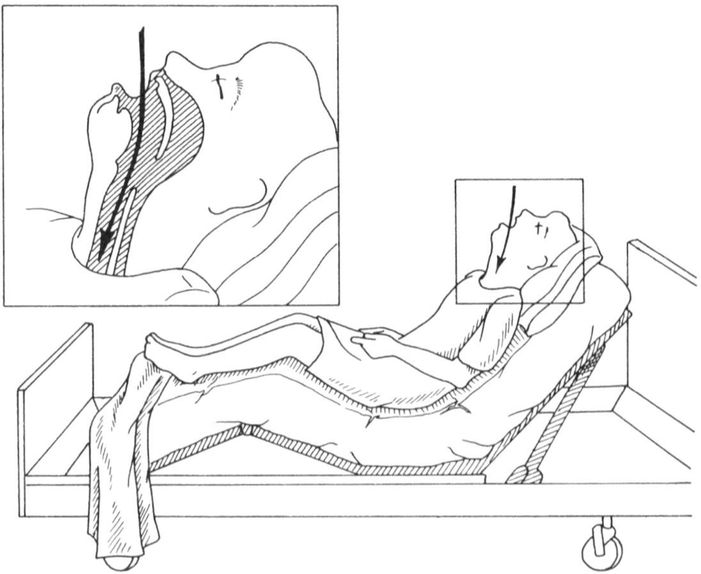

Fig. 11-2 Semi-Fowler's position with the head and neck hyperextended into the sniff position for keeping an open airway.

fants can have the first two fingers of the rescuer pressed up into the abdomen between the navel and xiphoid process. Each effort should be done with the intent to clear the obstruction.

A chest thrust can be performed on a victim who is too obese to wrap your arms around or who is in the later months of pregnancy. Wrap your arms around the victim's chest. Make a fist with one hand. Place its thumb side on the sternum where your hand would be placed to do cardiopulmonary resuscitation (CPR) chest compressions. Place the other hand over the first. Pull back into the victim's chest slowly and distinctly so as to loosen any obstruction. Repeat this as often as necessary until the foreign object is coughed out or the victim becomes unconscious. Each effort should be done with the intent to clear the obstruction.

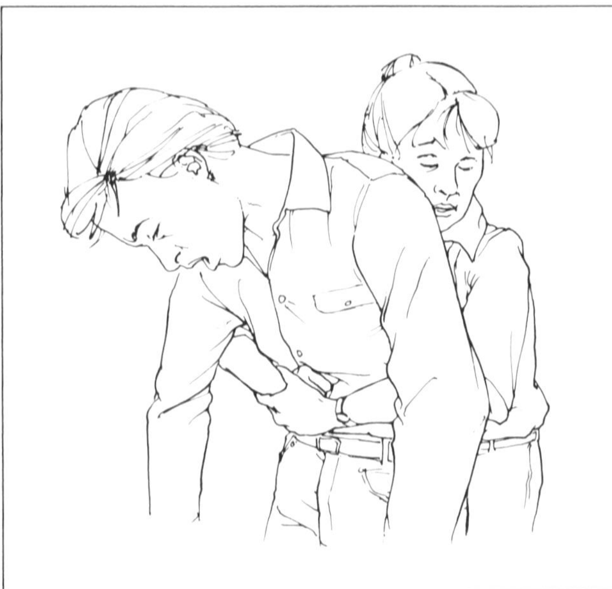

Fig. 11-3 Administering the Heimlich maneuver to a conscious victim of an upper airway obstruction. (From Standards and guidelines for cardiopulmonary resuscitation [CPR] and emergency cardiac care [ECC]. *JAMA* 1992; 268:2193. Used by permission.)

If the victim becomes unconscious, perform the following steps:

1. Lay the victim supine with the face turned up.
2. Call out for help.
3. Check for a foreign body by opening the victim's mouth with the cross-finger technique (see Fig. 10-5). In an adult, insert a finger to sweep out any foreign body. In a child or infant, *look* into the mouth. If anything is seen, sweep it out with a finger.
4. Attempt to ventilate the victim. Ventilate, if possible, at the normal rate.
5. Repeat the Heimlich maneuver if the victim's airway cannot be ventilated. This is done by kneeling next to the victim, placing the heel of one hand midline on the abdomen between the navel and the xiphoid process, placing the other hand on top, and quickly thrusting upward toward the chest (see Fig. 10-9).

   A markedly obese or obviously pregnant victim can have chest thrusts performed on him or her. The rescuer's hands should be placed on the sternum as they would for cardiac compressions. Perform compressions similarly to how a cardiac compression would be done. In either case, repeat the maneuver six to ten times.
6. Check for a foreign body as described earlier.
7. Attempt to ventilate the victim as described earlier.
8. Repeat steps 5, 6, and 7 as necessary.
9. If the airway is cleared, proceed with normal CPR steps. See Section 10 on cardiopulmonary resuscitation for details.

2. Humidify an artificial airway. (IIIB1b) [R, Ap]

Patients with an endotracheal or tracheostomy tube in place should ideally be provided 100% relative humidity at body temperature. If not, secretions in the airway may dry and result in mucous plugs. Patients with an oropharyngeal or nasopharyngeal airway may also be given supplemental humidity by a simple aerosol mask to help prevent drying of secretions. See Section 7, on humidity and aerosol therapy for a complete discussion of the subjects of humidity and aerosol therapy and administrative devices.

3. Oropharyngeal airways.

a. Get the necessary equipment. (IIA5a) [R, Ap]

The oropharyngeal airway (also known as a bite block) is made of plastic that is hard enough to withstand any patient's biting force. This airway is indicated in an unconscious patient who is experiencing upper airway obstruction because the tongue is falling back and blocking the oropharynx. This is commonly seen in a patient who is supine. A properly sized and placed oropharyngeal airway lifts the tongue forward. By separating the tongue from the soft palate and posterior portion of the oropharynx the airway is made patent. Suctioning out the patient's oral secretions is also made easier. It is helpful to also hyperextend the patient's head and place it in the sniff position described earlier. An oropharyngeal airway is poorly tolerated in a conscious patient and can cause gagging and even vomiting.

An oropharyngeal airway is sometimes used in a patient with an endotracheal tube. It is used to keep the tube from being bitten. A cooperative patient with an intubated airway usually does not need an oropharyngeal airway.

A third indication is to prevent a patient with seizures from biting his or her tongue. If the patient's jaw is clamped shut, wait for it to relax before placing the airway. Forcing the mouth open by prying on the teeth can cause them to be broken or knocked out.

A number of manufacturers make oropharyngeal airways. They fall into two basic types: hollow center and I-beam.

Hollow Center

Hollow center types have an oval or rectangular shape in cross section and are hollow in the center. A suction catheter can be easily placed through the hollow center so that the back of the throat can be cleared of secretions. Examples include the Guedel, Cath-Guide Guedel, Connel, Waters with an oxygen nipple adapter, Rosser, and Safar.

The Rosser and Safar airways have an outer tube that can be attached by a practitioner to provide a mouthpiece for rescue breathing. If rescue breathing must be performed, it is probably more effective to ventilate with a mask and manual resuscitator when one becomes available.

I-Beam

I-beam types are shaped like an I-beam in cross section. A suction catheter can easily be guided along the groove on either side of the I-beam to the back of the throat so that secretions can be cleared out. Examples include those produced by Berman.

See Figs. 11-4 and 11-5 for examples. Note that they all have a flange or widening at the outer end. This is placed against the patient's lips to prevent the whole airway from being inserted or drawn into the mouth. The body of the airway has a curve that supports and lifts the tongue so that the oropharynx is patent.

Oropharyngeal airways come in a variety of sizes from infant to adult. The proper

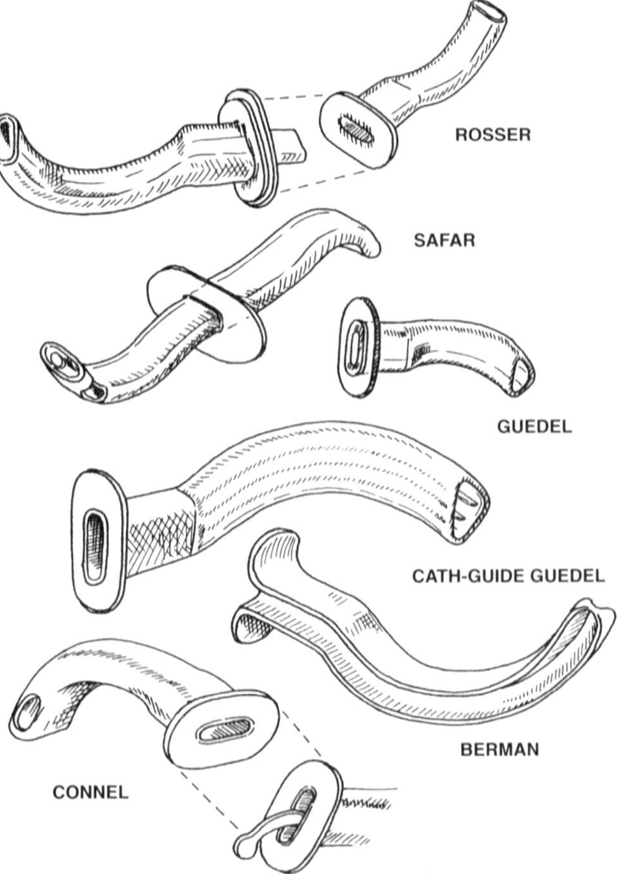

Fig. 11-4 Hollow and I-beam types of oropharyngeal airways.

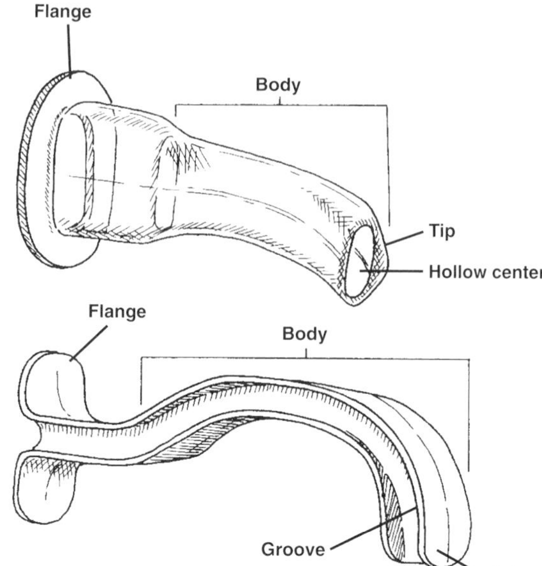

Fig. 11-5 Close-ups of hollow and I-beam types of oropharyngeal airways.

size is found by holding it against the patient's face with the flange against the lips. The end of the airway should reach the angle of the jaw (Fig. 11-6). It is important that the airway be properly sized to the patient. Too large an airway can block the oropharynx by extending past the tongue. Too small an airway can push the tongue back into the oropharynx rather than pulling the tongue forward as it should. A properly placed and sized oropharyngeal airway is shown in Fig. 11-7.

b. Put the equipment together, make sure that it works properly, and identify and fix any problems with it. (IIB6a) [R, Ap]

Most oropharyngeal airways are single units. There is nothing to assemble. Make sure that the channel in the hollow-center types is patent. If a unit is plugged by secretions, blood, or a foreign substance, the patient cannot breathe through the opening. A suction catheter cannot be passed through either.

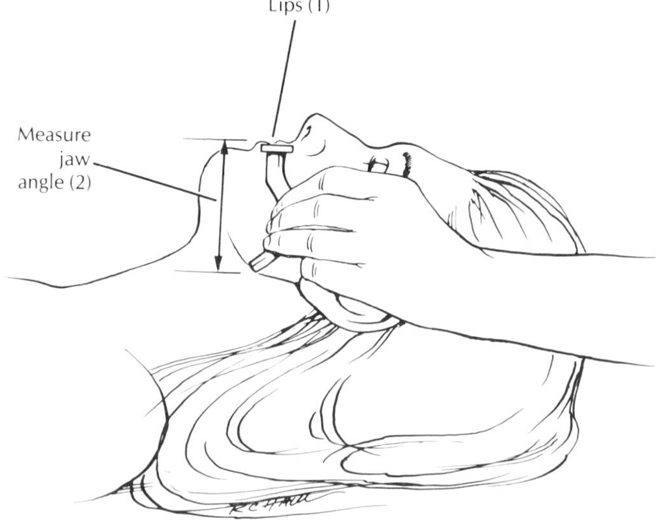

Fig. 11-6 Procedure for measuring the proper size of the oropharyngeal airway. (From Eubanks DH, Bone RC: *Comprehensive Respiratory Care,* ed 2. St Louis, Mosby, 1990. Used by permission.)

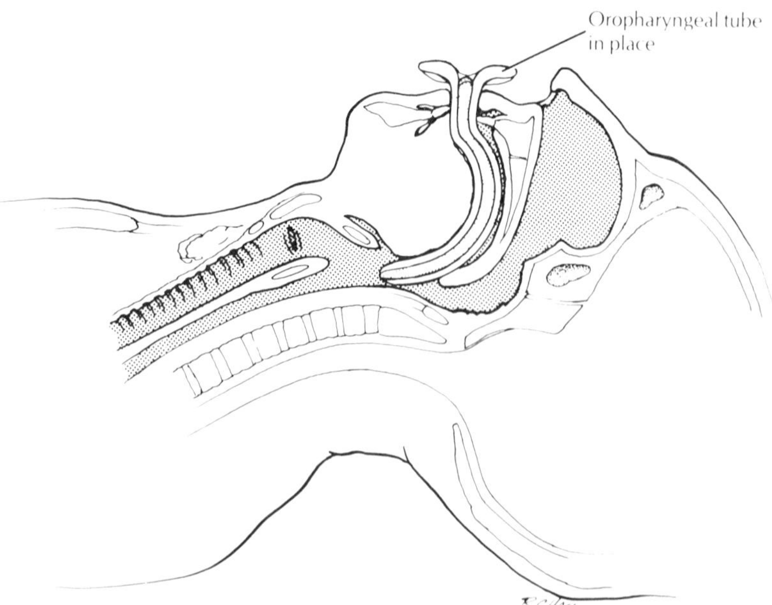

Fig. 11-7 Cross section through the head showing the proper position of an oropharyngeal airway. (From Eubanks DH, Bone RC: *Comprehensive Respiratory Care,* ed 2. St Louis, Mosby, 1990. Used by permission.)

There are hollow-center types, such as the Rosser, that have an attachable outer part. The outer part is snapped onto the oropharyngeal airway when the practitioner needs to perform rescue breathing. It has a wide flange so that the lips can be covered and sealed to prevent a leak.

c. Insert the correct oropharyngeal airway. (IIIB3) [R, Ap]

There are two widely used methods to insert an oropharyngeal airway.

A. First method:
   1. Open the patient's mouth with the cross-finger technique. Insert the airway backward into the patient's mouth until it reaches the palate. Some authors recommend inserting it past the uvula.
   2. Twist the airway 180 degrees, and insert it the rest of the way until the tongue is supported by the curved body.
   3. The flange should rest at the lips (Fig. 11-8).

B. Second method:
   1. Open the patient's mouth with the cross-finger technique. Insert the airway into the mouth with the curved body rotated toward a cheek.
   2. Twist the airway 90 degrees, and insert it the rest of the way so that the tongue is supported by the curved body.
   3. The flange should rest at the lips.

Some practitioners believe that the airway should not be secured in the patient's mouth. That way it can be quickly removed if the patient awakens and begins to gag. Sometimes the airway is taped across the flange and cheeks of an unconscious patient. Never block the patient's mouth with the tape. Be prepared to loosen the tape and remove it.

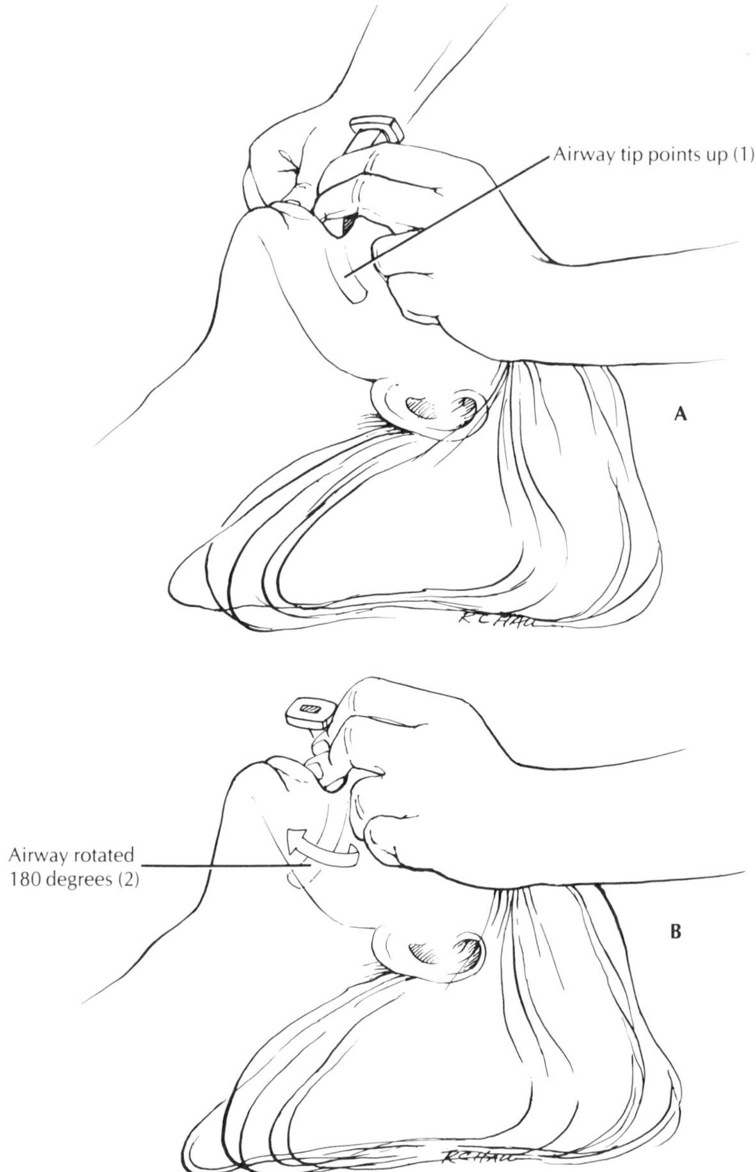

Fig. 11-8 A procedure for inserting an oropharyngeal airway. **A,** The airway is placed with the tip pointing toward the palate. **B,** The airway is rotated 180 degrees to support the tongue. (From Eubanks DH, Bone RC: *Comprehensive Respiratory Care,* ed 2. St Louis, Mosby, 1990. Used by permission.)

4. Nasopharyngeal airways.

a. Get the necessary equipment. (IIA5a) [R, Ap]

Nasopharyngeal airways (also known as nasal airways, nasal trumpets, or nasal stints) are made of a relatively soft and pliable plastic or rubber. This is to decrease the chances of damaging the delicate mucus membranes of the nose and nasopharynx.

A nasopharyngeal airway is often used to ensure a patent airway by pushing the patient's tongue forward off of the posterior portion of the oropharynx. As mentioned earlier, this is commonly a problem in a supine, unconscious patient. The nasopharyngeal airway is probably not as effective in keeping the tongue forward as the oropharyngeal airway. However, it has the advantage over an oropharyngeal airway in that it is better tolerated in a semiconscious or alert patient.

It is also commonly used to provide a secure channel through which to pass a suction catheter or bronchoscope. The nasopharyngeal airway protects the patient's mucous membranes from the trauma of repeatedly passed catheters.

A third use would be in a patient with trauma to the jaw or seizures with a tightly closed jaw. In these cases an oropharyngeal airway cannot be used. The nasopharyngeal airway can be passed into the patient's oropharynx to push the tongue forward and maintain an airway.

Several manufacturers make the two basic types of nasopharyngeal airways.

Blunt Tip

The Sakalad Airway is an example of a blunt tip. The hollow cannula has the usual distal and proximal openings.

Beveled Tip

The Rüsch Airway and Bardex Airway both have a beveled tip. These come with right-sided and left-sided cut bevels. If possible, get the airway with the bevel cut that opens toward the patient's oropharynx (toward the nasal septum). For example, if the airway is going to be inserted into the left naris, the bevel should be cut on the right side of the tube so that it is open to the patient's oropharynx. If you were inserting the tube into the right nostril, you would want the bevel cut on the left side of the tube.

See Fig. 11-9 for a close-up of a nasopharyngeal airway. All have a flange that fits up close to the patient's nostril. This prevents the entire tube from being pushed into the patient. All have a cannula with a channel for breathing or suctioning through.

Nasopharyngeal airways come in a variety of sizes for adults. They can be properly sized by measuring from the tip of the nose to the tragus of the ear and adding 2 to 3 cm (Fig. 11-10).

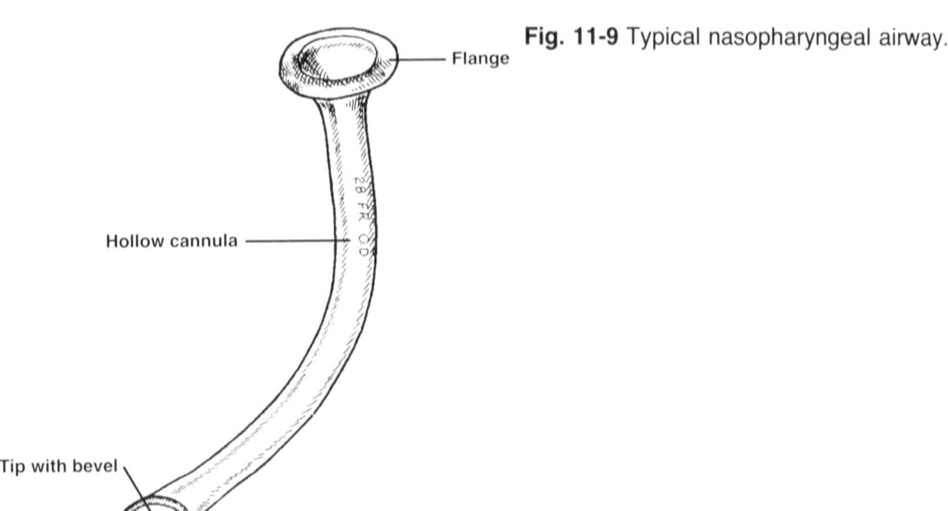

Fig. 11-9 Typical nasopharyngeal airway.

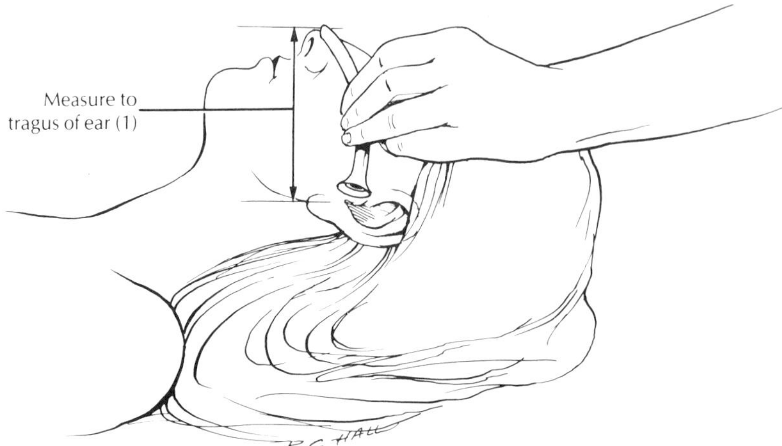

Fig. 11-10 Procedure for measuring the proper size of the nasopharyngeal airway. (From Eubanks DH, Bone RC: *Comprehensive Respiratory Care,* ed 2. St Louis, Mosby, 1990. Used by permission.)

b. Put the equipment together, make sure that it works properly, and identify and fix any problems with it. (IIB6a) [R, Ap]

All nasopharyngeal airways are made up of a single piece. There is nothing to assemble. Make sure that the tube is not plugged by dried secretions, blood, or a foreign body. If plugged, the patient cannot breath through it, and a suction catheter cannot be passed through it.

c. Insert the correct nasopharyngeal airway. (IIIB3) [R, Ap]

Steps in the Procedure

1. Select the most patent nostril. Check the patient's chart for a history of a broken nose, deviated septum, or current head cold. Interview the conscious patient to see whether one nostril is more open than the other. Place your finger in front of the patient's nostrils to feel which one has greater airflow. Avoid forcing the airway into a nostril and nasal passage that will be damaged by the procedure.
2. Lubricate the properly sized airway with a sterile, water-soluble lubricant such as K-Y jelly. Place the lubricant on a sterile, 4 by 4-inch gauze pad, and then smear it over the length of the airway.
3. Tell the patient what you are going to do.
4. Gently place the airway into the nostril. It should be directed straight back parallel to the hard palate. Stop if you feel any resistance. Try a different angle if resistance is felt. Do not force the airway. Try the other nostril if necessary.
5. Check the placement by looking into the patient's mouth with a flashlight and tongue depressor. A properly placed nasopharyngeal airway will be seen in the oropharynx and extend behind the tongue (Figs. 11-11 and 11-12).
6. Secure the airway by sticking a safety pin through the flange and taping the pin to the bridge of the patient's nose or cheek (see Fig. 11-11). This will help to prevent the airway from being accidentally pulled out or pushed in.
7. Rotate the airway to the other nostril, if possible, on a regular basis. This will help to prevent ulceration of the mucous membrane. Some authors recommend rotation at least every 48 hours, whereas others recommend rotation at much shorter time intervals.

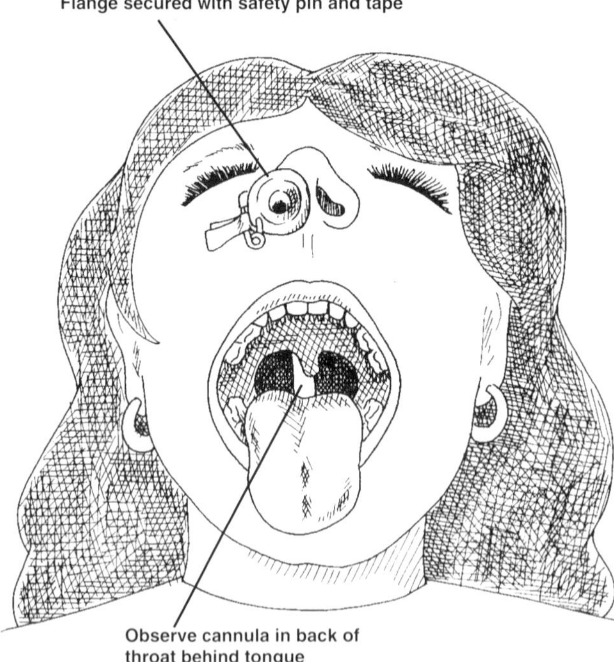

Fig. 11-11 Proper position of the nasopharyngeal airway behind the tongue can be determined by looking into the mouth. The tube is also secured by placing a safety pin through the flange and taping it to the cheek.

5. Oral and nasal endotracheal tubes.
a. Get the necessary equipment. (IIA5b) [R, Ap]

An endotracheal tube is the best emergency device for maintaining a secure airway. It also provides a direct suctioning route to the lungs and prevents aspiration. Mechanical ventilation can easily be provided through it. An endotracheal tube is meant to be a

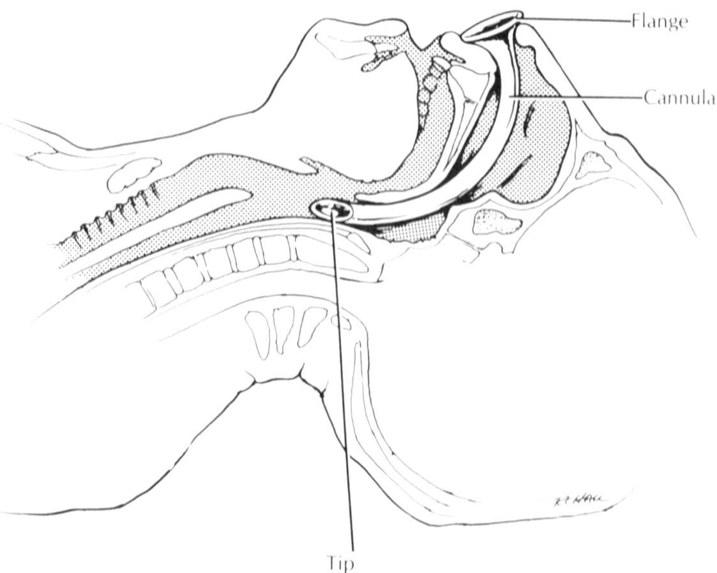

Fig. 11-12 Cross section of the head showing the proper position of the nasopharyngeal airway. (From Ellis PD, Billings, DM: *Cardiopulmonary Resuscitation: Procedures for Basic and Advanced Life Support.* St Louis, Mosby, 1980. Used by permission.)

temporary airway. However, it can be kept in patients for weeks if necessary. Meticulous mouth care must be given to these patients to prevent ulcerations from prolonged contact with the tube. Pliable plastic is used in these tubes so that it bends as the patient's head is turned.

For the most part, oral and nasal endotracheal tubes can be used interchangeably. They both serve the same purposes. In a side by side comparison, it will be noted that the nasal endotracheal tube is longer and more curved than an oral endotracheal tube. An anesthesiologist would request a nasal tube if he or she is going to place it by the nasal route. Oral tubes are used in the majority of patients.

It is extremely important to insert the properly sized tube into the patient's trachea. Table 11-1 lists the usual tube size to place into a patient based on his or her age.

b. Put the equipment together, make sure that it works properly, and identify and fix any problems with it. (IIB6b) [R, Ap]

Refer to Fig. 11-13 for these components of a standard endotracheal tube:

1. The hollow curved body is the main part of the tube. Through it the patient can breathe, or a suction catheter can be placed. Printing on the side will show the outer and inner diameters. Make sure that the central channel is not plugged by dried secretions, blood, or a foreign body.

2. The proximal end is left outside of the patient's nose or mouth. An adapter with a 15-mm-OD equipment connector is inserted into the tube. The other end of the adapter narrows and is individually sized to fit snuggly into the interior diameter (ID) of the endotracheal tube. The adapters cannot be cross-fitted to different sizes of endotracheal tubes.

3. The distal end is inserted into the patient's trachea. The tip is cut with either a right- or left-sided bevel. The bevel cut creates an oval-shaped opening that is less likely

Table 11-1. Endotracheal and Tracheostomy Tube Sizes Based on Patient Age*

Age	ID† (mm)	Approximate OD† (mm)	Fr† Size (OD)
Newborn			
<1000 g	2.5	4.0	12
1000-2000 g	3.0	5.0	14
2000-3000 g	3.5	5.5	16
>3000 g to 6 mo old	3.5-4.0		16-18
Pediatric			
18 mo	4.0	6.0	18
3 yr	4.5	6.5	20
5 yr	5.0	7.0	22
6 yr	5.5	8.0	24
8 yr	6.0	9.0	26
Adult			
16 yr	7.0	10.0	30
Normal-sized woman	7.5-8.0	11.0	32-34
Normal-sized man	8.0-8.5	12.0	34-36
Large adult	9.0-10.0	13.0-14.0	38-42

***Note 1:** It is important to always use the largest tube that can be placed into the patient without causing any harm during the intubation. This is because the larger the internal diameter of the tube, the less airway resistance it causes. Be prepared to insert a tube that is one size larger or smaller than anticipated based on individual variances. **Note 2:** The mathematical relationship between the outer diameter in millimeters and French size can be easily calculated. The French size is determined by multiplying the outer diameter in millimeters by 3. The outer diameter in millimeters is found by dividing the French size by 3.

†*ID,* internal diameter; *OD,* outer diameter; *Fr,* French.

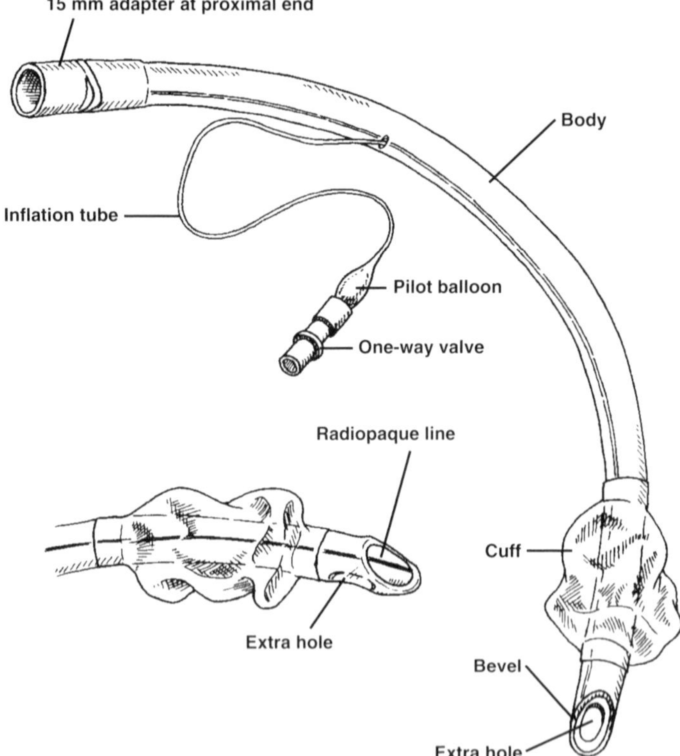

Fig. 11-13 Typical, modern endotracheal tube with its component parts. The insert shows the important features found at the distal end of the tube.

to become plugged with secretions than is a round opening. An extra hole (the Murphy eye) is cut in the tube on the opposite side of the bevel.

4. A line of radiopaque material is imbedded in the tube from the tip back to the cuff. This is important because it is seen as a white line on the chest x-ray film to show where the tip of the tube is located in the trachea (see the insert in Fig. 11-13).

5. A cuff (balloon) is located a few centimeters back from the tip of the tube. It is blown up with air to seal the trachea so that mechanical ventilation can be performed and aspiration is prevented. Most modern tubes have a large residual volume, low-pressure cuff. The cuff inflation and pressure-measuring techniques will be discussed later in this section. **Note:** All tubes with a 5-mm OD or greater have cuffs. Smaller neonatal and pediatric tubes are available with or without a cuff.

6. A cuff-filling inflation tube is connected about half way down the tube. The proximal end is left out of the patient's mouth, and the distal end goes to the cuff so that it can be inflated and deflated. A pilot balloon that inflates and deflates with the cuff is found in the middle of the capillary tube or connected with the one-way valve at the distal end. The one-way valve has an end that connects to any syringe. A 5- to 10-ml syringe is used to inflate or deflate the cuff. When the syringe is disconnected, the one-way valve seals to prevent the air in the cuff from escaping.

The cuff should be inflated and syringe disconnected from the one-way valve before the tube is placed in the patient. This is to make sure that the system works properly. The cuff should hold the air. Do not use any tube with a leaking cuff or one-way valve. Deflate the cuff before placing the tube in the patient.

There are a number of specialty endotracheal tubes that can be found in limited use. They all share the previously mentioned characteristics except for some special feature. It is beyond the scope of this book to describe all of these possible variations. If available, these tubes are worth looking over to become familiar with them.

6. Intubation equipment: laryngoscope and blades.
a. Get the necessary equipment. (IIA5d) [R, Ap]

The laryngoscope is made up of two basic parts: a handle and a blade. The most commonly seen handle is made of stainless steel; some newer units are made of plastic. The handle contains two C-size batteries to power the light source in the blade. They all have a common base with a hooking bar so that the blades can be attached (Figs. 11-14 and 11-15).

Blades come in a variety of sizes from pediatric to adult. They all have a common hook so that they can be snapped and locked in place on the handle. The stainless steel handles use stainless steel blades. The newer plastic handles use plastic blades. The two different sets of handles and blades are not interchangeable.

The blades come in two different shapes. The Miller blades are straight. MacIntosh blades are curved (see Fig. 11-14). The intubating person may specify a specific style of blade as well as blade size.

b. Put the equipment together, make sure that it works properly, and identify and fix any problems with it. (IIB6e) [R, Ap]

Check Fig. 11-15 for the steps in fastening the blade to the handle:

1. Hold the handle in the left hand and the blade in the right hand.
2. Place the hook on the blade over the hooking bar on the base of the handle.
3. Pull the blade down so that it snaps into place on the handle. The handle and blade should fit together at a 90-degree angle.
4. Make sure that the light bulb in the stainless steel blade is tight.

The light source will shine when the handle and blade are properly connected because an electrical circuit has been completed. Failure of the light source to shine could be from any of the following problems:

1. The handle and blade are not properly connected and snapped into place. Disconnect them by performing the opposite motions and reconnect them properly (listed earlier).

2. You have cross-connected stainless steel and plastic components. Only stainless steel handles go with stainless steel blades, and plastic handles with plastic blades.

3. The batteries are low as shown by the bulb failing to glow or glowing with a yellow instead of white light. Unscrew the cap from the handle. Replace the old batteries with two new C-size batteries. When reassembled, the bulb should glow with a white light.

4. The batteries are not placed properly. The positive poles (+) must be toward the base of the handle, and the negative poles (−) must be toward the cap of the handle. When reassembled, the bulb should glow with a white light.

5. The light bulb in the stainless steel blade is loose or defective. Tighten the light bulb by turning it clockwise. It should light up if it was just loose. Unscrew and throw away a defective light bulb. Replace it with a light bulb of the same size. When reassembled, the bulb should glow with a white light. The newer plastic laryngoscopes use a fiberoptic bundle as the light source. There is no light bulb to tighten or replace.

7. Tracheostomy tubes.
a. Get the necessary equipment. (IIA5c) [R, Ap]

The tracheostomy tube offers the same uses as the endotracheal tube such as maintaining a secure airway, providing a direct suctioning route to the lungs, preventing as-

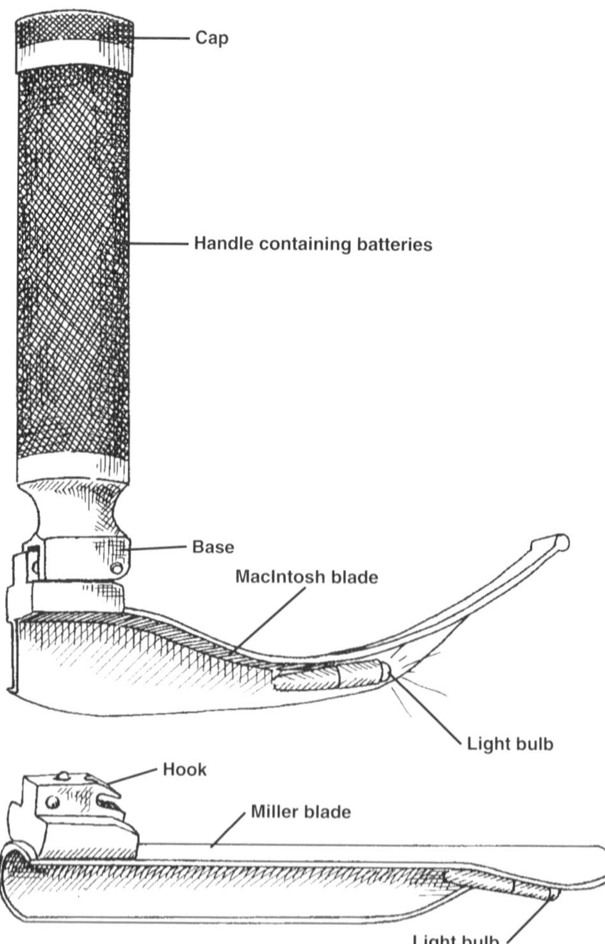

Fig. 11-14 Laryngoscope handle with a MacIntosh (curved) blade attached. A Miller (straight) blade is below for comparison. Note the component parts and features.

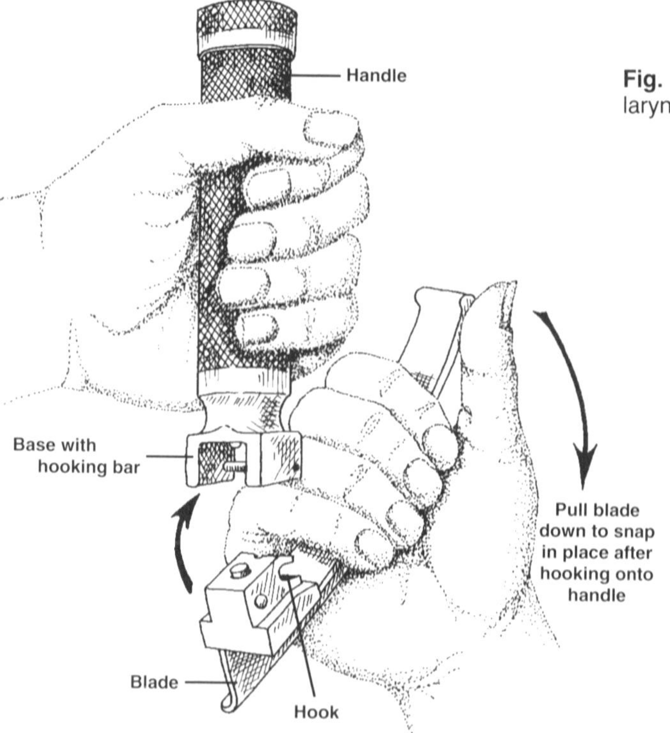

Fig. 11-15 Motions to attach a laryngoscope blade to a handle.

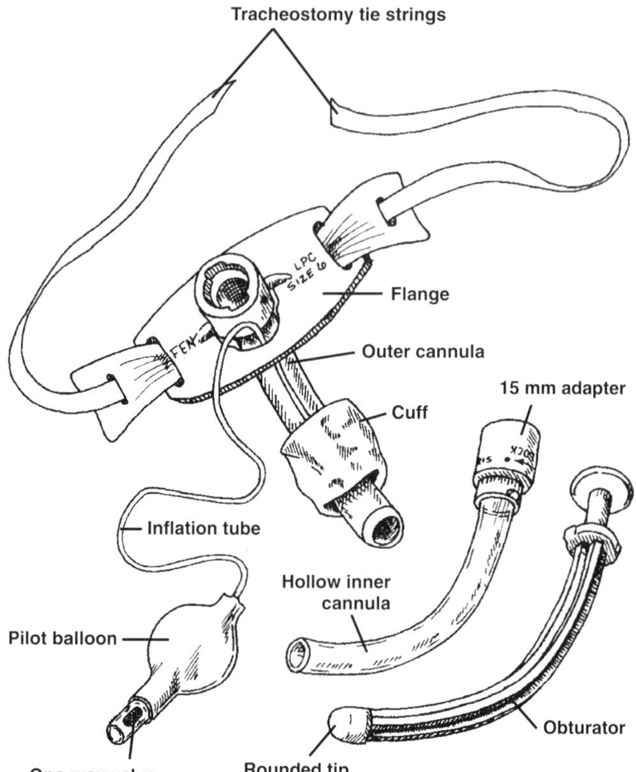

Fig. 11-16 Typical tracheostomy tube with its component parts and features.

piration, and assuring a safe route to provide mechanical ventilation. In addition, it is placed in the patient who has an upper airway obstruction or facial trauma that make intubation impossible. A tracheostomy tube is often placed in a patient who will require long-term mechanical ventilation or who needs a permanent artificial airway. In the long term, a tracheostomy is said to be more comfortable than an endotracheal tube even though it requires a surgical procedure. An additional advantage of a tracheostomy tube over an endotracheal tube is that it allows the patient to eat and drink.

These tubes come in a variety of sizes for patient's of all ages from neonatal to adult. See Table 11-1 for tracheostomy tube sizes for patients based on their age. Commonly, the outside diameter size of the tube should fill approximately two thirds of the patient's trachea. The trachea is sealed when the cuff is inflated. Most modern tracheostomy tubes are constructed of a hard PVC plastic and have a high-volume, low-pressure cuff. Some specialty tubes are made of silver, rubber, or latex. The older, silver tubes have a cuff that may be removed. It would be wise to work with as many different types of tracheostomy tube as possible. There are a number of manufacturers of these tubes just as there are of endotracheal tubes. Examples include Portex, National Catheter Corp., and Rüsch.

b. Put the equipment together, make sure that it works properly, and identify and fix any problems with it. (IIB6c) [R, Ap]

The following are commonly seen examples of tracheostomy tube styles:

Standard Tracheostomy Tube

The majority of patients will have this type of tube placed after the tracheostomy procedure. Refer to Fig. 11-16 for these features of a typical tracheostomy tube:

1. The outer cannula is the airway that the patient breathes through. The proximal end is outside of the patient's stoma and attached to an adjustable flange. The angle of the flange can be adjusted so that the distal end of the cannula fits properly into the patient's trachea. Soft, cloth tracheostomy tie strings are tied to the ends of the flange. The loose ends are tied behind the patient's neck to hold the tube in place. The distal end of the cannula has a small area where radiopaque material is imbedded into it. As with an endotracheal tube, this allows the end of the cannula to be seen on a chest x-ray film.

The cuff is a high–residual volume, low-pressure type. Air is put into and taken out of the cuff by an inflation tube with a pilot balloon and one-way valve. All of the cuff considerations discussed with the endotracheal tubes apply here also.

2. The obturator is slid into the outer cannula's opening before it is inserted into the patient's stoma. The obturator has a rounded end that protrudes from the end of the cannula. This prevents any tissue trauma during the insertion. The obturator is removed as soon as the cannula is in place.

3. An inner cannula is slid into the outer cannula's opening and locked into place with a clockwise twist. This completes the airway. The proximal end has a standard 15-mm-OD adapter so that all respiratory care equipment fits onto it. The distal end is flush with the end of the outer cannula. Some practitioners believe that the inner cannula should be periodically removed and cleaned so that secretions do not build up. Other practitioners believe that this is unnecessary if the airway is properly humidified and suctioning is performed as needed.

Fenestrated Tracheostomy Tube

Refer to Fig. 11-17 when reviewing these features of the fenestrated tracheostomy tube:

1. The outer cannula has an opening called the fenestration (Dutch for window). The rest of the cannula, cuff, inflation tube, and flange are the same as already discussed.

2. The inner cannula functions as discussed earlier. When it is in place, the tube functions as the standard model does.

3. The outer cannula plug is used to prevent the patient from breathing through the proximal end of the tube. The plug does not cover the fenestration; therefore, the patient is able to breathe through the upper airway. The patient can now talk and cough out any secretions.

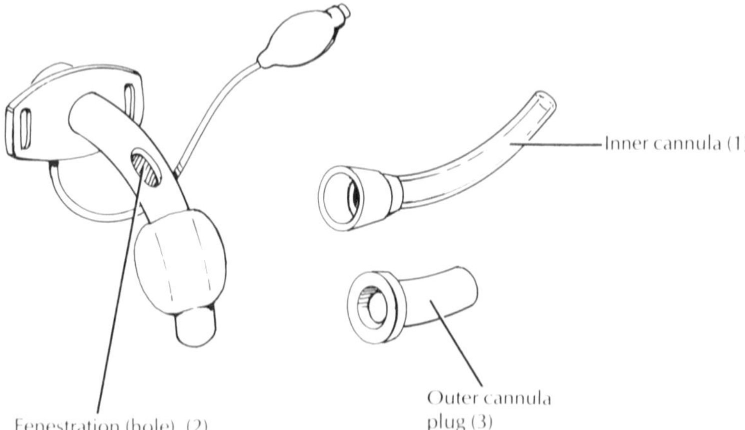

Fig. 11-17 Fenestrated tracheosotomy tube with its component parts and features. (From Eubanks DH, Bone RC: *Comprehensive Respiratory Care,* ed 2. St Louis, Mosby, 1990. Used by permission.)

This tube is often placed in a patient who can breathe spontaneously and who is being considered for a complete removal of the tracheostomy tube. If the patient does well with this tube, it can probably be removed safely. If the patient has difficulty, the plug can be removed, the inner cannula can be replaced, and the patient's airway can be suctioned or mechanically ventilated.

Speaking Tracheostomy Tube

Refer to Fig. 11-18 when reviewing these features of the speaking tracheostomy tube:

1. The cannula is the standard type except that an additional tube has been added to carry a compressed gas through a hole in the back of the cannula. This gas flows up through the vocal cords and allows the patient to speak. The voice will not be as strong as normal but is still a great help to the patient's psychological well-being. The patient can still be mechanically ventilated, be suctioned, and eat and drink as usual.
2. A Y-connector is added to the compressed gas tube. Usually about 4 to 6 L/min of compressed air or oxygen are set by a flowmeter to run to the Y. Closing off the other opening in the Y with a finger diverts the gas into the patient's larynx for speaking. A

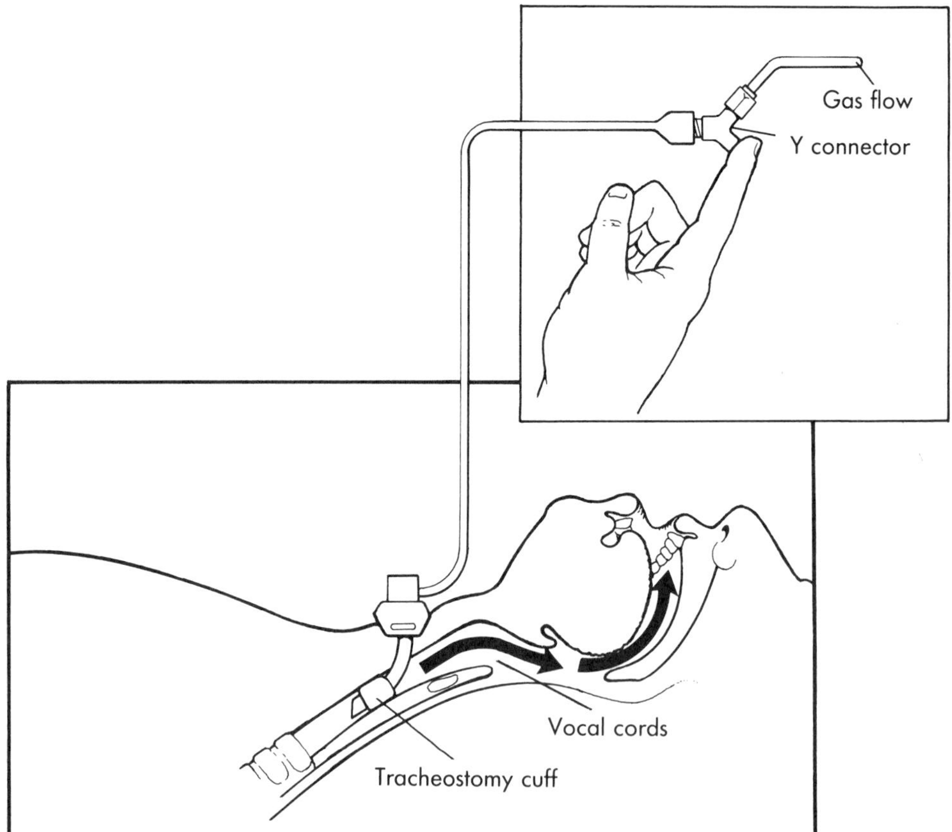

Fig. 11-18 Pitt tracheostomy tube permits the patient to speak. Note its special feature that directs an outside gas flow past the vocal cords. (From Simmons KF: Airway care, in Scanlan CL, Spearman CB, Sheldon RL [eds]: *Egan's Fundamentals of Respiratory Care,* ed 5. St Louis, Mosby, 1990. Used by permission.)

little experimentation with flows will help the patient find the flow that works best for speaking.

Most tubes have cuffs that must be inflated before insertion into the patient to make sure that the cuff is sealed and the one-way valve does not leak. Do not use a tube with a leaking cuff or one-way valve. Kamen-Wilkinson endotracheal and tracheostomy tubes are an exception because they have a self-inflating foam cuff. A syringe is used to *deflate* the cuff before placement into the patient. The cuff should stay deflated. A leaking cuff will reinflate and should be discarded. In a properly functioning cuff, removal of the syringe and opening the pilot balloon valve to room air pressure results in the cuff inflating.

Make sure that the obturator, inner cannula, and plug all fit properly into the outer cannula. They all should easily snap into place and be easily removable. Check this before inserting the tube into the patient.

Secretions or foreign matter can plug the lumen of the cannula. Suction to remove any obstruction. If the catheter cannot be inserted beyond the tube and the patient is having respiratory distress, the tube will have to be removed and replaced. A mucous plug or cuff that has herniated or slipped over the end of the tube can cause this.

8. Tracheostomy buttons.

a. Get the necessary equipment. (IIA5c) [R, Ap]

A tracheostomy button is a hard plastic tube that is placed into the patient's stoma to keep it open after the tracheostomy tube has been removed. The patient is able to eat, talk, and cough normally. Yet, in case the patient has difficulty or needs a breathing treatment, the airway can be reestablished quickly. In general, the patient sizes for tracheostomy buttons match the same sizes for tracheostomy tubes listed in Table 11-1.

b. Put the equipment together, make sure that it works properly, and identify and fix any problems with it. (IIB6c) [R, Ap]

Refer to Fig. 11-19 when reviewing these features of the tracheostomy button:

1. The hollow outer cannula has a slightly flared proximal end. This will keep it from slipping all of the way into the patient. The distal end is flanged and split into several flexible "grippers."
2. A closure plug fits into the outer cannula and snaps into the flexible grippers on the end of the outer cannula. This seals the button so that the patient breathes through the upper airway.
3. A hollow inner cannula can be inserted into the outer cannula instead of the plug. This inner cannula has a standard 15-mm OD so that a Briggs adapter or other respiratory care equipment can be attached if needed. The patient can also be suctioned.
4. Spacers of various widths are used to make sure that the inner cannula is placed in the patient to the right depth. The end of the tube should enter the trachea but not obstruct it. See the airway picture in Fig. 10-19 for the proper position.

There is a special type of tracheostomy button that is used with patients who are not to breathe in through their upper airway but may breathe out through it.

Refer to Fig. 11-20 when reviewing these features of the Kistner tracheostomy tube:

1. The hollow plastic cannula keeps the stoma open. The distal end is flanged so that it is not likely to be pulled out of the trachea accidentally.
2. The proximal end of the cannula is capped with a one-way valve. The valve allows

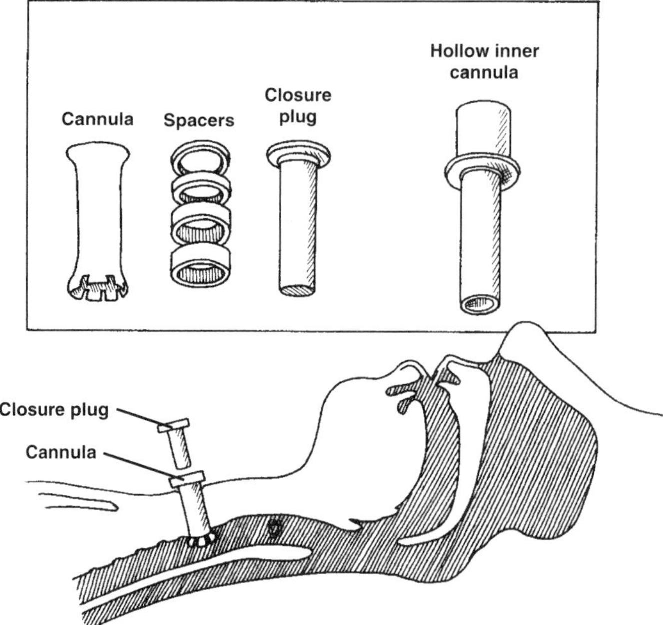

Fig. 11-19 Typical tracheostomy button with its component parts. The insert shows the tracheostomy button properly positioned in the patient.

the patient to breathe in room air or an oxygen- and aerosol-enriched gas source. Expiration is through the upper airway. The patient can talk, eat, and cough normally.

Make sure that all component pieces of these tracheostomy buttons fit together properly and can be easily disconnected if necessary. The cannula must be kept clear of any secretions, blood, or foreign debris. A suction catheter should be passable through the hollow opening in the cannula. If the button is obstructed and the patient is having trouble breathing through his or her upper airway, the button should be removed and replaced with another or a tracheostomy tube.

This ends the general discussion on specific airway management procedures and equipment. The entry level examination may ask questions on this material and the related materials that follow.

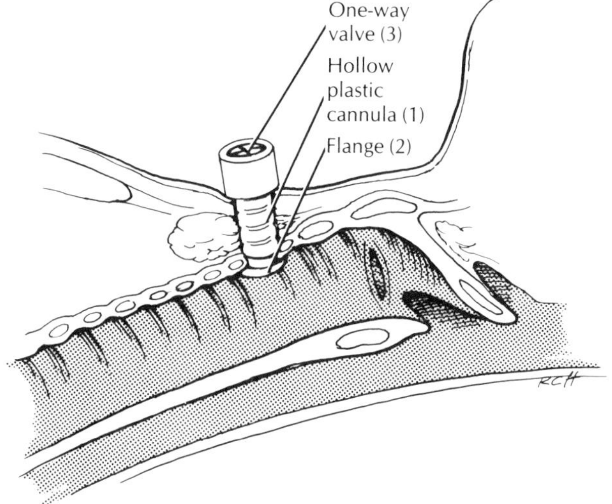

Fig. 11-20 Kistner tracheostomy button. (From Eubanks DH, Bone RC: *Comprehensive Respiratory Care,* ed 2, St Louis, Mosby, 1990. Used by permission.)

Module B. Ensure that the artificial airway is properly placed and maintained.

1. Palpate the endotracheal tube for proper placement. (IB2d) [R, Ap, An]

Often the endotracheal tube can be palpated in an infant as it is being inserted through the larynx. This is because the laryngeal structures are so pliable. Feeling the tube being inserted through the larynx would indicate that it is properly located within the trachea. If the tube cannot be palpated through the larynx, it has probably been inserted into the esophagus. It is more difficult to use this technique with confidence in adults because their laryngeal structures are more stiff. It may not be possible to tell by palpation if an adult has had the endotracheal tube inserted into the larynx and trachea or not.

2. Auscultate the patient's breath sounds and record any changes. (IB3a and b) [R, Ap]

Respiratory efforts without breath sounds would prove that a complete obstruction exists in the patient's airway. Inspiratory or expiratory stridor or wheezing would prove that a partial obstruction exists in the patient's airway. Listen for stridor over the larynx. Wheezing may be heard over the major airways. The restoration of the normal airway should result in the return of normal breath sounds over all areas of both lung fields (unless there is another, unrelated problem).

It is especially important to check for bilateral breath sounds after an endotracheal tube has been placed. If the tube has been inserted too far, it will enter a mainstem bronchus. No breath sounds would be heard in the opposite lung. The right mainstem bronchus is commonly accidentally intubated because it comes off of the trachea at a less acute angle than the left mainstem bronchus. No breath sounds would be heard over the left lung field. If both lung fields cannot be auscultated, at least listen to the right apical area. If breath sounds are heard here, the tube is most likely positioned properly in the trachea. This one site can be checked because the segmental bronchus to the right upper lobe comes off of the right mainstem bronchus in such a way that if the right mainstem bronchus is intubated, the upper lobe segmental bronchus will be blocked (see Fig. 9-1).

3. Make the recommendation for a chest x-ray film, as needed, to help determine the patient's condition. (IA2a) [R, Ap]

A chest x-ray film should always be taken to confirm the location of a newly placed endotracheal or tracheostomy tube. The chest x-ray film should be repeated if there has been a significant change in the patient's condition or if the tube has been pulled back or pushed deeper into the trachea.

A chest x-ray film will also confirm the presence and location of an opaque foreign body in the airway. Metallic objects, stones, and coins will be clearly seen. Less radiopaque objects will be barely seen, if at all. The chest x-ray film will also detect a pneumothorax related to the tracheostomy procedure or other pulmonary conditions.

4. View the chest x-ray film to see the position of the endotracheal or tracheostomy tube. (IB5) [R, Ap]

All modern endotracheal and tracheostomy tubes contain a strip of radiopaque material near the distal tip of the tube. This is easily noticed as the white line seen on the chest x-ray film and confirms the location of the tip of the tube in the airway (see Fig. 11-13).

The ideal location of the tip of the endotracheal tube is the middle third of the trachea. When the tube is positioned properly, it is less likely to have the tip pushed into the carina when the patient bends his or her head forward or to have the cuff hit the vocal cords if the patient's head is bent back. Both endotracheal and tracheostomy tubes should be positioned midline within the trachea. They should not be twisted laterally because the tip can cause damage to the tracheal wall.

5. Ensure that the endotracheal or tracheostomy tube stays properly positioned. (IIIC4) [R, Ap]

The endotracheal tube body has centimeter marks placed on it starting at the distal end and finishing at the proximal end. Check and record the centimeter mark at the patient's teeth or gums. The average adult's distance from the midtrachea to teeth is about 23 to 25 cm. The practitioner will be able to tell if the tube has been accidentally pulled out some or pushed further into the patient by looking at the current centimeter mark. If the tube is intentionally adjusted, the new centimeter mark should be checked and recorded.

A wide variety of handmade, as well as manufactured, devices are available to secure the endotracheal tube in the correct position. Fig. 11-21 shows one way to make a tube holder from adhesive tape. This has the advantages of being flexible when the patient moves and inexpensive. Tincture of benzoin can be applied to the patient's cheeks to make the tape hold more securely without tearing the skin. An oropharyngeal airway may or may not be needed.

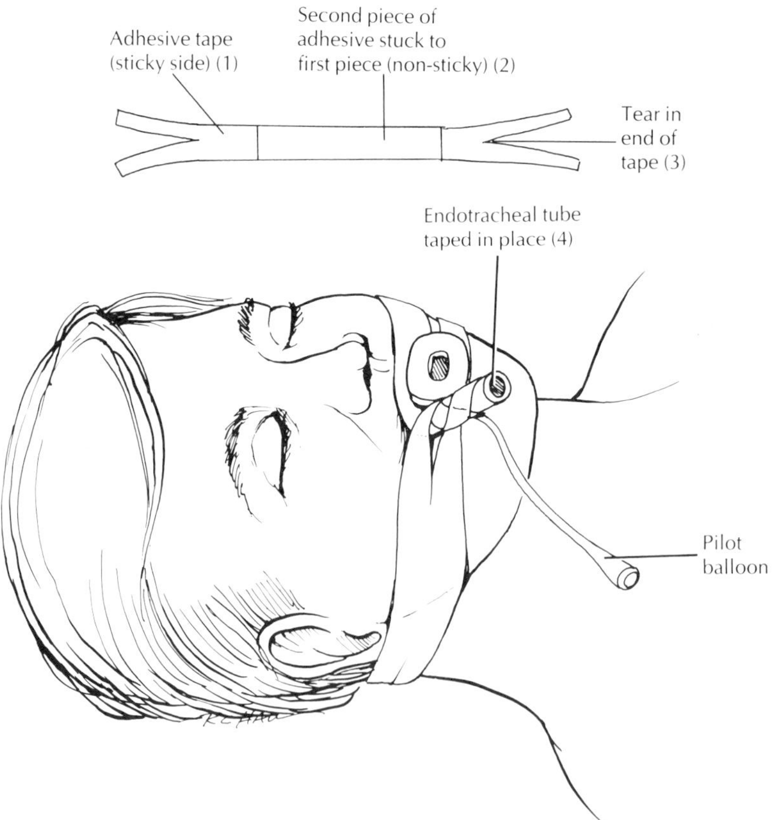

Fig. 11-21 Taping the endotracheal tube to secure it in the airway. (From Eubanks DH, Bone RC: *Comprehensive Respiratory Care,* ed 2. St Louis, Mosby, 1990. Used by permission.)

The manufactured tube holders are made of plastic with cloth ties and usually include a built-in bite block. Make sure that it is sized properly to the patient's mouth. Too large a bite block can injure the tongue, lips, and mouth. Watch for a gag reflex. This type of holder would be useful in the patient who is prone to seizuring.

6. Change the position of the endotracheal or tracheostomy tube. (IIIF3d) [R, Ap, An]

As mentioned earlier, an endotracheal tube is ideally located within the middle third of the trachea. Check the chest x-ray film for positioning. If the tube is too high within the trachea, it may be pulled up through the vocal cords if the patient's head is hyperextended. An air leak would likely be heard at the larynx if the patient is using a mechanical ventilator. In this case, the cuff should be deflated and the tube inserted deeper into the trachea.

Conversely, if the tip of the tube is inserted too deeply into the trachea, it may be pushed into a mainstem bronchus if the patient's head is moved toward the chest. In this situation no breath sounds would be heard in the opposite lung (usually the left). This problem would require that the cuff be deflated and the tube pulled up into the middle third of the trachea. In either case, reinflate the cuff after the tube is repositioned. A chest x-ray film should be taken to confirm the tube's position after it has been moved.

A tracheostomy tube should be positioned so that the flange is snug against the base of the neck and the outer cannula is within the trachea. If pulled out too far, the cuff will likely be seen at the stoma. An air leak may be heard or secretions may be seen to bubble out of the stoma. Correct the problem by deflating the cuff, inserting the tube so that the flange is against the base of the neck, and reinflating the cuff.

7. Keep an endotracheal or tracheostomy tube cuff properly inflated.
a. Get the necessary cuff pressure manometer. (IIA8c) [R, Ap]
b. Put the equipment together, make sure that it works properly, and identify and fix any problems with it. (IIB14c) [R]

A number of manufactured units are available for measuring cuff pressure. Only one is discussed here because it is widely used. The Cufflator is a convenient one-piece device that allows for the measurement of cuff pressure. The system consists of a pressure gauge calibrated in centimeters of water, hand pumped reservoir, internal one-way valve, pressure release valve, and adapter to fit into the one-way valve on the cuff inflating tube. A three-way stopcock can be added to the one-way valve adapter. This can be used to prepressurize the system before attaching it to the patient's one-way valve on the cuff inflating tube (Fig. 11-22). The pressure in the cuff can be measured as air is added by squeezing the hand pump or as air is removed by the pressure release valve. The volume of air added or removed cannot be measured.

A second system can be "home made," although it is also commercially available. It consists of a 5- to 10-ml syringe, three-way stopcock, and pressure gauge (either millimeters of mercury or centimeters of water). The syringe and pressure gauge are attached to two of the ports on the stopcock. The third port on the stopcock is connected to the one-way valve on the cuff inflating tube. When the stopcock handle is opened to all three ports, the pressure throughout the system and the cuff are the same. Air can be added or removed with the syringe. The pressure gauge shows the system and cuff pressure as the air volume is adjusted (Fig. 11-23). One advantage of this system over the Cufflator is that the volume of air that is added or subtracted can be measured. This system can also be prepressurized so that its pressure matches the pressure anticipated in the cuff.

With any of these systems, it is necessary to keep airtight connections. An air leak will be noticed as the pressure drops unexpectedly. Tighten the connections to create a seal so that the pressure is maintained.

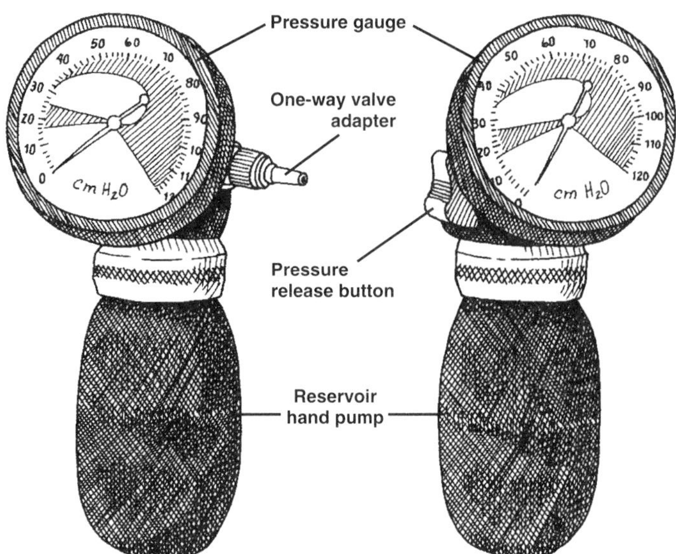

Fig. 11-22 Cufflator device use to measure the cuff pressure with its component parts.

c. Measure and maintain the proper cuff volume and pressure in the endotracheal or tracheostomy tube. (IIIB1d and IIIE14) [R, Ap]

All of the previously mentioned endotracheal and tracheostomy tubes have a cuff for sealing the airway. Most brands of modern tubes have cuffs that are designed to have a relatively large reservoir volume that fills at a relatively low pressure. The soft, flexible

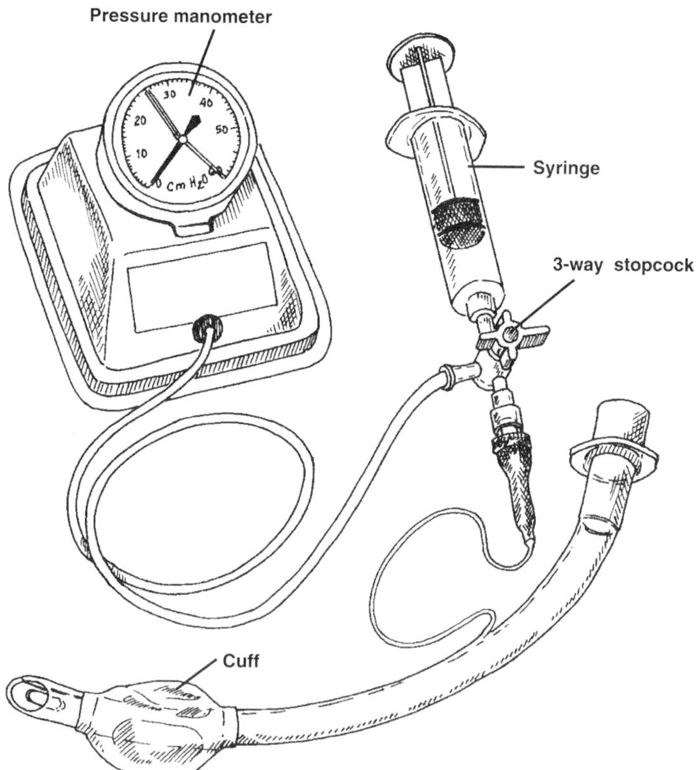

Fig. 11-23 Cuff measuring device made from a pressure manometer, three-way stopcock, and 10-ml syringe.

balloon seals the airway by having a large surface area that conforms to the shape of the trachea. Some reusable endotracheal tubes used in the operating room still have the older low–residual volume, high-pressure cuffs. See Fig. 11-24 for a comparison of the two types of cuffs.

All manufacturers (except Kamen-Wilkenson) have designed cuffs that must be actively filled with air by way of a one-way valve and syringe. These cuffs have greater than atmospheric pressure in them. That pressure is placed against the wall of the trachea. The greater the pressure on the wall of the trachea, the greater the disruption of normal lymphatic and blood flow. Shapiro et al. state that a patient with a normal blood pressure (120/80 mm Hg) will have the following effects at these cuff pressures:

a. Lymphatic flow blockage will occur at pressures greater than 5 mm Hg (8 cm H_2O). Edema of the tracheal mucosa will result.

b. Capillary blood flow blockage will occur at pressures greater than 18 mm Hg (24 cm H_2O). Venous (and lymphatic) drainage will be stopped as a result.

c. Arterial blood flow blockage will occur at pressures greater than 30 mm Hg (42 cm H_2O). Arterial (and lymphatic and capillary) flow will be stopped as a result.

In general, the clinical goal is to keep the cuff pressure as low as possible to make sure that the circulation through the tracheal wall is normal. It seems reasonable to try to keep the cuff pressure no greater than 15 mm Hg (21 cm H_2O). This would hold true for all normotensive patients.

d. Inflate and deflate the cuff as indicated. (IIIF3c) [R, Ap, An]

A spontaneously breathing patient must have the cuff inflated to prevent the aspiration of oral secretions into the lungs. In general, keep the pressure at about 15 mm Hg (21 cm H_2O), as discussed earlier. It may be necessary to keep a higher cuff pressure in a mechanically ventilated patient. High positive airway pressures can result in an air leak around the cuff if the endotracheal or tracheostomy tube is too small. Ideally the tube should be replaced with a larger one. However, some patients are too unstable to tolerate reintubation of their airways and must simply have the cuff pressure increased temporarily.

Hypertensive patients may be able to tolerate higher cuff pressures than normotensive patients before blood flow to the tracheal tissues is stopped. Hypotensive patients will suffer from the loss of blood flow to the tracheal wall at lower cuff pressures than those previously listed.

It is clear that a cuff pressure greater than the patient's mucosal capillary pressure will prevent the flow of blood through the area covered by the cuff. Tissue ischemia (hypoxemia) will result. If the ischemia is severe enough, tissue necrosis will follow. The higher the cuff pressure and the longer the high cuff pressure is maintained, the greater the likelihood of tissue necrosis. If the necrosis is circumferential (all the way around) to the trachea, tracheal stenosis will likely occur. Tracheal stenosis is found when the diameter of the trachea is narrowed because of scar tissue buildup after the normal mucosa

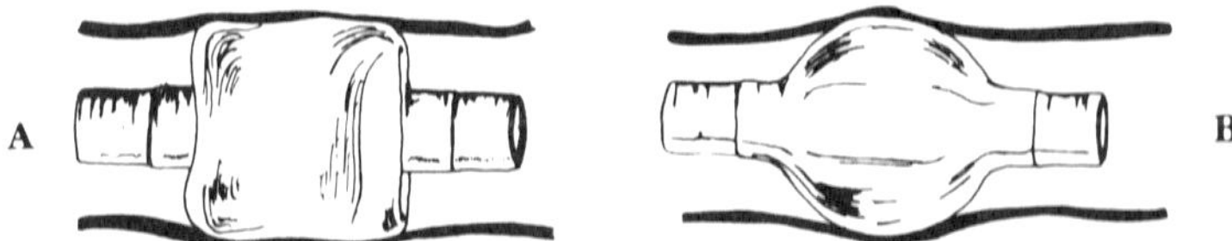

Fig. 11-24 A, Shape of an inflated high residual volume, low-pressure cuff seen in modern endotracheal and tracheostomy tubes. **B,** Shape of an inflated low residual volume, high-pressure cuff seen in esophageal obturator airways. (From McPherson SP: *Respiratory Therapy Equipment,* ed 4. St Louis, Mosby, 1990. Used by permission.)

and underlying tissues have died. The patient's airway is permanently narrowed and, if serious, must be surgically corrected. Another severe complication of high cuff pressures and tracheal necrosis is the development of a tracheoesophageal fistula. This is an opening between the trachea and esophagus. This is made more likely when the patient also has a nasogastric tube in place. The fistula will permit food to pass into the airway and lungs, causing pneumonia. Mechanical ventilation is made more difficult because of the air leak from the lungs to the esophagus. Surgical repair of the fistula is required.

As can be seen, it is very important that the cuff pressure be monitored and kept as low as possible. There are two slightly different ways to inflate the cuff and maintain a safe cuff pressure. It is recommended with either method that the cuff pressure be monitored at least every 8 hours or whenever air is put into or taken out of the cuff.

Minimal Leak

The minimal leak method can be used only with patients on a positive-pressure ventilator. Basically the purpose is to find the cuff pressure that results in *a small leak* at the cuff when the patient's airway pressure is greatest.

Steps in the procedure:

1. Connect the cuff pressure–measuring device (see earlier discussion) to the one-way valve on the cuff inflating tube.
2. Listen with a stethoscope over the patient's larynx.
3. Inflate or deflate the cuff as necessary while listening for an air leak.
4. Stop changing the air volume when a minimal leak is heard at the peak airway pressure in the breathing cycle. The tidal volume should still be delivered except for this minor leak.
5. Note the cuff pressure where the minimal leak was heard. Note the cuff volume, if possible.
6. Disconnect the cuff pressure–measuring device.
7. It may be necessary to add more volume and pressure to the cuff if the leak gets worse when the peak airway pressure increases.

Minimal Occluding Volume

The minimal occluding volume method can be used only with patients on a positive-pressure ventilator. Basically the purpose is to find the cuff pressure that results in *no leak* at the cuff when the patient's airway pressure is greatest.

Steps in the procedure:

1. Connect the cuff pressure–measuring device (see earlier discussion) to the one-way valve on the cuff inflating tube.
2. Listen with a stethoscope over the patient's larynx.
3. Inflate or deflate the cuff as necessary while listening for an air leak.
4. Stop changing the air volume when no leak is heard at the peak airway pressure in the breathing cycle.
5. Note the cuff pressure where the seal was heard. Note the cuff volume, if possible.
6. Disconnect the cuff pressure measuring device.
7. It may be necessary to add more volume and pressure to the cuff if a leak results when the peak airway pressure increases.

It must be reinforced that this discussion relates only to those tubes that must be actively filled with air and have variable intracuff pressures. Several manufacturers have developed endotracheal and tracheostomy tubes that have built-in cuff pressure limitations. These tubes have a pressure-relieving one-way valve that does not permit the cuff pressure to exceed safe levels. Pressures are limited to about 18 or 25 mm Hg, depending on the manufacturer. These tubes are produced by Lanz Medical Products Corporation, Extracorporeal Medical Specialties, Inc., and Shiley Laboratories, Inc.

The Foam Cuff developed by Kamen-Wilkinson is also designed to limit the intracuff pressure to about 20 mm Hg. This cuff is unique in that it is made of foam that is covered by a silicone sheath. Air is pulled out of the foam before intubation. The cuff is then allowed to refill with room air to its normal shape and seal the trachea. Air should never be injected into these cuffs.

Clinical experience has shown that these types of tubes have cuffs that seal well in the spontaneously breathing patient. Difficulty can arise when using these cuffs in patients who are undergoing positive-pressure ventilation. An airway pressure greater than the maximum cuff pressure can result in a leak and loss of tidal volume. Remember, these cuff pressures cannot be increased.

This discussion would not be complete without mentioning the recent manufacture of systems designed to raise the cuff pressure to match the peak airway pressure of a patient using a mechanical ventilator. A tube connects the inspiratory circuit to the one-way valve on the cuff inflating tube. As a positive-pressure breath is delivered, the pressure in the circuit is also applied to the patient's cuff. There should be no loss of tidal volume. When the patient exhales and the airway pressure drops to normal, the cuff pressure also drops back to its normal level.

Module C. Patient Assessment.

1. Determine and continue to monitor how the patient responds to the treatment or procedure.

The fear and hypoxemia caused by a sudden upper airway obstruction will result in a transient increase in the patient's heart rate, blood pressure, and attempted respiratory effort. Once the airway has been opened and normal breathing and oxygen levels are restored, the vital signs should return toward the baseline level.

If the airway cannot be quickly restored, and the patient becomes dangerously hypoxemic, the heart rate may slow or show dangerous dysrhythmias, blood pressure will drop, and respiratory efforts will become weaker and then stop. Death will result if the airway cannot be opened and the hypoxemia corrected.

The insertion of an endotracheal tube sometimes results in a slowing of the heart rate because of vagal nerve stimulation in the trachea. This is usually self-limiting, and the heart rate will return to baseline.

A conscious patient with a nasopharyngeal airway will be able to tell you how he or she is tolerating it. The conscious patient with an endotracheal tube or tracheostomy will be unable to speak. Alternative ways to communicate will have to be provided. Examples include alphabet boards and picture boards for pointing and pencil and paper for notes. Head nods for yes and no and lip reading are often used. It is important that questions are worded so that they can be answered with a yes or no answer. Avoid questions that require a lengthy written answer unless the patient seems ready and willing to do so.

2. Modify the treatment or procedure and recommend any changes in the patient's respiratory care plan, depending on response.

The indications or uses for the various airways are listed with the information on that airway. In general, the airway should be removed when it is no longer needed. Typically an oropharyngeal airway should be removed from a patient who has regained consciousness. A nasopharyngeal airway should be removed if the patient no longer needs it as an airway or for a suctioning route. Endotracheal and tracheostomy tubes can be removed when the patient does not need mechanical ventilation, a suctioning route, is no longer in danger of aspiration, or does not need a permanent artificial airway.

3. Change the humidification device and connector used with an artificial airway as needed. (IIIF3a) [R, Ap]

Typically an aerosol generator or humidifier warmed to provide 100% of the patient's humidity needs is connected to the endotracheal or tracheostomy tube. This should be provided to any patient with a problem of thick secretions or large amounts of secretions. A Briggs adapter/aerosol T-adapter with a reservoir tube can be used to humidify the airway (see Fig. 5-20). A tracheostomy mask can also be used to provide moisture to the patient with a tracheostomy. This mask does not add any weight to the tracheostomy tube and so may be more comfortable than a Brigg's adapter. It does have the drawback of not being a closed system so that some outside air may be breathed in by the patient (see Fig. 5-19). See Section 5 on oxygen therapy and Section 7 on humidity and aerosol therapy for other details.

It is acceptable to use a condensing humidifier if the patient does not have a problem with thick secretions, pneumonia, or bronchitis. The condensing humidifier makes use of a hygroscopic filter that removes the warmth and natural humidity from the patient's exhaled gas. This moisture evaporates from the filter on the patient's next breath in. Between 70% and 90% of the patient's body humidity can be met by using this device. Most commonly these devices are used with a patient who is breathing on a mechanical ventilator.

4. Recheck any math work and make note of incorrect data. (IIIA2c) [R, Ap, An]

There may be the need to convert the units used in the cuff pressure manometers from millimeters of mercury to centimeters of water. These proportional conversions are based on the masses of the two elements: 1 mm Hg = 1.36 cm H_2O.

Convert from mm Hg to cm H_2O with this equation:

$$\text{cm } H_2O = \text{mm Hg} \times 1.36$$

Example:

The patient's cuff pressure is measured at 10 mm Hg. What is the cuff pressure in cm H_2O?

$$\text{cm } H_2O = 10 \text{ mm Hg} \times 1.36$$

$$\text{Cuff pressure} = 13.6 \text{ cm } H_2O$$

Convert from cm H_2O to mm Hg with this equation:

$$\text{mm Hg} = \frac{\text{cm } H_2O}{1.36}$$

Example:

The patient's cuff pressure is measured at 15 cm H_2O. What is the cuff pressure in mm Hg?

$$\text{mm Hg} = \frac{15 \text{ cm } H_2O}{1.36}$$

$$\text{Cuff pressure} = 11 \text{ mm Hg}$$

BIBLIOGRAPHY

Caldwell SL, Sullivan KN: Artificial airways, in Burton GG, Hodgkin JE (eds): *Respiratory Care—a Guide to Clinical Practice*, ed 2. Philadelphia, Lippincott, 1984.

Eubanks DH, Bone RC: *Comprehensive Respiratory Care*, ed 2. St Louis, Mosby, 1990.

McPherson SP: *Respiratory Therapy Equipment*, ed 4. St Louis, Mosby, 1990.

Rarey KP, Youtsey JW: *Respiratory Patient Care*. Englewood Cliffs, NJ, Prentice-Hall, 1981.

Shapiro BA, Harrison RA, Kacmarek RM, et al: *Clinical Application of Respiratory Care*, ed 3. Chicago, Mosby, 1985.

Sills JR: An emergency cuff inflation technique. *Respir Care* 1986; 31:199-201.

Simmons KF: Airway care, in Scanlan CL, Spearman CB, Sheldon RL (eds): *Egan's Fundamentals of Respiratory Care*, ed 5. St Louis, Mosby, 1990.

Standards and guidelines for cardiopulmonary resuscitation (CPR) and emergency cardiac care (ECC). *JAMA* 1992; 268:2171-2295.

Stephenson Jr HE: Cardiopulmonary resuscitation, in Burton GG, Hodgkin JE (eds): *Respiratory Care—a Guide to Clinical Practice*, ed 2. Philadelphia, Lippincott, 1984.

Watson MA: Cardiopulmonary resuscitation, in Barnes TA (ed): *Respiratory Care Practice*. Chicago, Mosby, 1988.

SELF-STUDY QUESTIONS

1. Your conscious patient has a cervical spine injury. She is lying flat in bed on her back and is showing signs of an upper airway obstruction. How would you recommend that her airway be opened at this time?
   A. Hyperextend her neck and head.
   B. Perform the jaw-thrust maneuver.
   C. Perform a tracheostomy.
   D. Place an oropharyngeal airway.
   E. Place a nasopharyngeal airway.

2. You are preparing a stainless steel–type laryngoscope handle and blade for an anesthesiologist. The light will not shine. Which of the following would you do to fix the problem?
   I. Get a smaller blade to fit the handle.
   II. Get a larger blade to fit the handle.
   III. Tighten the light bulb.
   IV. Replace the handle with with a plastic one.
   V. Check the batteries and replace them if necessary.
   A. I
   B. II
   C. III, V
   D. IV
   E. I, II, IV

3. Clinical signs of a partial upper airway obstruction include all of the following *except:*
   A. Inability to make any sounds
   B. Suprasternal retractions
   C. Increased use of accessory muscles of ventilation
   D. Intercostal retractions
   E. Inspiratory stridor

4. Which of the following are considerations for the chest thrust Heimlich maneuver?
   I. It can be performed on a very obese victim.
   II. The rescuer places his or her hands between the victim's sternum and navel.
   III. Thrust quickly and firmly into the victim.
   IV. The rescuer places his or her first on the lower third of the sternum.
   V. It can be performed on a victim who is in the later months of pregnancy.
   A. I, IV
   B. II, III
   C. III, IV
   D. I, IV, V
   E. I, II, III

5. An oropharyngeal airway would be indicated under which of the following conditions:
   I. To maintain an airway before performing a tracheostomy.
   II. When seizure activity is expected or present.
   III. An unconscious patient who is lying supine and has a soft tissue upper airway obstruction.
   IV. To stabilize the mouth in a patient with a traumatic jaw injury.
   V. An orally intubated patient who is biting the tube.
   A. III, V
   B. I
   C. IV, V
   D. IV
   E. II, III, V

6. To minimize the risk of soft tissue injury to the trachea, how should the endotracheal tube cuff pressure be kept?
   A. At less than 30 mm Hg in a hypertensive patient
   B. At less than 20 cm H_2O in a normotensive patient
   C. At greater than 20 mm Hg in a hypertensive patient
   D. At greater than 30 cm H_2O in a hypertensive patient
   E. At less than 25 mm Hg in the normotensive patient

7. To ensure that the endotracheal tube is placed properly, you would recommend all of the following *except:*
   A. Listen to the right upper lobe if the left lung field is inaccessible.
   B. Listen for bilateral lung sounds.
   C. Have a lateral neck x-ray film taken.
   D. Have a chest x-ray film taken.

8. An endotracheal tube cuff pressure of greater than 30 mm Hg will likely cause which of the following?
   I. Loss of capillary flow through the tracheal soft tissues
   II. Loss of lymphatic flow through the tracheal soft tissues
   III. Tracheal wall damage
   IV. A tight seal of the airway to prevent the aspiration of oral secretions
   V. Loss of venous flow through the tracheal soft tissues
   A. I, II, III, V
   B. II, IV
   C. V
   D. I
   E. II

9. While assisting with a CPR attempt, the anesthesiologist asks you to get a properly sized endotracheal tube so that the patient's airway can be quickly intubated. The patient is an average-sized man. What would you get?
   A. An adult-sized oropharyngeal airway
   B. A 7.0-mm-ID oral endotracheal tube
   C. A 10.0-mm-ID nasal endotracheal tube
   D. An 8.0-mm-ID nasal endotracheal tube
   E. An 8.0-mm-ID oral endotracheal tube

10. You have just measured a tracheostomy tube's cuff pressure with a blood pressure–type mercury manometer. The pressure was 17 mm Hg. Your charting is supposed to show the pressure in centimeters of water pressure. What would you record in the patient's chart?
   A. 12.5 cm H_2O
   B. 0.08 cm H_2O
   C. 17 mm Hg
   D. 23 cm H_2O
   E. None of the above

Answer Key:

1. B; 2. C; 3. A; 4. D; 5. E; 6. B; 7. C; 8. A; 9. E; 10. D.

12 Suctioning the Airway

Module A. Suctioning Devices.

1. Oropharyngeal suction devices.

a. Get the necessary equipment for the procedure. (IIA6c) [R, Ap]

The most commonly used oropharyngeal suction device is called a Yankauer suction catheter. It is made of hard plastic and has an angled catheter to reach into the back of the mouth. The catheter comes packaged as sterile. It may be used more than once because suctioning the oropharynx is considered to be a clean (not sterile) procedure. There may be one large opening or several medium-sized openings at the tip of the catheter. The openings are large enough to permit easy suctioning of saliva, food, or vomitus. The handle is grooved to minimize slippage. Some handles include a thumb control valve so that suction can be applied to the tip only when wanted. When the valve is uncovered, no vacuum is applied to the catheter tip. Covering the opening with a thumb creates a vacuum at the tip for suctioning the patient's mouth (Fig. 12-1). The Yankauer may be discarded when no longer needed or sterilized for use with another patient.

A flexible plastic or rubber catheter can be used to suction the oropharynx when a Yankauer suction catheter is not available. It comes packaged as sterile but may used more than once to suction the oropharynx. The catheter should be of the largest diameter possible to reduce the chance of it becoming plugged. The opening at the catheter tip should be cut straight (perpendicular) across instead of at an angle. There should not be any side openings (Fig. 12-2). The catheter is discarded when no longer needed.

b. Put the equipment together, make sure that it works properly, and identify and fix any problems with it. (IIB8c) [R, Ap]

The catheters just mentioned are single pieces with nothing to assemble. They must be attached to a vacuum source by a length of soft rubber tubing. Both the Yankauer and plastic or rubber catheters have a connector for the vacuum tubing. While a clean glove is worn over the hand with the catheter, the vacuum tubing is held by the other hand and stretched over the end of the catheter connector so that it is sealed. The other end of the vacuum tubing is stretched over the connector at the vacuum source.

The vacuum must be applied to the tip of the catheter for oral secretions to be removed. Check for a vacuum at the tip by any of these methods:

a. Listen for the sound of air being drawn into the tip.

b. Put the tip into a container of sterile water. Close the thumb control opening. The water must be drawn up the catheter.

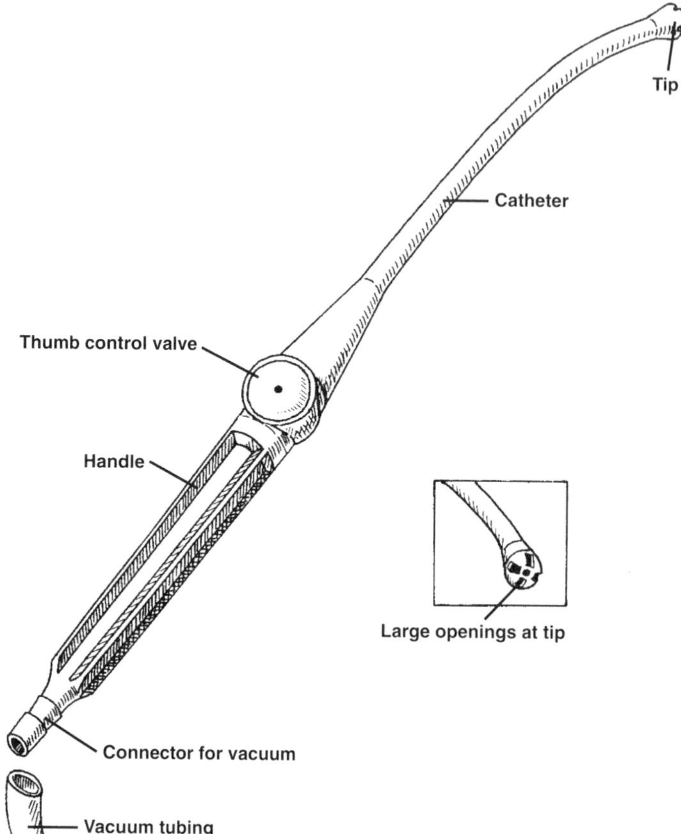

Fig. 12-1 Features of a Yankauer suction catheter.

c. Place a clean gloved hand placed over the tip if no water is available. Close the thumb control opening. The glove should be attracted to the catheter.

Failure to have a vacuum at the catheter tip can mean:

A. The vacuum is not turned on.

Some centralized vacuum systems have a dial that turns the system off and on and sets the vacuum level. Turn the dial to the right (clockwise) to turn on the system and set the vacuum level. Some other centralized vacuum systems have an on/off switch and a dial for the vacuum level. The vacuum level can be preset and the system turned on or off by flipping the switch.

Fig. 12-2 Features of a suction catheter with a cross-cut tip.

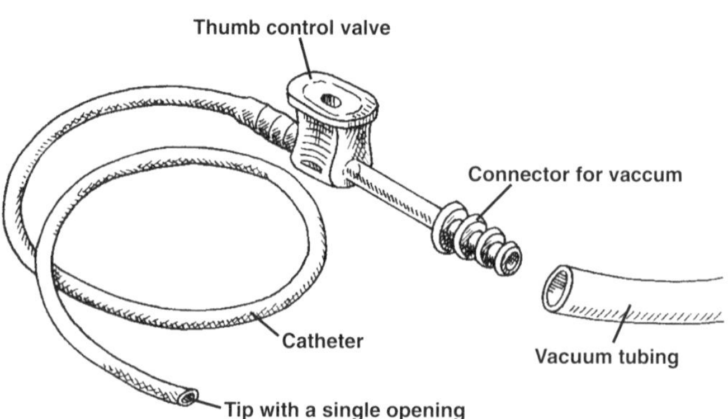

Free-standing vacuum systems can be moved from patient to patient. They use a pump to create the vacuum level and must be plugged into a working electrical outlet. The on/off switch must be turned on. The simpler systems have a preset vacuum level. Variable vacuum levels can be set with a dial in the more sophisticated systems.

The amount of vacuum that can be applied to the patient varies depending on the age of the patient, the thickness of the secretions, or the physician's order.

B. The system is not sealed, so the vacuum is lost to the atmosphere. Check the following:
   1. Make sure that the rubber vacuum tubing fits tightly over the connectors on the catheter and on the vacuum system.
   2. Make sure that the catheter is not cracked or defective with a hole. Check to make sure that the vacuum tubing is not defective or cut. Replace either a Yankauer, plastic, or rubber catheter or vacuum tubing that is defective.
   3. Close the thumb control if it has been left open.
   4. Check the central or free-standing vacuum system to make sure that the secretion collection jar is sealed properly.

C. The system is blocked, and no vacuum can get through to the tip. Check the following:
   1. Check for a knot in the vacuum tubing or soft catheter. Untie any knot in the vacuum tubing. Replace a knotted soft catheter.
   2. Check for a blockage in the catheter or vacuum tubing. Try to suction some sterile water to clear the blockage into the secretion collection jar. Replace the catheter, or vacuum tubing, or both if the blockage cannot be cleared.

2. Suction catheters.

a. Get the necessary equipment for the procedures (IIA6a) [R, Ap, An]

All of the following catheters are intended for suctioning the trachea. They come sterile and individually packaged. It is highly recommended that the outer diameter of the catheter be no more than one-half the inner diameter of the airway that it is passing through. For example, if the patient has an endotracheal tube that is 7-mm ID, the suction catheter should be no more than 3.5-mm OD. This guideline is intended to minimize the obstruction to the airway so that the patient can still breathe around the catheter. A thicker catheter may remove secretions more effectively, but it places the patient at greater risk for hypoxemia by blocking the airway and suctioning too much air out of the lungs.

See Table 12-1 for the recommended suction catheter sizes for the various endotracheal or tracheostomy tubes. The practitioner can also easily compare the relative sizes of the tube and suction catheter at the bedside before suctioning. Suction catheters are sized by the French (Fr or F) scale of their outer diameter. Endotracheal and tracheostomy tubes are sized by inner diameter and outer diameter in millimeters and often by outer diameter in French. Review Table 11-1 if necessary. The following formula and example will show how to calculate the outer diameter size of any suction catheter to know the endotracheal or tracheostomy tube with which it may be used.

Because each French unit is about 0.33 mm, the *outer* diameter in millimeters of a suction catheter can be found by multiplying the French size by 0.33. For example, calculate the outer diameter of a 12 Fr suction catheter:

$$12 \text{ Fr} \times 0.33 = 3.96 \text{ (about 4.0) mm OD of the catheter}$$

Table 12-1. Recommended Suction Catheter French Sizes for the Various Endotracheal and Tracheostomy Tube Sizes*

Age	ID† of Tube Sizes (mm)	Suction Catheter Size (Fr)
Newborn		
<1000 g	2.5	5
1000-2000 g	3.0	6
2000-3000 g	3.5	8
>3000 g to 6 mo old	3.5-4.0	8
Pediatric		
18 mo	4.0	8
3 yr	4.5	8
5 yr	5.0	10
6 yr	5.5	10
8 yr	6.0	10
Adult		
16 yr	7.0	10
Normal-sized woman	7.5-8.0	12
Normal-sized man	8.0-8.5	14
Large adult	9.0-10.0	16

*__Note:__ It is recommended to use a suction catheter with an outer diameter that is no more than half of the inner diameter of the endotracheal tube.
†*ID,* Inner diameter.

So, this sized catheter could be used on an 8.0-mm-ID endotracheal tube. See Figure 12-3 for the relative sizes of this endotracheal tube and catheter.

There may also be some clinical use in knowing the *inner* diameter of a suction catheter because it relates to the maximum particle size that can pass through it. The following formula can be used to interconvert from French to millimeters.

$$\text{mm} = \frac{\text{Fr} - 2}{4}$$

Example:
You have a 12 Fr suction catheter. What is its *inner* diameter in millimeters?

$$\text{mm} = \frac{12 - 2}{4}$$

$$\text{mm} = \frac{10}{4}$$

$$\text{mm} = 2.5 \text{ (See Fig. 12-3.)}$$

Catheters for Open Airway Suctioning

Open airway suctioning is used here to refer to having the patient breathe room air spontaneously after being disconnected from the source of supplemental oxygen. This happens to the patient with a normal upper airway when the oxygen mask is removed for nasotracheal suctioning. It also happens when the patient with an endotracheal or trache-

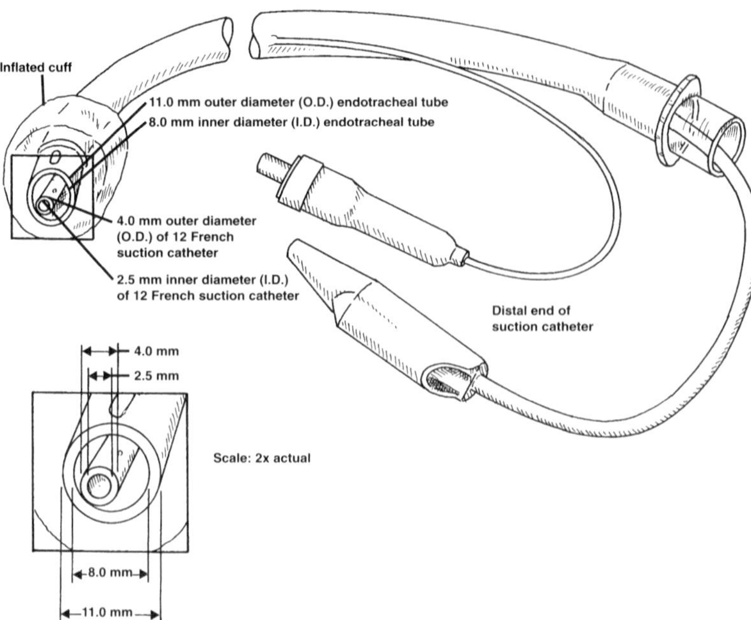

Fig. 12-3 No. 12 Fr suction catheter inside of an 8.0-mm-ID endotracheal tube. The outer diameter of the catheter should be no more than one half of the inner diameter of the tube so that the patient can still breathe around it.

ostomy tube has the aerosol T-adapter (Briggs' adapter) or ventilator circuit removed for suctioning purposes. It has been well shown that the patient's arterial oxygen pressure (Pao_2) and oxygen saturation (Spo_2) levels fall dramatically during open airway suctioning. This hypoxemia is caused by two factors. First, the patient will now inhale room air instead of the oxygen-enriched gas as before. Second, the vacuum applied to the lungs to remove secretions also removes gas (oxygen) from the lungs. Because of these factors, it is important to hyperoxygenate the patient before, during, and after all suctioning efforts.

These types of catheters have been in use for many years. There are two basic types, as shown in Fig. 12-4. Closing the thumb control, as shown in Fig. 12-5, allows the vacuum to be selectively applied to the secretions when desired. The tips of the catheters can vary greatly. This is because there has been a considerable amount of effort spent in recent years trying to develop a catheter tip that will most effectively remove secretions without damaging the tracheal mucosa. Fig. 12-6 shows some of the catheter tips that have been developed to minimize mucosal damage. Note that all feature at least one opening in the catheter that is back from the opening at the tip. Compare this with the single end opening found on the oral suction catheter shown in Fig. 12-2. The side openings are designed to prevent the vacuum from being applied to the tip when it makes contact with the mucosa. Examples include Aspir-Safe, Regu-Vac, Tri-Flo, and Aero-Flo.

Notice in Figs. 12-4 and 12-6 that most of the catheters are straight throughout their length. All of these catheters will tend to enter the right mainstem bronchus during deep suctioning. This is because its angle off of the trachea is less acute compared with the left mainstem bronchus. This results in it being difficult, if not impossible, for any of these catheters to suction the left mainstem bronchus. The Coudé catheter has been designed with an angled tip to better enable it to be guided into the left (or right) mainstem bronchus. See the far right example in Figure 12-6. When these catheters are used, the direction of the thumb control valve can help determine the angle of the bent tip.

Use of these traditional types of catheters during open airway suctioning always results in some level of hypoxemia. The use of a relatively new type of suction catheter may help to alleviate this problem. The insufflating suction catheter (ISC) is designed to alter-

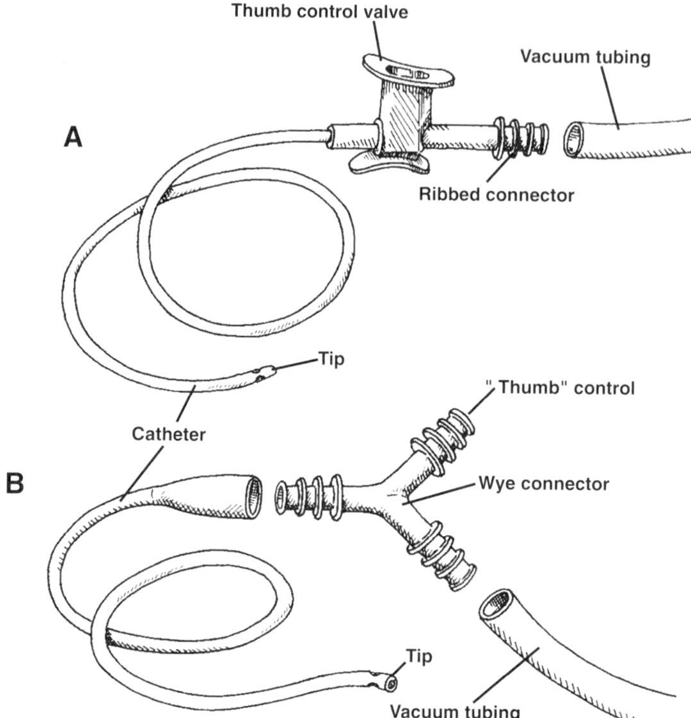

Fig. 12-4 Features of two types of suction catheters with angle-cut tips and side holes. Type **A** has its own thumb control valve. Type **B** needs to have a thumb control valve constructed from a Y connector.

natively provide oxygen through the catheter or vacuum for suctioning. The thumb control end of the catheter is modified with two male-type tubing connectors and a way to switch the lumen of the catheter between them. In clinical practice the smaller connector is attached to small-bore oxygen tubing. The larger connector is attached to a length of rubber vacuum tubing. Oxygen flow is set at 10 to 15 L/min. The thumb control is set to direct the oxygen through the catheter and into the patient as the catheter is advanced. After the catheter has been deeply placed into the trachea for suctioning, the thumb control is switched from delivering oxygen to applying suction. The catheter then functions just like all of the others to remove secretions. At least two studies have looked at the use of these catheters and have concluded that hypoxemia was reduced and the time taken to preoxygenate the patient could be reduced or eliminated. Manufacturers include American Pharmaseal Company with its Jinotti Catheter, VenTech Inc., with its VenTech ISC, and Genesis Medical, Ltd., with its Genesis insufflating suction catheter.

Catheters for Closed Airway Suctioning

Closed airway suctioning will be used here to refer to suctioning when the patient remains connected to the original source of oxygen. This may be done through a special

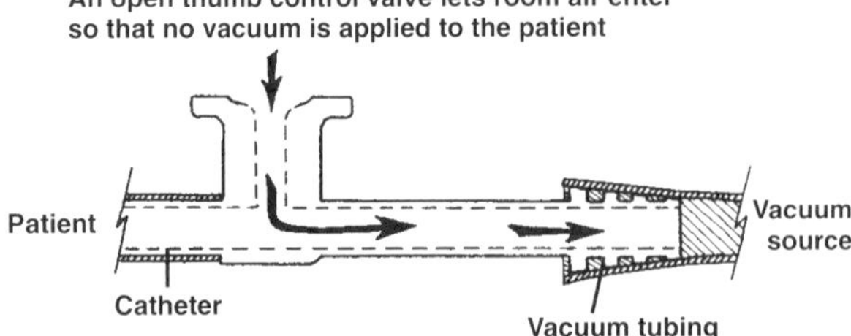

Fig. 12-5 Close-up of a thumb control valve showing how room air is drawn into the vacuum tubing when the valve is left open. Closing the valve applies vacuum to the catheter tip to suction secretions.

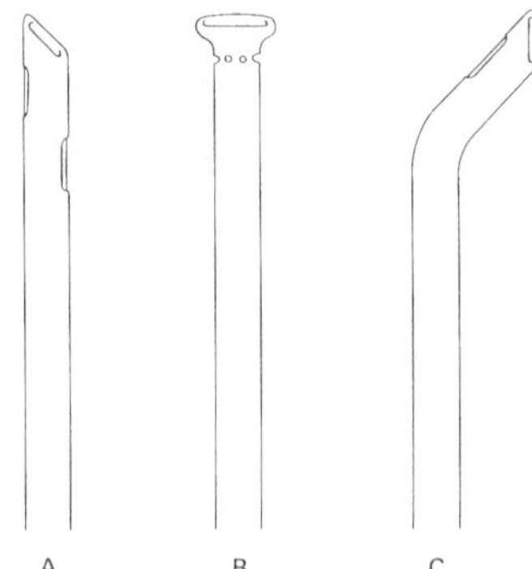

Fig. 12-6 Close-up of the ends of three different suction catheters. Catheter **A** shows a bevel cut of the tip with two offset side holes. Catheter **B** shows a ring tip with several side holes around it. Catheter **C** shows a Coudé (curved-tip) catheter, which may help in guiding it into either the left or right mainstem bronchus. (From Rarey KP, Youtsey JW: *Respiratory Patient Care.* Englewood Cliffs, NJ, Prentice-Hall, 1981. Used by permission.)

aerosol T-adapter or, more commonly, with the patient receiving mechanical ventilation. Spontaneously breathing patients are less likely to suffer hypoxemia with sealed airway suctioning because they can continue to inhale the prescribed oxygen percentage. In addition, if the patient is using a ventilator, tidal volume breaths can still be delivered and positive end-expiratory pressure (PEEP) levels maintained. If hypoxia does occur it will be less severe and of a shorter duration than with open airway suctioning.

Ballard Medical Products and Concord/Portex have made these units available as a self-contained sterile catheter and protective sheath suctioning system (Fig. 12-7). In these systems, a flexible, clear plastic sheath covers the catheter to maintain its sterility. Gloves are not needed by the practitioner. The self-contained systems have a financial advantage over the traditional catheter and gloves suctioning method in that they can be reused for up to 24 hours. A modified T-piece can be attached to the catheter and connected to a patient's endotracheal or tracheostomy tube. Aerosol tubing or a ventilator circuit can be attached to the T-piece. This has the clinical benefit of never disconnecting the patient from the source of supplemental oxygen or mechanical ventilation during the suctioning procedure.

One must completely withdraw the catheter from the endotracheal tube into the sheath, or it will act as a partial obstruction. These closed-system suction catheters come with either the traditional straight tip or the Coudé tip for selective bronchial suctioning.

Another device to create a sealed system for endotracheal tube suctioning consists of an elbow adapter that has an inner plastic sleeve or diaphragm. As the traditional catheter is inserted into the opening on the elbow adapter, the sleeve or diaphragm conforms to the catheter so that there is no air leak (Fig. 12-8). This ensures that the ventilator delivered volumes and pressures are not lost through a leak. Manufacturers include Marquest Medical Products, Inc., with its Trach Swivel Adaptor with Port that is used with adults and B + B Medical Technologies with its Neo_2Safe adapter that is used with neonates.

b. Put the equipment together, make sure that it works properly, and identify and fix any problems with it. (IIB8a) [R, Ap]

All of these suction catheters are intended for suctioning the trachea. They are sterile and individually packaged. They come as a single unit with no parts to put together. The tip has an opening, usually cut at an angle, and one or more side openings. Most catheters also have a built-in thumb control valve with a ribbed connector for the vacuum tubing. Closing the thumb control valve results in a vacuum at the tip of the catheter for suctioning secretions (see Figs. 12-4 and 12-5).

Some catheters do not have the thumb control valve. One can easily be made by using a Y-connector. The Y-connector should be clean but does not need to be sterile because it will not enter the patient's trachea or touch any sterile surface (see Fig. 12-4,B).

Only a hand covered by a sterile glove can be allowed to touch the area of the catheter that will enter the patient's trachea. The practitioner's other hand should also be gloved. A clean glove is acceptable because it will not touch the part of the catheter that will enter the patient's trachea.

While holding the body of the catheter and the thumb control valve and vacuum connector with the sterile gloved hand and the vacuum tubing with the clean gloved hand, slip the vacuum tubing overthe catheter's vacuum connector. The seal should be tight so that there is no vacuum leak.

From now on, only the sterile gloved hand may touch the patient contact part of the catheter. The clean gloved hand may touch only the thumb control valve and vacuum tubing. If the catheter is contaminated, it must be discarded.

The catheter can be tested for patency and vacuum at the tip by the three methods described earlier in the discussion on oropharyngeal suction devices. Note that only a *sterile* glove may be touched against the tip of the suction catheter to check for a vacuum.

Recently Ballard Medical Products and other manufacturers have made available self-contained sterile catheter and protective sheath suctioning systems (see Fig. 12-7).

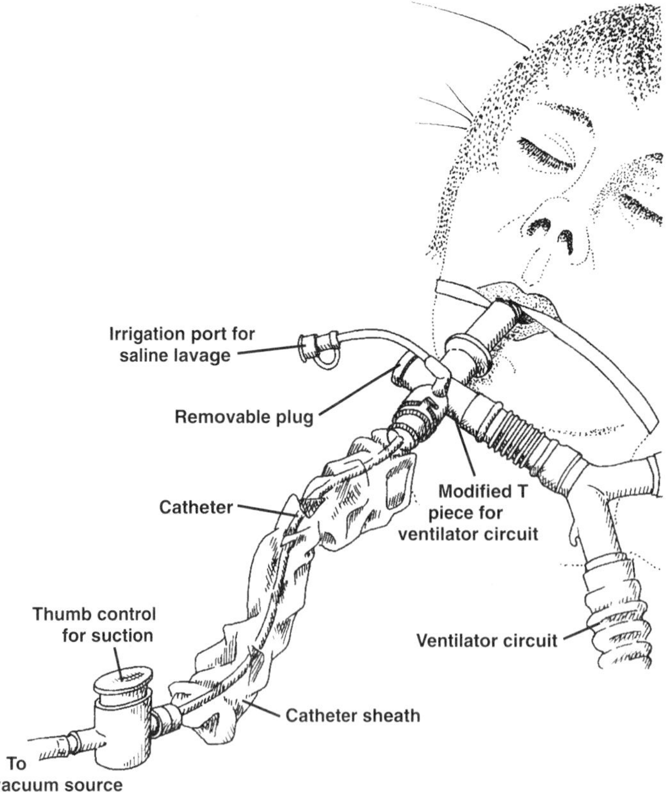

Fig. 12-7 Self-contained catheter and sheath suctioning system. (Based on the Ballard Medical Products suction system and the TRACH-CARE continuous use suction system.)

In these systems, a flexible, clear plastic sheath covers the catheter to maintain its sterility. Gloves are not needed by the practitioner. The self-contained system has a financial advantage over the traditional catheter-and-glove suctioning method in that it can be reused for up to 24 hours. A modified T-piece can be attached to the catheter and connected to a patient's endotracheal or tracheostomy tube. Aerosol tubing or a ventilator circuit can be attached to the T-piece. This has the clinical benefit of never disconnecting the patient from the source of supplemental oxygen or mechanical ventilation during the suctioning procedure.

The three common causes of an equipment failure and how to fix them are described in the earlier discussion on oropharyngeal suction devices.

3. Specimen collectors.

a. Get the necessary equipment for the procedure. (IIA6b) [R, Ap]

There are a variety of specimen collectors (commonly called Luken traps). They are packaged as sterile so that there will be no contamination of the sputum sample with nonpatient organisms. Figs. 12-8 to 12-11 show the key features and functions of several sputum sample collectors.

The specimen jar has volume markings and screws into either a special lid used to suction the specimen or a regular lid for shipment to the laboratory. The special lids used in the systems featured in Figs. 12-8 and 12-9 must be connected to a sterile catheter. Fig. 12-10 shows a system with its own catheter. The vacuum source is provided to these specimen collectors by a length of vacuum tubing as in the previously described suction catheter systems. Fig. 12-11 shows a DeLee system sometimes used in the delivery room. The physician, nurse, or practitioner uses mouth suction to remove secretions from the newborn. In all of these examples, after the sample has been collected, the special lid is unscrewed and replaced with the regular specimen jar lid.

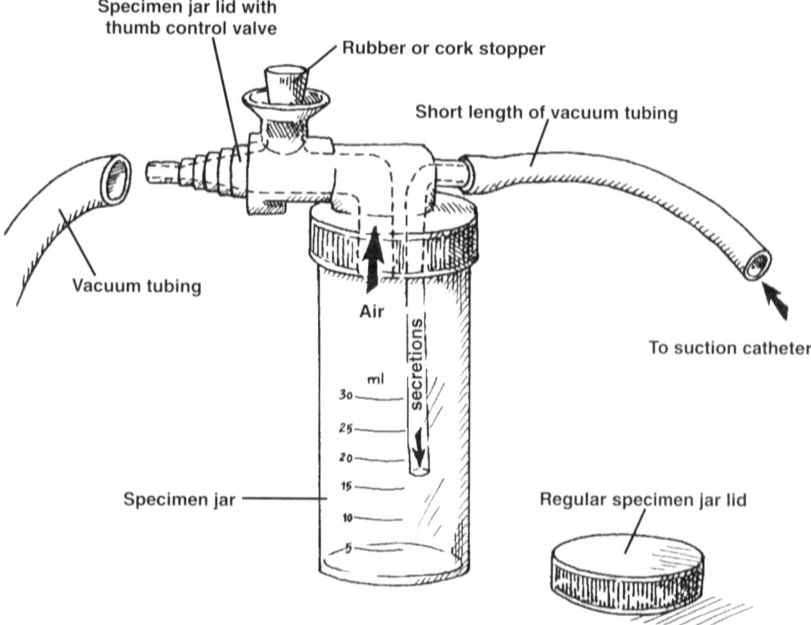

Fig. 12-8 Features of a sputum specimen collection system with a thumb control valve.

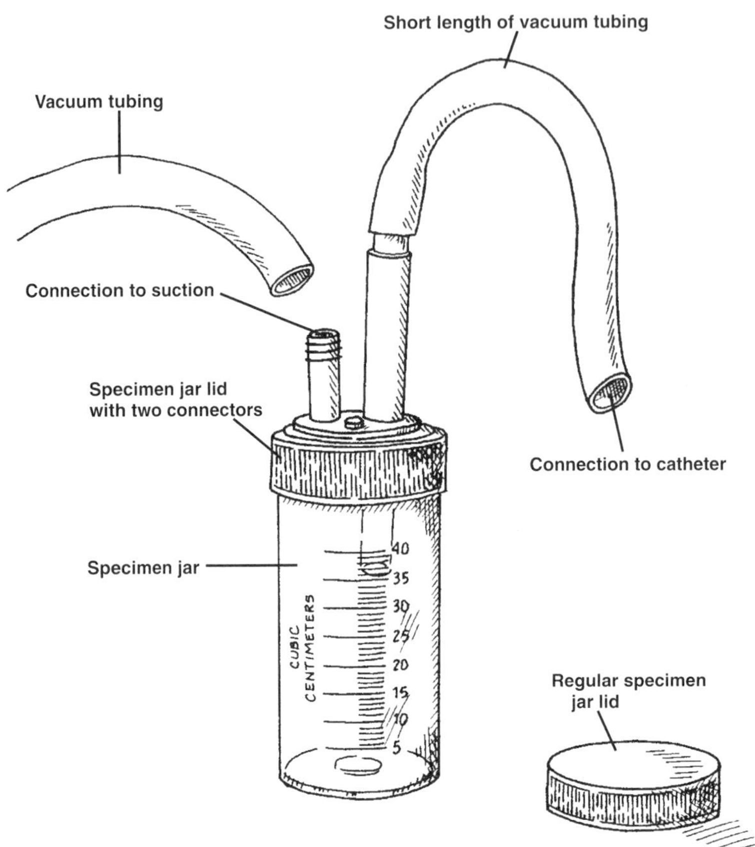

Fig. 12-9 Features of a sputum specimen collection system without a thumb control valve.

b. Put the equipment together, make sure that it works properly, and identify and fix any problems with it. (IIB8b) [R, Ap]

A properly working specimen collection system will provide a vacuum to the tip of the suction catheter when the thumb control valve or mouthpiece is sealed and vacuum applied. This is tested by dipping the catheter tip into a container of sterile water or saline solution. The liquid will be drawn up the catheter and deposited in the specimen jar. (The water can be emptied out of the jar by simply unscrewing the jar and discarding it.)

Failure to have a vacuum at the tip of the suction catheter could be caused by any of the previously mentioned possibilities. They can be checked and corrected by the methods listed earlier.

There are two likely causes of an inability to suction secretions. First, the jar is not screwed tightly into the special lid. This allows room air to be drawn in. Simply screw it in tightly. Second, the secretion channel is plugged. Discard it and replace it with a new specimen collector.

Module B. Initiate the suctioning procedures to remove tracheal and oral secretions. (IIIF3b) [R, Ap, An]

Tracheal or oral secretions must be actively removed by suctioning whenever the patient cannot clear them out and is at risk of obstructing the airway. Suctioning may be

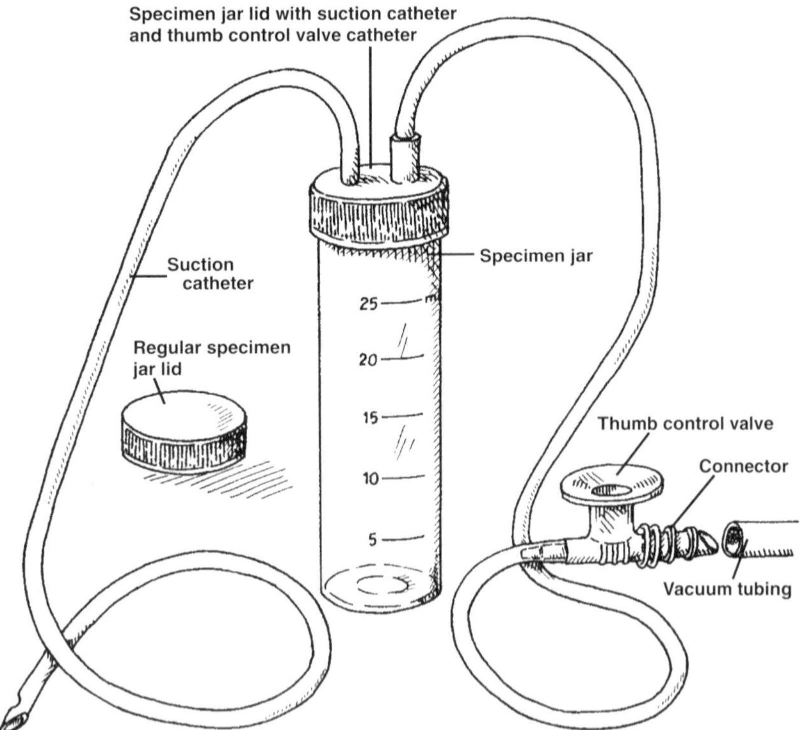

Fig. 12-10 Features of a sputum specimen collection system with a thumb control valve built into a catheter.

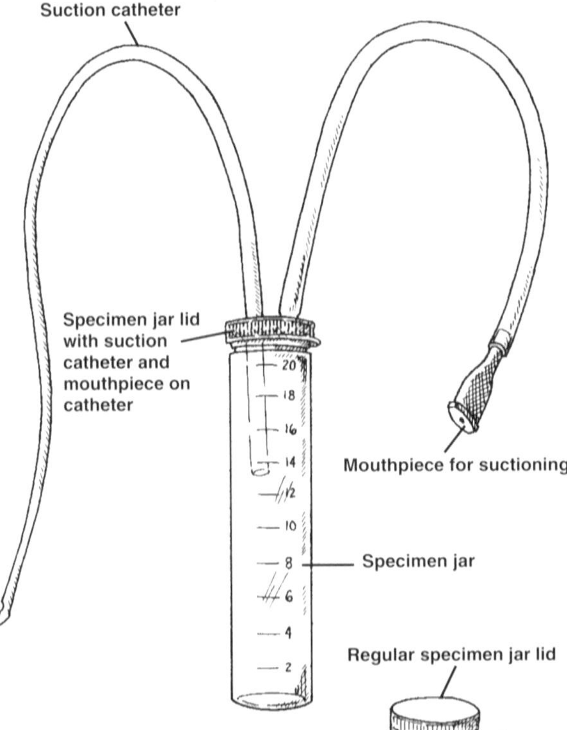

Fig. 12-11 Features of a DeLee sputum specimen collection system with a mouthpiece for the practitioner to apply suction through.

needed in patients who are unconscious and lack swallowing or coughing reflexes. Or, the patient may be too weak to cough effectively to remove tracheal secretions. Often the physician will write a standing order to suction the patient on a regular basis or as needed. However, in many institutions there is a protocol to suction any patient who is at risk of obstructing his or her airway. For example, the comatose patient who vomits should have the mouth suctioned out even though there is no specific physician's order to do so.

Suctioning secretions from a patient's trachea, by any of the following four methods, places the patient at risk. The following two factors must be understood, identified when they occur, and prevented or corrected.

Preventing Hypoxemia During the Suctioning Procedure (IIID3) [R, Ap]

Suctioning the trachea removes air (and oxygen), as well as secretions, from the lungs. Hypoxemia, however, can be minimized by hyperoxygenating the patient for 1 to 2 minutes before suctioning. It is generally recommended that the patient receive 100% oxygen, if possible. Infants younger than 6 months of age should be given a FIO_2 only 10% greater than their base level. This is because of the risk of retrolental fibroplasia/retinopathy of prematurity (ROP). For example, if the infant was inspiring 40% oxygen, it may be increased to 50% for the suctioning procedure.

Check the patient's arterial blood gas results or SpO_2 value to see whether the patient is hypoxic before beginning the procedure. SpO_2 values can also be monitored throughout the suctioning procedure to see how low the saturation drops and when the patient has been resaturated (> 90%) after suctioning is performed. The patient's chart should also be checked for any history of cardiac problems. Sudden hypoxemia from suctioning could result in life-threatening dysrhythmias such as premature ventricular contractions (PVCs). Check the patient's pulse rate and rhythm before and after suctioning. If the patient is using a cardiac monitor, it should be watched for rate and rhythm

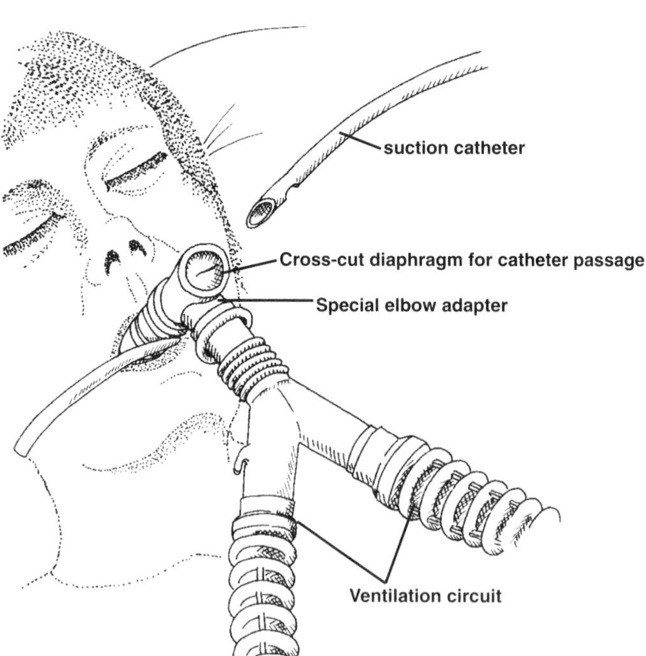

Fig. 12-12 Features and placement of a special elbow adapter that can be suctioned through without losing tidal volume or pressure when the patient's airway is being mechanically ventilated.

changes that are related to the suctioning procedure. Tachycardia is frequently seen with hypoxemia. Check the blood pressure of any patient who has suctioning-related dysrhythmias. The patient's vital signs should return to normal when oxygenation is restored.

Any modern mechanical ventilator can be set to deliver 100% oxygen. The most current ventilators have a 100% oxygen button designed just for this purpose. Pushing it results in the patient receiving pure oxygen for 1 to 2 minutes (depending on the manufacturer). Several sigh breaths can also be delivered. A special type of ventilator elbow adapter will allow for the passage of a suction catheter without removing the ventilator circuit from the patient's endotracheal or tracheostomy tube (see Fig. 12-12). The Ballard suctioning system can also be used, as shown in Fig. 12-7. These are especially useful in preventing hypoxemia in patients receiving high levels of PEEP, who should not be disconnected from the ventilator if at all possible.

A spontaneously breathing patient can have a non-rebreathing mask placed and set to deliver close to 100% oxygen. If a non-rebreathing mask is not available, turn up the oxygen flow or percentage to whatever appliance the patient is using. A spontaneously breathing patient with an endotracheal or tracheostomy tube can have 100% oxygen delivered through a Brigg's adapter/aerosol T. A manual resuscitation bag can also be used to give the patient several sigh breaths.

The patient must be reoxygenated before another attempt at suctioning is made. Giving 100% oxygen after the suctioning episode helps the patient to reoxygenate faster. Giving several sigh breaths will also help reoxygenation to occur faster than normal tidal volume breathing will.

Vagus/Vagal Nerve Stimulation

Vagal nerve endings are found in the hypopharynx and trachea. When they are mechanically stimulated by a suction catheter, any of the following may be seen:

a. The patient may have an induced bronchospasm.
b. The patient may become bradycardic.
c. The patient's blood pressure may drop because of the bradycardia.

Listen to the patient's breath sounds before and after suctioning to tell whether there is an increase in wheezing, which shows bronchospasm. Check the patient's heart rate and rhythm by palpation or cardiac monitor to tell whether he or she is becoming bradycardic. The blood pressure can also be measured to check for hypotension.

Further suctioning should be delayed, if possible, until the patient's wheezing and vital signs have returned to normal. It may be necessary to modify the suctioning procedure by not going as deeply and striking the carina, not twisting the catheter, or not suctioning for as long to reduce the risk of vagal stimulation. A local anesthetic such as lidocaine (Xylocaine) can be nebulized (with a physician's order) to reduce the local reaction to the catheter.

1. Perform endotracheal or tracheostomy tube suctioning on the patient. (IIIB2d) [R, Ap]

This procedure is the same for suctioning through both tubes except to note that the catheter will not need to be inserted as far into the tracheostomy tube before hitting the carina.

Generally Accepted Steps in the Procedure

A. Check the chart for specific orders, an order to suction as needed, or any special patient considerations.
B. Gather up the needed equipment:
   1. Suction catheter no larger than one half the interior diameter of the patient's endotracheal or tracheostomy tube.
   2. Two sterile gloves or one sterile glove and one clean glove. (This may be skipped if a self-contained system is used.)
   3. Specimen collector if ordered.
   4. Vacuum system.
   5. Sterile water or normal saline and sterile basin.
C. Tell the patient what is going to be done.
D. If possible, place the patient in semi-Fowler's and sniff positions.
E. Give the patient 100% oxygen for at least 30 seconds before suctioning and for at least 1 minute afterward until the patient is no longer hypoxemic. (The infant who is less than 6 months old can have the F_{IO_2} increased by 10%.)
F. Get help if necessary.
G. Wash your hands. (This may be skipped if a self-contained system is used or in an emergency.)
H. Using sterile technique, put on the gloves, get the catheter out of its packaging, and connect the vacuum tubing to the catheter.
I. Set the vacuum level the lowest possible that still effectively removes secretions. Plevak and Ward[1] and Eubanks and Bone[2] suggest the following ranges for vacuum:
   1. Adults: 100 to 120 mm Hg
   2. Children: 80 to 100 mm Hg
   3. Neonates: 60 to 80 mm Hg
J. Test that the vacuum is reaching the tip of the catheter.
K. Disconnect the ventilator circuit or oxygen appliance from the tube (except with a self-contained system).
L. Suction the tube:
   1. Without any vacuum, quickly pass the catheter down the tube until an obstruction is felt. Withdraw the catheter 2 cm.
   2. In the adult, the entire procedure from disconnection of the oxygen, suctioning, to reconnection of the oxygen and normal breathing should take no longer than 10 to 15 seconds. In the infant, the entire procedure should take no longer than 10 seconds.
   3. Withdraw the catheter with a twisting motion while suctioning intermittently. Suction to clear out any secretions. Typically, in the adult, suctioning may be applied for between 5 and 10 seconds. In the infant, suctioning may be applied for no more than 5 seconds.
   4. Turning the patient's head to the right might help direct the catheter down the left mainstem bronchus. The catheter will tend to enter the right mainstem bronchus if the head is in a neutral position or twisted to the left.
M. Reoxygenate the patient for at least 1 minute before suctioning again. Giving 100% oxygen (or 10% more than the base level in the infant) and several sigh breaths will help this happen faster.
N. Monitor the patient's vital signs, oxygen level, and breath sounds before suctioning again. Suction again, if needed, when the patient is stable.
O. Normal saline solution may be instilled into the tube if the secretions are too viscous (thick) to easily be suctioned out. The saline solution will help to loosen the secretions. The patient is also likely to cough vigorously. The amount of sa-

line solution to be instilled will vary with the size of the patient and the viscosity of the secretions.
General guidelines for the instillation of normal saline solution:
1. Neonates may be given a few drops to 0.33 ml at a time.
2. Adults may be given 5 to 10 ml at a time or in divided doses.
3. A physician's order may be needed to instill saline solution.

P. Dispose of the catheter and glove by pulling the glove inside out over the catheter. Self-contained systems may be left in place for up to 24 hours.
Q. Rinse the vacuum tubing clear of secretions.
R. Turn off the suction unit.

See Table 12-2 for hazards and complications of nasotracheal suctioning.

2. Perform nasotracheal suctioning on the patient. (IIIb2e) [R, Ap]

Generally Accepted Steps in the Procedure

A. Check the chart for specific orders, an order to suction as needed, or any special patient considerations.
B. Gather up the needed equipment:
1. Suction catheter no larger than one half the diameter of the patient's nostril.
2. Get an appropriately sized and type of nasopharyngeal airway to minimize nasal mucosal damage.
3. Use sterile, water-soluble, lubricant jelly.
4. Use a sterile 4 by 4 inch gauze pad.

C. Tell the patient what is going to be done.
D. If possible, place the patient in semi-Fowler's and sniff positions.
E. Give the patient 100% oxygen for at least 30 seconds before suctioning and afterward for at least 1 minute until the patient is no longer hypoxemic. (The infant who is less than 6 months old can have the F_{IO_2} increased by 10%.)
F. Get help if necessary.
G. Wash your hands. (This may be skipped in an emergency.)
H. Using sterile technique, put on the gloves, get the catheter out of its packaging, apply lubricant jelly to the catheter tip, and connect the vacuum tubing to the catheter. Add the steps that follow.

Table 12-2. Hazards and Complications of Endotracheal Suctioning

Cardiac arrest
Respiratory arrest
Hypoxemia
Cardiac dysrhythmias
Bronchospasm
Increased intracranial pressure
Hypertension
Hypotension
Apnea from interruption of mechanical ventilation
Pulmonary hemorrhage
Mechanical trauma to tracheal and bronchial mucosa
Infection to and/or from patient and respiratory care practitioner
Atelectasis

I. Set the vacuum level the lowest possible that still effectively removes secretions. Plevak and Ward and Eubanks and Bone suggest the following ranges for vacuum:
   1. Adults: 100 to 120 mm Hg
   2. Children: 80 to 100 mm Hg
   3. Neonates: 60 to 80 mm Hg

J. Test that the vacuum is reaching the tip of the catheter.

K. Remove the oxygen appliance from the patient so that the nose may be reached. Directing the end of the oxygen tubing or nasal cannula prongs toward the patient's mouth may help to prevent hypoxemia.

L. Suction the trachea:
   1. Without any vacuum, advance the catheter into the nasopharyngeal airway. If no nasopharyngeal airway is available, without any vacuum, advance the catheter into the most open nasal passage. The catheter should be advanced parallel to the turbinates to minimize tissue trauma. Never force the catheter. (The most patent nasal passage can be determined by checking the chart for a history of deviated septum, asking the patient if one side feels more open, or feeling which nostril has more airflow through it.)
   2. Have the cooperative patient stick his or her tongue out. The practitioner or assistant can grasp the uncooperative patient's tongue with a 4 by 4 inch gauze pad or gloved hand.
   3. Advance the catheter as the patient inspires. The epiglottis and vocal cords are open at this time, and it is easiest to slip the catheter into the trachea. The cooperative patient should be told to inhale slowly and deeply. Some practitioners find it helpful to disconnect the catheter from the vacuum tubing and listen to the end of the catheter for the sound of air movement. The patient will cough vigorously when the catheter is in the trachea (Fig. 12-13).
   4. Advance the catheter until an obstruction is felt. Then, pull the catheter back about 2 cm.
   5. Withdraw the catheter with a twisting motion while suctioning intermittently. Suction to clear out any secretions. Typically, in the adult, suctioning may be applied for between 5 and 10 seconds. Suctioning in the infant should be applied for no more than 5 seconds. If the secretions are cleared, the catheter is pulled out. There is a difference in technique between practitioners over whether the catheter should be withdrawn or left in place if the patient still has secretions. Some prefer to withdraw the catheter, let the patient rest and reoxygenate, and reinsert the catheter for more suctioning. Others prefer to leave the catheter in place to minimize tissue trauma from a reinsertion, let the patient rest and reoxygenate, then suction again.
   6. The entire procedure will probably take longer than 20 seconds, so it is important to keep the oxygen tubing directed toward the patient's mouth.
   7. Turning the patient's head to the right might help direct the catheter down the left mainstem bronchus. The catheter will tend to enter the right mainstem bronchus if the head is in a neutral position or twisted to the left.

M. Reoxygenate the patient for at least 1 minute before suctioning again. Giving 100% oxygen (or 10% more than the base level in the infant) will help this happen faster.

N. Monitor the patient's vital signs, oxygen level, and breath sounds before suctioning again. Suction again, if needed, when the patient is stable.

O. Normal saline solution may be instilled down the suction catheter by pulling off the vacuum tubing, inserting the tip of the syringe (not needle) into the end of the catheter, covering the thumb control valve, and squirting the saline solution into the catheter. The other considerations listed earlier would apply here.

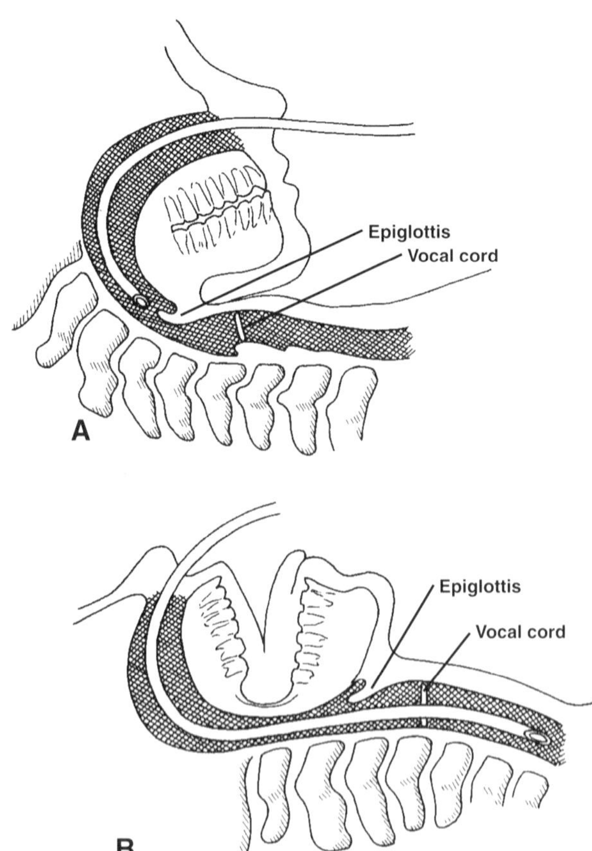

Fig. 12-13 Cross section through the airway showing nasotracheal suctioning. **A,** With the head in the sniff position, the catheter is advanced through a nostril to the level of the vocal cords. **B,** During an inspiration, the catheter is advanced into the trachea. The patient will cough, and secretions can be suctioned out.

P. Dispose of the catheter and glove by pulling the glove inside out over the catheter.
Q. Rinse the vacuum tubing clear of secretions.
R. Turn off the suction unit.

See Table 12-3 for contraindications and hazards and complications of nasotracheal suctioning.

3. Perform orotracheal suctioning on the patient. (IIIB2e) [R, Ap]

Orotracheal suctioning is a more difficult procedure than nasotracheal suctioning and not performed as often.

Generally Accepted Steps in the Procedure

A. Check the chart for specific orders, an order to suction as needed, or any special patient considerations.
B. Gather up the needed equipment:
   1. Suction catheter no larger than one half the diameter of the patient's nostril. Even though the catheter is going through the mouth, the critical diameter is the trachea. This guideline should help to prevent too large a catheter being forced into the trachea.

Table 12-3. Contraindications and Hazards and Complications of Nasotracheal Suctioning

Contraindications
- Absolute:
  - Epiglottitis
  - Laryngotracheobronchitis (croup)
- Relative:
  - Blocked nasal passages
  - Nasal bleeding
  - Acute facial, neck, or head injury
  - Bleeding disorder
  - Upper respiratory tract infection
  - Irritable airway
  - Laryngospasm

Hazards and complications
- Cardiac arrest
- Respiratory arrest
- Hypoxemia
- Cardiac dysrhythmias
- Bronchospasm
- Increased intracranial pressure
- Hypertension
- Hypotension
- Pulmonary hemorrhage
- Infection to and/or from patient and respiratory care practitioner
- Atelectasis
- Pain
- Catheter misdirected into esophagus
- Gagging and/or vomiting
- Uncontrolled coughing
- Mechanical trauma: nasal turbinates, perforation of pharynx, nasal bleeding, bleeding of the tracheal and bronchial mucosa

2. The nasopharyngeal airway is not needed.
3. The sterile, water-soluble lubricant jelly and 4 by 4 inch gauze may not be needed if the patient's mouth is moist. Some may always prefer to lubricate the catheter tip.
4. Use sterile water or normal saline solution and sterile basin. Pour some water or saline into the basin.

C. Tell the patient what is going to be done.
D. If possible, place the patient in semi-Fowler's and sniff positions.
E. Give the patient 100% oxygen for at least 30 seconds before suctioning and for at least 1 minute afterward until the patient is no longer hypoxemic. (The infant who is less than 6 months old can have the F_{IO_2} increased by 10%.)
F. Get help if necessary.
G. Wash your hands. (This may be skipped in an emergency.)
H. Using sterile technique, put on the gloves, get the catheter out of its packaging, and connect the vacuum tubing to the catheter. Add the following steps if necessary:
   1. With the clean gloved hand, squeeze some of the lubricant jelly on the 4 by 4 inch gauze pad.

   2. Lubricate the tip and first few centimeters of the catheter.

I. Set the vacuum level the lowest possible that still effectively removes secretions. Plevak and Ward[1] and Eubanks and Bone[2] suggest the following ranges for vacuum:
   1. Adults: 100 to 120 mm Hg
   2. Children: 80 to 100 mm Hg
   3. Neonates: 60 to 80 mm Hg

J. Test that the vacuum is reaching the tip of the catheter.

K. Remove the oxygen appliance from the patient so that the mouth may be reached. A nasal cannula may be placed on the patient to give supplemental oxygen. An assistant may be able to direct the end of the oxygen tubing toward the patient's mouth to help prevent hypoxemia.

L. Suction the trachea:
   1. Without any vacuum, advance the catheter into the oral pharynx.
   2. Have the cooperative patient stick his or her tongue out. The practitioner or assistant can grasp the uncooperative patient's tongue with a 4 by 4 inch gauze pad or gloved hand.
   3. Advance the catheter as the patient inspires. The epiglottis and vocal cords are open at this time, and it is easiest to slip the catheter into the trachea. The cooperative patient should be told to inhale slowly and deeply. Try to avoid stimulating the patient's gag reflex by not striking the oropharynx with the tip of the catheter. The patient will cough vigorously when the catheter is in the trachea.
   4. Advance the catheter until an obstruction is felt. Then, pull the catheter back about 2 cm.
   5. Withdraw the catheter with a twisting motion while suctioning intermittently. Suction to clear out any secretions. Typically, in the adult, suctioning may be applied for between 5 and 10 seconds. Suctioning in the infant may be applied for no more than 5 seconds. If the secretions are cleared, the catheter is pulled out. There is a difference in technique between practitioners over whether the catheter should be withdrawn or left in place if the patient still has secretions. Some prefer to withdraw the catheter, let the patient rest and reoxygenate, and reinsert the catheter for more suctioning. Others prefer to leave the catheter in place to minimize tissue trauma from a reinsertion, let the patient rest and reoxygenate, then suction again.
   6. The entire procedure will probably take longer than 20 seconds so it is important to keep the oxygen tubing directed toward the patient's mouth.
   7. Turning the patient's head to the right might help direct the catheter down the left mainstem bronchus. The catheter will tend to enter the right mainstem bronchus if the head is in a neutral position or twisted to the left.

M. Reoxygenate the patient for at least 1 minute before suctioning again. Giving 100% oxygen (or 10% more than the base level in the infant) will help this happen faster.

N. Monitor the patient's vital signs, oxygen level, and breath sounds before suctioning again. Suction again, if needed, when the patient is stable.

O. Normal saline solution may be instilled down the suction catheter by pulling off the vacuum tubing, inserting the tip of the syringe (not needle) into the end of the catheter, covering the thumb control valve, and squirting the saline into the catheter. The other considerations listed earlier would apply here.

P. Dispose of the catheter and glove by pulling the glove inside out over the catheter.

Q. Rinse the vacuum tubing clear of secretions.

R. Turn off the suction unit.

4. Perform oropharyngeal suctioning on the patient. (IIIB2e) [R, Ap]

Generally Accepted Steps in the Procedure

A. Check the chart for specific orders, an order to suction as needed, or any special patient considerations.
B. Gather up the needed equipment:
   1. Yankauer or regular suction catheter.
   2. One or two clean gloves, if desired.
   3. Vacuum system.
   4. Sterile water or normal saline solution and sterile basin.
C. Tell the patient what is going to be done.
D. If possible, place the patient in semi-Fowler's and sniff positions.
E. It is probably not necessary to give the patient supplemental oxygen before suctioning unless the patient is already using it.
F. Get help if necessary.
G. Wash your hands.
H. Using clean technique, put on the gloves, get the catheter out of its packaging, and connect the vacuum tubing to the catheter.
I. Set the vacuum level the lowest possible that still effectively removes secretions. Plevak and Ward[1] and Eubanks and Bone[2] suggest the following ranges for vacuum:
   1. Adults: 100 to 120 mm Hg
   2. Children: 80 to 100 mm Hg
   3. Neonates: 60 to 80 mm Hg
J. Test that the vacuum is reaching the tip of the catheter.
K. If the patient is wearing an oxygen mask, it must be removed to give access to the mouth. The oxygen tubing can be directed into the patient's mouth.
L. Suction the oropharynx:
   1. Gently direct the Yankauer or catheter along both sides of the tongue toward the throat. Clear out any secretions or vomitus.
   2. The conscious, spontaneously breathing patient should be able to tolerate suctioning for several seconds. Allow the patient to catch his or her breath as needed.
   3. The mouth can be suctioned for a longer time in the patient with an intubated airway because the procedure will not interfere with breathing.
   4. Avoid pushing the suction device into the posterior of the oropharynx. Retching and vomiting can result from a stimulated gag reflex. The spontaneously breathing patient would be at risk of aspirating vomitus.
M. Reoxygenate the patient for at least 1 minute before suctioning again. Giving 100% oxygen (or 10% more than the base level in the infant) will help this happen faster.
N. Monitor the patient's vital signs, oxygen level, and readiness before suctioning again. Suction again, if needed, when the patient is stable.
O. Dispose of the catheter and glove by pulling the glove inside out over the catheter. The Yankauer or regular catheter may be used more than once.
P. Rinse the vacuum tubing (and Yankauer or regular catheter if used more than once) clear of secretions.
Q. Turn off the suction unit.

This ends the general discussion on suctioning the airway. The entry level examination is known to ask direct questions over the previously mentioned and following aspects of suctioning. In general, Section 1 and the previous discussion covers Module C. A few additional comments are added as needed.

Module C. Patient Assessment.

1. Determine and continue to monitor how the patient responds to the treatment or procedure.

Hypoxemia and vagal stimulation can result in unstable vital signs and bronchospasm. Hearing coarse, intermittent expiratory sounds (rhonchi) indicate that there are secretions in the airway. Tracheal suctioning should clear these secretions and result in the return of normal breath sounds (or at least an improvement).

Pneumonia and bronchitis result in chest x-ray changes that show areas of infiltrate. Right or left lung involvement (or both), individual lobes, and segments with disease can be determined. If the left lung is involved, using a Coudé catheter with an angled tip or turning the patient's head to the right may help to direct the catheter down the left mainstem bronchus. As the patient's condition improves, the chest x-ray film should show clearing of infiltrates.

A conscious patient should be able to communicate with you about how he or she feels after the suctioning of secretions. Hopefully the feeling of dyspnea will be improved.

2. Modify the procedure and recommend any changes in the patient's respiratory care plan, depending on the response.

a. Make a change in the size and type of suction catheter. (IIIF7a) [R, Ap]

As discussed earlier, the outer diameter of the suction catheter should be no more than half the inner diameter of the patient's endotracheal tube. If the secretions are easy to suction out, a smaller catheter may be used. The spontaneously breathing patient is less likely to become hypoxic if the tube is less obstructed.

A catheter with a Coudé tip should be used if the catheter needs to be directed into one or the other mainstem bronchus. Closed-system catheters such as those made by Ballard Medical Products offer two advantages over single-use catheters. First, they are more economical if the patient needs frequent suctioning. Second, patients using mechanical ventilators will continue to be ventilated, oxygenated, and have PEEP maintained during the suctioning episode. The newer catheters that offer intermittent or continuous insufflation of oxygen may reduce the hypoxemia that many patients experience during the suctioning procedure. However, they are difficult to use and costly.

b. Change the level of vacuum used when suctioning. (IIIF7b) [R, Ap]

In general, the lowest possible vacuum level should be used that adequately removes secretions. Several authors have listed recommended maximum vacuum levels to be applied to adults, children, and neonates. These were listed earlier. However, the AARC Clinical Practice Guidelines[3,4] on suctioning state that there is a lack of experimental data to support these or any other written maximum pressures.

c. Instill an irrigating solution into the trachea. (IIIF7c) [R, Ap]

Sterile normal saline solution (0.9%) is widely accepted as useful to instill into the trachea to dilute and mobilize pulmonary secretions. It should be used whenever secretions are difficult to suction out. Also, by making the secretions easier to remove, one can use a lower vacuum level. In adults, about 5 to 10 ml are instilled into the trachea and then suctioned out with any secretions. Less is used with children, but no universal guidelines are available. Neonates have been reportedly given a few drops to 0.33 ml.

d. Change the frequency of suctioning. (IIIF7d) [R, Ap]

Secretions obstruct the airways and should be removed if possible. Often this requires more than one suctioning episode. There is no harm in repeatedly suctioning the patient as long as he or she is reoxygenated in between. Watch for any complications as listed in Tables 12-2 and 12-3. Also, listen to the patient's breath sounds for rhonchi, or palpate the chest for secretions in between suctioning efforts. Stop suctioning when it is no longer needed.

e. Change the duration of the suctioning procedure. (IIIF7e) [R, Ap]

Generally speaking, suctioning should take between 5 and 10 seconds; the entire procedure should take between 10 and 15 seconds. Some patients may not be able to tolerate this. Be prepared to suction for a shorter period. Suction repeatedly rather than increase the suctioning time.

As listed in Table 12-2 and 12-3, stop the procedure if the patient becomes hypoxic or has tachycardia, bradycardia, dysrhythmias, hypotension, or bronchospasm. Bloody secretions could indicate mucosal damage and would justify stopping the procedure.

Hypoxemia, tachycardia, bradycardia, dysrhythmias, hypotension, bronchospasm, pneumothorax, or pulmonary hemorrhage that place the patient's life in danger would indicate the cancellation of the suctioning order. Once the underlying problem has been corrected and safe suctioning can be performed, the order may be resumed.

BIBLIOGRAPHY

AARC Clinical Practice Guideline: Endotracheal suctioning of mechanically ventilated adults and children with artificial airways. *Respir Care* 1993; 38:500-504.

AARC Clinical Practice Guideline: Nasotracheal suctioning. *Respir Care* 1992; 37:898-901.

Caldwell SL, Sullivan KN: Artificial airways, in Burton GG, Hodgkin JE (eds): *Respiratory Care,* ed 2. Philadelphia, Lippincott, 1984.

Caldwell SL, Sullivan KN: Suctioning protocol, in Burton GG, Hodgkin JE (eds): *Respiratory Care,* ed 2. Philadelphia, Lippincott, 1984.

Burton GG: Patient assessment procedures, in Barnes TA (ed): *Respiratory Care Practice.* Chicago, Mosby, 1988.

Burton GG: Practical physical diagnosis in respiratory care, in Burton GG, Hodgkin JE (eds): *Respiratory Care,* ed 2. Philadelphia, Lippincott, 1984.

Eubanks DH, Bone RC: *Comprehensive Respiratory Care,* ed 2. St Louis, Mosby, 1990.

Frownfelter DL: Chest physical therapy and airway care, in Barnes TA (ed): *Respiratory Care Practice.* Chicago, Mosby, 1988.

Guidelines for the prevention of nosocomial infections, *AARTimes,* vol 7, issue 9, September 1983.

Lehrer S: *Understanding Lung Sounds.* Philadelphia, Saunders, 1984.

Nath AR, Capel LH: Lung crackles in bronchiectasis. *Thorax* 1980; 35:694.

Plevak DJ, Ward JJ: Airway management, in Burton GG, Hodgkin JE, Ward JJ (eds): *Respiratory Care,* ed 3. Philadelphia, Lippincott, 1991.

Rarey KP, Youtsey JW: *Respiratory Patient Care.* Prentice-Hall, Englewood Cliffs, NJ, 1981.

Scott AA, Koff PB: Airway care and chest physiotherapy, in Koff PB, Eitzmann DV, Neu J (eds): *Neonatal and Pediatric Respiratory Care.* St Louis, Mosby, 1988.

Shapiro BA, Harrison RA, Kacmarek RM, et al: *Clinical Application of Respiratory Care,* ed 3. Chicago, Mosby, 1985.

Simmon KF: Airway care, in Scanlan CL, Spearman CB, Sheldon RL (eds): *Egan's Fundamentals of Respiratory Care,* ed 5. St Louis, Mosby, 1990.

Wilkins RL, Hodgkin, JE, Lopez B: *Lung Sounds, a Practical Guide.* St Louis, Mosby, 1988.

Wojciechowski WV: Incentive spirometers and secretion evacuation devices, in Barnes TA (ed): *Respiratory Care Practice.* Chicago, Mosby, 1988.

SELF-STUDY QUESTIONS

1. While advancing a catheter into your patient's nasopharynx so that she can be nasotracheally suctioned, you notice that the cardiac monitor shows that her pulse rate has dropped from 105 to 70 beats/min. The most likely cause of this is:
   A. Transient hypoxemia
   B. Induced bronchospasm
   C. Stimulated gag reflex
   D. Vagal stimulation
   E. Too large a catheter for her nasal passage

2. Before suctioning a patient with an intubated airway for the first time, it is important to check the chart for:
   I. A history of cardiac disease or dysrhythmias
   II. A written order
   III. A history of a strong gag reflex
   IV. Blood gas results or pulse oximetry results
   V. A history of asthma or bronchospasm
   A. II, III
   B. IV, V
   C. I, II, IV, V
   D. III, V
   E. I, II, III, IV, V

3. The properly sized suction catheter should be no larger than _____ the interior diameter of a patient's endotracheal tube:
   A. ⅛
   B. ¼
   C. ½
   D. ⅔
   E. ¾

4. Placing a suction catheter into your patient's trachea and applying vacuum will result in:
   I. Transient hypoxemia
   II. Removal of secretions that are present
   III. Stopping of the hypoxic drive because of vagal stimulation
   IV. Removal of air from the lungs
   V. Insufflation of air into the esophagus and stomach
   A. III, IV, V
   B. I, II
   C. IV, V
   D. III, IV
   E. I, II, IV

5. If your patient has a room air arterial oxygen pressure of 65 mm Hg, the most important step to take to prevent hypoxemia during suctioning is:
   A. Give the patient 100% oxygen before and after the procedure.
   B. Use a large catheter so that the secretions can be pulled out quickly.
   C. Hyperextend the patient's neck and head.
   D. Use a small catheter so that the patient can breathe around it.
   E. Suction for no longer than 20 seconds.

6. The best position for a patient to be placed in before suctioning is:
   I. Neck and head bent forward
   II. Supine
   III. Trendelenburg
   IV. Neck and head hyperextended
   V. Semi-Fowler's
   A. I, V
   B. II, IV
   C. III, IV
   D. IV, V
   E. I, III

7. Aids to nasopharyngeal suctioning include:
   A. Lubricating the catheter in sterile water.
   B. Lubricating the catheter tip in a sterile, water-soluble lubricant jelly.
   C. Placing the catheter in the refrigerator so that it will be firmer and can be passed more easily.
   D. Lubricating the catheter in sterile normal saline solution.
   E. Measure the needed length of catheter by placing it next to the nose and measure to the angle of the jaw.

8. You are using a Yankauer suction catheter when you notice that is cracked. The best thing to do is:
   A. Continue to use it.
   B. Tape over the crack.
   C. Put lubricating jelly in the crack to seal it.
   D. Replace the catheter.
   E. Send it back to central equipment processing to be resterilized.

9. You are preparing to suction a patient for a mucous sample when you notice that the vacuum is not reaching the end of the catheter. All of the following are possible causes of this problem *except:*
   A. The vacuum is not turned on to the proper level.
   B. The vacuum tubing is knotted.
   C. The vacuum tubing, specimen collector, and catheter system are connected so that they are airtight.
   D. The catheter is plugged with foreign matter.
   E. The specimen jar is not screwed tightly into the special lid.

10. While connecting the suction catheter to the vacuum tubing, you accidentally touch the tip of the catheter with your clean-gloved hand. You would proceed to:
    A. Discard the clean glove and start over.
    B. Suction the patient.

C. Put a sterile glove over the clean glove and suction the patient.
D. Ask the nurse's opinion.
E. Discard the catheter and start over.

Answer Key:

1. D; 2. C; 3. C; 4. E; 5. A; 6. D; 7. B; 8. D; 9. C; 10. E.

13 Intermittent Positive-Pressure Breathing

Module A. Initiate Intermittent Positive-Pressure Breathing (IPPB) therapy to achieve adequate spontaneous ventilation.

The contents of this module are covered for the sake of understanding and completeness. These topics are not listed in the National Board for Respiratory Care's (NBRC's) examination content outline. They must be understood to provide quality and safe patient care and to enable the learner to comprehend the following modules, which are tested by the NBRC.

1. Description.

The Respiratory Care Committee of the American Thoracic Society published the following definition in its *Guidelines for the Use of Intermittent Positive Pressure Breathing (IPPB)*, in 1980*;

> "IPPB treatments" refers to the use of a pressure-limited respiratory to deliver a gas with humidity and/or aerosol to a spontaneously breathing patient for periods of time that are generally no greater than 15 to 20 minutes each.

A pressure-limited respirator may be powered by compressed gas or electricity. The patient's tidal volume should be greater than normal when it is enhanced by IPPB. This greater than normal tidal volume is caused by the use of positive pressure against the lungs. Pressure is also directed against the airways and, through contact with the airways and lungs, the entire chest. The patient's exhalation is usually passive but can be slowed by modifying the exhalation valve.

Shapiro et al. list the following as the physiologic effects of IPPB:

a. Increased mean airway pressure.

By definition, the patient is receiving a positive airway pressure instead of generating a negative intrathoracic pressure to create the tidal volume. Most authors recommend that patients with heart disease be monitored closely for the effects of the increased mean airway pressure. It is possible to decrease the normal return of venous blood to the heart and therefore decrease the cardiac output. They recommend an expiratory time that is long enough to allow for normal venous return before the next positive pressure breath is given. The patient's heart rate and blood pressure can be monitored to ensure that they stay in the normal range. Realey lists IPPB as a beneficial treatment in patients with car-

*Respiratory Care Committee of the American Thoracic Society: Guidelines for the use of intermittent positive pressure breathing (IPPB). *Respir Care* 1980; 25:365.

diogenic pulmonary edema because the pressure reduces the venous return to the heart. Their breathing is improved by reducing the amount of blood (and the resulting edema) in the lungs.

Pulmonary barotrauma is the second concern raised by the use of positive airway pressure. It is possible for patients with small airways disease to trap air in the alveoli. This can lead to the rupture of a bleb, resulting in a pneumothorax. Care must be taken with the patient with bullous emphysema to ensure that the tidal volume is exhaled completely.

b. Increased tidal volume.

The primary goal of IPPB is to increase the patient's assisted tidal volume to greater than the spontaneous tidal volume. Indeed, if the spontaneous tidal volume is greater than the assisted tidal volume, IPPB is not needed for lung expansion.

c. Decreased work of breathing.

A properly coached passive treatment with the controls set to meet the patient's inspiratory needs will result in a decrease in the work of breathing. This requires considerable skill on the part of the practitioner. The sensitivity, inspiratory flow, and peak pressure must be frequently adjusted to minimize the patient's work. The patient must be asked if the control adjustments make it easier or harder for him or her to breath in. Failure to tailor the breathing treatment to the patient's needs may actually increase the work of breathing.

d. Alteration of the inspiratory/expiratory (I/E) ratio.

Patients with high airway resistance or low lung compliance will often change their breathing pattern to reduce the work of breathing (see Section 1). These breathing patterns may lead to a worsening of the patient's condition. Alteration of normal ventilation and perfusion ratios in the lungs may worsen hypoxemia. Properly administered and coached IPPB can be used to adjust the I/E ratio to the benefit of the patient. The patient can be taught how to breathe in a more physiologically normal pattern.

Because the delivered tidal volume gas is dry, it must be humidified. All authors state that one or a combination of the following must be used to assure that the patient receives humidified gas: a nebulizer or ultrasonic unit to produce a bland aerosol or a cascade type of humidifier. All can be placed in line with the circuit.

2. Indications.

The following are listed in the AARC Clinical Practice Guideline on IPPB:

1. To treat atelectasis when other deep breathing methods are ineffective. Patients who are uncooperative, unconscious, or physically incapable of being coached in deep breathing and coughing techniques or performing incentive spirometry may be helped by IPPB. As presented in Section 6, the patient who cannot generate an inspiratory capacity (IC) of greater than 12 ml/kg, a vital capacity (VC) of greater than 15 ml/kg, or who has a postoperative IC less than 33% of the preoperative value will be benefitted by IPPB rather than incentive spirometry. An inspiratory pause at the end of the IPPB breath will help to better distribute the gas to open atelectatic areas.

The AARC Guideline lists the following poor pulmonary function values as supporting the need for IPPB. This is because they suggest that the patient would have an ineffective cough: VC less than 70% of predicted or less than 10 ml/kg, forced expiratory volume in 1 second (FEV_1) less than 65% of predicted, or maximum voluntary ventilation (MVV) less than 50% of predicted.

2. To more effectively deliver aerosolized medications. If the patient cannot coordinate his or her breathing pattern to make use of a metered dose inhaler or hand-held nebulizer, IPPB may be used. Examples of when IPPB would be better include any situation when the patient is unconscious, uncooperative, or physically incapable.

These patients are physically unable to make effective use of simpler methods of lung inflation (incentive spirometry) or to take an aerosolized medication (metered dose inhaler or hand-held nebulizer). Examples of these types of patients include the elderly, chronically debilitated, those with neuromuscular diseases, and those with kyphoscoliosis. It may also be used to provide temporary support to home care patients.

3. To enhance the patient's cough effort and sputum clearance. The combination of aerosolized saline, with or without a bronchodilator or mucolytic, and deeper tidal volumes may help the patient to cough more productively. The practitioner must stop the treatment periodically to coach the patient's cough effort.

The following additional indications were listed in *Guidelines for the Use of Intermittent Positive Pressure Breathing (IPPB):*

1. To treat impending ventilatory failure as seen by an increased arterial carbon dioxide pressure ($Paco_2$). It may be possible to delay or avoid intubation and mechanical ventilation in the deteriorating chronic obstructive pulmonary disease (COPD) patient. The patient would be able to relax and reduce the work of breathing during a passive IPPB treatment. It may be necessary to give IPPB for 5 to 10 minutes as often as every one-half to 1 hour. The treatment should also be given with the intention of helping the patient's cough and sputum clearance.

2. To treat the patient with acute pulmonary edema. Realey recommends the use of IPPB with 100% oxygen and peak pressures of 40 cm H_2O or higher in these patients. This is to temporarily reduce the venous return to the heart. Some authors recommend the nebulization of ethyl alcohol in approximately a 30% to 50% concentration to reduce the surface tension of pulmonary edema froth so that the bubbles burst. This procedure will not correct the underlying cardiac problem, which must be treated by other means.

3. To induce a sputum sample for culture and sensitivity or other diagnostic studies. This would be indicated only if simpler methods did not work.

4. To deliver medications for special purposes when simpler methods do not work. For example, to deliver a local anesthetic such as lidocaine (Xylocaine) before a bronchoscopy procedure.

3. Contraindications.

Untreated pneumothorax is listed by all authors and the AARC Guidelines as an absolute contraindication. An increased intrathoracic pressure will convert a simple pneumothorax into a tension pneumothorax. The consequences could be fatal. Once a chest tube has been inserted into the pleural space and a pleural drainage system set up, IPPB could be administered. There may be an increase in the air leak, but it will not be life threatening.

The AARC Guidelines[3] list the following as relative contraindications. Any patient with one of these should be carefully evaluated to make a wise decision about the clinical use of IPPB:

1. Active hemoptysis. Coughing up blood indicates that a tear has occurred in the airway or lung tissues. The IPPB treatment should be stopped if there is a large amount

of hemoptysis. Certainly massive hemoptysis (defined as greater than 600 ml of blood coughed out in a 16-hour period) would contraindicate IPPB.

2. Hemodynamic instability.
3. Intracranial pressure greater than 15 mm Hg.
4. Chest x-ray film that shows a bleb.
5. Tracheoesophageal fistula.
6. Recent surgery on the esophagus, skull, face, or mouth.
7. Untreated, active tuberculosis. (Hazard to the practitioner.)
8. Nausea, air swallowing, or hiccups (singulation).

4. Hazards and Precautions.

The AARC Guidelines list these items:

1. Pneumothorax
2. Barotrauma
3. Increased airway resistance from a bronchospastic reaction to the positive pressure or an adverse reaction to a medication. This can result in alveolar overdistention, air trapping, and auto–positive end-expiratory pressure (PEEP)
4. Hyperoxia when 100% oxygen is delivered to the patient. Some COPD patients who are hypercarbic and breathing on hypoxic drive may hypoventilate as a result
5. Secretions that may become impacted when the inhaled gas is not humidified adequately
6. Nosocomial infection
7. Decreased venous return (According to Realey, this would be helpful in a patient with pulmonary edema.)
8. Increased ventilation to perfusion mismatch. This could worsen any hypoxemia.
9. Hyperventilation.
10. Psychological dependence. This may be seen in the long-term home care patient who does not want to switch to another method of taking inhaled medications.

5. Initiation of therapy.

a. Steps in the basic procedure.

A. Check for a complete and proper order specifying the patient, oxygen percentage, frequency of treatment, medication, and any special considerations.
B. Gather the necessary equipment, medication, and so on.
C. Set up the equipment outside of the patient's room.
D. Introduce yourself, the department, and your purpose to the patient.
E. Confirm the patient's identity.
F. Have the patient sit up in bed or a chair; an obese patient may stand.
G. Interview the patient.
H. Assess the patient's vital signs.
I. Assess the patient's breath sounds.
J. Prepare the IPPB unit for operation:
   1. If the unit is electrical, plug into a working outlet.
   2. If the unit is pneumatic, plug into either a compressed air or oxygen outlet as ordered.
   3. Set the following controls:
      a. Set sensitivity at -1 cm H_2O pressure.
      b. Set nebulizer to run on inspiration only.
      c. Adjust the flow as necessary.
      d. Set the peak pressure at about 10 to 15 cm H_2O.

4. Test the nebulizer by turning on the machine.
5. Cover the mouthpiece with a clean tissue to ensure that it cycles off at the preset pressure.

K. Instruct the patient to sip on the mouthpiece like a straw to turn the machine on. Have the patient relax and let the machine fill his or her lungs with air. The patient should hold his or her breath in for 2 to 3 seconds and exhale slowly.

b. Giving a passive treatment.

Most authors describe the patient taking this kind of treatment. With a passive treatment, the patient relaxes and lets the machine fill the lungs until the preset pressure is reached. As mentioned earlier, the patient is then told to hold in his or her breath before exhaling passively. This treatment is given with the intent of minimizing the patient's work of breathing. As slow a flow rate as possible is used so that any nebulized medication will be deposited deeply into the small airways and lungs.

c. Giving an active treatment.

Several authors advocate having the patient take an active treatment where he or she interacts with the IPPB machine to get as deep a breath as possible.

Welch et al. have found that the patient's posttreatment inspiratory capacity is greatest when the practitioner (1) uses as high a peak pressure as the patient can tolerate and (2) coaches the patient to inhale as deeply as possible with the IPPB machine. They and others believe that this is the best way to treat or prevent atelectasis.

6. Initial settings on the Bird Mark 7.

The older version of the Mark 7 is used as the model respirator of the Bird series. The current Mark 8 has similar features. Other Bird units will have slightly different controls and features.

Refer to Fig. 13-1 for the following:

1. Adjust the *air-mix* knob to the desired gas mix.

2. Sensitivity should be set so that the patient has to generate about −1 cm H_2O pressure to cycle the unit on. Set the *sensitivity* control (on the left-hand side of the unit when facing it) to the reference number 15. This is at approximately the 2 o'clock position. Turning the control lever counterclockwise will make the unit more sensitive. Push in the hand timer rod to note that the unit cycles on easily.

3. Flow should be set so that the patient feels comfortable with the inspiratory time. Set the *flow rate* knob so that the reference number 15 is at the 12 o'clock position; the *off* sign will be at the eight o'clock position. Turning the *flow rate* knob more counterclockwise will increase the flow.

4. Peak pressure should be set at about 10 to 15 cm H_2O pressure. Set the *pressure* control (on the right-hand side of the unit when facing it) to the reference number 15. This is at approximately the 10 o'clock position. Turning the control lever more clockwise increases the peak pressure. Hold a clean tissue against the patient's mouthpiece to see that the unit cycles off at the desired peak pressure.

7. Initial settings on the Bennett PR-II.

The PR-II is used as the model respirator of the Bennett series. Other Bennett units will have slightly different controls and features.

Refer to Figs. 13-2 and 13-3 for the following:

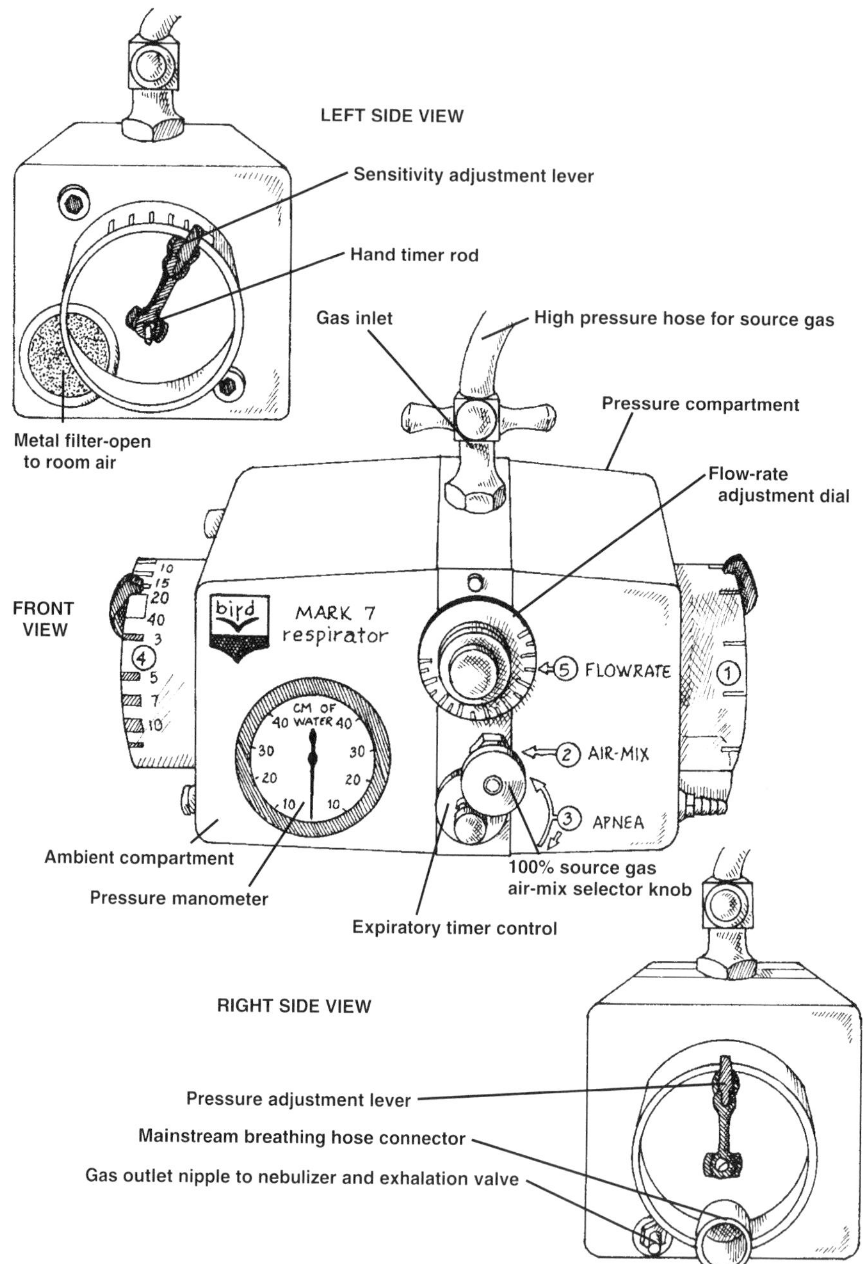

Fig. 13-1 Controls and features of the Bird Mark 7 IPPB unit.

1. Adjust the *air dilution* knob to the desired gas mix.
2. Sensitivity should be set so that the patient has to generate about −1 cm H_2O pressure to cycle the unit on. Turning the control lever counterclockwise will make the unit more sensitive. Push up on the Bennett valve strut to note that the unit cycles on easily.
3. Flow should be set so that the patient feels comfortable with the inspiratory time. The Bennett valve is designed to automatically open and close itself to allow the patient as much flow as desired. Set the *peak flow* control knob as counterclockwise as possible

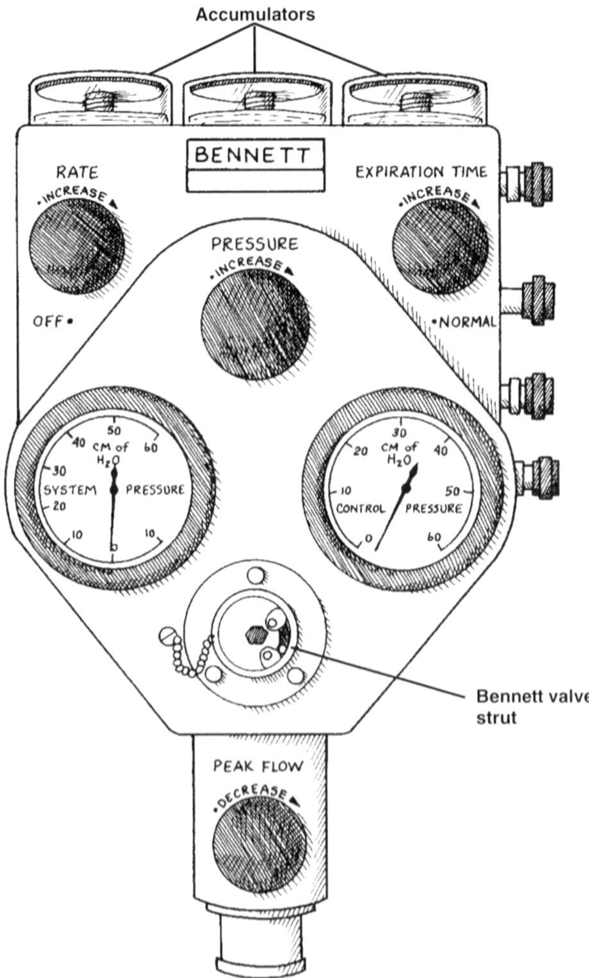

Fig. 13-2 Front controls and features of the Bennett PR-II IPPB unit.

so that it is at the maximum setting. Turning the *peak flow* knob more clockwise will decrease the patient's peak flow.

4. Peak pressure should be set at about 10 to 15 cm H_2O pressure. Dial the *pressure* control clockwise until the *control pressure* gauge shows the desired peak pressure. Hold a clean tissue against the patient's mouthpiece to see that when the unit cycles off the *system pressure* gauge reads the same as the *control pressure gauge*.

5. Turn the *inspiration nebulization* control counterclockwise for medication to be nebulized only during an inspiration. Some practitioners believe that the *expiration nebulization* control should be turned on slightly so that the mouthpiece and circuit dead space is filled with medication before the next breath. Others are opposed to this because it wastes medication when the patient stops the treatment.

6. A small leak in the circuit, mouthpiece, or face mask can be overcome by adding some additional flow by turning on the *terminal flow* control. It is normally left off. Turn the control counterclockwise to add as much additional flow as necessary to overcome the leak.

Details on the design and control specifications for the various Bird and Bennett models can be found in the manufacturers' literature and McPherson's book *Respiratory Therapy Equipment*.

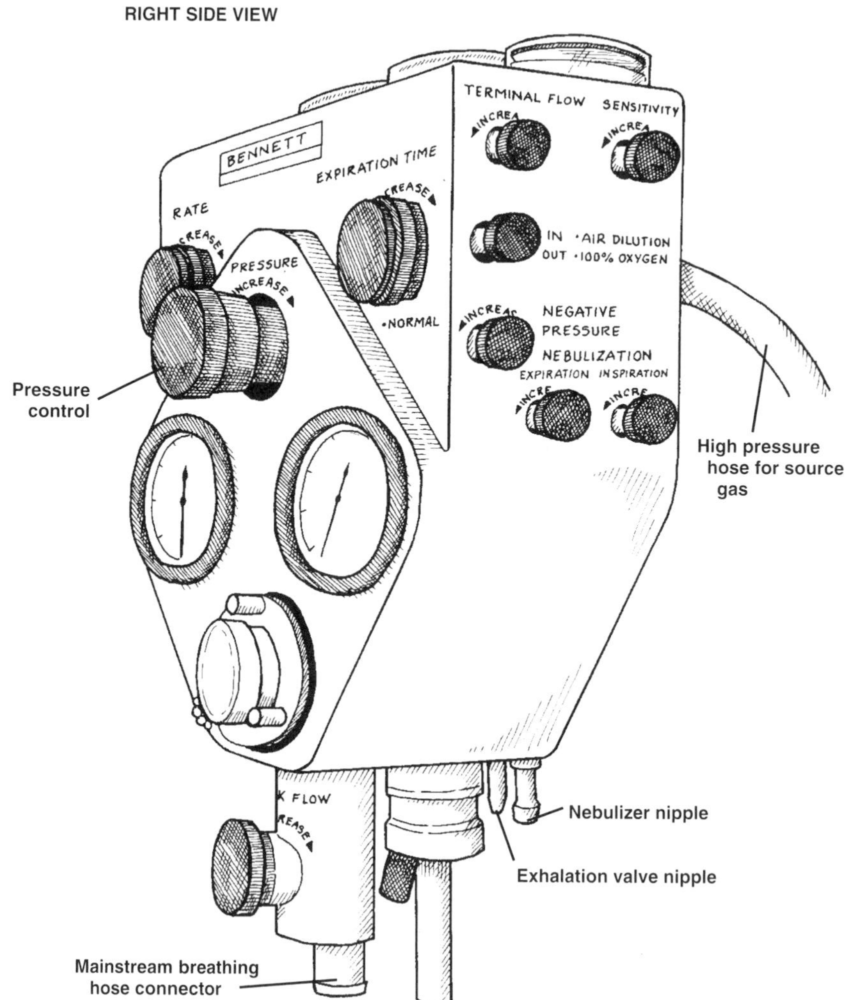

Fig. 13-3 Right side controls and features of the Bennett PR-II IPPB unit.

Module B. Adjust IPPB therapy to achieve adequate spontaneous ventilation.

1. Change the patient-machine interface (IIIC5c) [R, Ap]:
a. Mouthpiece.

A conscious, cooperative patient can take a treatment with a mouthpiece. He or she must be instructed to place it between the teeth (or gums) and seal the lips around it so that there is no leak. Instruct the patient to sip gently on it to turn on the IPPB machine. As long as the lips are sealed and there are no other leaks, the positive-pressure breath will stop when the preset pressure is reached. Nose clips are often helpful to prevent a leak through the nose as the patient is learning how to take the treatment. The nose clips can be removed after the patient has learned how to seal the nasopharynx with the soft palate.

Quite a variety of mouthpieces are available. All share the common features of a raised edge so that the teeth will not slip off and a 22 mm–outer diameter (OD) connector end to insert into the IPPB circuit (Fig. 13-4).

b. Mouth seal (Bennett seal).

An unconscious, uncooperative, or aged patient who cannot seal his or her lips can be aided by placing a soft rubber seal around the mouthpiece. The most commonly used seal is made by Puritan-Bennett and is called the Bennett seal. The practitioner gently holds the seal around the patient's lips to seal the airway so that the patient can trigger the breath and cycle the machine off (Fig. 13-5). Nose clips are also commonly needed.

c. Face mask.

The face mask can be used if the mouth seal does not provide an airtight seal. This might be because of the patient's facial structure or lack of teeth. Mouth trauma, surgery, or lip sores would be other reasons to use a face mask.

The mask should be clear and properly sized to fit comfortable over the patient's nose and mouth. The practitioner should be able to get a seal with a minimum amount of hand pressure (Fig. 13-6). The equipment connection opening in the mask has a 22-mm inner diameter (ID) so that it will connect directly to the IPPB circuit. A 22-mm-OD male adapter and short length of aerosol tubing can be added for flexibility and patient comfort. The clear mask is important so that the practitioner can see whether the patient has vomited or has a large amount of secretions or saliva in his or her mouth. The mask should never be strapped to the patient's face so that the practitioner can attend to another patient.

This is the least effective patient attachment device if the therapeutic goal is to deliver an aerosolized medication. Much of the medication will rain out on the patient's face or in the nasal passages if he or she is a nose breather.

d. Tracheostomy/endotracheal tube (elbow) adapter.

The elbow adapter is designed to connect the patient's tracheostomy or endotracheal tube to the IPPB circuit (or other respiratory care equipment). The IPPB end has a 22-mm-ID connector. The tracheostomy/endotracheal tube end has a 15-mm-ID connector (Fig. 13-7). Most elbow adapters have an opening for passing a suction catheter directly into the tube without having to disconnect the IPPB circuit. Simply pull off the cap to pass the catheter, and replace the cap to seal the airway and circuit. If the patient has had the cuff deflated, it will have to be reinflated to seal the airway. An unsealed cuff will result in an air leak, and the gas flow will not turn off.

2. Adjust the sensitivity. (IIIC5a) [R, Ap]

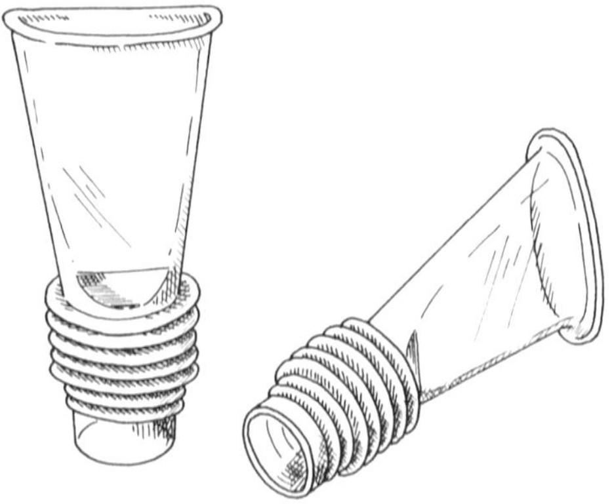

Fig. 13-4 Universal IPPB mouthpiece with a tapered 22- to 18-mm machine connector.

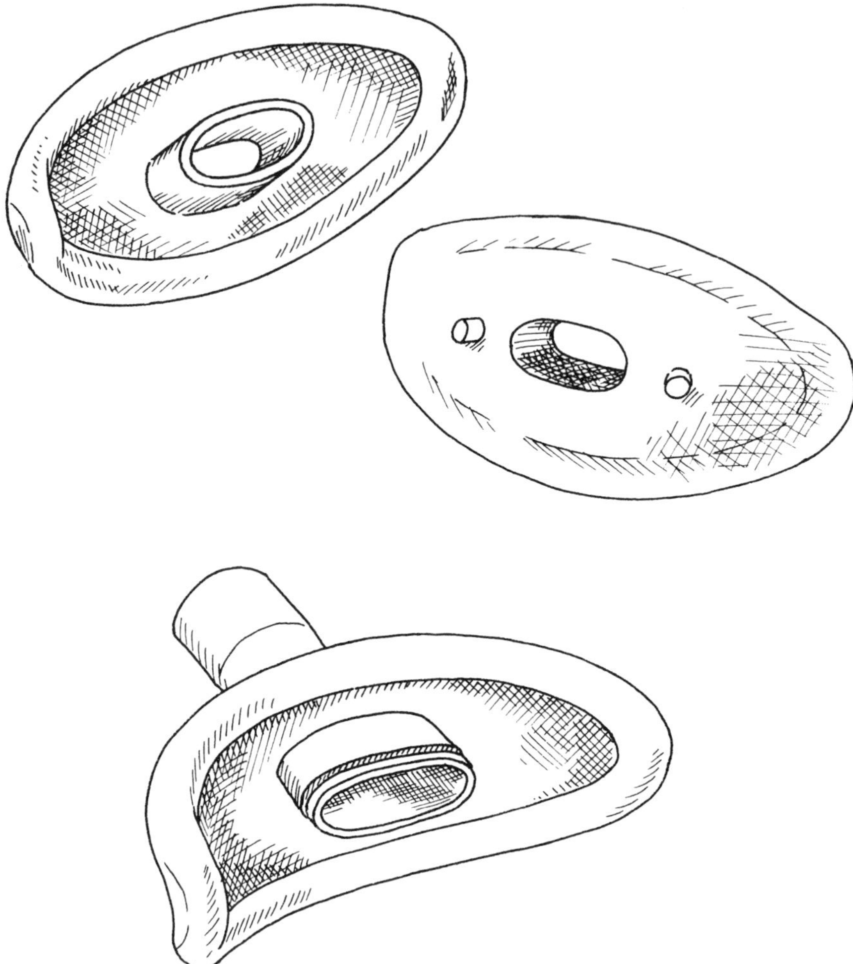

Fig. 13-5 *Top,* Bennett or mouth flange seal. *Bottom,* IPPB mouthpiece inserted into the seal.

The sensitivity of the IPPB unit refers to how much effort or work the patient will have to perform to turn the unit on for a breath. Commonly the sensitivity is set so that the patient has to generate a negative pressure of only about -1 cm H_2O pressure to begin an inspiration. This can be seen by looking at the needle deflecting into the negative range on the pressure manometer. Ask the patient whether the machine can be easily turned on to get a breath. The IPPB unit should not be set so sensitive that it self-cycles.

The sensitivity range on the Bird series is -0.01 to -5 cm H_2O. Turning the *sensitivity/starting effort* adjustment lever counterclockwise toward the smaller reference numbers makes the unit more sensitive. The sensitivity range on the Bennett series is -0.5 to -1 cm H_2O. Turning the *sensitivity* control counterclockwise makes the unit easier to turn on.

3. Adjust the F_{IO_2}. (IIIC5b) [R, Ap]

Both the Bird and Bennett units can be powered by compressed air or oxygen. The decision as to what oxygen percentage to give depends on the patient's condition. The

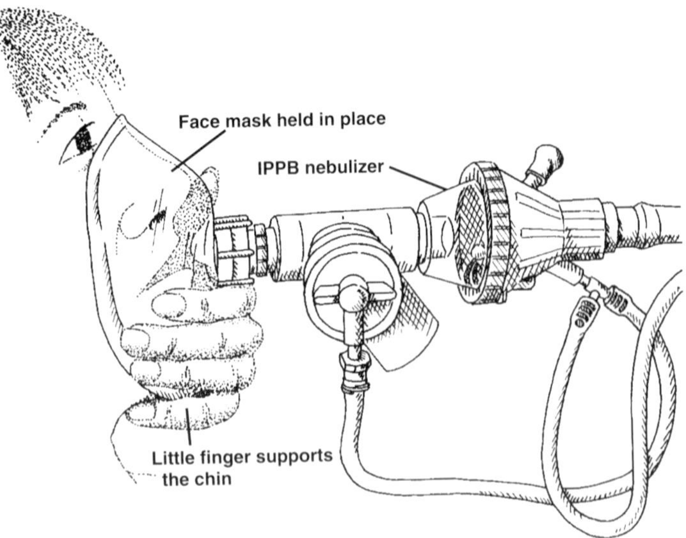

Fig. 13-6 Giving an IPPB treatment with the use of a face mask.

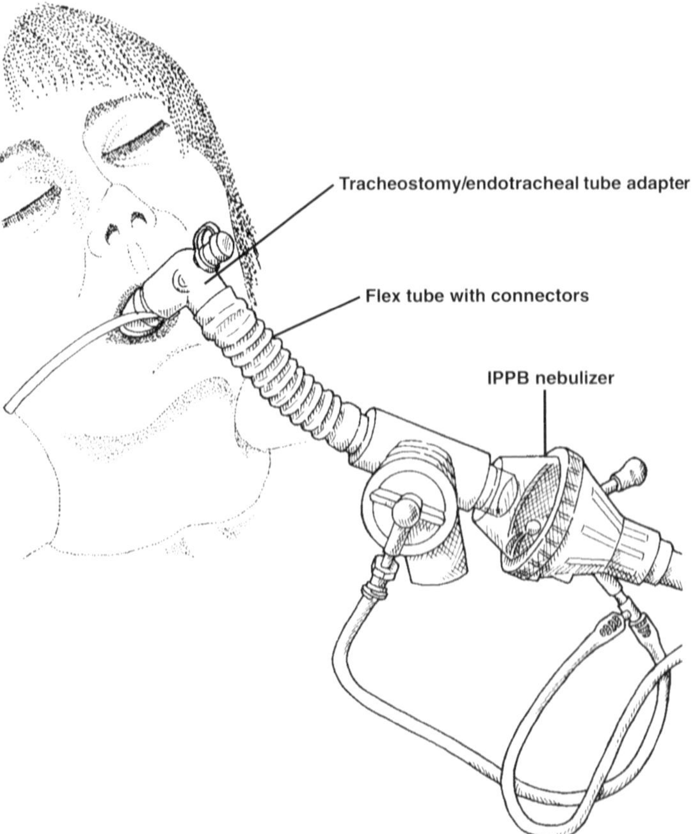

Fig. 13-7 Giving an IPPB treatment with the use of a tracheostomy/endotracheal tube adapter.

physician may include the oxygen percentage in the treatment order. Some departments have oxygen protocols in their treatment procedure. Generally compressed air (21% oxygen) should be used whenever the patient does not need supplemental oxygen.

A patient with COPD who is retaining carbon dioxide and breathing on hypoxic drive should also be given room air via the IPPB unit. The patient may be allowed to keep wearing a nasal cannula with oxygen during the treatment so that the blood oxygen level will be kept normal. Remember that the delivery of a larger than normal tidal volume will, by itself, increase the patient's Pa_{O_2} level. Giving this patient a high oxygen percentage by IPPB may result in the slowing down or stopping of spontaneous ventilation. The unavailability of piped-in compressed air should not be an excuse to give a patient a high oxygen percentage when it may be harmful. IPPB can be given through a gas-powered unit powered by a compressed air cylinder or an electrically powered unit.

Supplemental oxygen will be given if either unit is powered by oxygen and the *air-mix/air dilution* knobs are set to dilute the source gas with room air. This would be appropriate for patients who require supplemental oxygen and are not at risk of stopping their spontaneous ventilation. Most practitioners use this method of giving IPPB because piped oxygen is usually available in all patients' rooms.

Pure oxygen should be given to the patient who is severly hypoxemic. Examples include acute pulmonary edema, respiratory failure, and carbon monoxide poisoning. The *air-mix/air dilution* knobs must be set so that only the source gas (oxygen) is delivered to the patient.

A. Varying oxygen percentage on the Mark 7:
   1. Pushing the *air-mix* knob into the center body results in pure source gas. This could be either air or oxygen.
   2. Pulling the *air-mix* knob out of the center body results in a dilution of the source gas with room air. If oxygen is the source gas, the room air will dilute the delivered gas to between 60% and 90% (or more) oxygen.

B. Varying oxygen percentage on the PR-II:
   1. Pulling the *air dilution* knob out of the body results in pure source gas. This could be either air or oxygen.
   2. Pushing the *air dilution* knob into the body results in a dilution of the source gas with room air. If oxygen is the source gas, the room air will dilute the delivered gas to between 40% and 80% oxygen.
   3. Turning on the *terminal flow* control results in the dilution of source gas with room air. This will dilute the final percentage if the source gas is oxygen.

4. Adjust the flow. (IIIC5a) [R, Ap]

The patient should initially feel comfortable with the flow rate and the inspiratory time. Ask the patient a simple question, such as, "Is the breath coming too fast or too slow?" He or she will be able to give you a short answer or even a hand gesture in response. As the treatment progresses, the practitioner may be able to adjust the flow to modify the patient's breathing pattern to better achieve the therapeutic goal, for example:

1. Anxious patients may initially need a fast flow. As they are coached to relax and get used to the treatment, the practitioner should try to reduce the flow.

2. Slower flows result in medications being deposited deeper into the lungs. This is important if the patient is having a bronchodilator, mucolytic, or antibiotic nebulized.

3. Faster flows result in the deposition of medications in the upper airways. This is important if the patient is receiving racemic epinephrine for laryngeal edema or lidocaine for a local anesthetic of the upper airway before bronchoscopy.

Turning the *inspiratory time/flow rate* control counterclockwise increases the flow rate on the Bird series. Pulling the *air-mix* knob out from the center body increases the total flow by allowing room air to be entrained along with the source gas.

Flow rate in the PR-II is determined by the patient's inspiratory effort and how open the Bennett valve is. Flow can be decreased somewhat by turning the *peak flow* control clockwise. Flow is not affected by the position of the *air dilution* knob.

5. Adjust the volume, pressure, or both. (IIIC5a) [R, AP]

A review of the current respiratory care textbooks reveals that all authors agree that the basic goal of IPPB is to increase how deeply the patient inspires. Unfortunately, there is considerable difference about what inspiratory volume is being measured or by how much that breath should be increased for therapeutic goals to be achieved. Rather than choose one author over the others, all recommendations will be listed:

1. Rarey and Youtsey: IPPB volume should be either (a) 3 to 4 ml times ideal body weight in pounds or (b) 10 ml times weight in kilograms.
2. Eubanks and Bone: IPPB volume should be either (a) greater than the spontaneous tidal volume, (b) at least 10% greater than the spontaneous inspiratory capacity (IC), or (c) at least 10% greater than the spontaneous vital capacity (VC).
3. Realey: IPPB volume should be either (a) at least 15 ml/kg of ideal body weight or (b) at least one third of the predicted IC.
4. Ziment IPPB volume should be at least 25% greater than the spontaneous tidal volume.
5. Shapiro et al: IPPB volume should be greater than the spontaneous VC.
6. Respiratory Care Committee of the American Thoracic Society: IPPB volume should be either (a) at least 25% greater than the spontaneous tidal volume or (b) at least as great as the spontaneous IC.

If the therapeutic goal is to prevent or treat atelectasis, having the patient inspire a deeper than spontaneous breath should help. Because all of the current IPPB units are pressure cycled, the only way to increase the inspired volume during a passive treatment is to increase the peak pressure. Coaching the patient during an active treatment will result in a larger volume without the need for as great a peak pressure. Decrease the peak pressure if the patient complains of discomfort or cannot hold that much pressure without loosing the lip seal.

Module C. IPPB equipment.

1. Get the necessary equipment for the procedure. (IIA11a) [R, Ap]

The two most widely used IPPB machines are the Bird Mark 7/8 (or a variation on it found in the series) and the Bennett PR-II. Both are pneumatically powered and found in most hospitals. Bennett makes a home care unit that is electrically powered.

2. Put the equipment together, make sure that it works properly, and identify and fix any problems with it. (IIB9a) [R, Ap]

See Fig. 13-8 for the Bird setup and Fig. 13-9 for the Bennett setup.

A. General setup procedures:
   1. Check for plentiful source gas. Make sure that the oxygen or air tank has the proper regulator. Check the pressure in the gas cylinder.

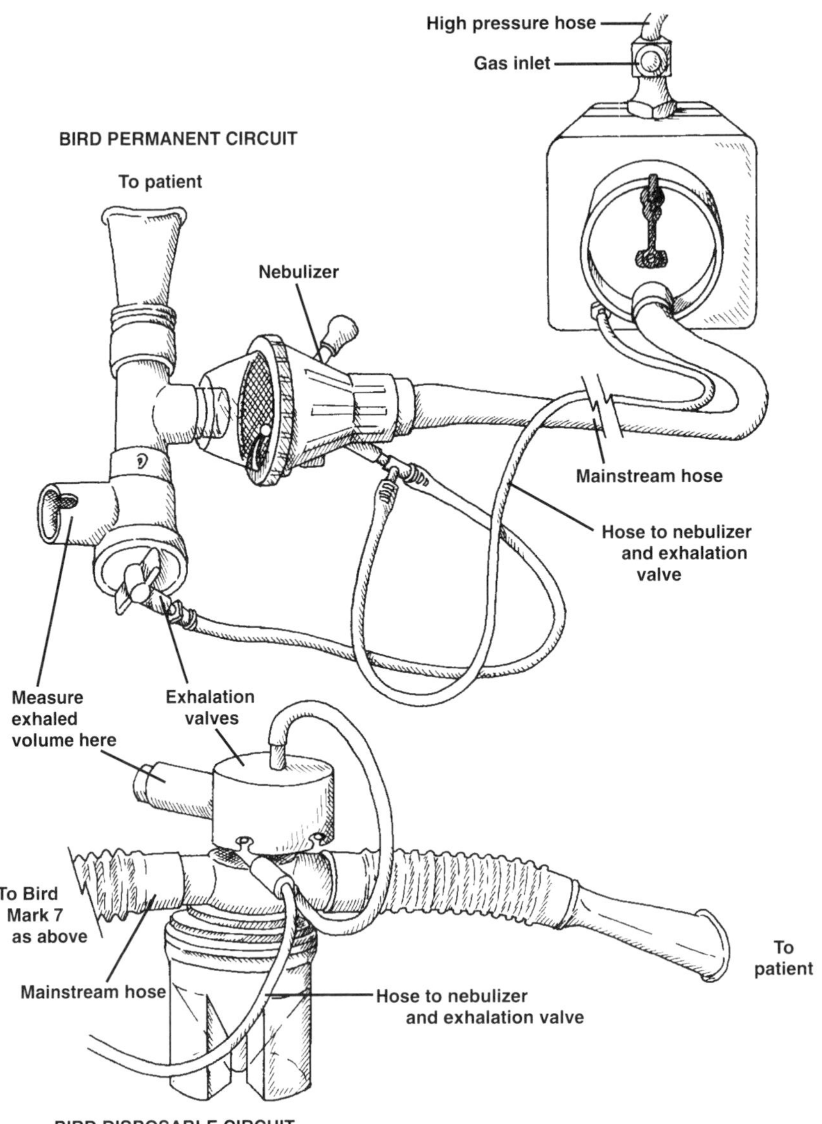

Fig. 13-8 Features of permanent and disposable Bird IPPB circuits.

2. Attach the high-pressure hose to the source gas and the IPPB unit at the gas inlet. Make sure that the connections are tight.
3. Bacteria filters are optional. They are inserted between the IPPB unit gas outlets and the mainstream and nebulizer hoses.
4. A cascade-type humidifier is optional. Some practitioners prefer to warm and humdify the mainstream gas before it reaches the patient.
5. Check to see that the IPPB circuit is put together properly and that all of the connections are tight.
6. Set the initial treatment parameters for sensitivity, flow, and peak pressure. Manually cycle the unit on. Cover the mouthpiece to see that the unit cycles off at the preset pressure.
7. Add any medication to the nebulizer. Check to see that the nebulizer is producing a mist.

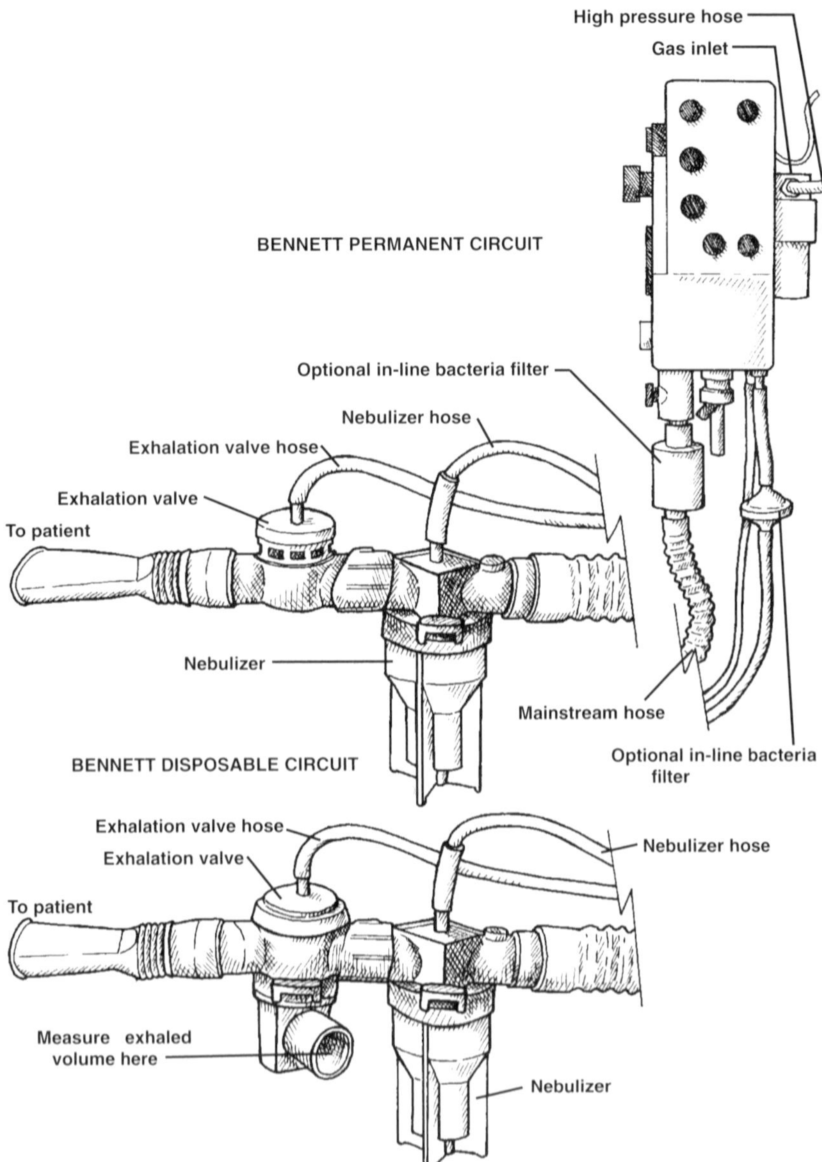

Fig. 13-9 Features of permanent and disposable Bennett IPPB circuits.

B. Bird setup:

1. One end of the mainstream (large-bore) hose is connected to the mainstream breathing hose connector on the right side of the unit. The other end is connected to the nebulizer.
2. One end of the nebulizer (small-bore hose is connected to the small nipple on the right hand side of the unit. The other end is connected to a T-piece at the nebulizer.
3. A piece of small-bore hose is used to connect one limb of the T-piece and the exhalation valve. Gas flowing through this hose powers both the nebulizer and the exhalation valve.

C. Bennett setup:
   1. One end of the mainstream (large-bore) hose is connected to the mainstream breathing hose connector on the underside of the unit. The other end is connected to the nebulizer.
   2. One end of the nebulizer (medium-bore) hose is connected to the larger of two nipples on the underside of the unit. The other end is connected to the nebulizer nipple.
   3. One end of the exhalation (small-bore) hose is connected to the smaller of two nipples on the underside of the unit. The other end is connected to the exhalation valve nipple.

Fixing a problem is only possible after the problem has been identified. The practitioner should be familiar with both permanent and disposable types of Bird and Bennett circuits. Leaks of any sort in the circuit will prevent the unit from cycling off so that the patient can exhale. Tighten up any friction fit or screw-type connections to stop the leak.

A leak at the source gas connection or high-pressure hose gas inlet connection will result in a rather loud hissing sound. When connections are tightened properly, the hissing and leak will stop.

Debris such as mucus or blood will plug the nebulizer capillary tube and prevent any mist from being formed. Disassemble the nebulizer and rinse it under running water to try to clear the capillary tube. Replace the nebulizer if necessary.

This ends the general discussion on IPPB. The following topics may also be tested on the entry level examination. Review the previous discussion and Sections 1 and 4 for more details.

Module D. Patient Assessment.

1. Determine and continue to monitor how the patient responds to the treatment.

The patient's heart and respiratory rates should be determined before, at least once during, and after the treatment. Patients with unstable heart disease or hypotension may need to also have their blood pressure measured. The patient's heart rhythm should be monitored if the heart rate changes by 20 beats/min or more or the blood pressure changes significantly.

Breath sounds should be heard more clearly to the bases of the lungs. One of the goals of IPPB is to give the patient larger tidal volumes than normal. More secretions may be heard in the airways if the larger tidal volumes result in their mobilization. However, if the deeper breaths enable the patient to cough more effectively, more secretions should be coughed out. Wheezing should be diminished if a bronchodilator medication is nebulized to a patient with bronchospasm.

Check the chest x-ray film to identify if the patient has atelectasis or another specific lung problem that would be helped by IPPB. A chest x-ray film should be obtained if a pneumothorax is suspected.

As discussed earlier, all authors agree that some form of bedside spirometry must be performed to determine that the IPPB volume is greater than the patient's IC or VC. The AARC Guideline is that the IPPB volume should be at least 25% greater than the patient's spontaneous tidal volume. Some authors recommend the monitoring of other bedside respiratory parameters. They state that the passively taken IPPB treatment will rest the patient so that the lung mechanics tests should be improved. The patient's peak flow or FEV_1 value should be improved after a properly administered treatment with a nebulized bronchodilator.

Ask about the patient's feelings toward the treatment and write them in the chart. Note any significant comments made by the patient. Note the patient's preferred flow and pressure or volume settings.

2. Modify the treatment and recommend any changes in the patient's respiratory care plan depending on the response.

As already mentioned, the general treatment length is 15 to 20 minutes. The patient may not be able to tolerate that length of time because of fatigue. This is often seen in aged or debilitated patients.

Stop the treatment if the patient has a pulse change of 20 beats/min or more. It is most common to see the pulse increase because of a nebulized bronchodilator drug. A decreased venous return to the heart may be shown by an increased heart rate or drop in blood pressure.

The contraindications, hazards, and precautions to IPPB were discussed earlier. The treatment should be canceled if the patient has an untreated pneumothorax or massive hemoptysis. Other serious problems would also justify the cancellation of the order.

BIBLIOGRAPHY

AARC Clinical Practice Guideline: Intermittent positive pressure ventilation. *Resp Care* 1993:38:1189-1195.

Eubanks DH, Bone RC: *Comprehensive Respiratory Care*, ed 2. St Louis, Mosby, 1990.

Fluck Jr, RJ: Intermittent positive-pressure breathing devices, in Barnes TA (ed): *Respiratory Care Practice*. Chicago, Mosby, 1988.

McPherson SP: *Respiratory Therapy Equipment*, ed 3. St Louis, Mosby, 1985.

McPherson SP: *Respiratory Therapy Equipment*, ed 4. St Louis, Mosby, 1990.

Miller WF: Intermittent positive pressure breathing (IPPB), in Kacmarek RM, Stoller JK (eds): *Current Respiratory Care*. Philadelphia, BC Decker, 1988.

Realey AM: Hyperinflation therapy, in Scanlan CL, Spearman CB, Sheldon RL, (eds): *Egan's Fundamentals of Respiratory Care*, ed 5. St Louis, Mosby, 1990.

Welch MA, Shapiro BJ, Mercurio P, Wagner W, et al: Methods of intermittent positive pressure breathing. *Chest* 1980; 78:463-467.

Weizalis CP: Intermittent positive-pressure breathing, in Barnes TA (ed): *Respiratory Care Practice*. Chicago, Mosby, 1988.

Wilkins RL, Hodgkin JE, Lopez B: *Lung Sounds, a Practical Guide*. Mosby, St Louis, 1988.

Respiratory Care Committee of the American Thoracic Society: Guidelines for the use of intermittent positive pressure breathing (IPPB). *Respir Care* 1980; 25:365-370.

Shapiro BA, Harrison RA, Kacmarek RM, et al: *Clinical Application of Respiratory Care*, ed 3. Chicago, Mosby, 1985.

Ziment I: Intermittent positive pressure breathing, in Burton GG, Hodgkin JE (eds): *Respiratory Care*, ed 2. Philadelphia, Lippincott, 1984.

SELF-STUDY QUESTIONS

1. Your patient complains that it is difficult for her to start the IPPB treatment. You would adjust which of the following controls?
   A. Pressure
   B. Flow

C. Sensitivity
D. Terminal flow
E. Expiratory retard

2. Your patient is having a difficult time keeping a tight seal around the mouthpiece. He complains that the breath is too long and takes the mouthpiece out. To help the PR-II cycle off, you would adjust which of the following?
   A. Pressure
   B. Flow
   C. Sensitivity
   D. Terminal flow
   E. Expiratory retard

3. Your patient is going into pulmonary edema. She has rales in both lung fields and is coughing up pink, frothy sputum. What oxygen percentage would you recommend for her IPPB treatment?
   A. 21%
   B. 40%
   C. 80%
   D. 100%
   E. None of the above

4. All of the following are indications for IPPB *except:*
   A. To deliver medications to a patient who cannot coordinate the use of a metered dose inhaler or hand-held nebulizer
   B. To treat a patient with acute pulmonary edema.
   C. To treat a comatose patient with atelectasis.
   D. As a substitute for incentive spirometry in a patient with an inspiratory capacity that is 60% of predicted.
   E. To treat a cooperative patient with atelectasis.

5. You are ordered to give an IPPB treatment to a comatose patient who has lip ulcers. What patient-machine connection would you use?
   A. Mouthpiece
   B. Face mask
   C. Bennett seal with mouthpiece
   D. Intubation of the patient with an endotracheal tube adapter
   E. None of the above

6. The sensitivity control should be set at what level at the start of the IPPB treatment?
   A. 0 cm H_2O
   B. −1 cm H_2O
   C. −3 cm H_2O
   D. −5 cm H_2O
   E. −7 cm H_2O

7. While coaching an active IPPB treatment, you notice that the needle on the pressure manometer bounces around as the pressure increases. To better adjust the treatment to the patient's needs, you would do which of the following?
   A. Increase the flow.
   B. Decrease the flow.
   C. Increase the peak pressure.
   D. Decrease the sensitivity.
   E. Decrease the expiratory retard.

8. You are asked to evaluate a patient for the need for IPPB or incentive spirometry. She weighs 125 pounds. IPPB would be indicated if her bedside spirometry values showed which of the following?
   I. Tidal volume of 400 ml
   II. Inspiratory capacity of 610 ml
   III. Inspiratory capacity of 720 ml
   IV. Vital capacity of 780 ml
   V. Vital capacity of 1030 ml
   A. II, IV
   B. I, III, V
   C. II, V
   D. III, IV
   E. I, V

9. You are giving an IPPB treatment on a Bird Mark 7 unit. To give the patient a 100% source gas of oxygen, you adjust the air mix control knob. What effect will this adjustment have on the flow rate to the patient?
   A. No effect
   B. Increased flow
   C. Decreased flow

10. You would stop the IPPB treatment under which of the following conditions?
   I. You suspect the patient has just developed a pneumothorax.
   II. The patient has a difficult time keeping his lips sealed.
   III. The patient's wheezing gets worse, and he complains of dyspnea.
   IV. The patient says that his lungs feel full of air.
   V. The patient coughs up a large amount of blood.
   A. I, II
   B. III, IV
   C. IV, V
   D. II, IV
   E. I, III, V

Answer Key:

1. C; 2. D; 3. D; 4. E; 5. B; 6. B; 7. A; 8. A; 9. C; 10. E.

14 Mechanical Ventilation

All publicly available versions of the entry level examination feature mechanical ventilation questions specifically about adults or questions that could apply to either adults or pediatric patients. There are very few questions that relate specifically to pediatric patients. The National Board for Respiratory Care (NBRC) has developed a pediatric/perinatal respiratory care specialty examination that deals exclusively with neonates and children. This section is written with the adult patient in mind except when neonatal or pediatric patients are specified.

The NBRC is known to ask questions about using and troubleshooting problems with specific ventilators. It is beyond the scope of this book to cover all possible mechanical ventilators. That information is available in the manufacturers' literature or equipment books such as McPherson's *Respiratory Therapy Equipment*. The NBRC has asked specific questions on the Bennett MA-1 and PR-2, the Bird series, and BEAR 1 and 2. It would seem wise for the learner to become familiar with the workings of the newer ventilators such as the Servo 900 B and C, Bear 1000, and Puritan-Bennett 7200, and Respironics Adult Star. In addition, it would be wise to become familiar with the function of the more common pediatric ventilators such as the Bourns BP200, Bear Cub, Sechrist IV-100 and IV-100B, and Infant Star.

Module A. Ventilatory support.

The decision to place a patient on ventilatory support should not be taken without due consideration of its need. A number of physiologic criteria have been compiled to help the clinician determine when a patient is in respiratory or ventilatory failure. These are listed in Table 14-1. Remember that the patient may not fail each and every criteria. However, it is likely that the patient will fail one or more of the criteria in each category.

1. Perform the following therapeutic procedures to adequately support the patient using mechanical ventilation.

a. Choose the best ventilator. (IIIC6) [R, Ap, An]

Pressure-cycled ventilators such as the Bird series or Bennett PR-2 may be acceptable for use with patients who have and are expected to keep a normal airway resistance and lung-thoracic compliance. Examples would include an unconscious patient from a drug overdose or under anesthesia or a patient with a neuromuscular disease such as myasthenia gravis or Guillain-Barré syndrome. As long as these patients are stable, the preset pressure will deliver the intended tidal volume.

If the patient's airway resistance increases from bronchospasm, secretions, or kinking

Table 14-1. Indications for Ventilatory Support*

Ventilation
1. Apnea
2. $Paco_2$ > 55 mm Hg in a patient who is not ordinarily hypercapneic
3. V_D/V_T ratio > 0.55-0.6 (55%-60%)

Oxygenation
1. Pao_2 < 80 mm Hg on 50% O_2 or more
2. $P(A\text{-}a)O_2$ > 300-350 mm Hg on 100% O_2
3. Intrapulmonary shunt > 20%

Pulmonary mechanics
1. Spontaneous tidal volume < 3-4 ml/lb or 7-9 ml/kg of ideal body weight
2. Vital capacity < 10-15 ml/kg
3. MIP > −20 to −25 cm H_2O
4. FEV_1 less than 10 ml/kg
5. Respiratory rate < 12 breaths/min or > 35 breaths/min in an adult

Miscellaneous
1. Unconscious patient
2. Unstable and unacceptable vital signs
3. Unstable cardiac rhythm due to hypoxemia and/or acidosis
4. Worsening cardiopulmonary or other major organ system

*$Paco_2$, Arterial CO_2 pressure; V_D/V_T, dead space/tidal volume; Pao_2, Arterial O_2 pressure; $P(A\text{-}a)O_2$, difference in the partial pressure of O_2 in alveolar gas and arterial blood; *MIP,* maximum inspiratory pressure; FEV_1, forced expi ratory volume in 1 sec.

of the endotracheal tube, the tidal volume will decrease. The tidal volume will also decrease if the patient's lung-thoracic compliance decreases. The reason is the same in both cases. These ventilators are pressure cycled or pressure limited. Once the preset pressure is reached, the ventilator cycles into exhalation. As a result, any condition that results in a higher airway resistance or decreased compliance will result in a lower tidal volume because less volume is delivered per unit of pressure.

Conversely, if the patient's airway resistance decreases or compliance increases, the delivered tidal volume will increase. More volume will be delivered per unit of pressure. In either case, the practitioner would have to make frequent adjustments in the preset pressure to hope to keep a stable tidal volume. This is not practical or safe.

A volume-cycled ventilator such as a Bennett MA-1, Puritan-Bennett 7200, BEAR 1000, or Servo 900 B or C is indicated whenever the patient's airway resistance or lung-thoracic compliance is expected to change. These types of ventilators will deliver a preset tidal volume to the patient, at whatever pressure is needed, despite changing patient conditions. Because of this, volume-cycled ventilators are recommended in the majority of patients who need ventilatory support.

In addition, these types of ventilators come with a built-in alarm system for detecting patient problems, can be used in a variety of modes, can deliver positive end-expiratory pressure (PEEP), and can generate more pressure to deliver the tidal volume than can the pressure-cycled ventilators. Even among these types of ventilators there is considerable variation in what can be done. The learner is encouraged to become familiar with their control functions, modes, pressure limits, alarms, and so forth.

One of the most fundamentally important decisions that the physician and practitioner must make in the care of a patient is what method will be used to ventilate the patient. The method or mode of ventilation is determined by the patient's condition and the limitations of the ventilator and breathing circuit.

Modes of Ventilation

1. Control (C). Control is the simplest method of providing ventilatory support and is used on an apneic patient. The ventilator is set with a mandatory respiratory rate and

tidal volume. The machine is incapable of allowing any patient interaction. For example, the ventilator might be set to deliver a tidal volume of 700 ml at a rate of 14 times/min. Because of this limitation, it is rarely, if ever, used in modern medicine except when the patient must be kept sedated or pharmacologically paralyzed (see Fig. 14-1,A for the pressure/time curve). These ventilators, as with the others below, have additional controls for determining oxygen percentage, inspiratory flow, inspiratory/expiratory (I/E) ratio, sigh breaths, and alarm settings.

2. Assist/control (A/C). This mode has a set backup respiratory rate but allows the patient to trigger additional machine-delivered breaths. A sensitivity control is adjusted to allow the patient to easily start a breath as needed. All tidal volumes are the same. For example, the ventilator might be set to deliver the same tidal volume of 700 ml with a backup rate of 14 times/min. Yet, if the patient makes a respiratory effort 20 times/min, the machine will deliver the 700-ml tidal volume that often (see Fig. 14-1,B for the pressure/time curve).

3. Intermittent mandatory ventilation (IMV). IMV has a set backup respiratory rate and tidal volume that will be delivered to the patient. In addition, in between the mandatory breaths, the patient can breathe spontaneously as frequently as desired. The patient can also take in as large a spontaneous tidal volume as needed. The sensitivity control is set so that the patient cannot trigger any extra ventilator tidal volumes. For example, the ventilator might be set to deliver a 700-ml tidal volume 8 times/min. Let us say that the patient breathes spontaneously 10 more times and has an average tidal volume of 400 ml. The total rate would be counted at 18. The total minute volume would be the combination of the machine's volume and the patient's volume (see Fig. 14-1,C for the pressure/time curve).

4. Synchronous intermittent mandatory ventilation (SIMV). SIMV is similar to IMV except that the sensitivity control is functional. The patient can trigger a machine-delivered tidal volume during a preset time interval. The timing of the backup rate is such that the patient can get only as many ventilator breaths as are set. The total respiratory rate and total minute volume would be calculated as discussed earlier (see Fig. 14-1,D for the pressure/time curve).

5. Pressure support ventilation (PSV). PSV is similar to intermittent positive-pressure ventilation (IPPB) in that when the patient initiates a ventilator breath, a preset pressure is delivered to the airway. The patient has the flexibility to determine the respiratory rate. The physician orders a PSV level that is enough to either overcome the patient's calculated airway resistance or to deliver a minimum tidal volume, depending on the clinical goal. The tidal volume will be stable if the patient passively takes the PSV breath, or it can be larger if the patient interacts actively with the pressure that is delivered (see Fig. 14-1,E for the pressure/time curve).

6. PEEP. An American College of Chest Physicians and American Thoracic Society (ACCP-ATS) joint committee defined PEEP as a residual pressure above atmospheric maintained at the airway opening at the end of expiration.

PEEP is administered through a mechanical ventilator and is not a mode by itself. Rather, it is used in conjunction with any of the previously mentioned modes. PEEP is set to prevent the patient from exhaling back to ambient (atmospheric) pressure. The higher the level of PEEP, the more progressively the patient's functional residual capacity (FRC) is increased. The therapeutic goal of this is to increase the patient's arterial oxygen pressure (Pa_{O_2}) (see Fig. 14-1,F for the pressure/time curve).

7. Continuous positive airway pressure (CPAP). An ACCP-ATS joint committee defined CPAP as a pressure above atmospheric maintained at the airway opening throughout the respiratory cycle during spontaneous breathing.

CPAP is similar to PEEP in purpose and effect. It is different from the previously mentioned modes in that the patient does not receive any ventilator-delivered tidal volume breaths. The patient must be capable of providing all of the minute ventilation for carbon dioxide removal. CPAP can be delivered through some mechanical ventilators or through a free-standing system (see Fig. 14-1,G for the pressure/time curve).

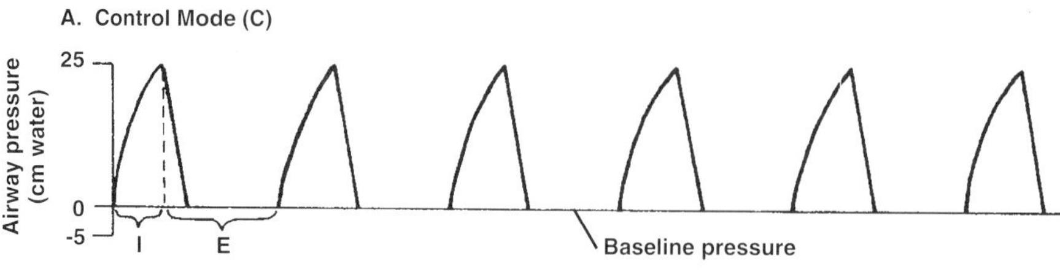

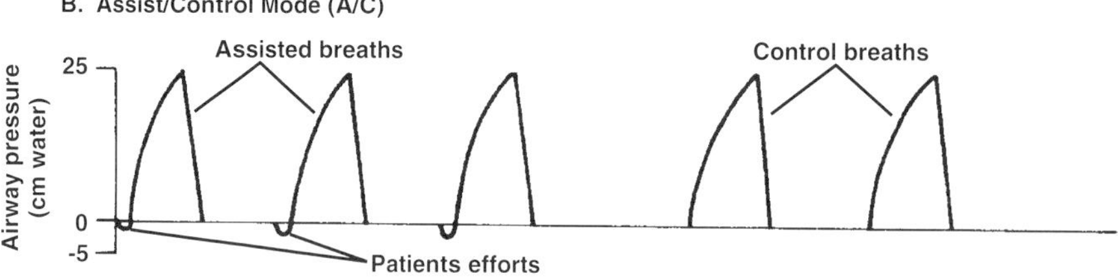

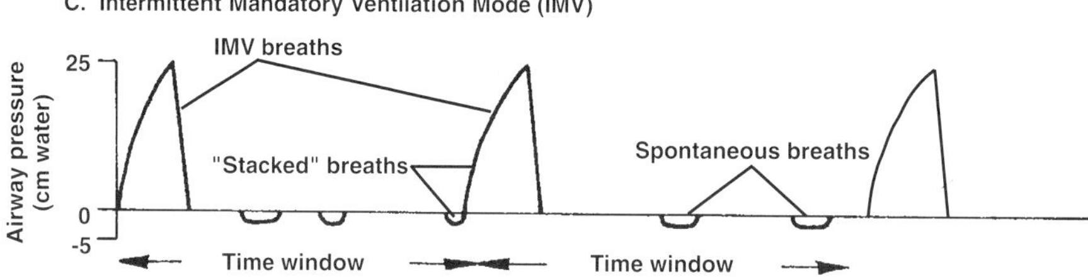

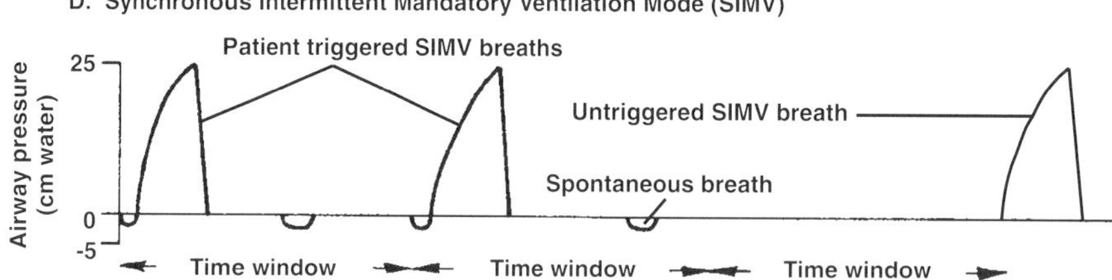

Fig. 14-1 Pressure vs. time waveforms for the various modes of mechanical ventilation. **A,** Control mode *(C)* shows no patient effort and consistent I/E ratios. **B,** Assist/control mode *(A/C)* shows that the patient's initial effort triggers a machine tidal volume breath. **C,** Intermittent mandatory ventilation mode *(IMV)* shows spontaneous tidal volume breaths occurring between predetermined machine tidal volume breaths. Note the "stacked" breaths that happen when the patient takes in a breath that is then supplemented by a machine breath. **D,** Synchronous intermittent mandatory ventilation mode *(SIMV)* shows that a patient effort within a time window results in the delivery of a machine tidal volume. Any other patient efforts within the time window result in a spontaneous tidal volume. If no patient efforts occur within the time window, a machine tidal volume will be automatically delivered.

Continued.

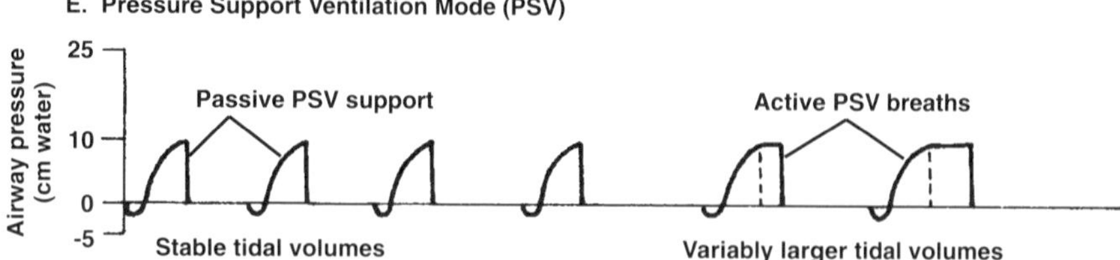

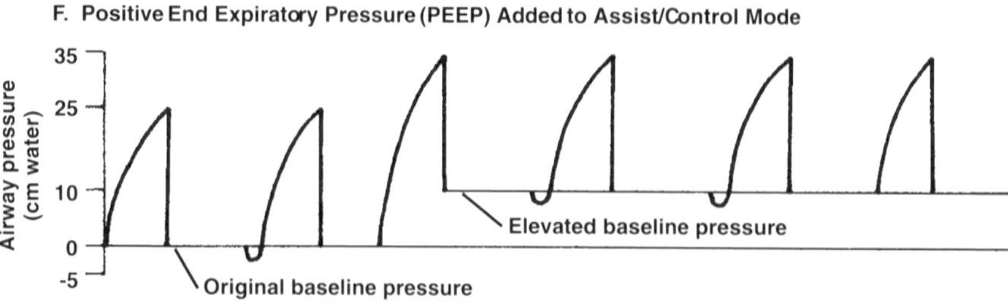

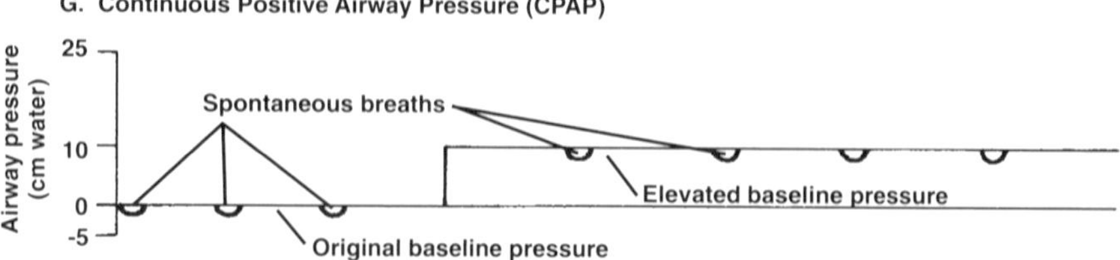

Fig 14-1 cont'd E, Pressure support ventilation *(PSV)* mode shows how the patient must initiate all breaths, which are then supported to a predetermined airway pressure. Stable tidal volumes will be seen if the patient inhales passively. Variably larger tidal volumes will result if the patient inhales more actively. **F,** Positive end-expiratory pressure *(PEEP)* therapy can be added to the assist/control mode (as shown) or any other. The elevated baseline pressure prevents alveolar collapse. The sensitivity control must be set at −1 to −2 cm H_2O so that the patient is able to trigger a breath without undue effort. **G,** Continuous positive airway pressure (*CPAP)* shows that the patient takes spontaneous tidal volumes while exhaling against an elevated baseline pressure.

b. Choose the appropriate tidal volume for mechanical ventilation. (IIIC7) [R, Ap, An]

A spontaneously breathing 70-kg (154-lb) adult with normal lungs and metabolism needs a tidal volume in the following range to adequately remove carbon dioxide:

- 6 to 9 ml/kg of ideal body weight, *or*
- 3 to 4 ml/lb of ideal body weight

Example:

6 ml × 70 kg = 420 ml
9 ml × 70 kg = 630 ml

3 ml × 154 lb = 462 ml
4 ml × 154 lb = 616 ml

Splitting the differences, a spontaneous tidal volume of about 500 ml is considered normal.

Fig 14-2 shows the Radford nomogram for predicting normal spontaneous tidal volumes based on body weights. It can be used to establish an initial tidal volume for most patients. Chronically hypercapneic (high carbon dioxide level) patients must be ventilated with some caution. It is not uncommon for these patients to have a lower than normal tidal volume. To give this type of patient a ventilator-delivered tidal volume in the normal range may result in blowing off too much carbon dioxide and causing a respiratory alkalosis. Care must be taken to ensure that the patient's tidal volume, rate, and minute volume (see later discussion) are such that the chronically high arterial carbon dioxide pressure ($Paco_2$) is maintained.

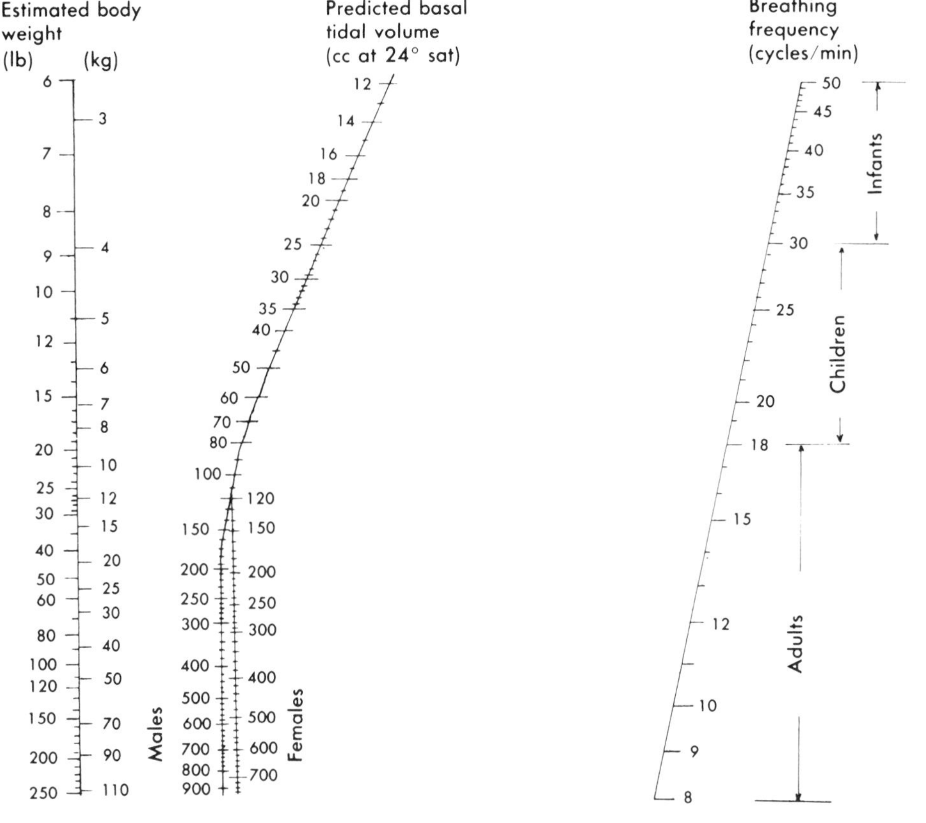

Corrections of predicted basal tidal volumes.
For patients not in coma: add 10%
Fever: add 5% for each °F above 99 (rectal)
add 9% for each °C above 37 (rectal)
Altitude: add 5% for each 2000 feet above sea level
add 8% for each 1000 meters above sea level
Intubation: subtract volume equal to one-half body weight in pounds
subtract 1 cc/kg of body weight
Dead space: add equipment dead space

Fig. 14-2 The Radford nomogram can be used to predict a basal tidal volume and respiratory rate based on the patient's body weight. (From Williams-Colon S, Thalken FR: Management and monitoring of the patient in respiratory failure, in Scanlan CL, Spearman CB, Sheldon RL [eds]: *Egan's Fundamentals of Respiratory Care,* ed 5. St Louis, Mosby, 1990. Used by permission.)

Most authors recommend a set ventilator tidal volume of 10 to 15 ml/kg of ideal body weight. This volume is higher than spontaneous for two reasons: (1) some of the set volume is lost to the patient because of gas compression and tubing stretch/compliance (covered later), and (2) most patients need larger than normal tidal volumes because their lungs are not functioning normally. Exceptions are patients with severe chronic restrictive lung disease or those who have had a pneumonectomy. Their tidal volume should be set at about 5 to 10 ml/kg of ideal body weight to avoid excessive ventilating pressure.

For example, our 70-kg (154-lb) adult with normal lungs would need a mechanical ventilator–set tidal volume in the following range:

- 10 ml × 70 kg = 700 ml
- 15 ml × 70 kg = 1050 ml

It is common practice to get a set of arterial blood gas values after the patient is stable on the ventilator. The tidal volume can be adjusted within the range depending on whether the patient's Pa_{CO_2} value is too high or low for the therapeutic goal. The most direct way to change alveolar ventilation is to modify the delivered tidal volume. A larger tidal volume, while everything else remains the same, will result in a lower Pa_{CO_2} value. Conversely, a smaller tidal volume, while everything else remains the same, will result in a higher Pa_{CO_2} value.

The following formula can be used to help predict what tidal volume will produce a desired Pa_{CO_2} value:

$$[V_T - (V_{D_{anat}} + V_{D_{mech}})] \times f \times Pa_{CO_2} = [V_T' - (V_{D_{anat}} + V_{D_{mech}})] \times f \times Pa_{CO_2}'$$

where

- V_T = current tidal volume.
- $V_{D_{anat}}$ = anatomic dead space. This is calculated at 1 ml/lb or 2.2 ml/kg of ideal body weight.
- $V_{D_{mech}}$ = added mechanical dead space.
- f = ventilator rate.
- Pa_{CO_2} = actual patient Pa_{CO_2} value.
- V_T' = desired tidal volume.
- Pa_{CO_2}' = desired patient Pa_{CO_2} value.

Note: Other, simpler formulas are available for calculating a change in minute volume or tidal volume. This one is presented because it takes into account more factors and can be used to calculate a change in tidal volume, rate, or mechanical dead space.

Example:

The patient is a 70-kg (154-lb) man who is being ventilated on the control mode (he is apneic). His ventilator settings are a tidal volume of 1000 ml, rate of 12 times/min, fractional inspired oxygen concentration (F_{IO_2}) of 0.3, and no added mechanical dead space. His arterial blood gas values are an arterial oxygen pressure (Pa_{O_2}) of 90 mm Hg, Pa_{CO_2} of 30 mm Hg, pH of 7.48, Sa_{O_2} of 95%, and a base excess (BE) of 0.

The clinical goal is to adjust the patient's tidal volume as needed to produce a Pa_{CO_2} value of 40 mm Hg. In summary:

V_T = 1000 ml current tidal volume.

$V_{D_{anat}}$ = 154 ml of anatomic dead space. This is calculated at 1 ml/lb or 2.2 ml/kg of ideal body weight.

$V_{D_{mech}}$ = no added mechanical dead space.

f = 12 times/min for the ventilator rate.
Pa_{CO_2} = 30 mm Hg actual patient Pa_{CO_2} value.
V_T' = desired tidal volume.
Pa_{CO_2}' = 40 mm Hg desired patient Pa_{CO_2} value

Placing the data and goal into the formula results in the following:

$$[V_T - (V_{D_{anat}} + V_{D_{mech}})] \times f \times Pa_{CO_2} = [V_T' - (V_{D_{anat}} + V_{D_{mech}})] \times f \times Pa_{CO_2}'$$
$$[1000 - (154 + 0)] \times 12 \times 30 = [V_T' - (154 + 0)] \times 12 \times 40$$

Simplifying produces the following:

$$[846] \times 12 \times 30 = [V_T' - 154] \times 480$$
$$304{,}560 = 480\ V_T' - 73{,}920$$
$$378{,}480 = 480\ V_T'$$
$$788\text{ ml} = V_T'$$

The solution is to reduce the patient's tidal volume from 1000 to 788 ml.

c. Choose the appropriate rate for mechanical ventilation. (IIIC7) [R, Ap, An]

See Table 1-2 for a listing of the normal resting respiratory frequencies based on age. If the patient is apneic and has a normal temperature and an appropriately set tidal volume, the respiratory rates in the indicated ranges will produce a normal Pa_{CO_2} level. This must be confirmed by arterial blood gas measurements. If the tidal volume cannot be changed, adjusting the respiratory rate will modify alveolar ventilation. A higher respiratory rate, while everything else remains the same, will result in a lower Pa_{CO_2} level. Conversely, a lower respiratory rate, while everything else remains the same, will result in a higher Pa_{CO_2} level.

See Fig. 14-2 for the Radford nomogram for predicting a normal respiratory rate and tidal volume based on body weights. It can be used to establish an initial rate for most patients. As mentioned earlier, chronically hypercapneic patients must be ventilated with some caution. It is not uncommon for these patients to have a higher than normal respiratory rate. To give this type of patient a higher ventilator-delivered rate and larger tidal volume may result in blowing off too much carbon dioxide and causing a respiratory alkalosis. Care must be taken to ensure that the patient's tidal volume, rate, and minute volume (see later discussion) are such that the chronically high Pa_{CO_2} level is maintained. This elevated carbon dioxide level may be gradually decreased over a period of hours by adjusting the tidal volume or rate. Adult patients with severe chronic restrictive lung disease or those who have had a pneumonectomy may need respiratory rates of 20 to 30 per minute or greater to meet their minute volume needs. This is because their delivered tidal volume must be smaller than normal because of their condition.

The same formula can be used to help predict what respiratory rate will produce a desired Pa_{CO_2} value:

$$[V_T - (V_{D_{anat}} + V_{D_{mech}})] \times f \times Pa_{CO_2} = [V_T - (V_{D_{anat}} + V_{D_{mech}})] \times f' \times Pa_{CO_2}'$$

where

- V_T = current tidal volume.
- $V_{D_{anat}}$ = anatomic dead space. This is calculated at 1 ml/lb or 2.2 ml/kg of ideal body weight.
- $V_{D_{mech}}$ = added mechanical dead space.
- f = the ventilator rate.
- f' = desired ventilator rate.
- Pa_{CO_2} = actual patient Pa_{CO_2} value.
- Pa_{CO_2}' = desired patient Pa_{CO_2}' = value.

Example:

The patient is the same 70-kg (154-lb) man who is being ventilated on the control mode (he is apneic). His ventilator settings are a tidal volume of 1000 ml, rate of 12 times/min, F_{IO_2} of 0.3, and no added mechanical dead space. His arterial blood gas values are a Pa_{CO_2} of 90 mm Hg, Pa_{CO_2} of 30 mm Hg, pH of 7.48, Sa_{O_2} of 95%, and a BE of 0.

The clinical goal is to adjust the patient's ventilator rate as needed to produce a Pa_{CO_2} of 40 mm Hg. In summary:

V_T = 1000 ml current tidal volume.
$V_{D_{anat}}$ = 154 ml anatomic dead space. This is calculated at 1 ml/lb or 2.2 ml/kg of ideal body weight.
$V_{D_{mech}}$ = no added mechanical dead space.
f = 12 for the current ventilator rate.
f' = desired ventilator rate.
Pa_{CO_2} = 30 mm Hg actual patient Pa_{CO_2} value.
Pa_{CO_2}' = 40 mm Hg desired patient Pa_{CO_2} value.

Placing the data and goal into the formula results in the following:

$$[V_T - (V_{D_{anat}} + V_{D_{mech}})] \times f \times Pa_{CO_2} = [V_T - (V_{D_{anat}} + V_{D_{mech}})] \times f' \times Pa_{CO_2}'$$

$$[1000 - (154 + 0)] \times 12 \times 30 = [1000 - (154 + 0)] \times f' \times 40$$

Simplifying produces:

$$[846] \times 12 \times 30 = [846] \times f' \times 40$$

$$304{,}560 = 33{,}840\, f'$$

$$9 = f'$$

The solution is to reduce the patient's respiratory rate from 12 to 9 breaths/min.

d. Choose the appropriate minute ventilation for mechanical ventilation. (IIIC7) [R, Ap, An]

The subjects of minute ventilation and alveolar minute ventilation were covered in Section 4—pulmonary function testing.

Normal minute volume is based on a normal metabolism, cardiopulmonary system, tidal volume, and respiratory rate. A man's minute ventilation is usually four times his body surface area. A woman's minute ventilation is usually 3.5 times her body surface

DUBOIS BODY SURFACE CHART

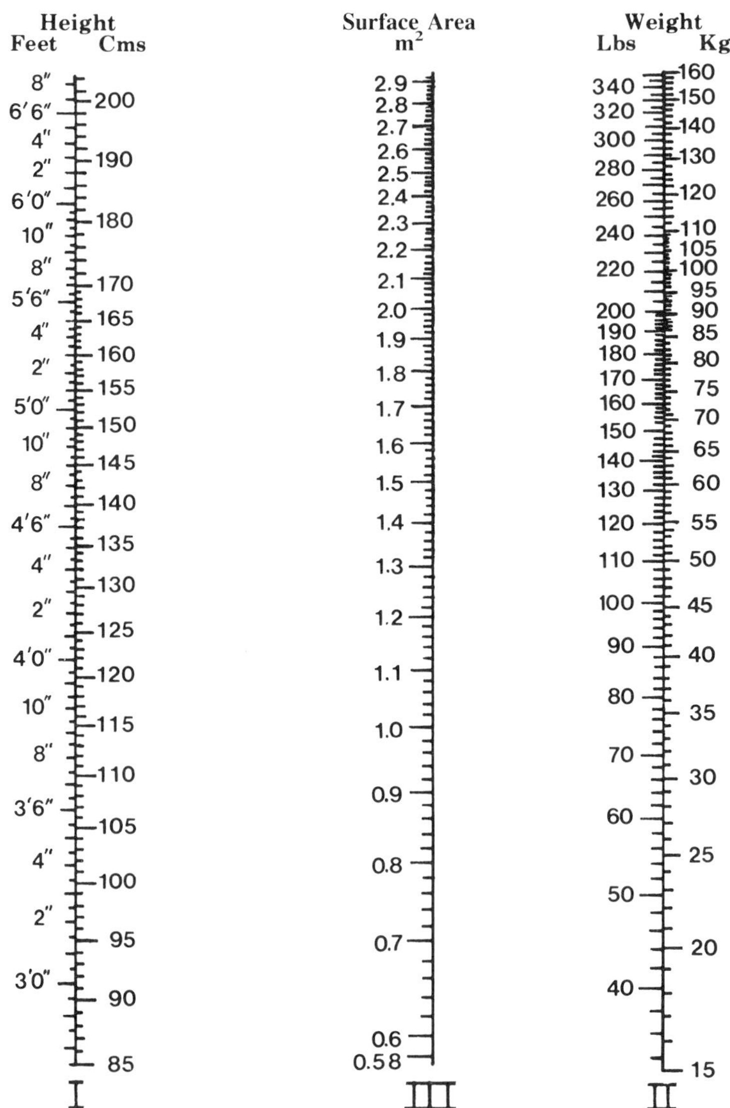

Fig. 14-3 DuBois body surface chart (as prepared by Bothby and Sandlford of the Mayo Clinic). Directions: To find body surface of a patient, locate the height in inches (or centimeters) on scale I and weight in pounds (or kilograms) on scale II and place a straight edge (ruler) between these two points, which will intersect scale III at the patient's surface area. (From Pilbeam SP: *Mechanical Ventilation: Physiological and Clinical Applications.* St Louis, Mosby, 1986. Used by permission.)

area. Body surface area (BSA) is calculated by using either the DuBois Body Surface Area chart seen in Fig. 14-3 or the following formula:

$$\text{BSA} = 0.007184 \times \text{height in centimeters} \times \text{weight in kilograms}$$

The following factors can cause a patient to have a *larger* than normal minute ventilation:

- Increased anatomic or alveolar dead space
- Increased temperature
- Increased metabolism
- Metabolic acidosis
- Increased shunt
- Pain or anxiety

The following factors can cause a patient to have a *smaller* than normal minute ventilation:

- Decreased anatomic or alveolar dead space
- Decreased temperature
- Decreased metabolism
- Metabolic alkalosis
- Sedation

The previously mentioned patient data would result in the following minute volume calculation:

- Minute volume = $V_T \times f$ (**Note:** Corrected tidal volume should be used if the patient is on a mechanical ventilator.)
- Minute volume = 1000 ml × 12
- Minute volume = 12,000 ml

Remember that tidal volume can be found by dividing minute volume by rate.
The previous patient data would result in the following minute alveolar volume calculation:

- Minute alveolar volume = $(V_T - V_{D_{anat}}) \times f$
- Minute alveolar volume = (1000 ml − 154 ml) × 12
- Minute alveolar volume = 846 × 12
- Minute alveolar volume = 10,152 ml

Blood gases must always be evaluated for the Pa_{CO_2} level to tell whether the patient's minute ventilation is adequate. A high carbon dioxide level indicates a need to increase the tidal volume, respiratory rate, or both. A low carbon dioxide indicates a need to decrease the tidal volume, respiratory rate, or both. In both cases, the key to modifying the carbon dioxide level is to modify the alveolar ventilation. That is best accomplished by changing the tidal volume rather than the rate.
The following formula can be used to calculate a change in the minute volume:

$$\dot{V}_E' = \frac{Pa_{CO_2} \times \dot{V}_E}{Pa_{CO_2}'}$$

where

- $\dot{V}_E'$ = unknown desired minute volume.
- $\dot{V}_E$ = current minute volume.
- Pa_{CO_2} = current carbon dioxide level.
- Pa_{CO_2}' = desired carbon dioxide level.

Example:

The patient is the same 70-kg (154-lb) man who is being ventilated on the control mode (he is apneic). His ventilator settings are a tidal volume of 1000 ml, rate of 12 times/min, F_{IO_2} of 0.3, and no added mechanical dead space. His arterial blood gas values are a Pa_{O_2} of 90 mm Hg, Pa_{CO_2} of 30 mm Hg, pH of 7.48, Sa_{O_2} of 95%, and a BE of 0.

The clinical goal is to adjust the patient's minute volume as needed to produce a Pa_{CO_2} value of 40 mm Hg. In summary:

V_T = 1000 ml current tidal volume.
f = 12 times/min for the current ventilator rate.
$\dot{V}_E$ = 12,000 ml current minute volume.
Pa_{CO_2} = 30 mm Hg actual patient Pa_{CO_2} value.
Pa_{CO_2}' = 40 mm Hg desired patient Pa_{CO_2} value.

Placing the data and goal into the formula results in the following:

$$\dot{V}_E' = \frac{Pa_{CO_2} \times \dot{V}_E}{Pa_{CO_2}'}$$

$$\dot{V}_E' = \frac{30 \times 12,000}{40}$$

$$\dot{V}_E' = \frac{360,000}{40}$$

$$\dot{V}_E' = 9000 \text{ ml}$$

The goal can be accomplished by reducing the minute volume from 12,000 to 9000 ml. As mentioned earlier, this is best done by reducing the tidal volume. Remember that the tidal volume must be kept at no less than 10 ml/kg of ideal body weight to avoid the development of atelectasis. The respiratory rate may be decreased, if necessary, to provide this reduced minute volume.

e. Begin and modify continuous mechanical ventilation when the settings are ordered by the physician. (IIIC9) [R, Ap, An]

Typical ventilator orders include the following:

- Mode such as control, assist/control, IMV, SIMV, or pressure support
- Oxygen percentage
- Respiratory rate
- Tidal volume or minute volume
- Sigh volume and frequency
- Special settings such as mechanical dead space, PEEP, or CPAP

The respiratory care practitioner is commonly asked to set the following ventilator controls based on department protocol or the patient's condition and response to the ventilator.

Sensitivity

Sensitivity is usually set at about −1 to −2 cm H_2O pressure. The patient should not have to work very hard to trigger a machine tidal volume.

Flow

Flow is adjusted to set the inspiratory time and inspiratory/expiratory (I/E) ratio to meet the patient's needs.

I/E Ratio

The I/E ratio is adjusted to ensure that the patient can inhale in as physiologically appropriate a manner as possible and completely exhale the inspired tidal volume.

Alarms

Alarm systems are different for each type of ventilator. Generally speaking, they are set with a safety margin of ± 10% from the patient's normal ventilator settings. A variation of greater than 10% results in an audible or visual alarm condition.

Gas Temperature

The goal for most patients is to minimize their humidity deficit by giving gas that is humidified and warmed to near body temperature. It is common to see the gas warmed to 90 to 95° F (35° C). This decreases the patient's humidity deficit to a miniscule level and reduces the "rainout" of water vapor condensing in the ventilator circuit. A temperature probe should be placed in the inspiratory tubing as close to the patient as possible to monitor the inspired gas temperature. This goal can be accomplished by either a cascade- or wick-type humidifier or a heat moisture exchanger.

f. Begin and modify intermittent mandatory ventilation (IMV), synchronous intermittent mandatory ventilation (SIMV), and pressure support ventilation (PSV) modes. (IIIC10) [R, Ap, An]

IMV came into use in 1971 as a modification of the ventilator circuit in an attempt to better ventilate neonates. Because of the rapid respiratory rate and small tidal volumes of newborns, the existing assist/control-type ventilators were unable to meet their needs. IMV is designed to give the patient a set, timed machine respiratory rate and tidal volume. The patient can breathe at any spontaneous rate and tidal volume desired in between the machine-delivered breaths. IMV has been used for adults since 1973 and has been shown to be an effective mode of ventilation for them as well.

IMV is most successful on patients who have the ability to take in a breath at least as deep as their anatomic dead space and those who have a moderate spontaneous respiratory rate and have fairly normal airway resistance and lung compliance. These patients are able to ventilate alveoli, prevent atrophy of the diaphragm and other muscles of ventilation, and not have an exhausting work of breathing. IMV has been shown, in these types of patients, to be an excellent mode of ventilation when weaning the patient off of the ventilator. The patient is able to rest during mechanical breaths and gradually take over more of the work of breathing as the machine rate is reduced. The mechanical tidal volume breath should be large enough to prevent atelectasis and acts like a sigh.

An additional benefit of IMV is that it reduces the negative effects of mechanical ventilation on the return of venous blood to the heart. As with IPPB, the positive-pressure breath delivered by the ventilator may decrease venous return to the heart and decrease cardiac output. An IMV patient who takes a spontaneous breath restores the normal venous return to the heart.

SIMV was designed into the next generation of ventilators with a demand valve for the additional flow. It was also designed into these units as a standard ventilating mode. This was accomplished by designing a special timing feature into the SIMV control. A "time window" was created in which the patient can take a spontaneous breath and trigger the machine to deliver the set tidal volume. Any other spontaneous breaths in that time window were totally determined by the patient.

SIMV has all of the benefits of IMV, and, in addition, it avoids the occurrence of "breath stacking" that is seen with some patients on IMV systems. This term was coined to describe what happened when the patient took in a spontaneous tidal volume and then had the IMV breath "stacked" on top of it. Some practitioners believed that this was a problem because patients would sometimes find the extra large volume uncomfortable or would be induced to cough. Other practitioners believed that breath stacking could actually be beneficial because it gave the patient a large sigh volume. A discussion of equipment and circuit specifications is found below:

A. Indications for IMV or SIMV:
   1. The patient has the ability to provide some but not all of the minute volume needs.
   2. The patient's cardiopulmonary condition that necessitated mechanical ventilation is at least stable if not improving.
   3. Optimally, the patient is conscious and cooperative and wishes to breathe spontaneously.

B. Initiation of IMV or SIMV:
   1. Prepare the circuit. Make sure that the oxygen percentage is the same for both the ventilator and the IMV/SIMV breaths.
   2. Commonly the sigh control is turned off when IMV/SIMV is used.
   3. Remove any mechanical dead space. It is not needed and may actually force the patient to work harder to breath more deeply to overcome its effect.
   4. With IMV, the sensitivity control must be turned off because the patient

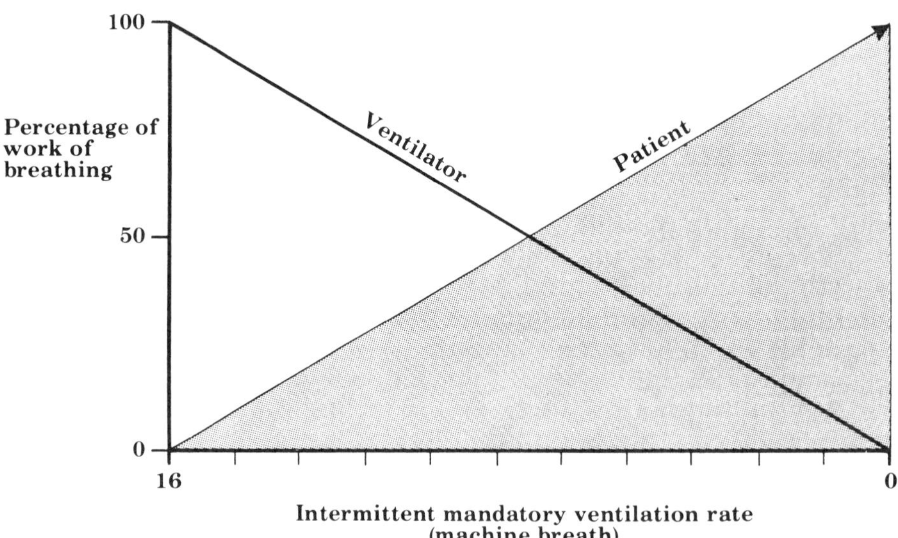

Fig. 14-4 The percentage of work of breathing and minute volume varies inversely between the ventilator and the patient when the IMV mode is used. As the IMV rate and minute volume fraction is reduced, the patient must make up the difference. (Adapted from Pilbeam SP: *Mechanical Ventilation: Physiological and Clinical Applications.* St Louis, Mosby, 1986. Used by permission.)

should not trigger any more machine breaths than ordered. With SIMV, the sensitivity control must be set so that the patient has to generate only about −1 to −2 cm H_2O pressure to trigger an SIMV breath. Make sure that the demand valve is functioning properly.
5. Inform the patient of what you are doing before starting IMV/SIMV.

The patient receiving IMV or SIMV has a ventilator rate (and tidal volume) that is intended to provide some fraction of the patient's total minute volume needs. It is especially important to closely observe these patients for signs of fatigue. Blood gas values must be obtained on a regular basis to document the patient's success or failure at the ventilator settings. Be prepared to decrease the ventilator rate (providing less support) if the patient is getting stronger. Conversely, be prepared to increase the ventilator rate (providing more support) if the patient is becoming weaker. Commonly, IMV/SIMV rate changes are made in steps of about two per minute depending on the patient's condition and response (Fig. 14-4). See Table 14-2 for factors that indicate the patient's tolerance of IMV/SIMV.

As stated earlier, pressure support ventilation (PSV) is similar to IPPB in that when the patient initiates a ventilator breath, a preset pressure is delivered to the airway. That pressure and the patient's cardiopulmonary condition determine the tidal volume. In addition, the patient has the flexibility to determine the respiratory rate, minute volume, inspiratory flow through a demand valve, and I/E ratio. PSV can be used as a mode by itself or combined with IMV/SIMV or pressure control ventilation in some current generation ventilators. There are two PSV options depending on the clinical goal: (a) deliver a desired tidal volume or (b) overcome the patient's calculated airway resistance.

When the pressure support level is adjusted to deliver a tidal volume, it is called

Table 14-2. Indications of IMV/SIMV Tolerance*

Indications IMV/SIMV is being well tolerated
Stable spontaneous respiratory rate
Stable heart rate
Stable spontaneous tidal volume
Stable vital capacity, MIP, and or FEV_1
No use or stable use of accessory muscles of ventilation
Patient indicates he is comfortable
Stable blood gases
Indications IMV/SIMV is not being well tolerated
Increased spontaneous respiratory rate
Tachycardia or dysrhythmias such as premature ventricular contractions
A drop in the spontaneous tidal volume
A drop in the vital capacity, MIP, and or FEV_1
Beginning or increased use of accessory muscles of ventilation
Patient complains of dyspnea
Deterioration of blood gases as seen by a falling Pao_2 or Spo_2 level and a rapidly falling or rising $Paco_2$ level

**IMV*, Intermittent mandatory ventilation; *SIMV*, synchronous intermittent mandatory ventilation; *MIP*, maxium inspiratory pressure; *FEV_1*, forced expiratory volume in 1 sec; *Pao_2*, arterial O_2 pressure; *Spo_2*, pulse oximetry.

PSV_{max} (for maximum pressure support ventilation). The clinical guidelines for PSV_{max} are:

a. Use enough pressure to deliver a tidal volume of 10 to 12 ml/kg of ideal body weight.
b. The patient should have to not assist the ventilator at a rate greater than 20 times/min to achieve acceptable arterial blood gas values.

PSV_{max} has been used in patients who have had acute respiratory failure that is resolving. Usually these patients have been maintained on the assist/control mode for several days to minimize their work of breathing while undergoing treatment for their condition. It is believed that PSV_{max} is ideal for reconditioning their diaphragm and other respiratory muscles. Reconditioning occurs when the assist or "trigger" pressure for the breathe is kept at low as possible (-1 to -2 cm H_2O pressure) and the tidal volume large. This pattern results in a low respiratory muscle work load. As the patient continues to improve, the PSV level is reduced. The patient's tidal volume will be stable if the patient passively takes in the PSV supported breath. Or, the tidal volume can be larger if the patient interacts actively with the pressure that is delivered. See Fig. 14-1, E for the pressure/time curve.

The pressure support level has also been used as a way to overcome the airway resistance caused by the patient's endotracheal tube. It has been believed that too small an endotracheal tube prevents some patients from successfully weaning by the IMV/SIMV mode. The addition of enough pressure support to overcome the additional work of breathing caused by the tube enables the patient to wean successfully and airway to be extubated. The patient's total airway resistance (airways and endotracheal tube) can be determined by this formula:

$$\text{Airway resistance } (R_{aw}) = \frac{\text{peak airway pressure} - \text{plateau pressure}}{\text{flow (in L/sec)}}$$

Flow in liters per second is found by taking the inspiratory flow in liters per minute and dividing it by 60 seconds.

For example, determine the pressure support level to set to overcome the airway resistance of a mechanically ventilated patient with the following parameters: inspiratory flow of 40 L/min, peak airway pressure of 40 cm H_2O, and plateau pressure of 30 cm H_2O.

$$\text{Flow} = \frac{40 \text{ L/min}}{60 \text{ seconds}} = 0.67 \text{ L/sec}$$

$$\text{Airway resistance } (R_{aw}) = \frac{\text{peak airway pressure} - \text{plateau pressure}}{\text{flow (in L/sec)}}$$

$$R_{aw} = \frac{40 - 30}{0.67} = \frac{10}{0.67} = 15 \text{ cm } H_2O\text{/L/sec}$$

Set the pressure support level at 15 cm H_2O to overcome the resistance of the endotracheal tube. Any greater pressure is delivering some tidal volume. It could be argued that using a pressure to match a resistance is like comparing "apples to oranges." They are not the same. However, the practice seems to be widely accepted clinically.

The pressure support level is reduced, as tolerated, when the patient's lung-thoracic compliance or airway resistance improves. As both return toward normal, the only barrier to extubation is the resistance offered by the endotracheal tube. Some practitioners advocate extubation when the PSV level is 10 cm H_2O or less. This is probably the pressure level needed to overcome the tube's resistance. So, the patient should tolerate extubation without any increase in the work of breathing.

2. Perform the following procedures to make sure that the patient is adequately oxygenated.

a. Minimize hypoxemia by positioning the patient properly. (IIID1) [R, Ap]

This was discussed in Section 5 on oxygen therapy.

b. Administer oxygen, as needed, to prevent hypoxemia. (IIID2) [R, Ap]

Oxygen administration and adjustment were discussed in Sections 3 and 5. Briefly, the goal of oxygen administration is to keep the Pa_{O_2} level of most patients between 60 and 90 mm Hg and the Sp_{O_2} level greater than 90%. Exceptions are the patient who is breathing on hypoxic drive and the patient who is in a cardiac arrest situation. The chronic obstructive pulmonary disease (COPD) patient who has a chronically low Pa_{O_2} level and chronically high Pa_{CO_2} level may be allowed to have a Pa_{O_2} as low as 50 to 55 mm Hg; Sp_{O_2} level as low as 85%. The patient in cardiac arrest must be given 100% oxygen. The following formula can be used to help guide the use of supplemental oxygen in most stable patients. Those patients who have refractory hypoxemia (e.g., adult respiratory distress syndrome [ARDS]) will not respond with a normal increase in Pa_{O_2} level as the oxygen percentage is increased.

$$\text{Desired } F_{IO_2} = \frac{\text{desired } Pa_{O_2} \times \text{current } F_{IO_2}}{\text{current } Pa_{O_2}}$$

Example:

Your patient has a Pa_{O_2} level of 55 mm Hg on 30% oxygen. The clinical goal is a Pa_{O_2} level of 90 mm Hg. What oxygen percentage should the patient have?

$$\text{Desired } F_{IO_2} = \frac{\text{desired } Pa_{O_2} \times \text{current } F_{IO_2}}{\text{current } Pa_{O_2}}$$

$$\text{Desired } F_{IO_2} = \frac{90 \text{ mm Hg} \times 0.3}{55}$$

$$\text{Desired } F_{IO_2} = \frac{27}{55}$$

$$\text{Desired } F_{IO_2} = 0.49 \text{ or } 49\% \text{ oxygen}$$

In the short term, use whatever oxygen percentage is needed to achieve the clinical goal. The risk of oxygen toxicity increases when the F_{IO_2} is greater than 0.5 for periods of more than 48 hours. Always recheck the patient's arterial oxygen level after a change has been made in the F_{IO_2}.

Either of the following formulas can be used in the special situation of determining the flows of air and oxygen into a "bleed in" type of IMV or CPAP system to obtain an ordered F_{IO_2}. Either version can also be used for determining the gas flows, total flow, and oxygen/air ratio through an air entrainment (venturi) mask.

First version:

$$(\text{L/min air} \times F_{IO_2} \text{ of air}) + (\text{L/min } O_2 \times F_{IO_2} \text{ pure } O_2) = \text{total flow} \times \text{desired } F_{IO_2}$$

Second version:

$$F_1C_1 + F_2C_2 = F_TC_T$$

where

F_1 = flow of first gas (oxygen)
C_1 = concentration of oxygen in the first gas (1.0 for pure oxygen)
F_2 = flow of second gas (air)
C_2 = concentration of oxygen in the second gas (0.21 for air)
F_T = total flow of both gases
C_T = concentration of oxygen in the mix of both gases

Algebraic manipulation enables the practitioner to solve for the unknown.

Example:

Determine the oxygen percentage through a bleed in system that has an oxygen flow of 10 L/min and an air flow of 15 L/min. Determine the total flow through the system. Determine the ratio of oxygen to air.
First version:

$$(\text{L/min air} \times F_{IO_2}) + (\text{L/min } O_2 \times F_{IO_2}\ O_2) = \text{total flow} \times \text{desired } F_{IO_2}$$

$$(15 \times 0.21) + (10 \times 1.0) = (15 + 10) \times \text{desired } F_{IO_2}$$

$$(3.15) + (10) = (25) \times \text{desired } F_{IO_2}$$

$$13.15 = 25 \text{ desired } F_{IO_2} \text{ (Divide both sides by 25.)}$$

$$0.526,\ 52.6\% = F_{IO_2}$$

$$\text{Total flow} = 15 + 10 = 25 \text{ L/min}$$

$$\text{Ratio} = \frac{10 \text{ L/min oxygen}}{15 \text{ L/min air}}$$

c. Adequately oxygenate the patient before and after suctioning, changing the ventilator circuit or performing other procedures where the patient is disconnected from the ventilator to prevent accidental hypoxemia. (IIID3) [R, Ap]

Ensuring adequate oxygenation was discussed in Sections 5 and 12. Briefly, remember to give the adult patient 100% oxygen for at least 30 seconds before suctioning. Perform the task as quickly and safely as possible to minimize time off of the ventilator. Leave the patient on 100% oxygen for at least 1 minute after the procedure or until he or she returns to a stable condition as before. Children younger than 6 months of age can have the F_{IO_2} increased by 10% for the procedure. It is acceptable to increase the inspired oxygen up to 100% before and after a procedure that requires disconnection from the ventilator. The goal is to prevent hypoxemia. The patient should be manually ventilated with a resuscitation bag if indicated. Always remember to return the patient to the original oxygen percentage when clinically indicated.

d. Begin and modify PEEP therapy. (IIID5) [R, Ap]

PEEP has been used since 1969 as a means to increase a patient's functional residual capacity (FRC) and thereby increase the Pa_{O_2} level. The FRC is important because it is the volume of air left in the lungs at the end of a normal exhalation. It keeps the alveoli open and helps to moderate the arterial oxygen levels throughout the respiratory cycle.

PEEP is generally indicated in any bilateral, generalized pulmonary condition where the FRC is decreased. Examples include generalized atelectasis, pulmonary edema, and conditions where surfactant is diminished or absent as in adult respiratory distress syndrome (ARDS) and infant respiratory distress syndrome (IRDS). All of these patients show a decreased lung compliance as measured by their static compliance (C_{st}).

Specific indications for PEEP include:

- Intrapulmonary shunt greater than 15%.
- Refractory hypoxemia (Pao_2 <60 mm Hg despite an Fio_2 of up to 0.8 to 1.0).
- The patient has had an Fio_2 of greater than 0.5 for 48 to 72 hours and shows no indication of a rapidly improving Pao_2, so that the Fio_2 can be lowered to a safer level.

Before PEEP is begun, the patient should be carefully monitored to establish the baseline condition. The same parameters should be monitored after each change in the PEEP level to determine how the patient is tolerating it. The best or optimal level of PEEP is the level that results in the best delivery of oxygen to the tissues (not necessarily the arterial blood). Often, a secondary goal is to reduce the inspired oxygen to a safe level. The patient is at risk of oxygen toxicity if more than 50% oxygen is inhaled for more than 48 to 72 hours. See Table 14-3 for recommendations on what to monitor during the application of PEEP and how to evaluate the data.

Table 14-3. Patient Monitoring During PEEP or CPAP Therapy*

Good tolerance of PEEP/CPAP therapy:

- Increased Pao_2 level
- Increased static lung compliance
- Stable cardiac output as shown by
  - Stable heart rate without rhythm disturbances
  - Stable blood pressure
  - The following can be measured only through a Swan-Ganz/pulmonary artery catheter:
    - Stable or increased $P\bar{v}o_2$
    - Stable cardiac output
    - Decreased pulmonary vascular resistance
    - Decreased intrapulmonary shunt

Poor tolerance of PEEP/CPAP therapy:

- Increased Pao_2 level (This can be deceiving if it is all you look at.)
- Decreased static lung compliance
- Decreased cardiac output as shown by
  - Increased heart rate and/or rhythm disturbances
  - Decreased blood pressure
  - The following can be measured only through a Swan-Ganz/pulmonary artery catheter:
    - Decreased $P\bar{v}o_2$
    - Decreased actual cardiac output
    - Increased pulmonary vascular resistance
    - Increased intrapulmonary shunt

**PEEP,* Positive end-expiratory pressure; *CPAP,* continuous positive airway pressure; *Pao_2;* arterial O_2 pressure; *$P\bar{v}o_2$,* mixed venous O_2.

The application of PEEP is not without risks. Like many situations where good and bad can come from something, these risks are weighted against the potential benefit to the patient. In the profoundly hypoxemic patient, PEEP can be a lifesaver. In the patient whose lungs are recovering, excessive levels of PEEP can result in the problems on the list that follows. PEEP is *never* indicated in a patient with normal lungs or overly complaint lungs (e.g., in emphysema). These problems can be fatal if severe enough.

Hazards of PEEP include:

- Pulmonary barotrauma:
  - Pneumothorax
  - Tension pneumothorax
  - Mediastinal emphysema
  - Pulmonary interstitial emphysema (PIE) in the neonate
  - Subcutaneous emphysema
- Decreased venous return to the heart, causing a decreased cardiac output and:
  - Tachycardia
  - Decreased blood pressure
  - Decreased tissue perfusion as measured by a decreased mixed venous oxygen ($P\bar{v}O_2$) level
  - Decreased urine output

PEEP therapy is usually begun at initial levels of 2 to 5 cm H_2O. After the patient's response is determined, 2 to 5 cm more PEEP may be applied. The patient is reevaluated. This process goes on until the best or optimal level of PEEP is determined (Fig. 14-5).

As the patient begins to recover, the PEEP level may be reduced in steps of 2 to 5 cm H_2O. Again, the patient is evaluated after every change in the PEEP level. If the patient's cardiovascular status is normal, the following are recommendations for how to decrease PEEP and oxygen levels:

- Decrease PEEP first if the PaO_2 level is greater than 60 mm Hg and the FIO_2 is less than 0.5.
- Decrease oxygen first if the PaO_2 level is greater than 60 mm Hg and the FIO_2 is greater than 0.5.

e. Begin and modify continuous positive airway pressure (CPAP). (IIID4) [R, Ap]

CPAP has the same indications, hazards, and patient evaluation processes discussed earlier in PEEP therapy. One possible physiologic benefit of CPAP over PEEP is that there is less reduction in the venous return to the heart. This is because with CPAP the patient is breathing spontaneously. During inspiration the airway pressure level becomes less positive than the baseline pressure. With PEEP, the baseline pressure is stable. Overall, a patient receiving control or assist/control ventilation with PEEP has a higher intrathoracic pressure than does a patient undergoing CPAP therapy. Therefore, patients treated by CPAP may be able to tolerate higher pressure levels than those patients being ventilated with PEEP therapy.

CPAP is usually increased and decreased in steps of 2 to 5 cm H_2O. As with PEEP, the patient is evaluated before CPAP is begun and again after every pressure change. See Table 14-3 for recommendations on what to monitor during the application of CPAP and how to evaluate the data.

Before a patient receives CPAP therapy, the practitioner and physician must be assured that the patient has the ability to breathe adequately to eliminate carbon dioxide. CPAP is contraindicated in an apneic patient or one who may become apneic. (This pa-

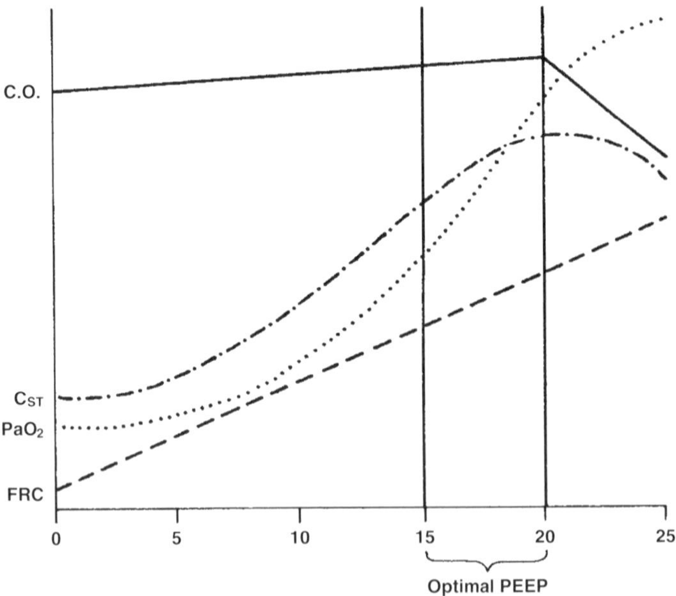

Fig. 14-5 The optimal or best positive end-expiratory pressure (PEEP) level is determined by monitoring arterial oxygen pressure (Pa_{O_2}) levels, static compliance *(C_{st})*, and cardiac output *(C.O.)*. As the functional residual capacity (FRC) is increased by PEEP, lung compliance is improved and ventilation and perfusion are better matched. Cardiac output should remain stable. It can be measured by the use of the proper pulmonary artery (Swan-Ganz) catheter or indirectly followed by monitoring the patient's heart rate and blood pressure. As can be seen, the optimal PEEP is found between 15 and 20 cm H_2O. Excessive PEEP is seen by the resulting drop in static compliance and cardiac output (rising heart rate and falling blood pressure). (Adapted from Pilbeam SP: *Methanical Ventilation: Physiological and Clinical Applications.* St Louis, Mosby, 1986.)

tient needs to undergo ventilation in the control or assist/control mode.) The patient must have an adequate respiratory rate, tidal volume, and minute volume. The heart rate and blood pressure should be stable. Negative inspiratory force and vital capacity values may be acceptable or low. Blood gas analysis typically shows refractory hypoxemia but a normal or low Pa_{CO_2} level. This shows that the patient would benefit from an elevated baseline pressure to increase the FRC but is quite capable of ventilating.

The patient must be carefully monitored for fatigue because the patient is providing all of the minute ventilation. Signs of fatigue include increasing respiratory rate, decreasing tidal volume or vital capacity, decreasing negative inspiratory force, and tachycardia. Blood gas measurement may show a stable or decreasing Pa_{O_2} value. A rising Pa_{CO_2} level is a definite sign of fatigue. The patient may complain of dyspnea. The practitioner will notice the patient is working harder than normal to breathe, as shown by the increased use of the accessory muscles of ventilation and heavy perspiration. When these signs occur, CPAP therapy should be discontinued and mechanical ventilation instituted in a mode that best fits the patient's needs.

3. Recommend and administer the following types of prescribed medications to mechanically ventilated patients so that they can be effectively ventilated and airway secretions can be removed: aerosolized bronchodilators, corticosteroids, saline solution, mucolytics, and cromolyn sodium. (IIIB2g and IIIF9d) [R, Ap, An]

See Section 8 for details on the various medications. They can be administered either by a metered dose inhaler or nebulizer as used with IPPB.

Usually the nebulizer is placed in line with the inspiratory tubing at least 18 inches back from the Y or at the manifold of the circuit. This position prevents the nebulizer from acting as mechanical dead space in the circuit. The inspiratory tubing also acts as a medication reservoir for the next inspiration (Fig. 14-6).

If a metered dose inhaler is used, a T-piece (e.g., a Briggs adapter) will have to be fitted into the circuit as described earlier. The practitioner must carefully time when to activate the dispenser so that the medication is inhaled at the start of the next tidal volume breath. A sigh volume would deliver the medication ever deeper into the lungs.

An IPPB-like nebulizer (as shown in Fig. 14-6) will need to be powered by a high-pressure gas source. Most modern ventilators (Puritan-Bennett 7200, BEAR 1000, etc.) are designed to power the nebulizer by diverting part of the tidal volume through the nebulizer when the nebulizer control is turned on. There is no change in the patient's oxygen percentage, tidal volume, or other ventilator parameters.

Some modern ventilators such as the Servo 900 B and C do not have this feature. Medications should be administered only by a metered dose inhaler with spacer as described in Section 7. Indeed, powering an IPPB-like nebulizer with an outside flowmeter will result in the Servo reading abnormally high volumes. An alarm condition could re-

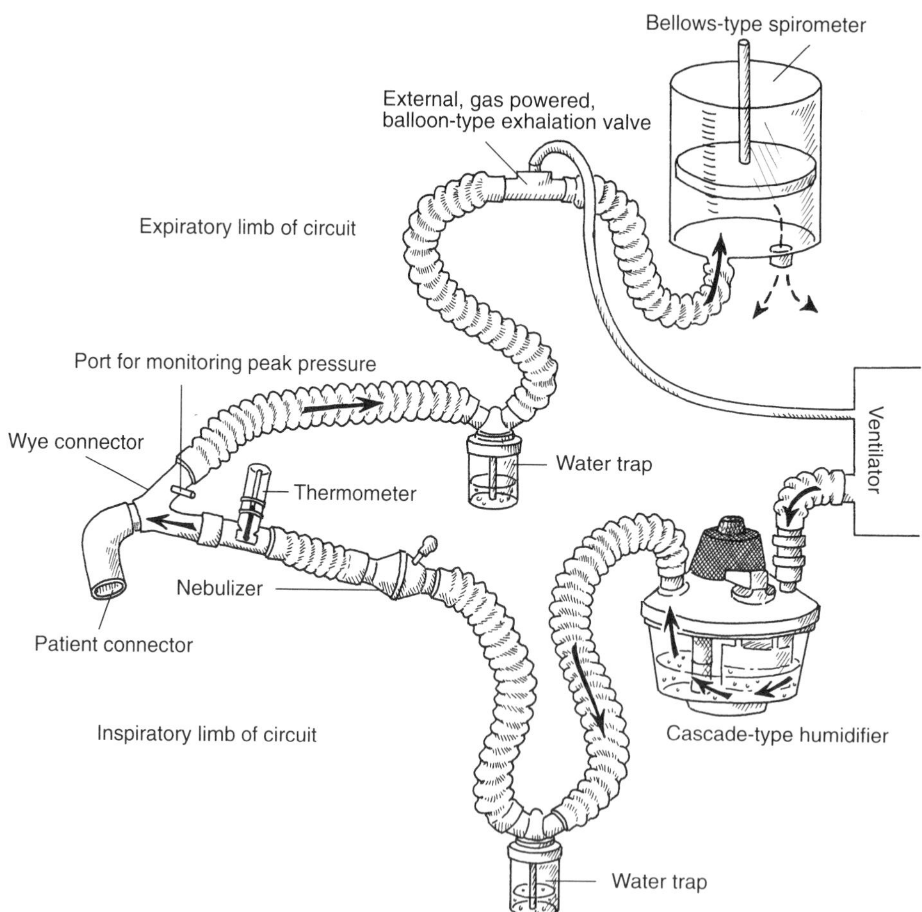

Fig. 14-6 Patient breathing circuit for continuous mechanical ventilation.

sult, or it could deliver smaller than preset volumes to compensate for the added flow. In addition, most of the medication will be wasted and will foul the internal exhalation valve and volume-measuring system.

Module B. Mechanical ventilation equipment.

Note: The literature produced by the manufacturers and the descriptions used in many standard texts break down the various ventilators into more catagories than used by the NBRC. To avoid confusion, this text uses the NBRC's more simplified terminology. A pneumatically powered ventilator will be defined here as powered by compressed gas and without any electrically powered control systems (electrically powered alarm systems may or may not be added on). An electrically powered ventilator will be defined here as being either electrically powered or controlled. Most volume cycled ventilators fall into this catagory. Microprocessor ventilators are electrically powered but controlled by one or more microprocessors (computers). Many of the most current volume cycled ventilators have microprocessors to control their functions.

1. Pneumatically powered ventilators.

a. Get the necessary equipment for the procedure. (IIA4a) [R, Ap]

The only commonly used pneumatically powered ventilators are the Bird series and the Bennett PR 2. A control or backup rate can be set on these units in case the patient is apneic. All other controls and functions are the same as discussed in Section 13. See Fig. 13-1 for the Bird Mark 7 and Fig. 13-2 and 13-3 for the Bennett PR 2 controls.

The following equipment and procedures are necessary:

1. Bennett PR 2 or Bird ventilator with an air/oxygen blender and hoses.
2. Bennett or Bird breathing circuit.
3. Bacteria filters.
4. Get the proper humidification system: either a passover- or cascade-type humidifier or a heat-moisture exchanger (discussed later on). Put sterile, distilled water in the passover- or cascade-type humidifier.
5. Get one or two water traps for condensation from the circuit.
6. Add on alarm system(s) such as a low-volume bellows spirometer or a low-pressure/disconnection alarm.
7. If a low-volume bellows spirometer alarm is used, a length of large-bore tubing will be needed to connect the exhalation valve to the bellows.

b. Put the equipment together, make sure that it works properly, and identify and fix any problems with it. (IIB5a) [R, Ap]

Refer to Figs. 13-8 and 13-9 for the IPPB circuits. The ventilator and circuits are similar to those used in IPPB therapy with the following exceptions:

a. Set the ordered oxygen percentage on the blender; set the Bird *air-mix* and Bennett *air dilution* selection controls to pure source gas from the blender. Analyze the F_{IO_2} through a port in the inspiratory limb of the circuit.

b. If a passover or cascade humidifier is used, a short length of large-bore tubing is connected between the outlet of the mainstream in-line bacteria filter and the inlet of the humidifier. The inspiratory limb of the circuit is connected to the outlet of the humidifier.

If a heat-moisture exchanger is used, it will be added between the circuit and the tracheostomy/endotracheal tube adapter (see Fig. 14-18).

c. A tracheostomy/endotracheal tube adapter will always be used to connect the circuit to the patient (see Fig. 14-18).

d. If a low-volume bellows spirometer alarm (e.g., on the MA-1 ventilator) is used, it needs to be connected to the circuit. An expiratory limb of the circuit is made by attaching one end of a length of large-bore tubing to the outlet port on the exhalation valve. (This is where the IPPB volume is measured.) The other end of the tubing is connected to the alarm. The bellows is "dumped" during inspiration by tapping into the small-bore tubing with a T-piece and connecting a length of small-bore tubing between the T and the dump mechanism on the spirometer. If a low-pressure or disconnection alarm is added, it is spliced into the inspiratory limb of the circuit with a Briggs adapter/T-adapter. The alarm is set to sound if the pressure drops about 5 cm H_2O below the peak pressure (see Module C, 4 for details).

e. Water traps are placed in the lowest part of the inspiratory and expiratory limbs of the circuit to hold any condensed water vapor.

Fig. 14-6 shows a complete circuit to a volume cycled ventilator. It is essentially the same circuit as used on a pressure cycled ventilator.

Setting the Backup Rate for Controlled Breaths

Bird Mark 7

Turn the expiratory timer control counterclockwise to decrease the expiratory time and therefore increase the backup rate. While looking through the green plastic cover to the left of the center body, it will be noticed that the stainless steel lever arm moves to the right and pushes the clutch plate. When the clutch plate contacts the center body, internal openings are lined up to allow gas to pass through to start a mechanical breath. If the lever arm does not move when the expiratory timer control is turned counterclockwise, the ventilator is defective and should not be used.

Bennett PR 2

Turn the *rate* control clockwise from the *off* position to decrease the expiratory time and therefore increase the backup rate. The ventilator will cycle on when the left accumulator reaches the bottom of its movement. The right accumulator moves down during the inhalation. If the accumulators do not cycle properly with the inspiration, the equipment is defective and should not be used. The I/E ratio is preset at 1: 1.5 when the unit is time-cycling on and off. The expiratory time can be increased by turning the *expiratory time* control clockwise.

In both the Bennett and Bird units, the backup rate must be timed and adjusted by means of a stopwatch or wristwatch with a sweep second hand. The I/E ratio may be manually adjusted by the previously mentioned controls and flow control (Bird only).

Both of these types of ventilators will send gas through the circuit during an inspiration and will not cycle off until the preset pressure is reached. Test the tightness of the circuit, backup rate, and delivered tidal volume by placing a test lung on the patient connection of the circuit. Set the controls to deliver the prescribed order. Be prepared to make final adjustments once either unit has been placed on the patient. The patient's airway resistance and lung compliance will greatly affect the functioning of both units.

Troubleshooting problems with these units were discussed in Section 13. Make sure that all connections are tight; there are more now with the addition of the humidification system and expiratory limb to the bellows spirometer.

A defective exhalation valve or one in which the small-bore tubing has popped off will send gas through the circuit and not to the patient. If a bellows spirometer is being used, you will notice that it fills during inspiration instead of during expiration as normal.

2. Electrically powered ventilators.

a. Get the necessary equipment for the procedure. (IIA4b) [R, Ap]

The majority of mechanical ventilators are electrically powered or controlled. They all are classified as volume cycled, meaning that a preset volume will be delivered from the ventilator with each breath regardless of the patient's condition. Each ventilator is unique in its abilities, modes, and so forth. It is beyond the scope of this book to discuss each and every volume-cycled ventilator. They will be presented in a generic manner. It is recommended that the learner become familiar with the functions of the Bennett MA-1, BEAR 1 and 2, and Servo 900 B and 900 C because they are widely used.

b. Put the equipment together, make sure that it works properly, and identify and fix any problems with it. (IIB5b) [R, Ap]

Each ventilator must be learned for its specifics. Generally speaking, the following steps should be taken to ensure that the ventilator is functioning properly:

1. Select the proper ventilator for the physician's orders and patient's needs.
2. Attach the circuit properly and make sure that all connections are tight (see Fig. 14-6).
3. Select the appropriate humidification device: a passover-type, cascade-type, or heat-moisture exchanger. Put sterile, distilled water in the passover or cascade unit.
4. Preset all of the physician-ordered parameters and any other settings that are needed to make the ventilator fully functional.
5. Place a test lung on the circuit at the patient connection.
6. Make sure that the ventilator delivers the preset rate, volume, oxygen percentage, I/E ratio, and so forth.

A low volume could be from a leak; check all connections, and tighten them as needed. The volume can be measured directly as it leaves the ventilator to see whether it is accurate or whether the unit is delivering the wrong volume. If the unit shows a volume entering the spirometer instead of the test lung during inspiration, the exhalation valve is broken, or the high-pressure line to it has popped off. All alarms must be working properly. Some are powered by batteries that need to be replaced when discharged.

3. Microprocessor ventilators.

a. Get the necessary equipment for the procedure. (IIA4c) [R, Ap]

The microprocessor ventilators are the most current generation of mechanical ventilators. They are electrically powered but controlled by one or more microprocessors (minicomputers). Examples include the Bennett 7200, BEAR 5 and 1000, Respironics Adult Star, Drager ERISA, and Hamilton Veolar. They all offer many modes of ventilation, including volume cycled assist/control and SIMV, pressure support, pressure control, PEEP, and CPAP. What makes these units unique compared with the electrically powered ventilators is that these modes can be added as needed by inserting a computer chip containing that feature. So, if a patient needs a particular mode not found on the ventilator, it can be easily added without changing the unit. In addition, many of these machines offer computer software for measuring bedside spirometry for weaning, work of breathing, and other parameters that give the clinician much valuable information. Airway resistance and static and dynamic lung compliance can be automatically calculated. Flow, volume, and pressure tracings are graphically displayed on the computer screen. Auto-PEEP can be documented and measured. These units offer the greatest amount of patient data and clinical flexibility of all currently available ventilators. The most challenging patients can probably be best cared for one one of these machines.

b. Put the equipment together, make sure that it works properly, and identify and any problems with it. (IIB5c) [R, Ap]

All of the previous general discussion on electrically powered ventilators applies to the microprocessor ventilators as well. An additional advantage to these units is that they self-diagnose most problems and display the problem for you. If a microprocessor should fail, the unit should be removed from the patient. The biomedical department or manufacturer will have to replace the computer chip.

4. Continuous mechanical ventilation (CMV) breathing circuits.

a. Get the necessary equipment for the procedure. (IIA11b) [R, Ap]

Either a permanent or a disposable circuit may be selected based on the type of ventilator on which it must be placed. A circuit with an external exhalation valve must be used with ventilators such as the Bennett MA-1 and MA-2 and BEAR 1 and 2. The Puritan-Bennett 7200, BEAR 5 and 1000, and Servo 900 B and C, and Respironics Adult Star feature internal exhalation valves and do not need a circuit with one. If the patient needs to receive aerosolized medications, the circuit should either include a nebulizer or be able to accept one. If not included, the nebulizer or metered dose inhaler adapter will have to added into the inspiratory limb of the circuit.

The compression factor and internal resistance of the circuit should also be considered. The compression factor is a main determinant of how much compressed volume is lost. Remember that the compressed volume is subtracted from the set tidal volume to determine the actual, delivered tidal volume. The compression factor varies with the material used to construct the circuit, the temperature of the inhaled gas, and the peak inspiratory pressure placed against the circuit. Permanent circuits have a slightly lower compression factor than disposable circuits. Some circuits have a smooth rather than a corrugated interior surface. The smooth surface causes less turbulence and results in less back pressure. So, more of the peak pressure is directed to deliver the tidal volume. A smooth bore circuit is required with the BiPAP Ventilatory Support System by Respironics, Inc. It is recommended that a low compressed volume and low resistance circuit be used whenever high pressures are required to deliver low tidal volumes. This is usually the case during high-frequency ventilation. (**Note:** Neither BiPAP nor high-frequency ventilation is listed as testable on the entry level examination. They are listed as testable on the registry examinations for therapists. They are included here only for the sake of completeness.)

A third consideration is whether to use an unheated or heated circuit. Usually the circuit is unheated. With these, a cascade-type humidifier or heat-moisture exchanger is used to warm and humidify the inspired gas. However, some practitioners prefer to use a heated circuit in the care of neonates. These circuits either have heated wires loosely running through the lumen of the tubing or have a wire embedded within the tubing itself. A heated-wire circuit offers finer control over the temperature of the inspired gas and minimizes condensation. Follow the manufacturer's guidelines to make sure that the system can adequately humidify the minute volume that is being used.

b. Put the equipment together, make sure that it works properly, and identify and fix any problems with it. (IIB9b) [R, Ap]

A number of companies produce circuits for the various types of ventilators, including the ventilator manufacturers. There is considerable variation based on the manufacturer and the type of ventilator it is designed for. Common, but not universal, features of the inspiratory limb of the circuit include:

- Water trap
- Humidification system
- Nebulizer
- Thermometer or temperature probe
- Pressure monitoring port
- Oxygen monitoring port

Common, but not universal, features of the expiratory limb of the circuit include:

- Exhalation valve
- Water trap

The heated-wire circuits must be used only with the humidifier that they are specifically designed to work with. The humidifier has a thermostat that regulates warming the humidifier water and heated wires to the same temperature. There are several other considerations when a heated-wire circuit is used. Never cover a heated-wire circuit with a patient's sheets or blanket or any other material. Do not rest the circuit on anything such as the bedrail, patient's body, or medical equipment. These circuits should always be supported on a boom arm or tube-tree.

All circuits use a Y connector to tie the inspiratory and expiratory limbs together and attach the circuit to the patient. See Fig. 14-6 for a generic CMV ventilator circuit. Make sure that the water level is properly maintained in the humidifier. Check the circuit and connections for leaks if the volume is low. Check the volume leaving the ventilator if it does not match the set and returned volume. The volume control or spirometer may be out of calibration. If the unit shows a volume entering the spirometer instead of the test lung during inspiration, the exhalation valve is broken. Replace it as needed.

c. Change the patient's ventilator circuit as needed. (IIIF8b) [R, Ap]

A circuit needs to be replaced if it is damaged in a way that prevents the patient from being ventilated. This is most commonly seen in circuits with external exhalation valves. If the valve is damaged and will not close, the circuit needs replacement.

Routine circuit changes are done for infection control purposes. It is generally recommended that the circuit and cascade-type humidification system be changed every 24 hours to minimize the chance of pathogens growing in it. Many departments are now using heat-moisture exchangers for humidification. Often departments are leaving these units and the circuit intact for several days before changing it. Infection control studies should be performed on these extended use systems to prove that they are not contaminated.

5. Ventilator breathing circuits: PEEP valve assembly.

a. Get the necessary equipment for the procedure. (IIA11d) [R, Ap]

There are a variety of PEEP systems that can be added to a ventilator or CPAP circuit (Figs. 14-7 to 14-12). Their features are discussed in the CPAP section later on.

A number of the newest generation of ventilators such as the Servo 900 B and 900 C, BEAR 5 and 1000, and Puritan-Bennett 7200 have internal exhalation valves and PEEP generating venturi systems (see Fig. 14-12). There is nothing to assemble at the bedside. Failure to generate PEEP indicates that the exhalation valve or PEEP-generating venturi system has failed in some manner.

Most other current ventilators use a balloonlike exhalation valve similar to that found

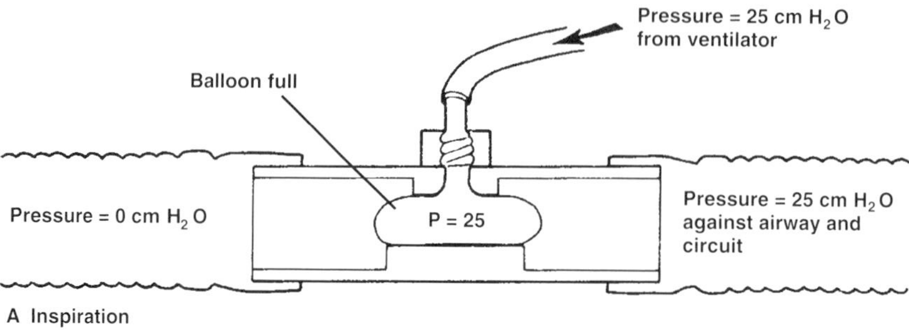

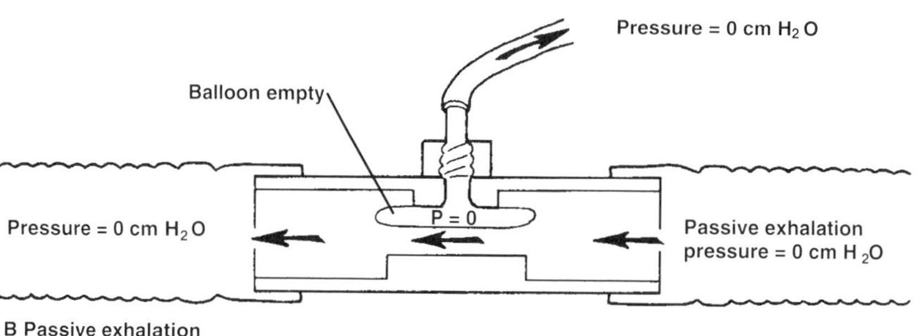

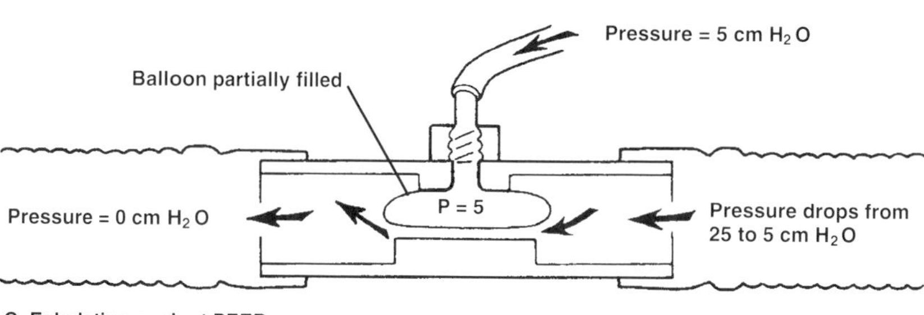

Fig. 14-7 Details of a balloon-type exhalation valve. **A,** The balloon is inflated during inspiration to block the escape of gas. **B,** The balloon is deflated during a passive exhalation to allow the escape of tidal volume gas from the patient. **C,** With exhalation against PEEP, the balloon is partially inflated with a pressure that creates the PEEP level.

in the Bennett MA-1 and BEAR 1 and 2 (see Fig. 14-7). PEEP is generated by keeping some gas in the balloon to act as a resistance to the patient's exhaled volume. There is a direct relationship between the volume of gas that is kept in the balloon, the pressure and resistance that it creates, and the PEEP level that is generated.

b. Put the equipment together, make sure that it works properly, and identify and fix any problems with it. (IIB9d) [R, Ap]

The key thing to check with any PEEP-generating system is that the proper level of PEEP is generated and maintained. This is determined by looking at how many centimeters of water pressure are seen on the ventilator's pressure manometer. Adjust the PEEP system gradually as the manometer pressure is checked. Once the ordered PEEP level is set, it should be stable throughout the respiratory cycle. Sensitivity should be set (as dis-

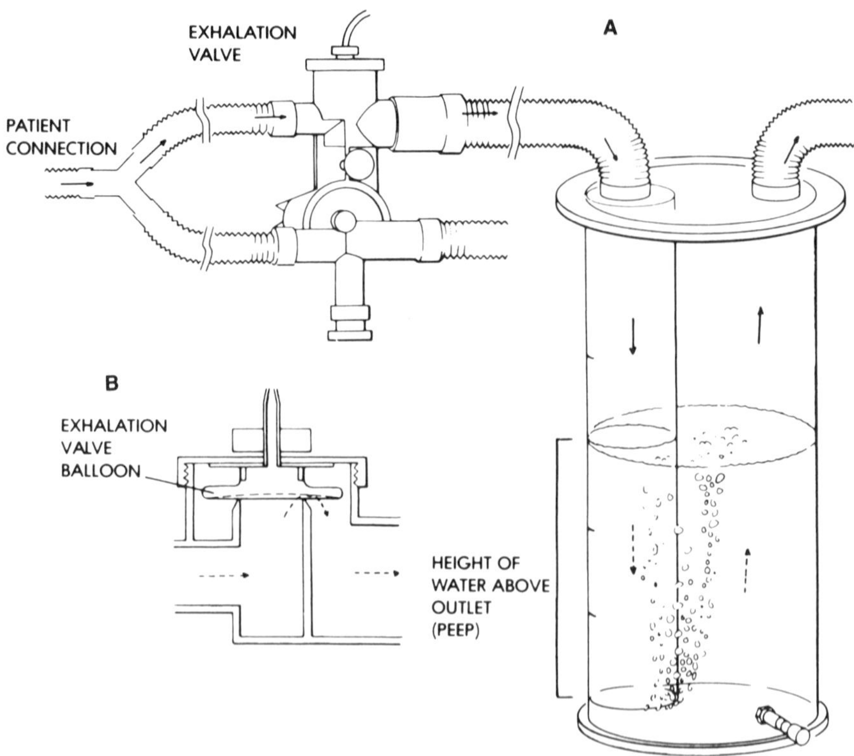

Fig. 14-8 Water-column PEEP device. Exhaled gas must bubble through the water column to escape. The height of the water determines the PEEP level. (From Kirby RR, Smith RA, Desautels DD [eds]: *Mechanical Ventilation.* New York, Churchill Livingstone, 1985. Used by permission.)

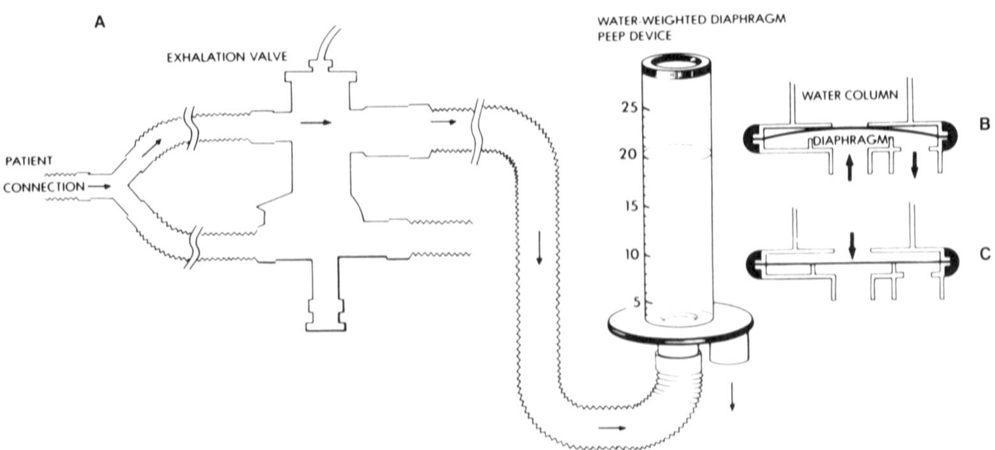

Fig. 14-9 Water-weighted diaphragm PEEP device. **A,** Expiratory limb of ventilator circuit attached to PEEP device. **B,** Exhaled gas forces the diaphragm up so that it can escape. **C,** At the end of expiration, the force of the weight of the water column is greater than the force of gas coming from the patient. As a result, exhalation stops and a PEEP level is maintained. (From Kirby RR, Smith RA, Desautels DD [eds]: *Mechanical Ventilation.* New York, Churchill Livingstone, 1985. Used by permission.)

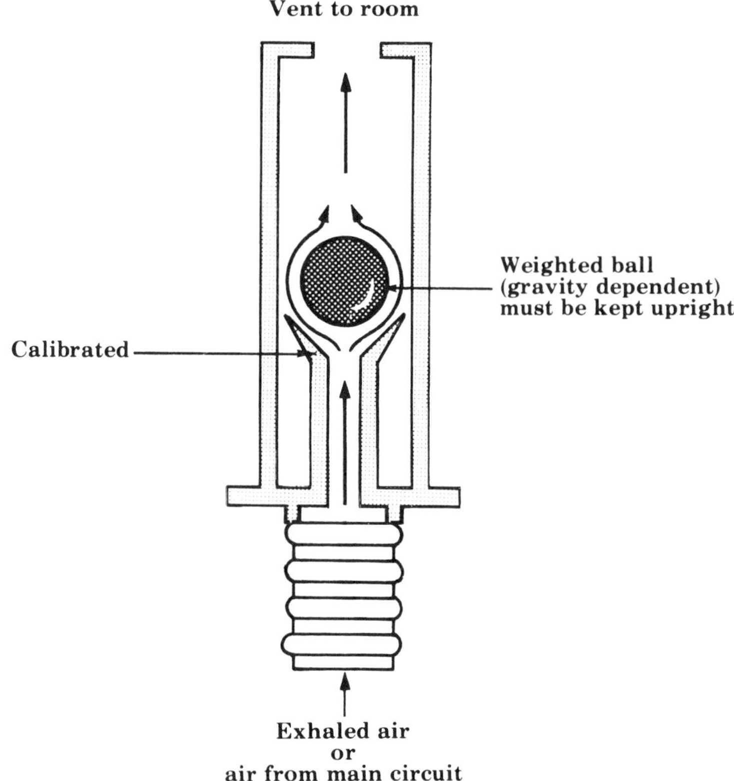

Fig. 14-10 Threshold resistor (weighted ball) positive end-expiratory pressure (PEEP) valve. (From Pilbeam SP: *Mechanical Ventilation: Physiological and Clinical Applications.* St Louis, Mosby, 1986. Used by permission.)

cussed earlier) at no more than −1 to −2 cm H_2O. That way, the PEEP level will be maintained at close to the ordered level even during an assisted breath. For example, PEEP is set at 10 cm, and the sensitivity is set at −1 cm. So, when the patient triggers a breath, it will occur at 9 cm PEEP.

Malfunctioning internal exhalation valves or PEEP-generation venturi systems cannot be easily repaired at the bedside. The ventilator will need to be replaced.

Balloon-type exhalation valves are prone to two problems:

a. The small-bore tube carrying gas from the ventilator to the balloon valve is pulled off. Reconnect the tubing to either the ventilator nipple connection or exhalation valve nipple connection.

Fig. 14-11 Spring-loaded disk positive end-expiratory pressure (PEEP) valve. (From Kirby RR, Smith RA, Desautels DD [eds]: *Mechanical Ventilation.* New York, Churchill Livingstone, 1985. Used by permission.)

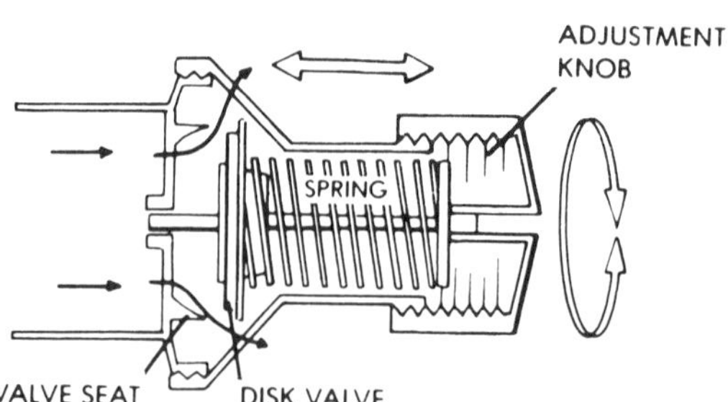

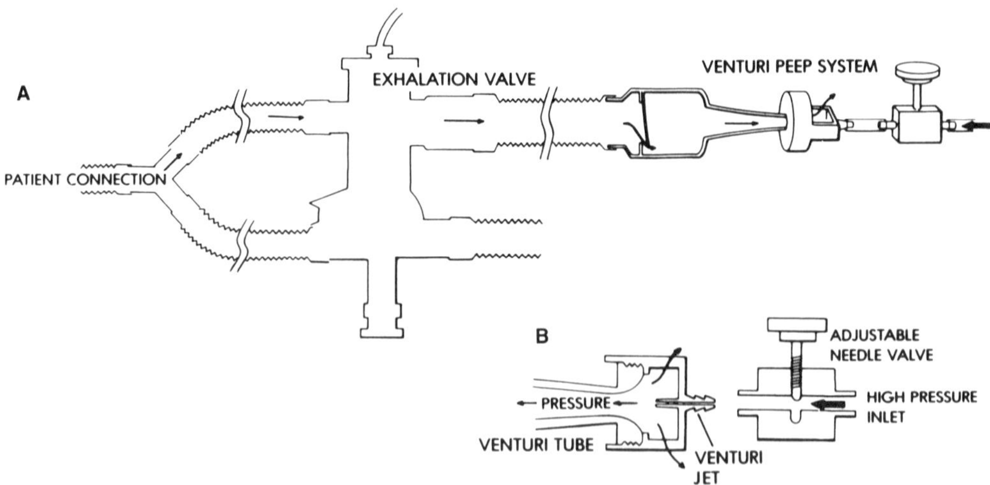

Fig. 14-12 Venturi PEEP system. **A,** Connected to the expiratory limb of a ventilator circuit. Arrows show escape of exhaled gas. **B,** Detail of the adjustable needle valve and venturi. (From Kirby RR, Smith RA, Desautels DD [eds]: *Mechanical Ventilation.* New York, Churchill Livingstone, 1985. Used by permission.)

b. The balloon is torn, and the gas leaks out. This can be confirmed by disassembling the exhalation valve assembly. Replace the balloon and reassemble the exhalation valve.

Both of these problems demonstrate themselves when the inspiratory tidal volume flows past the patient and directly into the exhaled tidal volume–measuring device. If the ventilator is a Bennett MA-1, the bellows spirometer will be seen to rise on inspiration instead of expiration, as normal. Little or no airway pressure is generated. The patient is poorly ventilated, if at all. This problem must be corrected immediately while the patient is being manually ventilated.

6. CPAP systems: breathing circuits.

a. Get the necessary equipment for the procedure. (IIA11c) [R, Ap]

Most current generation ventilators have a built-in CPAP mode. No additional circuitry is needed. After switching to the CPAP mode, set the desired level by adjusting the PEEP/CPAP dial and watch the reading on the pressure manometer.

Free-standing CPAP breathing circuits vary considerably. No manufacturer has developed a system that dominates the marketplace. Most commonly, each respiratory care department develops its own breathing circuit to meet its own needs. Traditionally, the complete circuit is changes after 24 hours of use to minimize the risk of infection.

b. Put the equipment together, make sure that it works properly, and identify and fix any problems with it. (IIB9c) [R, Ap]

Fig. 14-13 shows the typical components used in a CPAP breathing circuit. The components include:

- Air/oxygen blender
- Pediatric or adult flowmeter on the blender
- Cascade-type humidifier

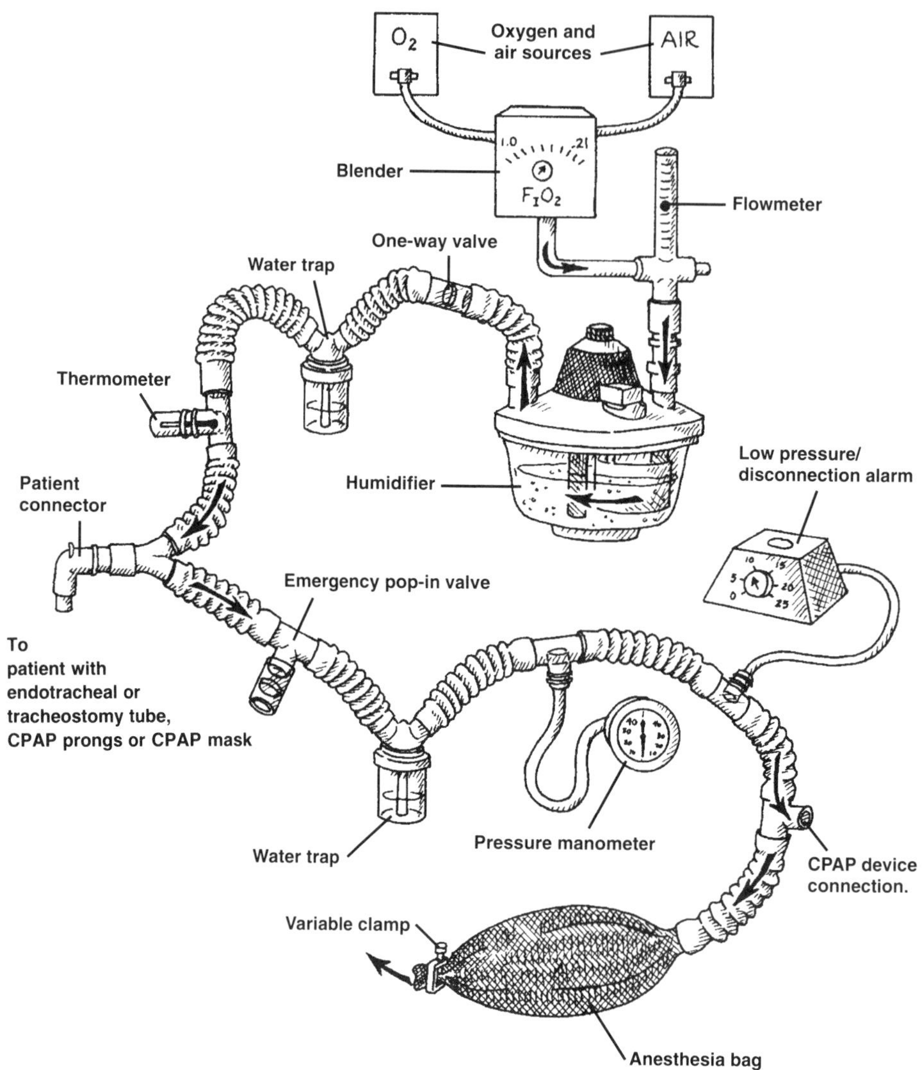

Fig. 14-13 Patient breathing circuit for continuous positive airway pressure (CPAP).

- Inspiratory circuit of large-bore/aerosol tubing with the following additions:
  - Water trap
  - One-way valve
  - Thermometer
- Y (wye) to connect the inspiratory and expiratory limbs of the circuit
- Patient connector (elbow adapter) to endotracheal/tracheostomy tube, CPAP prongs, or CPAP mask
- Expiratory circuit of large-bore/aerosol tubing with the following additions:
  - Water trap
  - One-way valve
  - Pressure manometer for measuring the CPAP level
  - Low-pressure/disconnection audible alarm
  - CPAP device (see later discussion)
  - Anesthesia bag as a reservoir
  - Variable resistance clamp on the tail of the anesthesia bag

Brigg's adapters/T-adapters for connecting the various features
Emergency pop-in valve in case gas flow is stopped

The CPAP level is adjusted by means of a variety of threshold resistors. Fig. 14-8 shows a column of water with a length of expiratory tubing inserted below the surface. When working properly, air bubbles will be seen as they come out of the end of the tubing. Fig. 14-9 shows another type of water column system. It features a rubber diaphragm that is forced down by the weight of the water against the expiratory limb of the circuit. The more water there is, the higher the CPAP level is. Fig. 14-10 shows a vertically mounted ball bearing. It creates a resistance as gas flows up past it. These ball bearing resistors come in weights of 2.5, 5, and 10 cm H_2O. They can be used individually or stacked and combined into a variety of CPAP levels. When working properly, air can be felt to escape out of the open end of the device. Fig. 14-11 shows a spring-loaded resistor that is adjusted to apply the desired CPAP level against the airway. When it is working properly, air can be felt as it escapes out of the vents on the device. Fig. 14-12 shows a free-standing venturi PEEP system. Gas from the venturi jet creates backpressure against the escaping patient tidal volume. Air can be felt as it exits from the vents when it is working properly.

All CPAP systems must be adjusted by checking the pressure level on the manometer. Set the low-pressure/disconnection audible alarm to sound at a few centimeters below the CPAP level. For example, if 10 cm CPAP is ordered, set the alarm to sound if the pressure drops below 8 cm of CPAP.

Flow through the CPAP breathing circuit must be sufficient to meet the patient's needs. Adjust the flowmeter setting and clamp on the anesthesia bag so that it is somewhat inflated with excess air escaping out past the clamp. With all of the devices, gas will escape through the path of least resistance. All or some may escape through the anesthesia bag, CPAP device, or both. The bag should collapse somewhat during the patient's inspiration and expand somewhat during the expiration. The CPAP level should not drop more than 1 or 2 cm from the baseline during an inspiration.

Make sure that the water level is properly maintained in the humidifier. Fill it with sterile, distilled water as often as necessary.

A sudden drop in the CPAP level to zero indicates a disconnection at the patient or somewhere in the breathing circuit. Check all connections and reassemble the break. The patient may need to be manually ventilated while the problem is corrected.

If the CPAP level drops more than 2 cm H_2O during an inspiration, the flow is inadequate and should be increased. Flow is also inadequate if the patient shows an increased use of accessory muscles of respiration or complains of increased work of breathing. Too high a flow is seen by an inadvertently high level of CPAP or the patient complaining of it being difficult to exhale.

Water column systems must be frequently monitored because of water loss caused by evaporation. The actual CPAP level will be progressively less than desired as the water is gradually lost. This system must regularly have water added to it or have the expiratory tubing inserted deeper to keep the desired CPAP level.

The ball bearing resistor system must be mounted vertically for gravity to keep the desired weight against the circuit. If it falls over and is horizontal, the CPAP pressure will be lost.

7. Masks for CPAP systems.

a. Get the necessary equipment for the procedure. (IIA1d) [R, Ap]

A CPAP mask and breathing circuit are used for patients who have obstructive sleep apnea. This condition is seen occasionally in children but most commonly in obese men who, when sleeping on their back, suffer an obstruction of the upper airway. The obstruction seems to be caused by the posterior collapse of the tongue and soft tissues of the throat when the patient is unconscious. The obstruction causes apnea with hypoxemia and hypercapnea. As the hypoxemia becomes dangerously low, the patient awakens with a start to take several deep breaths before falling asleep again. This scene repeats itself many times during the night. As a result, the patient never gets a good night's sleep and has many episodes of dangerous hypoxemia. CPAP, by means of the mask, forces the soft tissues open to the point that the airway is never obstructed (Fig. 14-14). The patient is now able to sleep normally and remain oxygenated.

These patients must have a thorough workup and a sleep study performed to confirm that this is their problem. A CPAP mask for home care would be indicated in such a patient if the patient has a diagnosed obstructive sleep apnea disorder and is found to have normal sensorium, airway reflexes, and spirometry when awake. The patient should have the CPAP mask, breathing circuit, and proper CPAP level determined by a sleep study in the hospital. The patient can use the system at home once it is set up properly and he or she has been trained in its use.

CPAP masks come in different sizes for children older than 3 years of age and adults. There are two different types of CPAP masks. Nose masks are designed to cover only the nose. They allow the patient to speak and offer the mouth as a second airway for breathing in case there is a malfunction of the CPAP system. The mouth also acts as a pressure relief route if the CPAP pressure should become too great. Pressures of up to 15 cm H_2O can usually be maintained (see Fig. 14-15).

Face masks are designed to cover the nose and mouth. They are transparent and similar to the mask used during bag-mask ventilation. The face mask must be used if the patient has persistent mouth breathing and cannot use a nose mask. With a good seal, pressures of greater than 15 cm H_2O can be maintained.

Both types of CPAP mask have a soft, very compliant seal to closely fit the contours of the face. Straps are needed to hold the mask in place. It is imperative that the mask properly fit the patient's face. Too large a mask will not seal and will allow gas and pres-

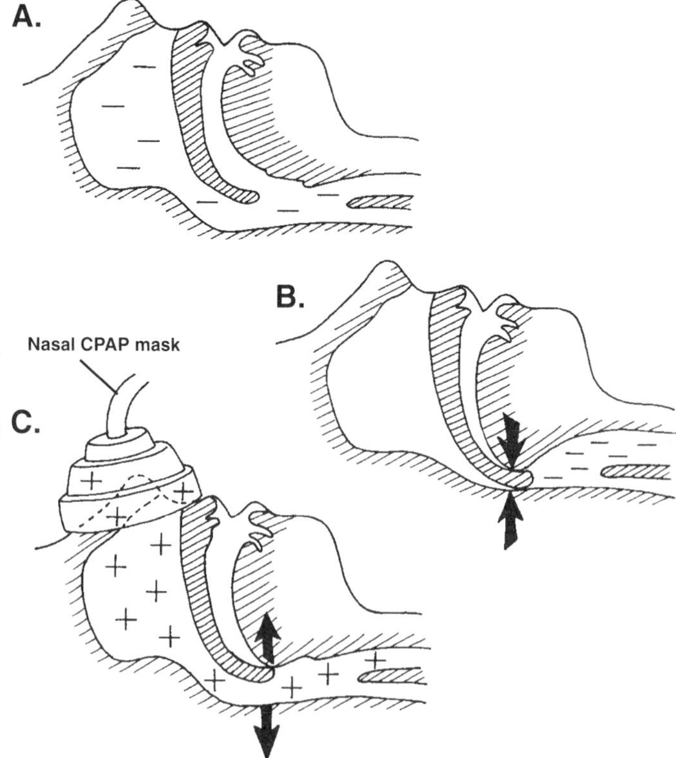

Fig. 14-14 Effect of a nasal continuous positive airway pressure (CPAP) mask. **A,** The normal upper airway remains patent during sleep. **B,** The abnormal upper airway of a patient with obstructive apnea collapses on inspiration during sleep. **C,** The pressure from a nasal CPAP mask keeps the abnormal upper airway patent during sleep. (Adapted from Scanlan CL: Respiratory failure and the need for ventilatory support, in Scanlan CL, Spearman CB, Sheldon RL [eds]: *Egan's Fundamentals of Respiratory Care,* ed 5. St Louis, Mosby, 1990.)

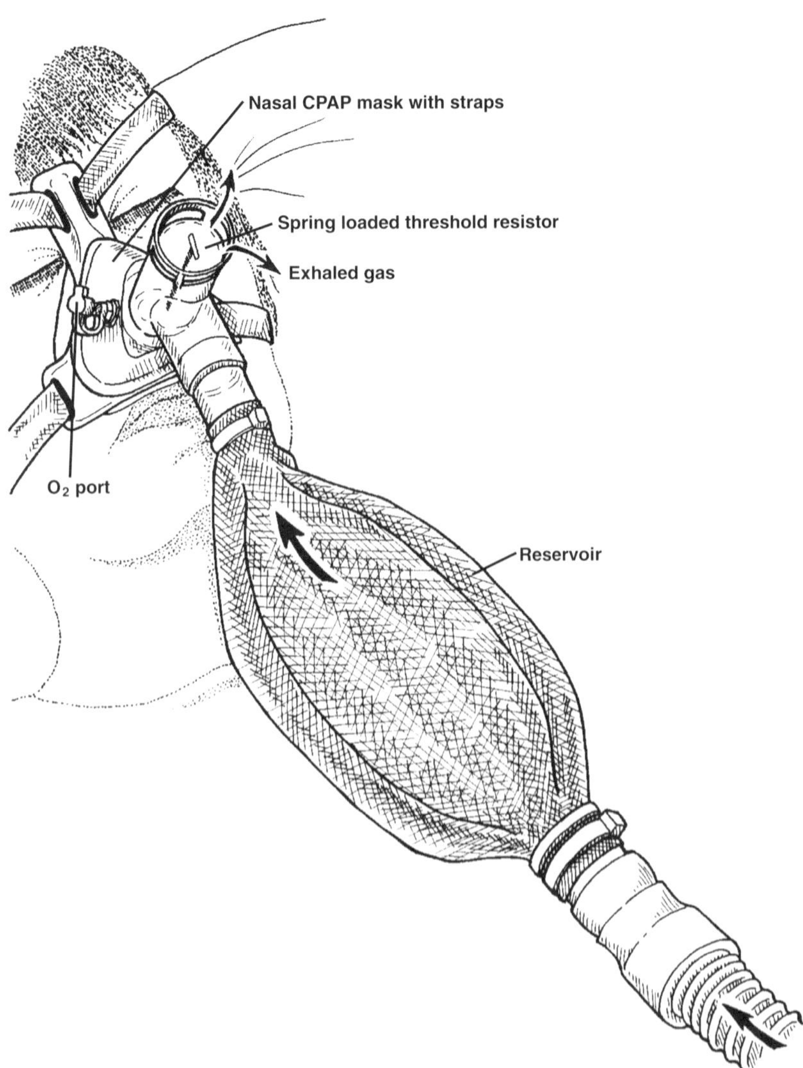

Fig. 14-15 Nasal continuous positive airway pressure (CPAP) mask in place on an adult patient.

sure to leak out. This will be seen as a decreased CPAP pressure on the manometer. The patient may show increased snoring or airway obstruction with periods of apnea. Too small or a misfitting mask could cause an uneven distribution of pressure on the face. This could lead to abrasions or pressure sores and ulcers on the face.

b. Put the equipment together, make sure that it works properly, and identify any problems with it. (IIB1e) [R, Ap]

Several companies manufacture mask CPAP systems. Respironics makes the Sleep-Easy III. Briefly, it consists of an electrically powered blower to generate gas flow and a spring-loaded threshold resistor that the patient exhales through to set the CPAP level. A single, large-bore hose carries gas from the blower to the mask (see Fig. 14-15). Vital Signs makes the Downs CPAP Generator. Briefly, it consists of a gas-powered venturi to generate flow. As mentioned earlier, a single, large-bore hose carries flow from the venturi to the mask. The patient exhales through a spring-loaded threshold resistor.

These are relatively simple circuits and do not have a humidification system, alarm system, or the other attachments seen in the hospital. Check the manufacturer's literature for specific directions on their application to the patient. Any mask CPAP system must be able to generate enough flow to meet the patient's minute volume and peak flow needs. The CPAP level must be stable throughout the breathing cycle.

A sudden drop in the CPAP level to zero indicates a disconnection at the patient or somewhere in the breathing circuit. Check all connections and reassemble the break.

If the CPAP level drops more than 2 cm H_2O during an inspiration, the flow is inadequate and should be increased. Flow is also inadequate if the patient shows an increased use of accessory muscles of respiration or complains of increased work of breathing. Too high a flow is seen by an inadvertently high level of CPAP or the patient complaining of it being difficult to exhale.

8. Nasal CPAP devices.

a. Get the necessary equipment for the procedure. (IIA1d) [R, Ap]

Nasal CPAP devices are used exclusively with neonates. These infants commonly have been born prematurely and have IRDS. Their immature lungs lack sufficient surfactant and need CPAP treatment to keep the alveoli open. Often nasal CPAP will meet the patient's needs so that endotracheal intubation and mechanical ventilation can be avoided. Nasal CPAP works with neonates because they are obligate nose breathers.

Nasal CPAP therapy is associated with the hazards of gastric distention and reflux aspiration. These occur when the airway pressure forces air into the stomach. A gastric tube is usually inserted to vent the air out.

There are two different devices for administering nasal CPAP: nasopharyngeal tube and nasal prongs.

Nasopharyngeal Tube

A nasopharyngeal tube is actually an endotracheal tube that has been cut shorter (Fig. 14-16,C). Select a tube that is the largest that can be easily inserted into the patient. Estimate the needed length by lying the tube along the patient's face and measur-

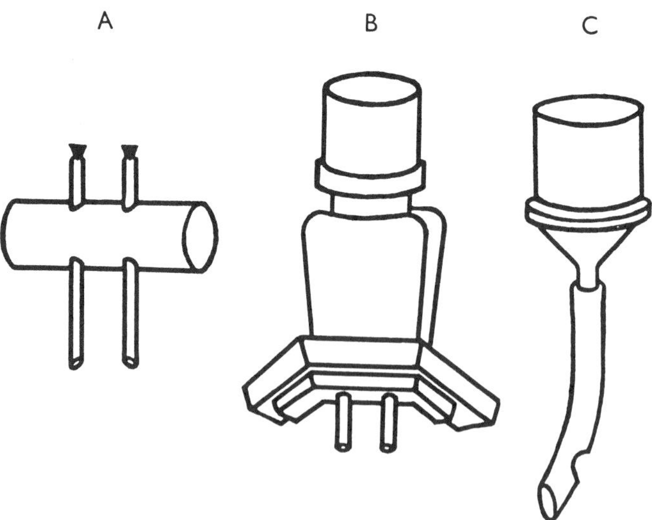

Fig. 14-16 Nasal continuous positive airway pressure (CPAP) devices for infants. **A,** Jackson-Reese tubes. **B,** Argyle nasal cannula (prongs). **C,** Endotracheal tube cut shorter for nasopharyngeal insertion (NP tube). (From Blodgett D: *Manual of Pediatric Respiratory Care Procedures.* Philadelphia, Lippincott, 1982. Used by permission.)

ing from the earlobe to the tip of the chin. It is inserted into either naris and advanced until the tip can be seen behind the uvula. This position can be confirmed by x-ray films of the chest and upper airway. The tube marking for length at the nostril should be recorded.

When properly positioned, CPAP is applied over the epiglottis. It is usually possible to keep pressure of about 10 cm H_2O. Excessive pressures will be vented out of the mouth. Try to prevent the infant from crying because this will result in a loss of pressure. A gastric tube is commonly inserted in through the other naris to vent any air from the stomach.

Nasal Prongs

Nasal prongs come in short and long versions (see Fig. 14-16,A and B). Both types involve prongs that fit into both nostrils. The prongs come in different diameters so that the proper size can be found to fit the internal diameter of the infant's nares. The short prongs are inserted 0.5 to 1.0 cm. Manufacturers include Argyle and Novametrix. The long prongs are inserted until the tip can be seen behind the uvula. Vesta and Jackson-Reese are manufacturers. As with the nasopharyngeal tube, CPAP is applied over the epiglottis.

In both types of prongs it is usually possible to keep pressures of about 10 cm H_2O. Excessive pressures will be vented out of the mouth. Try to prevent the infant from crying because this will result in a loss of pressure. A gastric tube is commonly inserted in through the mouth to vent any air from the stomach.

b. Put the equipment together, make sure that it works properly, and identify and fix any problems with it. (IIB1e) [R, Ap]

All of these patient connection devices fit into either the elbow adapter on the CPAP breathing circuit or directly into the circuit if the Y is removed. All must be secured to the patient in some fashion. A nasopharyngeal tube or long nasal prongs that extend beyond the nose usually need to be taped or tied like an endotracheal tube. If the patient is

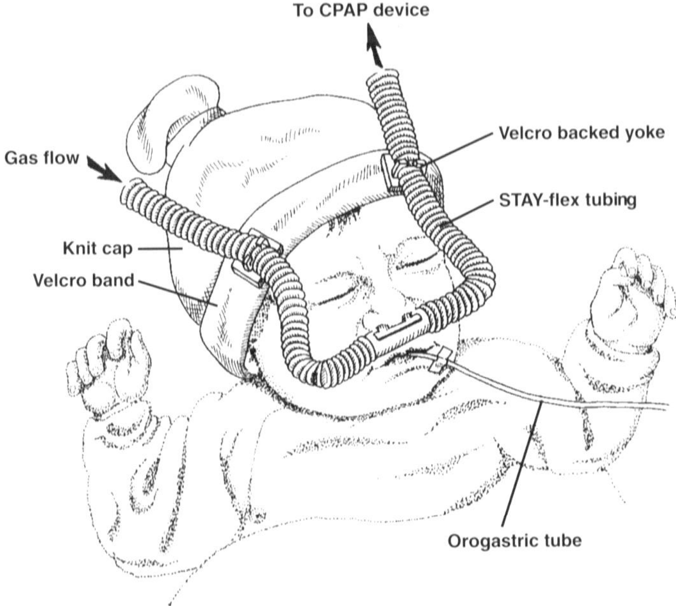

Fig. 14-17 An assembly for supporting nasal continuous positive airway pressure (CPAP) prongs in an infant. (Modified from an advertisement of the Stayflex tubing system from Ackrad.)

lying quietly, no securing may be needed at all. The short nasal prongs usually need a securing device because they are easily dislodged from the nostrils. A variety of devices are available, including Ackrad's Stayflex tubing and knit cap with Velcro tube holders (Fig 14-17). It is important that any securing system fit loosely enough so that the infant's circulation to the scalp or head is not constricted.

A sudden drop in the CPAP level to zero indicates a disconnection at the patient or somewhere in the breathing circuit. Check all connections and reassemble the break. The patient may need to be manually ventilated while the problem is corrected.

If the CPAP level drops more than 2 cm H_2O during an inspiration, the flow is inadequate and should be increased. Flow is also inadequate if the patient shows an increased use of accessory muscles of respiration or appears to have an increased work of breathing. Too high a flow is shown by a high level of CPAP or it appearing that the patient is having a difficult time exhaling. A common problem with small-diameter tubes like these is mucous plugging. A plugged tube will result in the backing up of gas and an increase in the CPAP values seen on the manometer. The patient would show distress at the increased work of breathing. Suction to clear out the mucous plug or remove the tube and place a new one.

9. Humidifiers: passover and cascade type.

a. Get the necessary equipment for the procedure. (IIA2a) [R, Ap]

b. Put the equipment together, make sure that it works properly, and identify and fix any problems with it. (IIB2a) [R, Ap]

The general discussion of this equipment was presented in Section 7. See Figs. 14-6 and 14-13 for setups in ventilator and CPAP breathing circuits. Both types are capable of providing 100% relative humidity. Passover-type systems are preferred with neonates.

The humidifier's temperature is usually maintained between 31° to 35° C. The temperature should never be greater than 37° C at the patient's airway. Normally a temperature probe is added into the inspiratory limb of the circuit near the Y. If a heated-wire circuit is being used with an infant, the temperature probe should be outside of the incubator and away from a radiant warmer's direct heat. The humidifier should provide at least 30 mg/L of water vapor. (Remember that saturated air at normal body temperature contains 44 mg/L of water vapor.)

Make sure that the water level is kept in the recommended range to properly humidify the gas. Avoid being sprayed with any circuit water during disconnections from the patient. It is considered contaminated and should be disposed of like any other contaminated fluid from the patient.

10. Humidifiers: heat and moisture exchangers.

a. Get the necessary equipment for the procedure. (IIA2b) [R, Ap]

Heat and moisture exchangers (HME) are designed to be warmed by the patient's exhaled breath and absorb the water vapor from the gas. The next inspired volume is then warmed and humidified by evaporation. The key element in the exchanger is a hygroscopic filter medium. Under ideal conditions, the units can achieve up to 70% to 90% body humidity. They should minimally provide 30 mg/L of water at 30° C.

A heat and moisture exchanger is also known as a heat-moisture exchanger, artificial nose, condensing humidifier, heat and moisture exchanging humidifier, and hygroscopic condenser humidifier. The manufacturer may have a term that it has coined for its particular unit and recommends for its ventilator.

Questions to ask when considering which heat and moisture exchanger to use include:

a. How much mechanical dead space does it add? All of these units are inserted into the circuit between the Y and the patient and create mechanical dead space. Select a unit with the smallest possible dead space volume. Watch for an increase in the patient's $Paco_2$ if the heat-moisture exchanger adds too much dead space or the patient's tidal volume is too small.

b. How efficient is the unit at humidifying the dry inspiratory gas? Pick the unit that provides the greatest percentage of body humidity. Do not use one that cannot meet these minimal standards.

c. Does the patient need a unit that acts as a bacterial filter? This would be important if the patient had a known bacterial infection and the staff wished to be protected from its airborne spread. The HME 15-22 Heat and Moisture Exchanging Filter made by Pall Biomedical Products Corporation is also a bacteria filter and can be used for infection control purposes, as well as for humidification of dry inspired gas.

d. Is the unit disposable or reusable? Many units are thrown away after 24 to 48 hours' use on a single patient. Disposable units are made by AirLife, Terumo, NCC, Pall Biomedical Products, and Engstrom. Siemens units are reusable. Staffing, infection control, and equipment processing considerations would make a difference in choosing which unit to use.

b. Put the equipment together, make sure that it works properly, and identify and fix any problems with it. (IIB2b) [R, Ap]

Most of these units are preassembled by the manufacturer. There is nothing to add. An exception is the Siemens unit, which has a replaceable filter. It may be necessary to attach a length of large-bore/aerosol tubing or an elbow adapter to make the unit fit onto the Y or endotracheal tube. All come with standard 15- or 22-mm connector ends. Air should flow easily through them with little resistance (Fig. 14-18).

Any disconnections can be easily noticed and reconnected. Replace any unit that has a mucous plug or other debris obstructing the channel. This might be demonstrated by the patient's peak airway pressure suddenly rising. Typically, these units are replaced every 24 to 48 hours when the breathing circuit is replaced.

11. Change the type of humidification equipment and patient connector as needed. (IIIF3a) [R, Ap]

A heat moisture exchanger is indicated in the following situations:

a. The patient has few, if any, secretions.
b. The patient will probably be weaned within 96 hours.
c. The patient is not on the IMV mode.
d. The patient is being transported on mechanical ventilation.

A heat and moisture exchanger is contraindicated in the following situations:

a. The patient has viscious, bloody, or large amounts of secretions.

b. The patient has a large air leak such that the exhaled volume is less than 70% of the inhaled tidal volume. This would result in a relatively dry hygroscopic filter. (Patients with uncuffed or torn cuffs on their endotracheal tubes or large bronchopleuralcutaneous fistulas would have large tidal volume leaks.)

c. The patient's temperature is less than 32° C.

d. The patient's spontaneous tidal volume is greater than 10 L/min.

e. Always remove the heat-moisture exchanger when delivering nebulized medications through the circuit.

A cascade-type humidifier is indicated in these situations:

a. The patient has viscous or copious secretions. An increase in the amount or viscosity of secretions or a change from white to yellow or green justifies the switch to a

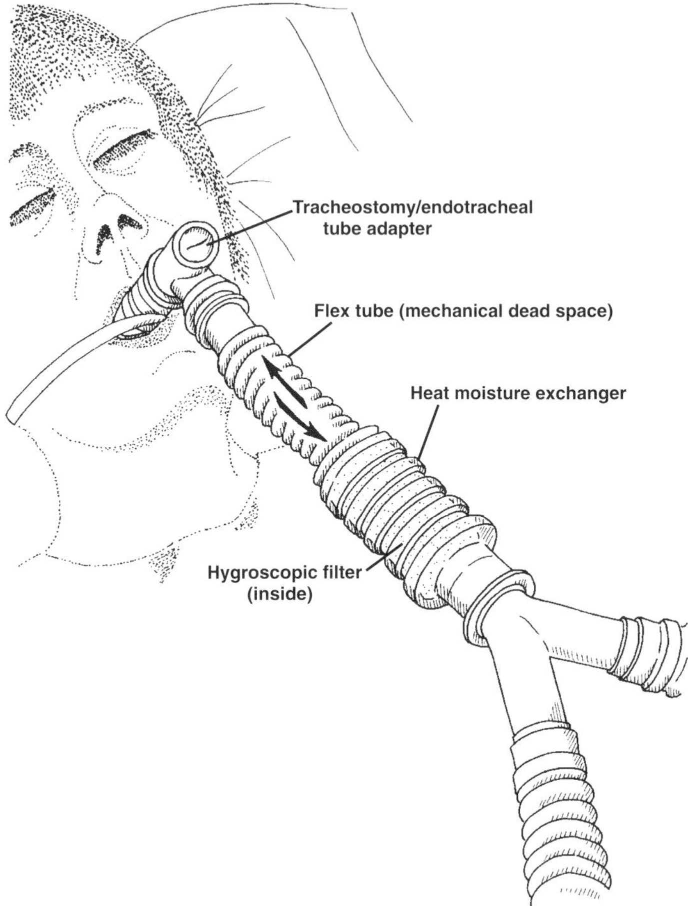

Fig. 14-18 Heat-moisture exchanger inserted into a patient's breathing circuit. Any extra tubing inserted between the wye and the endotracheal tube acts as mechanical dead space.

cascade-type humidifier. When secretions are coughed into a heat-moisture exchanger, it will become obstructed. This will be seen as a rapid increase in the peak pressure seen during an inspiration.

b. The patient will probably require mechanical ventilation for more than 96 hours.

c. The patient cannot have mechanical dead space added to the breathing circuit. If the patient's tidal volume is smaller (especially a child's) than the heat-moisture exchanger's dead space, it should not be used. IMV systems typically are set up without mechanical dead space, so a heat-moisture exchanger should not be used.

d. A heat-moisture exchanger should not be used with a patient receiving very large tidal volumes. This is because the filter's ability to hold moisture will be exceeded and the patient will breathe in some dry air. Check the manufacturer's literature for the maximum tidal volume that is recommended.

e. If the patient has a large air leak, as seen with a deflated cuff or bronchopleural fistula, a heat-moisture exchanger should not be used. With a large air leak, more air is inspired than expired and the exchanger will not be able to fully humidify the inspired tidal volume.

The patient connector can be a standard endotracheal/tracheostomy adapter, one designed to allow a suction catheter to pass through, or a Ballard-type self-contained suctioning system.

Module C. Patient assessment.

1. Determine and continue to monitor how the patient responds to the treatment or procedure.

Review Sections 1, 3, and 4, and earlier in this section as needed to go over the details of how a patient should be monitored. Briefly, determine the patient's vital signs and record them in the chart. Monitor the patient's heart rhythm. Auscultate the patient's breath sounds and record any changes. Make the recommendation for a chest x-ray film, as needed, to help determine the patient's condition.

2. Measure the following: (IIIE13) [R, Ap]

a. Tidal volume.

The patient's exhaled tidal volume is usually measured and recorded in his or her chart. Some of the newer ventilators also display an inhaled tidal volume. Actually, this is the tidal volume sent from the unit to the patient. Assuming no leaks, it is delivered to the patient. If possible, compare the two volumes. If they do not match closely, check for a leak or other reason for the difference. The patient on an IMV, SIMV, or pressure support mode should have both the machine delivered and spontaneous tidal volumes measured and recorded.

The weaning patient needs to have his or her spontaneous tidal volume measured along with the vital capacity. They and other parameters are used to judge weanability (see later discussion and Table 14-4 for more information).

b. Respiratory rate.

Count and record the machine delivered respiratory rate. If the patient is on an IMV, SIMV, or pressure support mode, count and record both the machine and spontaneous rates. The weaning patient should have his or her spontaneous rate counted and recorded (see later discussion and Table 14-4).

c. I/E ratio.

The I/E ratio should be calculated and recorded. Some newer ventilators will display it. Others will show inspiratory time and expiratory time. The I/E ratio can then be calculated as shown in Table 14-5. The discussion on modifying I/E ratio based on the patient's conditions is presented later on.

d. Maximum inspiratory pressure (MIP)

The discussion on MIP was presented in Section 4 on pulmonary function testing. It is further discussed later on and in Table 14-4 in terms of it being used as a weaning parameter.

e. Airway pressures

The following airway pressures should be observed and recorded if available:

1. Peak pressure (P_{peak}). The peak pressure reached during the delivery of a tidal volume is the pressure required to push the gas through the circuit, endotracheal tube, and the patient's airways and to expand the lungs. The sigh volume will require a greater pressure because it is a larger volume. These pressures should be recorded regularly

Table 14-4. Indications That the Patient Can Probably Be Weaned From the Ventilator*

Oxygenation
1. Pa_{O_2} value = 80 mm Hg or Sp_{O_2} value > 90% on 50% oxygen or less
2. $P(A\text{-}a)O_2$ < 300-350 mm Hg on 100% oxygen
3. Intrapulmonary shunt < 20%

Ventilation
1. Pa_{CO_2} value < 55 mm Hg in a patient who is not ordinarily hypercapneic
2. V_D/V_T ratio < 0.55-0.6 (55%-60%)

Pulmonary mechanics
1. Spontaneous tidal volume of 3-4 ml/lb or 7-9 ml/kg of ideal body weight
2. Vital capacity of at least 10-15 ml/kg
3. MIP > −20 to −25 cm H_2O
4. FEV_1 > 10 ml/kg
5. Respiratory rate of 12-35/min (adult). It is common to see an increase in the respiratory rate.

Miscellaneous
1. Conscious and cooperative patient who wants to breathe spontaneously
2. Stable and acceptably normal blood pressure and temperature
3. Stable cardiac rhythm. The heart rate should not increase by more than 15% -20%.
4. Corrected underlying problem that led to ventilatory support
5. Normal fluid balance and electrolyte values
6. Proper nutritional status

*Pa_{O_2}, arterial oxygen pressure; Sp_{O_2}, pulse oximetry; $P(A\text{-}a)O_2$, difference in the partial pressure of oxygen in alveolar gas and arterial blood; V_D/V_T, dead space/tidal volume; *MIP*, maximum inspiratory pressure; FEV_1, forced expiratory volume in 1 second.

Table 14-5. Time Variables in Mechanical Ventilation

Term	Symbol	Formula for Calculation
Frequency (rate)	f	Count breaths/min or $\frac{60}{t_I + t_E}$
Cycle time	$t_I + t_E$	Add $t_I + t_E$ or $\frac{60}{f}$
Inspiratory time	t_I(I)	$t_I = \frac{60}{f} - t_E$ or $t_I = \%t_I \times (t_I + t_E)$
Expiratory time	t_E(E)	$t_E = \frac{60}{f} - t_I$
Inspiratory/expiratory time ratio	I/E or t_I/t_E	$I/E = \frac{t_I}{t_E}$, usually numerator
Percent inspiratory time	$\%t_I$	$\%t_I = \frac{t_I}{t_I + t_E} \times 100$

From Scanlan CL: Physics and physiology of ventilatory support, in Scanlan CL, Spearman CB, Sheldon RL (eds): *Egan's Fundamentals of Respiratory Care,* ed 5. St Louis, Mosby, 1990. Used by permission.

whenever the patient and machine are checked. The importance of peak pressure in calculating dynamic compliance is discussed later on.

2. Plateau pressure (P_{plat}). The plateau pressure is found when the tidal volume has been delivered to the lungs and is temporarily held within them. The importance of plateau pressure in calculating static compliance is discussed later on.

3. Baseline pressure. The baseline pressure is the pressure measured at the end of exhalation. Normally it is seen as zero on the ventilator's pressure manometer. (Remember that in this case "zero" is actually local barometric pressure.) If the patient has therapeutic PEEP or CPAP, the baseline pressure will be greater than zero.

4. Mean airway pressure (P_{aw}). Mean airway pressure is the average pressure over an entire breathing cycle. Most of the newer ventilators will display a mean airway pressure. This pressure results from the patient's peak and baseline pressures plus the I/E ratio.

The ventilator's pressure limits and alarms are set based on the peak pressures delivered to the patient (discussed later on).

3. Observe how the patient responds to being mechanically ventilated. (IIIE12) [R, Ap, An]

Because a patient with an intubated airway cannot speak, it is necessary to communicate by asking simple questions that can be answered in a "yes" nod or "no" shake of the head. Other methods of communication are a pad of paper and pencil or picture boards.

It is not possible to predict how a patient will react to the initiation of mechanical ventilation or its prolonged need. Some patient's react with relief and relax when the work of breathing is reduced. Others may become angry at the limitations imposed on them. Still others may become depressed. The issue of a patient's emotional reaction to illness was discussed in detail in Section 1.

Physical responses to mechanical ventilation, as measured by the vital signs, can vary considerably. A patient who is anxious, angry, or in pain will have an increase in the vital signs. A patient who is relaxed, has a reduced work of breathing, and whose blood gas values are now normal will have a return to normal vital signs. Watch carefully for the patient whose drop in blood pressure coincides with a tachycardia. This patient may be having decreased venous return to the heart from an increased intrathoracic pressure.

4. Test the alarm systems and adjust them as needed. (IIIE11) [R, Ap, An]

All alarm systems must function properly. Test all audible and visual alarms. The practitioner should be familiar with the most widely used adult and infant ventilators and their alarm systems. It is common practice to set most alarms at ± 10% from the set value. For example:

a. The tidal volume is 1000 ml. Set the low volume alarm at 900 ml and the high-volume alarm at 1100 ml.

b. The minute volume is 10,000 ml. Set the high-volume alarm at 11,000 ml and the low volume at 9000 ml.

c. The oxygen percentage is set at 40%. Set the high-percentage alarm at 45% and the low-percentage alarm at 35%.

d. The low-pressure/disconnection alarm is set to sound if the ventilator delivered pressure is about 5 cm H_2O below the peak pressure. For example, if the peak pressure has been about the 40 cm H_2O, the low-pressure/disconnection alarm should be set at 35 cm H_2O. If a leak or disconnection occurs, the alarm will sound when the peak pressure does not reach 35 cm H_2O. If the patient is on a CPAP system, the low-pressure/disconnection alarm should be set to sound if the pressure drops about 2 to 3 cm H_2O below the set level. For example, if the patient is on 10 cm H_2O CPAP, the alarm should be set to alarm if the pressure drops to less than 7 cm H_2O.

These types of alarms usually have a timer that can be set to delay when the alarm sounds. If the alarm is on a ventilator, the delay should be set for about 3 to 5 seconds longer than the cycling time. For example, if the patient has a back-up rate of 10 times/min, the cycling time between mandatory breaths will be 6 seconds. Set the timer to delay the alarm sounding for about 10 seconds. So, if the patient is disconnected from the ventilator and the peak pressure does not reach 35 cm H_2O, the alarm will sound in 10 seconds. If the patient is on a CPAP system, the timer may be set for no delay or a short delay.

Adjust all the alarms to fit the clinical setting and the patient's condition. Some may need tighter limits, and others may need wider limits than those just discussed.

5. Lung mechanics.

a. Review the patient's chart for information on airway resistance and lung compliance. (IAlf3) [R, Ap]

These values may have been measured earlier in either the pulmonary function laboratory or on the ventilator. Compare any earlier values with those that will be measured. This is important for understanding the patient's trends toward an improving or worsening pulmonary condition.

b. Calculate the patient's airway resistance, dynamic lung compliance, and static lung compliance values on the ventilator. (IC1j) [R, Ap, An]

These calculations are important because they provide valuable information on the patient's pulmonary condition. The airway resistance (R_{aw}) value indicates how difficult it is to move the tidal volume through the patient's airways and if aerosolized bronchodilating medications are effective. The compliance values indicate how easily the tidal volume can be delivered into the lungs.

Static compliance (C_{st}) is the measurement of work required to overcome the elastic resistance to ventilation. It is a measurement of the compliance of the lungs and thorax (C_{LT}). Static compliance is measured in units of milliliters per centimeters of water pressure. The normal adult's static compliance is 100 ml/cm H_2O; the normal 3-kg infant's static compliance is 5 ml/cm H_2O. See later discussion for the procedure of its measurement.

Dynamic compliance (C_{dyn}) is the measurement of the combination of the patient's static compliance and airway resistance. Dynamic compliance is sometimes called dynamic characteristic. Airway resistance is the pressure required to move a tidal volume through the airways. It is also known as nonelastic resistance to ventilation. Airway resistance is measured in units of centimeters of water per liter per second at a standard flow rate of 0.5 L/sec (30 L/min). The normal adult's Raw is 0.6 to 2.4 cm H_2O/L/sec; the normal 3-kg infant's Raw is 30 cm H_2O/L/sec. Do not forget that this procedure is being performed on a patient with an intubated airway on a ventilator. The endotracheal tube adds to the patient's total Raw. The smaller the tube is, the greater resistance it offers to gas flowing through it. Altering inspiratory flow has an influence on the peak pressure measured for the calculation. The lower the flow, the less gas turbulence there is, and the lower the peak pressure is. Conversely, a higher flow will create more turbulence, and a higher peak pressure will be seen (see later discussion for the procedures for measuring airway resistance and dynamic compliance).

It is important to know that most of the microprocessor ventilators offer software for calculating all of these values. However, it is necessary to be able to calculate them manually for any other situation.

Procedure for Calculating Airway Resistance

1. Cycle a tidal volume. The patient should be breathing passively; fighting the breath will result in an erroneously high peak pressure and assisting with the breath will result in an erroneously low peak pressure.
2. Note the peak airway pressure on the manometer.
3. Briefly prevent the tidal volume from being exhaled. No air should be moving. Note that the pressure manometer shows a peak pressure and then a static or plateau pressure that is stable as long as the tidal volume is held in the lungs. Record the plateau pressure.
4. Calculate the flow in liters per second by taking the flow in liters per minute and dividing it by 60 seconds.
5. Place the peak airway pressure, plateau pressure, and flow into this formula and solve for airway resistance:

$$R_{aw} = \frac{\text{peak airway pressure} - \text{plateau pressure}}{\text{flow in L/sec}}$$

Example:

A mechanically ventilated patient has a peak airway pressure of 30 cm H_2O and plateau pressure of 20 cm H_2O. The peak flow is set at 60 L/min.

Calculate peak flow in liters per second:

$$\frac{60 \text{ L/min}}{60 \text{ seconds}} = 1 \text{ L/sec}$$

Calculate airway resistance:

$$R_{aw} = \frac{\text{peak airway pressure} - \text{plateau pressure}}{\text{flow in L/sec}}$$

$$R_{aw} = \frac{30 \text{ cm } H_2O - 20 \text{ cm } H_2O}{1 \text{ L/sec}} = 10 \text{ cm } H_2O\text{/L/sec}$$

This value is greater than normal for a patient breathing spontaneously. However, remember that the patient's airway is intubated. This results in a smaller airway and more resistance. Some practitioners use the calculated airway resistance as the basis for setting the pressure support ventilation level (discussed earlier). An increased airway resistance could indicate bronchospasm or secretions in the airways. Delivering an aerosolized bronchodilator or suctioning should result in the resistance returning to the original level.

Procedure for Calculating the Compliance Factor

Before the actual calculation of the patient's static and dynamic compliance can be performed, the static compliance of the breathing circuit must be determined. This is because some of the set tidal volume never reaches the patient because it is "lost" in the circuit. To be as accurate as possible in the calculation of static and dynamic compliance and the calculation of actual tidal and sigh volumes, this lost volume must be subtracted

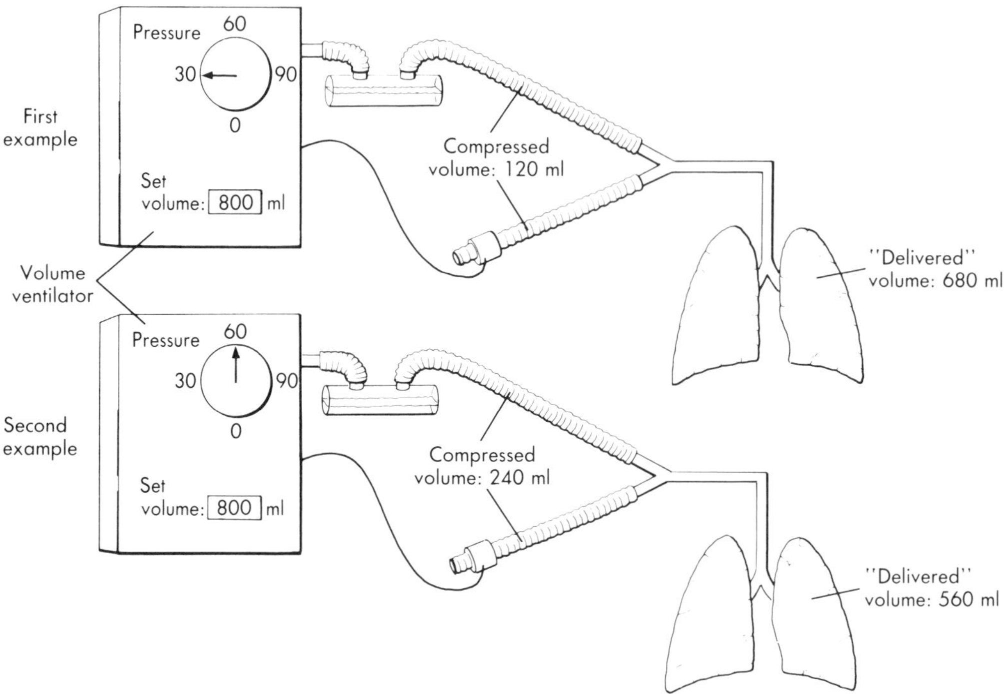

Fig. 14-19 Compressed volume is subtracted from the set tidal volume to determine the delivered tidal volume. Note how when the peak pressure doubles, the compressed volume doubles. The delivered tidal volume is reduced by a greater amount when the peak pressure is higher. (From Scanlan CL: Selection and application of ventilatory support devices, in Scanlan CL, Spearman CB, Sheldon RL [eds]: *Egan's Fundamentals of Respiratory Care,* ed 5. St Louis, Mosby, 1990. Used by permission.)

from the exhaled tidal volume (Fig. 14-19). The phrase compressed volume is commonly used to describe this lost volume. These three factors have an influence on the compressed volume:

a. Charles' law describes how as a gas is warmed it expands in volume. This occurs as the tidal volume is warmed by the cascade-type or heat-moisture exchanger humidification system. This would tend to expand the volume that is sent from the ventilator. The gas is also warmed by the patient and further expanded. This factor is more than offset by the following factors.

b. Boyle's law describes how as a gas is pressurized it is compressed in volume. The greater the pressure, the more the compression. Peak pressure is measured to calculate the amount of gas compression in the breathing circuit and internal circuit of the the ventilator. This factor will reduce the amount of tidal volume delivered to the patient's lungs.

c. The breathing circuit and internal ventilator circuit will stretch out in response to the pressure applied against it. Peak pressure is measured in order to calculate the amount of circuit stretch. This factor will also reduce the amount of tidal volume delivered to the patient's lungs.

Procedure

1. Remove the patient from the ventilator and manually ventilate him or her during the remainder of this procedure.

2. Set the pressure limit as high as possible.
3. Block the breathing circuit at the patient connector.
4. Cycle a tidal volume.
5. Perform either of the following: (a) note the peak pressure developed in the circuit as the tidal volume stretches out the circuit; or (b) if the ventilator's peak pressure hits the pressure limit, note the delivered tidal volume and the pressure limit. **Note:** If the patient is on PEEP therapy, subtract the PEEP level from the measured peak pressure to find the true peak pressure.
6. The compliance factor is found by dividing the measured tidal volume by the peak pressure.

Example:

The patient has a set tidal volume of 600 ml. Using step 5b, the peak pressure is found to be 80 cm H_2O, and the measured tidal volume is found to be 320 ml.

$$\text{Compliance factor} = \frac{320 \text{ ml}}{80 \text{ cm}} = 4 \text{ ml/cm } H_2O$$

The compressed volume is found by multiplying the compliance factor by either the peak or plateau pressure. The compressed volume is then subtracted from the exhaled tidal volume to determine the patient's actual tidal volume.

It may be possible to estimate the amount of gas compression and circuit stretch by adding together the compressed volume values provided by the manufacturers of the breathing circuit and ventilator and multiplying that number by the peak pressure. However, it is usually considered to be clinically most accurate to actually determine the value of all three factors at the bedside under real patient conditions.

Procedure for Calculating Static Compliance

1. Determine the compliance factor of the breathing circuit (as described earlier).
2. Reattach the patient to the ventilator. Reset all controls to their ordered or preset positions.
3. Cycle a tidal volume. The patient should be breathing passively; fighting the breath will result in an erroneously high peak pressure and assisting with the breath will result in an erroneously low peak pressure.
4. Briefly prevent the tidal volume from being exhaled. No air should be moving. Note that the pressure manometer shows a peak pressure and then a static or plateau pressure that is stable as long as the tidal volume is held in the lungs. Record the plateau pressure.
5. Calculate the static pressure using this formula:

$$C_{st} = \frac{\text{exhaled tidal volume} - \text{compressed volume}}{\text{plateau pressure} - \text{PEEP}}$$

where compressed volume = compliance factor × plateau pressure.

Procedure for Calculating Dynamic Compliance

1. Determine the compliance factor of the breathing circuit (as described earlier).
2. Reattach the patient to the ventilator. Reset all controls to their ordered or preset positions.

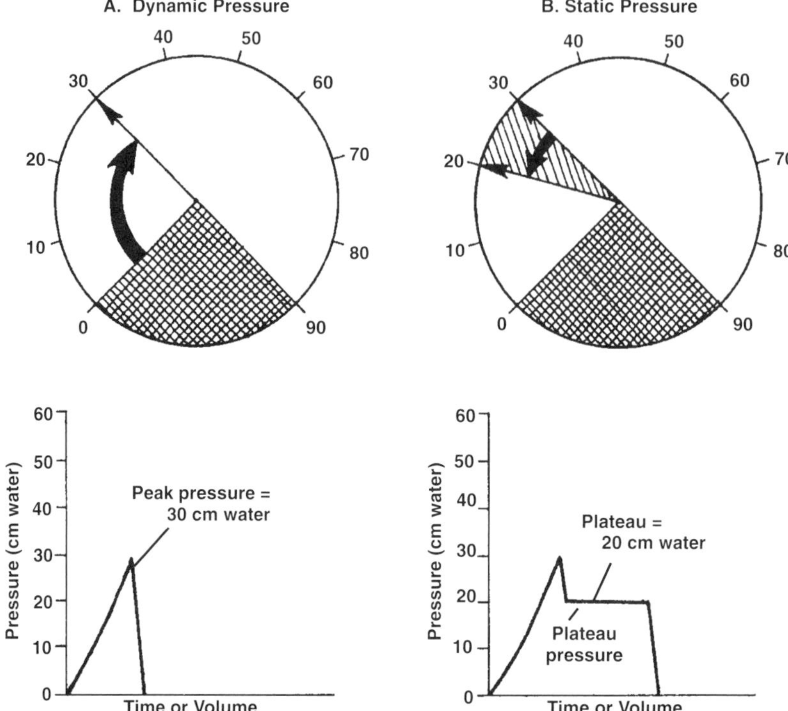

Fig. 14-20 Peak and static pressures without positive end-expiratory pressure (PEEP). **A,** Pressure manometer reading and pressure/volume curve for dynamic pressure. **B,** Pressure manometer reading and pressure/volume curve for static pressure. See the text for details.

3. Cycle a tidal volume. The patient should be breathing passively; fighting the breath will result in an erroneously high peak pressure and assisting with the breath will result in an erroneously low peak pressure.

4. Note the peak pressure on the manometer. If the pressure at the end of inspiration is less than peak pressure, the pressure at the end of inspiration should be used in the calculation.

5. Calculate the dynamic pressure using this formula:

$$C_{dyn} = \frac{\text{exhaled tidal volume} - \text{compressed volume}}{\text{peak pressure} - \text{PEEP}}$$

where compressed volume = compliance factor × peak pressure.

Example:

Calculate the static and dynamic compliance on a ventilated patient without PEEP therapy.

The patient has an exhaled tidal volume of 600 ml. The peak pressure is 30 cm H_2O and the static or plateau pressure is 20 cm H_2O (Fig. 14-20). The compliance factor has been determined to be 4 ml/cm H_2O.

$$C_{st} = \frac{\text{exhaled tidal volume} - \text{compressed volume}}{\text{plateau pressure} - \text{PEEP}}$$

where compressed volume = compliance factor × plateau pressure
= 4 ml/cm × 20 cm = 80 ml

$$C_{st} = \frac{600 \text{ ml} - 80 \text{ ml}}{20 \text{ cm} - 0}$$

$$= \frac{520 \text{ ml}}{20 \text{ cm}}$$

$$= 26 \text{ ml/cm } H_2O$$

$$C_{dyn} = \frac{\text{exhaled tidal volume} - \text{compressed volume}}{\text{peak pressure} - \text{PEEP}}$$

where compressed volume = compliance factor × peak pressure
= 4 ml/cm × 30 cm = 120 ml

$$C_{dyn} = \frac{600 \text{ ml} - 120 \text{ ml}}{30 \text{ cm} - 0}$$

$$= \frac{480 \text{ ml}}{30 \text{ cm}}$$

$$= 16 \text{ ml/cm } H_2O$$

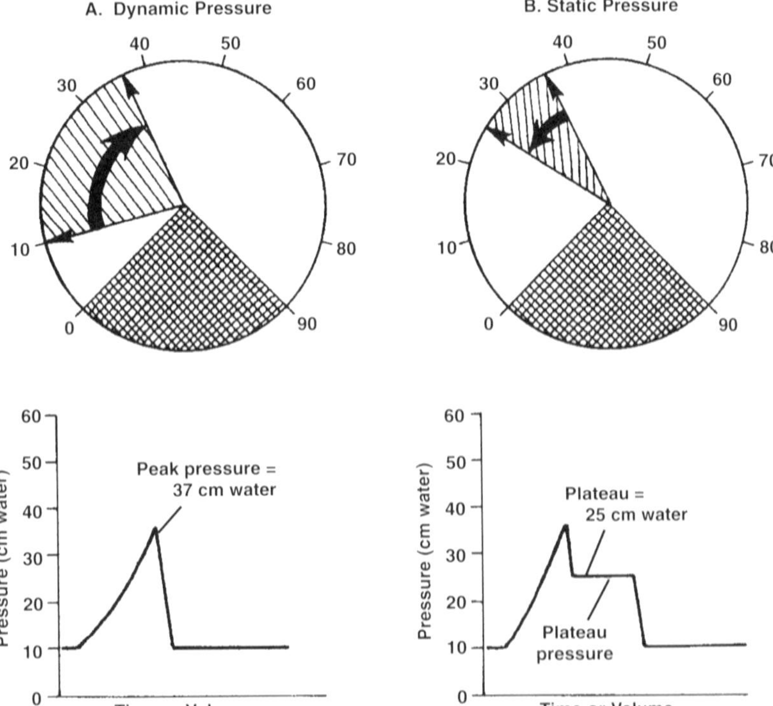

Fig. 14-21 Peak and static pressures with positive end-expiratory pressure (PEEP). **A,** Pressure manometer reading and pressure/volume curve for dynamic pressure. **B,** Pressure manometer reading and pressure/volume curve for static pressure. See the text for details.

Example:

Calculate the static and dynamic compliance on a ventilated patient with PEEP therapy.

The same patient has an exhaled tidal volume of 600 ml. Because of refractory hypoxemia, 10 cm of PEEP therapy is started. The peak pressure is now 36 cm H_2O, and the static or plateau pressure is now 25 cm H_2O (Fig. 14-21). The compliance factor has been determined to be 4 ml/cm H_2O.

$$C_{st} = \frac{\text{exhaled tidal volume} - \text{compressed volume}}{\text{plateau pressure} - \text{PEEP}}$$

where compressed volume = compliance factor × plateau pressure
= 4 ml/cm × (25 cm − 10 cm) = 60 ml

$$C_{st} = \frac{600 \text{ mL} - 60 \text{ ml}}{25 \text{ cm} - 10 \text{ cm}}$$

$$= \frac{540 \text{ ml}}{15 \text{ cm}}$$

$$= 36 \text{ mL/cm } H_2O$$

$$C_{dyn} = \frac{\text{exhaled tidal volume} - \text{compressed volume}}{\text{peak pressure} - \text{PEEP}}$$

where compressed volume = compliance factor × peak pressure
= 4 ml/cm × (36 cm − 10 cm) = 104 ml

$$C_{dyn} = \frac{600 \text{ ml} - 104 \text{ ml}}{36 \text{ cm} - 10 \text{ cm}}$$

$$= \frac{496 \text{ ml}}{26 \text{ cm}}$$

$$= 19 \text{ ml/cm } H_2O$$

c. Interpret the patient's airway resistance, dynamic lung compliance, and static lung compliance values on the ventilator. (IC1j) [R, Ap, An]

Any increase in airway resistance greater than normal creates an increase in the patient's work of breathing. Examples of conditions or situations where there will be an increased airway resistance include bronchospasm, secretions, mucosal edema, airway tumor, placement of a small endotracheal tube, and biting or kinking of the endotracheal tube. To breathe, the patient must consume more calories and oxygen. This can be exhausting and limit the patient's ability to do anything else. Correction of the problem should result in the airway resistance returning to normal.

There are six possible combinations of increasing or decreasing static and dynamic lung compliances. Each has its own possible causes and are covered in turn. The example discussed earlier and illustrated in Fig. 14-20 are used as a starting point for these variations.

It must be remembered that the patient must be passive on the ventilator for the measured values to be accurate. If the patient is assisting with the breath, the pressures will be too low. If the patient is fighting the breath, the pressures will be too high. Check two or three breaths for increased accuracy. Let the patient have a normal breath or two between each of the peak and plateau pressure measurement breaths.

Decreased Dynamic Compliance With Stable Static Compliance

Decreased dynamic compliance with stable static compliance is noticed as an *increase* in the peak pressure with an unchanged plateau pressure (Fig. 14-22). Causes include bronchospasm, coughing by the patient, secretions in the airways, water or kinking in the inspiratory limb of the circuit, or the patient biting the endotracheal tube. Correcting the underlying problem by aerosolizing a bronchodilator, suctioning, and so on results in the peak pressure returning to the original level.

Note that the inspiratory resistance has doubled from the original 10 to 20 cm while the plateau pressure has not changed. This confirms that the problem originates in the airway or breathing circuit. The patient's lung compliance has not changed.

Increased Dynamic Compliance With Stable Static Compliance

Increased dynamic compliance with stable static compliance is noticed as a *decrease* in the peak pressure with an unchanged plateau pressure (Fig. 14-23). This represents an improvement in the patient's airway resistance from the original condition. Secretions could be diminished, mucous plugs cleared, or bronchospasm corrected.

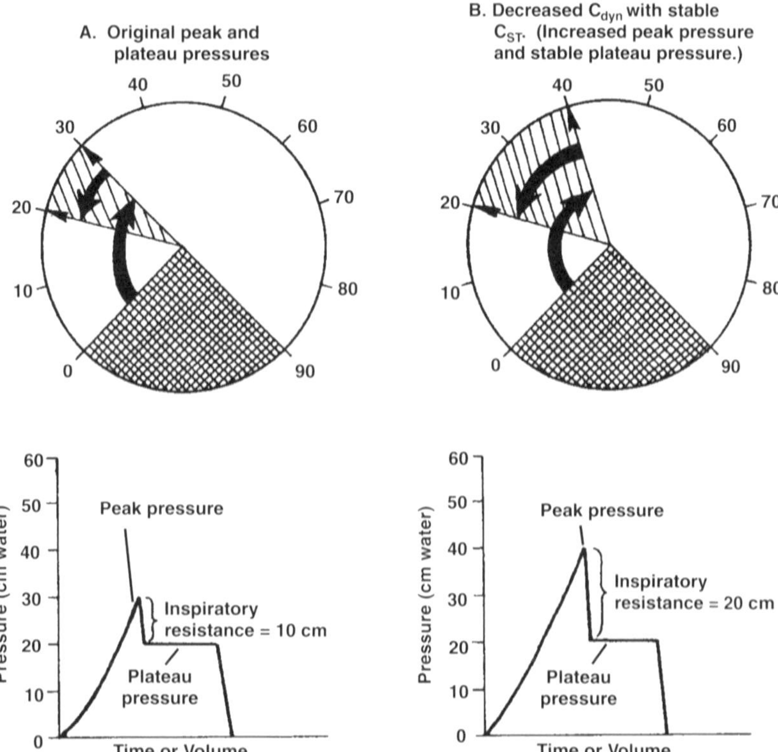

Fig. 14-22 Decreased dynamic compliance *(C_{dyn})* with a stable static compliance *(C_{st})*. **A,** Original pressure manometer reading and pressure/volume curve. **B,** Altered pressure manometer reading and pressure/volume curve.

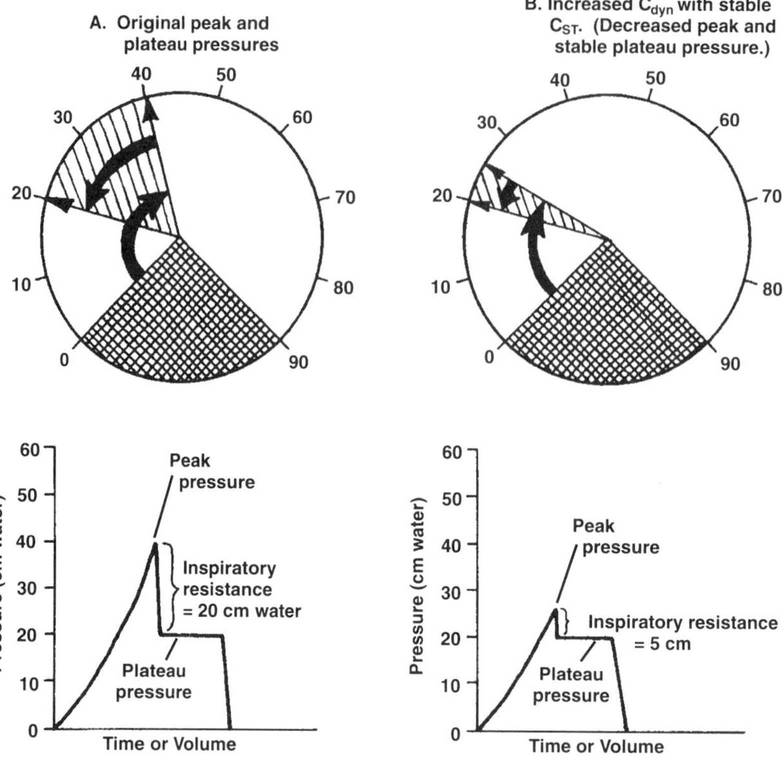

Fig. 14-23 Increased dynamic compliance (C_{dyn}) with a stable static compliance (C_{st}). **A,** Original pressure manometer reading and pressure/volume curve. **B,** Altered pressure manometer reading and pressure/volume curve.

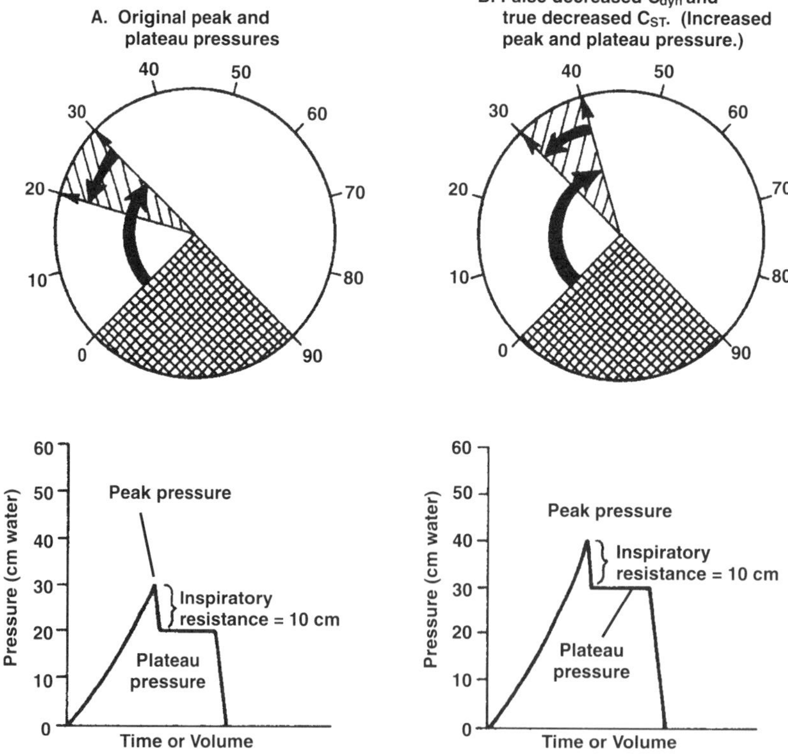

Fig. 14-24 False decreased dynamic compliance (C_{dyn}) with true decreased static compliance (C_{st}). **A,** Original pressure manometer reading and pressure/volume curve. **B,** Altered pressure manometer reading and pressure/volume curve.

Note that the inspiratory resistance has decreased from the original level of 20 to just 5 cm. This confirms that the patient's airway resistance has decreased. The patient's lung compliance has not changed.

False Decreased Dynamic Compliance With True Decreased Static Compliance

False decreased compliance with true decreased static compliance is noticed as an *increase* in *both* the peak and plateau pressures (Fig. 14-24). This is seen when the patient's lung-thoracic compliance worsens. The plateau pressure is elevated and the static compliance is decreased. Pulmonary conditions that result in a lowered compliance include ARDS and IRDS, pneumonia, pulmonary edema, atelectasis, consolidation, hemothorax, pleural effusion, air trapping, pneumomediastinum, and pneumothorax. Examples of chest wall and abdominal conditions that lower compliance include the various chest wall deformities, circumferential chest or abdominal burns, enlarged liver, pneumoperitoneum, peritonitis, abdominal bleeding, herniation, and advanced pregnancy.

As an artifact of the stiffer lungs, the peak pressure is also elevated, and the dynamic compliance is decreased. However, the difference between the peak and plateau pressures remains 10 cm H_2O. This demonstrates that there is no real increase in the patient's airway resistance.

True Decreased Dynamic Compliance With True Decreased Static Compliance

True decreased dynamic compliance with true decreased static compliance is also noticed as an *increase* in *both* the peak and plateau pressures (Fig. 14-25). This is seen with the combination of a decreased lung compliance and an increased airway resistance. Causes of both of these problems were discussed earlier.

False Increased Dynamic Compliance With True Increased Static Compliance

False increased dynamic compliance with true increased static compliance is noticed as a *decrease* in *both* the peak and plateau pressures (Fig. 14-26). This will be seen when the patient's lung-thoracic compliance improves. The plateau pressure decreases, and as an artifact, the peak pressure also decreases.

Notice that the difference between the peak and plateau pressures remains 10 cm H_2O. This indicates that the patient's airway resistance is unchanged.

True Increased Dynamic Compliance With True Increased Static Compliance

True increased dynamic compliance with true increased static compliance is also noticed as a *decrease* in *both* the peak and plateau pressures (Fig. 14-27). This is seen when both the patient's airway resistance and lung-thoracic compliance improve.

Notice that the plateau pressure has decreased, thus indicating more compliant lungs. Also notice that the difference between the peak and plateau pressures has decreased from 20 to 10 cm H_2O. This demonstrates that the airway resistance has also decreased.

All of the previous examples make use of a single tidal volume that is analyzed for peak and plateau pressures. Some practitioners advocate using several different tidal vol-

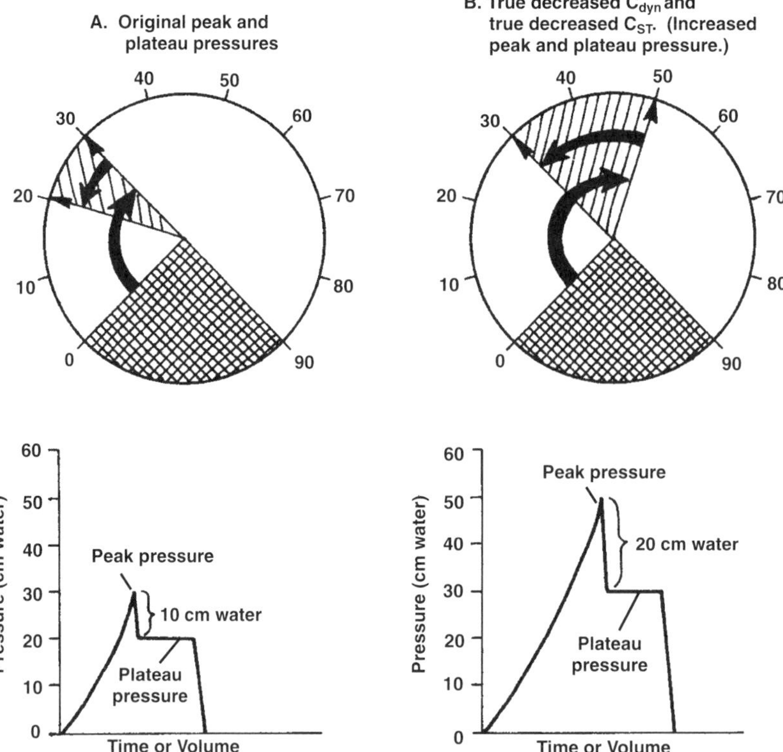

Fig. 14-25 True decreased dynamic compliance *(C_{dyn})* with true decreased static compliance *(C_{st})*. **A,** Original pressure manometer reading and pressure/volume curve. **B,** Altered pressure manometer reading and pressure/volume curve.

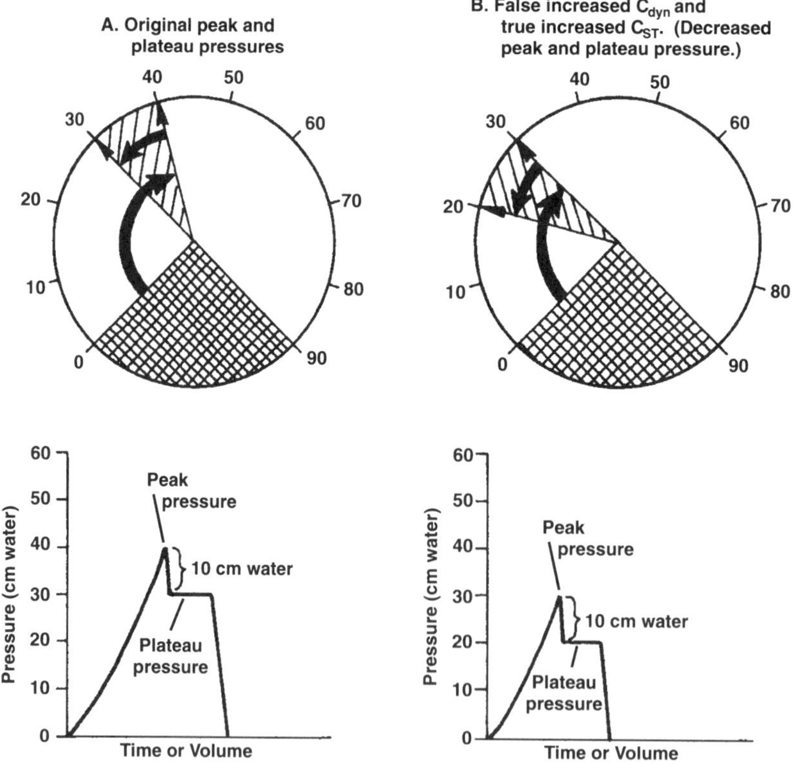

Fig. 14-26 False increased dynamic compliance *(C_{dyn})* with true increased static compliance *(C_{st})*. **A,** Original pressure manometer reading and pressure/volume curve. **B,** Altered pressure manometer reading and pressure/volume curve.

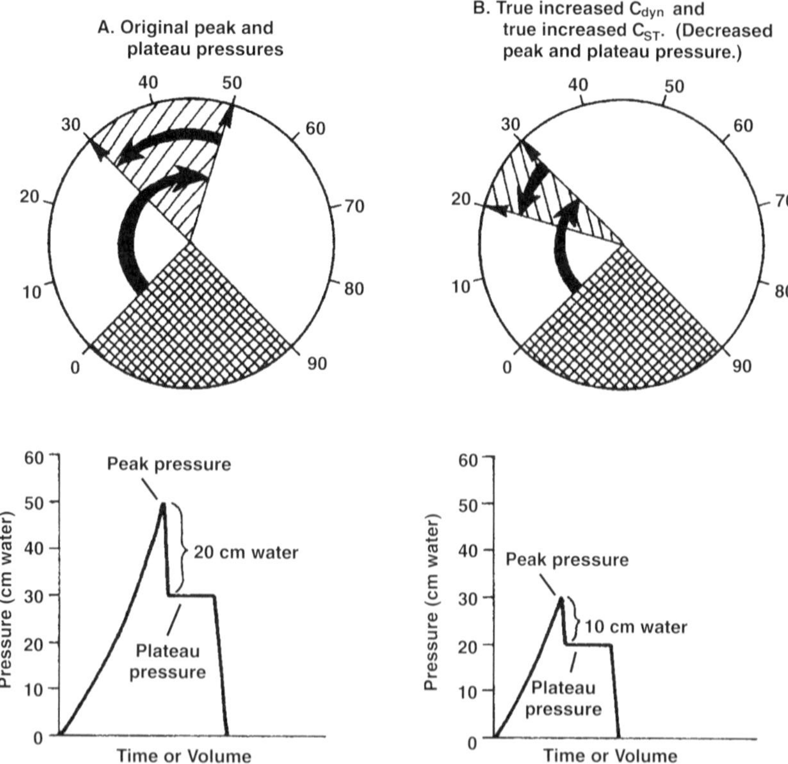

Fig. 14-27 True increased dynamic compliance *(C_{dyn})* with true increased static compliance *(C_{st})*. **A,** Original pressure manometer reading and pressure/volume curve. **B,** Altered pressure manometer reading and pressure/volume curve.

umes when measuring dynamic and static pressures. The procedure involves delivering a series of tidal volumes, determining the static and dynamic pressures at each volume, and then dividing the tidal volumes by the respective pressures. The various values are plotted on a graph to find the patient's optimal tidal volume (Fig. 14-28). The optimal tidal volume is found to result in the highest compliance values. Of the two, static compliance is preferred because it represents the resistance of only the lungs and thorax. If the tidal volume is too large and the lungs are overly stretched, the compliance values will decrease. In the example given, the best tidal volume is about 1.0 L (1000 ml). The optimal sigh volume can be found in the same way.

This procedure can also be used to help identify airway resistance and lung-thoracic compliance problems as shown earlier. Fig. 14-29 shows examples. Pulmonary embolism should be considered if the patient's condition deteriorates rapidly and there is no change in the dynamic and static compliance values.

6. Recommend changes in the respiratory care plan or make changes in mechanical ventilation based on the patient's response.

a. Make a recommendation to change the patient's position. (IIIF9h) [R, Ap, An]

Changing the patient's position was discussed in Section 5. Briefly, place a patient in Fowler's or semi-Fowler's position for weaning if tolerated.

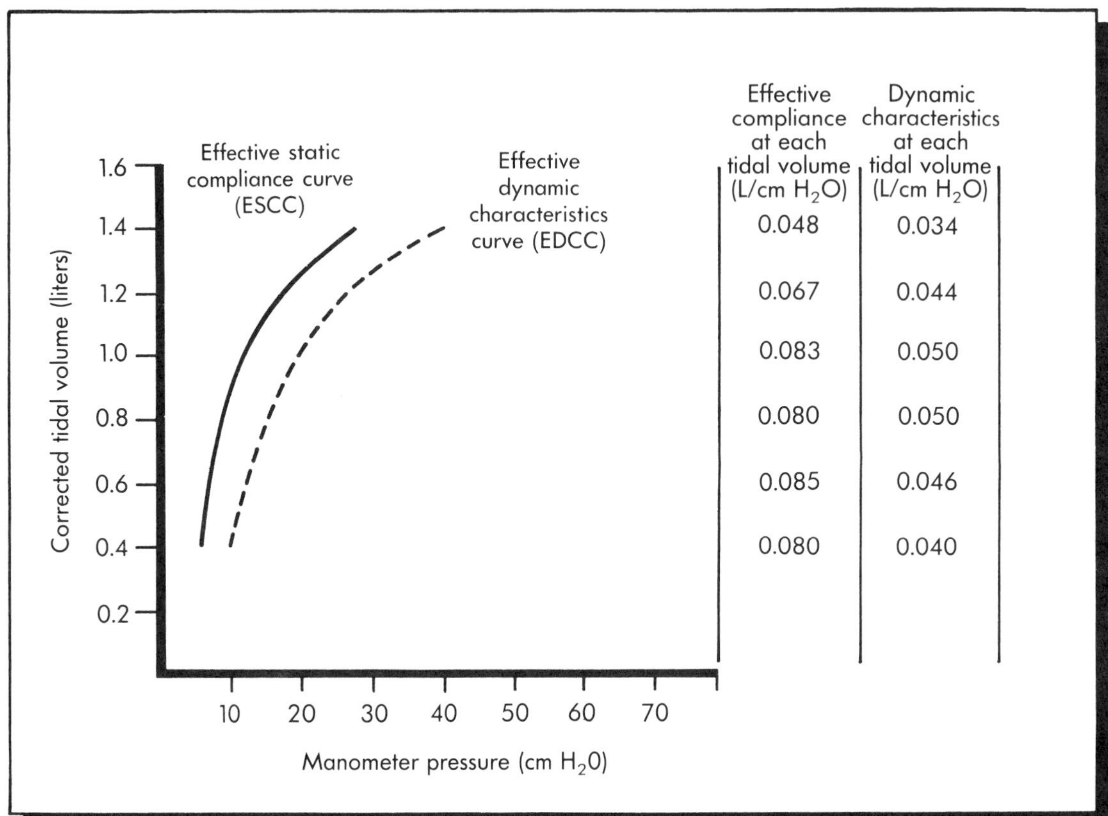

Fig. 14-28 Static and dynamic compliance curves and values. (Adapted from Williams-Colon S, Thalken FR: Management and monitoring of the patient in respiratory failure, in Scanlan CL, Spearman CB, Sheldon RL [eds]: *Egan's Fundamentals of Respiratory Care,* ed 5. St Louis, Mosby, 1990.)

b. Change the type of mechanical ventilator. (IIIF8i) [R, Ap, An]

Changing the type of mechanical ventilator is discussed earlier in this section. Briefly, a pressure cycled unit can be used with a patient without cardiopulmonary disease. Most patients with conditions that cause abnormal airway resistance or lung compliance should be placed on electrically powered volume cycled units. The microprocessor ventilators offer more ventilating options and monitoring of clinical information. They are best for the most critical patients.

c. Oxygen percentage.

i. Make a recommendation to change the oxygen percentage. (IIIF9g1) [R, Ap, An]

ii. Change the oxygen percentage. (IIIF8a) [R, Ap, An]

As discussed earlier, the goal of oxygen administration is to keep the Pa_{O_2} level of most patients between 60 and 90 mm Hg and the Sp_{O_2} level greater than 90%. Exceptions are the patient who is breathing on hypoxic drive and the patient who is in a cardiac arrest situation. The COPD patient who has a chronically low Pa_{O_2} level and chronically high Pa_{CO_2} level may be allowed to have a Pa_{O_2} value as low as 50 to 55 mm Hg and an Sp_{O_2} value as low as 85%. The patient in cardiac arrest must be given 100% oxygen.

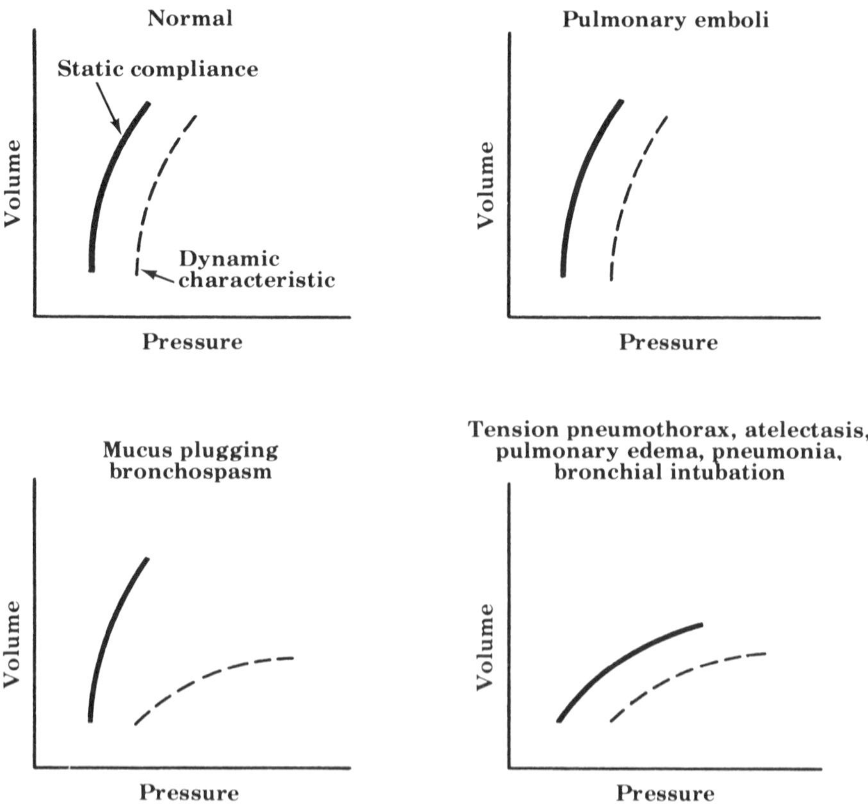

Fig. 14-29 Pressure/volume curves for normal airways and lungs, pulmonary embolism (no change in airway resistance or lung compliance), increased airway resistance, and decreased lung compliance. (From Pilbeam SP: *Mechanical Ventilation: Physiological and Clinical Applications.* St Louis, Mosby, 1986. Used by permission.)

Those patients who have refractory hypoxemia (e.g., ARDS) will not respond with a normal increase in Pa_{O_2} levels as the oxygen percentage is increased.

d. Make a recommendation to change the sensitivity. (IIIF9e) [R, Ap, An]

As discussed earlier, the sensitivity should be set so that the patient has to generate a negative pressure of about −1 to −2 cm H_2O to trigger the ventilator. Make a recommendation to change the sensitivity to minimize the patient's work of breathing.

e. Inspiratory flow.
- **i. Make a recommendation to change the inspiratory flow. (IIIF9o) [R, Ap, An]**
- **ii. Change the inspiratory flow. (IIIF8a) [R, Ap, An]**

See later discussion.

f. I/E ratio.
- **i. Make a recommendation to change the I/E ratio. (IIIF9s) [R, Ap, An]**
- **ii. Change the I/E ratio. (IIIF8a) [R, Ap, An]**

The topics of inspiratory flow and I/E ratio are considered together because they are interrelated. Table 14-5 shows the various formulas for calculating inspiratory time, expiratory time, I/E ratio, and related time variables.

It is possible to calculate the necessary flow rate to deliver a set tidal volume within the desired inspiratory time period. For example, if the patient has an ordered tidal volume of 500 ml, rate of 12 times/min, and I/E ratio of 1:2, calculate the required inspiratory flow as:

1. $\text{Cycle time} = \dfrac{60 \text{ seconds}}{\text{rate}} = \dfrac{60}{12} = 5 \text{ seconds}$

2. $\text{Inspiratory time} = \dfrac{\text{cycle time}}{\text{I} + \text{E}} = \dfrac{5 \text{ seconds}}{1 + 2} = \dfrac{5 \text{ seconds}}{3} = 1.67 \text{ seconds.}$

3. $$\begin{aligned}\text{Mean inspiratory flow} &= \frac{\text{tidal volume in L} \times 60 \text{ seconds/min}}{\text{inspiratory time}} \\ &= \frac{0.5 \text{ L} \times 60 \text{ sec/min}}{1.67 \text{ seconds}} \\ &= \frac{30 \text{ L/min}}{1.67 \text{ seconds}} \\ &= 18 \text{ l/min } (300 \text{ ml/sec})\end{aligned}$$

One basis for changing the inspiratory flow is to meet the patient needs. Commonly, the inspiratory flow for an adult will be initially set between 40 and 60 L/min (0.67-1.0 L/sec). An anxious patient often wants a faster flow rate when breathing rapidly. A patient who is resting comfortably may be able to have the flow rate reduced, which results in a lower peak pressure because there is less gas turbulence.

The inspiratory flow is also adjusted to set an I/E ratio. As a starting point, it is common to set the inspiratory flow so that the I/E ratio is 1:2. This is close to physiologically normal in a patient with normal airway resistance and lung-thoracic compliance. Having an expiratory time that is twice as long as the inspiratory time allows for a normal venous return to the heart.

The decision to change the I/E ratio is based upon the patient's pulmonary condition. The airway resistance and compliance determine how easily air flows into and out of the lungs and how much of the pressure applied to the lungs is transmitted throughout the chest. The product of the patient's airway resistance and lung-thoracic compliance is call the time constant of ventilation and is calculated as:

$$\text{Time constant of ventilation} = R_{aw} \times C_{LT}$$

Increased Inspiratory Time and Decreased Expiratory Time

This method of ventilation should be used in any condition where the patient has a small time constant of ventilation. This would be seen clinically as a normal airway resistance but a low lung-thoracic compliance. Examples of conditions where this is seen include IRDS, ARDS, pulmonary edema, pneumonia, and an enlarged abdomen.

The increased inspiratory time keeps the lungs inflated longer to provide more time for oxygen diffusion. This technique is commonly used with neonates with IRDS. At times an inverse I/E ratio as great as 4:1 (also seen as 1:0.25) is employed. Even if a high peak pressure is developed, the pressure is contained within the stiff lungs and not transmitted to the heart. As the lungs become more compliant, the inspiratory time must be reduced toward normal to prevent the pressure from compressing the heart. Full exhalation of the tidal volume must be assured. It is not usually a problem because the stiff lungs rapidly recoil to the resting level.

Decreased Inspiratory Time and Increased Expiratory Time

This method of ventilation should be used in any condition where the patient has a large time constant of ventilation. This would be seen clinically as an increased airway resistance but a normal lung-thoracic compliance. Examples of conditions where this is seen include asthma, bronchitis, large amounts of secretions, meconium or other aspiration, and airway tumor.

The increased expiratory time allows for a complete exhalation of the tidal volume. Care must be taken to measure both the inspired and expired volumes to make sure that they are equal and that the patient is not air trapping. Increase the expiratory time as needed until the tidal volume is completely exhaled. A second risk seen with these conditions is the development of inadvertent PEEP. Make sure that the manometer pressure returns to the baseline value at the end of expiration. As the airway resistance returns to normal, the expiratory time can be reduced to result in a more normal I/E ratio.

g. Flow pattern.

i. Make a recommendation to change the flow pattern. (IIIF9p) [R, Ap, An]

ii. Change the flow pattern. (IIIF8a) [R, Ap, An]

Most current generation ventilators offer more than one inspiratory flow pattern (Fig. 14-30). The sine wave is the most physiologically like a normal, spontaneous inspiration. The other wave forms can be compared with the sine wave to determine which one best meets the patient's needs. Each should be tried out in turn and these parameters evaluated:

Measured Parameter	Ideal Response
Peak pressure	Lowest
Mean airway pressure	Lowest
Blood pressure	Stable or improved
Heart rate	Stable or improved
Inspiratory and expiratory tidal volumes	Identical
Breath sounds	Improved
Patient's personal preference	Most comfortable

Ideally the best flow pattern is one in which the patient's airway pressures are lowest, the blood pressure is stable, the exhalation is complete, breath sounds are improved bilaterally, and the patient feels the most comfortable.

h. Tidal volume.

i. Make a recommendation to change the tidal volume. (IIIF9k) [R, Ap, An]

ii. Change the tidal volume. (IIIF8a) [R, Ap, An]

The specific tidal volume to select was discussed earlier in this section. Conditions where the tidal volume should be increased include atelectasis, consolidation, and when the present tidal volume is at the small end of the normal range and the patient has an

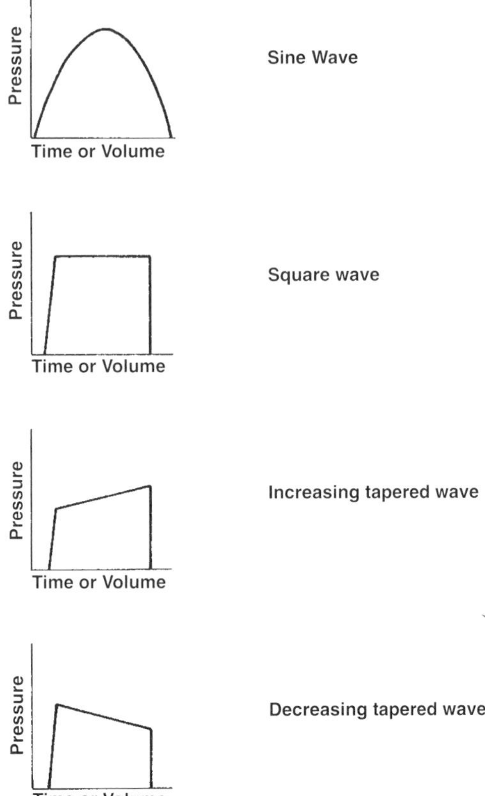

Fig. 14-30 Inspiratory waveforms.

elevated carbon dioxide level or low oxygen level. The upper level for a set tidal volume in the adult is 15 ml/kg of ideal body weight.

Conditions where the tidal volume should be decreased include air trapping, hyperinflated lungs as seen on the chest x-ray film by wide intercostal margins or flatten hemidiaphragms, and when the present tidal volume is at the large end of the normal range and the patient has a decreased carbon dioxide level. The lower level for a set tidal volume in the adult is 10 ml/kg of ideal body weight.

i. Respiratory rate.

i. Make a recommendation to change the respiratory rate. (IIIF91) [R, Ap, An]

ii. Change the respiratory rate. (IIIF8a) [R, Ap, An]

Respiratory rate was discussed earlier in this section. Increase the backup rate on the ventilator if the patient has an elevated carbon dioxide level and the tidal volume is at the high end of the normal range. Decrease the backup rate on the ventilator if the patient has a decreased carbon dioxide level and the tidal volume is at the low end of the normal range.

j. Change the sigh volume and frequency. (IIIF8a) [R, Ap, An]

People normally sigh every few minutes. A sigh is a volume larger than the normal tidal volume. It serves the purpose of opening up atelectatic alveoli and reorienting the surfactant in the alveoli so that they are stable.

Most ventilator-dependent patients receive a ventilator sigh volume just as they do a tidal volume. A sigh volume is typically 1.5 to 2 times the tidal volume if the tidal volume is in the low to middle range of normal. If the patient has a problem of atelectasis or consolidation, a larger sigh volume may be indicated. The patient may not need a sigh volume at all if the uncorrected tidal volume is at the 15 ml/kg upper limit. A patient with bullous emphysema, a pneumothorax, or cardiac status that is sensitive to high peak pressures may be contraindicated for a sigh volume. The patient who is air trapping the tidal volume should have a smaller (possibly no) sigh volume. Compare the inspired and expired volumes to ensure that there is no air trapping. Most current ventilators allow the clinician to tailor the sigh frequency to best meet the patient's clinical needs. The sigh frequency should be increased in patients with atelectasis or consolidation. The sigh frequency may need to be decreased or eliminated in patients who are air trapping the tidal or sigh volume. Sighs are usually not given when the patient is on the IMV/SIMV mode.

k. Pressure limits.

i. Make a recommendation to change the pressure limits. (IIIF9q) [R, Ap, An]

ii. Change the pressure limits. (IIIF8a) [R, Ap, An]

Set the high pressure limit for the tidal and sigh volumes so that they are delivered under normal conditions. Yet if the patient should cough, have secretions, or any other problem that would result in a sudden increase in the peak pressure, the pressure limit will be reached and the audible alarm will sound. Typically the pressure limit is set 5 to 10 cm H_2O greater than the peak pressure. The pressure limit may be set closer to the peak pressure with neonatal ventilation.

A low pressure or disconnection alarm should be set about 3 to 5 cm H_2O below the peak pressure or CPAP level. The alarm setting may be set closer to the peak pressure with neonatal ventilation (discussed earlier in this section).

Some ventilators such as the Servo 900 C have a separate high-pressure limit for use whenever PEEP therapy is applied. This would limit any inadvertent PEEP resulting from a mechanical failure or circuit obstruction. Set this high pressure limit at 1 to 2 cm H_2O greater than the ordered PEEP level.

l. Change the alarm settings. (IIIF8c) [R, Ap, An]

Alarm settings were discussed earlier in this module. Be prepared to adjust the alarm settings based on the patient's clinical situation.

m. Change the mechanical dead space. (IIIF8d) [R, Ap]

Mechanical dead space is added to increase the patient's $Paco_2$ level by making him or her rebreathe some exhaled carbon dioxide. The last part of the tidal volume to be exhaled came from the alveoli and is high in carbon dioxide. This last portion of the tidal volume is exhaled into the dead space tubing. This high CO_2 gas is then inhaled back to the alveolar level and increases the patient's $Paco_2$ level. The more dead space tubing there is, the more carbon dioxide is retained. It is important to realize that this same rebreathed volume of gas is lower in oxygen because of its diffusion into the patient's pulmonary circulation. If a large amount of mechanical dead space is added, it will be necessary to increase the Fio_2 to keep the ordered level. Measure the oxygen percentage between the dead space and the endotracheal/tracheostomy tube adapter.

Mechanical dead space is used only in the control and assist/control modes. It should not be used in IMV/SIMV, pressure support, or CPAP modes. Typically, a length of large-bore/aerosol tubing is added into the breathing circuit between the Y and the patient's endotracheal or tracheostomy tube (see Fig. 14-18). The following formula can be used to predict what amount of mechanical dead space will produce a desired Pa_{CO_2} level:

$$[(V_T - V_{D_{anat}}) - V_{D_{mech}}] \times f \times Pa_{CO_2} = [(V_T - V_{D_{anat}}) - V_{D_{mech}}'] \times f \times Pa_{CO_2}'$$

where

- V_T = current tidal volume
- $V_{D_{anat}}$ = anatomic dead space. This is calculated at 1 ml/lb or 2.2 ml/kg of ideal body weight.
- $V_{D_{mech}}$ = current mechanical dead space
- f = ventilator rate
- Pa_{CO_2} = actual patient Pa_{CO_2} value
- $V_{D_{mech}}'$ = desired mechanical dead space
- Pa_{CO_2}' = desired patient Pa_{CO_2} value

Example:

Your patient is a 70-kg (154-lb) man who is being ventilated on the control mode (he is apneic). His ventilator settings are tidal volume of 1000 ml, rate of 12 times/min, F_{IO_2} of 0.3, and no added mechanical dead space. His arterial blood gas values are Pa_{O_2} of 90 mm Hg, Pa_{CO_2} of 30 mm Hg, pH of 7.48, Sa_{O_2} of 95%, and BE of zero.

The clinical goal is to adjust the patient's mechanical dead space as needed to produce a Pa_{CO_2} level of 40 mm Hg. In summary:

V_T = 1000 ml current tidal volume
$V_{D_{anat}}$ = 154 ml anatomic dead space. This is calculated at 1 ml/lb or 2.2 ml/kg of ideal body weight.
$V_{D_{mech}}$ = no added mechanical dead space
f = 12 times/min for ventilator rate
Pa_{CO_2} = 30 mm Hg actual patient Pa_{CO_2} value
$V_{D_{mech}}'$ = desired amount of mechanical dead space
Pa_{CO_2}' = 40 mm Hg desired patient Pa_{CO_2} value

Placing the data and goal into the formula results in:

$$[(V_T - V_{D_{anat}}) - V_{D_{mech}}] \times f \times Pa_{CO_2} = [(V_T - V_{D_{anat}}) - V_{D_{mech}}'] \times f \times Pa_{CO_2}'$$
$$[(1000 - 154) - 0] \times 12 \times 30 = [(1000 - 154) - V_{D_{mech}}'] \times 12 \times 40$$

Simplifying produces the following:

$$[846] \times 12 \times 30 = [846 - V_{D_{mech}}'] \times 480$$
$$304{,}560 = (846 \times 480) - V_{D_{mech}}' \times 480$$
$$304{,}560 = 406{,}080 - 480\ V_{D_{mech}}'$$
$$-101{,}520 = -480\ V_{D_{mech}}'$$
$$211.5 \text{ ml} = V_{D_{mech}}'$$

The solution is to increase the patient's mechanical dead space from zero to 212 ml.

n. Make a recommendation to change the mode of ventilation. (IIIF9r) [R, Ap, An]

Changing the mode of ventilation is discussed earlier in this section.

o. PEEP therapy.

i. Make a recommendation to begin using PEEP therapy. (IIIF9f1) [R, Ap, An]

ii. Make a recommendation to change the level of PEEP. (IIIF9n) [R, Ap, An]

iii. Change the level of PEEP. (IIIF8f) [R, Ap, An]

PEEP therapy was discussed earlier in this section. Remember that therapeutic PEEP is indicated in situations where the patient has bilaterally small lungs with a reduced FRC. This results in atelectasis and hypoxemia. The proper level of PEEP will restore the FRC and improve oxygenation. Watch for side affects of barotrauma or decreased cardiac output from too much pressure. The patient should be carefully monitored with blood gas analyses and vital sign checks before starting PEEP and after each change.

p. CPAP therapy.

i. Make a recommendation to begin using CPAP. (IIIF9f2) [R, Ap, An]

ii. Make a recommendation to change the level of CPAP. (IIIF9m) [R, Ap, An]

iii. Change the level of CPAP. (IIIF8g) [R, Ap, An]

CPAP therapy was discussed earlier in this section. Briefly, all of these considerations for PEEP apply to CPAP except that the patient must be able to breath spontaneously.

q. IMV.

i. Make a recommendation to begin using IMV. (IIIF9f3) [R, Ap, An]

ii. Make a recommendation to change the IMV rate. (IIIF9j) [R, Ap, An]

IMV is discussed earlier in this section. Briefly, the patient must be able to provide some spontaneous breathing but still needs support by the ventilator. As the patient improves, the IMV rate is reduced.

r. Change the inspiratory plateau. (IIIF8e) [R, Ap, An]

Inspiratory plateau (also known as inflation hold) is a technique whereby the patient is temporarily prevented from exhaling the ventilator delivered tidal volume. It is added therapeutically to improve the distribution of the tidal volume. Patients with ARDS and pulmonary edema can benefit from it. Oxygenation should improve in direct proportion to the duration of the inspiratory plateau. The duration of inspiratory plateau is measured in different ways, depending on the ventilator. For example, the BEAR 5 and 1000 and Puritan-Bennett 7200 can have it added in steps of 0.1 second up to several seconds total. The Servo 900 B and C can have it added as a variable percentage of the total duration of the breathing cycle. It is important to reduce the inspiratory plateau as the patient's ventilation and lung compliance improve. Patient's with normal ventilation and compliance should not receive any inspiratory plateau.

Notice that the use of an inspiratory plateau increases the inspiratory phase of the breathing cycle. This results in a shorter expiratory time if the rate is kept the same. Or, the rate must be reduced to keep the same I/E ratio. Again, as discussed earlier, make sure that the tidal volume is completely exhaled. The patient's condition should be monitored closely to determine if the level of inspiratory plateau is appropriate.

Nontherapeutic inspiratory plateau is added temporarily to determine the plateau pressure on the ventilator. This is considered to be the pressure needed to deliver the tidal volume. See Fig. 14-20 for an example. With this information, the patient's effective static compliance can be calculated. Its calculation and interpretation were discussed earlier in this section. An inspiratory plateau of 0.5 to 1.0 second is usually long enough to find the plateau pressure. Remember to turn off the inspiratory plateau afterward.

s. Change the pressure support level. (IIIF8j) [R, Ap, An]

See the earlier discussion in this section for full details. As a brief review, remember that pressure support is used either to deliver a desired tidal volume or overcome the resistance of the patient's endotracheal tube. More pressure support would tend to deliver a larger volume and reduce the patient's work of breathing. Less would deliver a smaller volume and require the patient to contribute more effort toward the total minute volume.

t. Wean the patient from the ventilator.

i. Make a recommendation to begin weaning from the ventilator. (IIIH4f4) [R, Ap, An]

Indications that the patient will tolerate weaning usually include some, if not all, of the criteria listed in Table 14-4. It is not necessary that the patient pass each and every criteria. However, the more the patient can attain, the more likely he or she is to successfully wean. Individual physicians and practitioners may favor some of these conditions over others and may include other factors not listed.

There are patients who will not wean successfully even though objective criteria indicated that they should. Conversely, some patients can wean successfully even when objective criteria indicate that the patient will not succeed. The key point to keep in mind is that each patient must be evaluated individually. Look at the objective criteria, as well as how the patient actually performs during weaning.

ii. Recommend changes in the weaning procedures. (IIIF9i) [R, Ap, An]

iii. Make changes in the weaning procedures. (IIIC81 and IIIF8h) [R, Ap, An]

Weaning must be individualized to best meet the patient's needs. There is no best method for all patients. Each of the five methods presented here has its advocates and a body of clinical evidence to show that it is a valid weaning technique. The practitioner must evaluate the patient before recommending any particular weaning method. The patient must also be evaluated during the weaning trial to determine if the method chosen is meeting his or her needs. The practitioner needs to be prepared to discontinue weaning if the patient is failing and be ready to try another weaning approach to help ensure success.

Ventilator Discontinuance

Ventilator discontinuance is one of two methods used to originally wean patients who had been ventilated by the assist/control mode (see Fig. 14-1,A). It is still used today with patients who have been ventilated for a short period and are now fully prepared to stop ventilator treatment. Examples include continued prophylactic ventilation after surgery and because of an unreversed anesthesia or a narcotic overdose with respiratory center depression.

When the patient is stable, awake, and alert and meets the criteria listed in Table

14-4, he or she can be prepared for weaning. The patient should be instructed about the weaning, suctioned, and put in Fowler's or semi-Fowler's position if possible. The ventilator circuit is disconnected, and an aerosol and oxygen mix is breathed in via a Brigg's adapter/aerosol T adapter. The oxygen percentage should be the same as originally inspired or up to 10% higher, depending on the patient's Pa_{O_2} level on the ventilator.

Ventilator discontinuance and weaning begin at the same moment (Fig. 14-31,A). The patient goes from having the ventilator provide 100% of the minute volume needs to providing none of it. The patient should be watched continuously because he or she is now breathing totally independently. Vital signs and respiratory mechanics should be measured every 5 to 10 minutes throughout the procedure. If the patient deteriorates, ventilator therapy is reestablished. After a rest period, intermittent ventilator discontinuance or another mode of weaning might be tried. If the patient is stable, an arterial blood

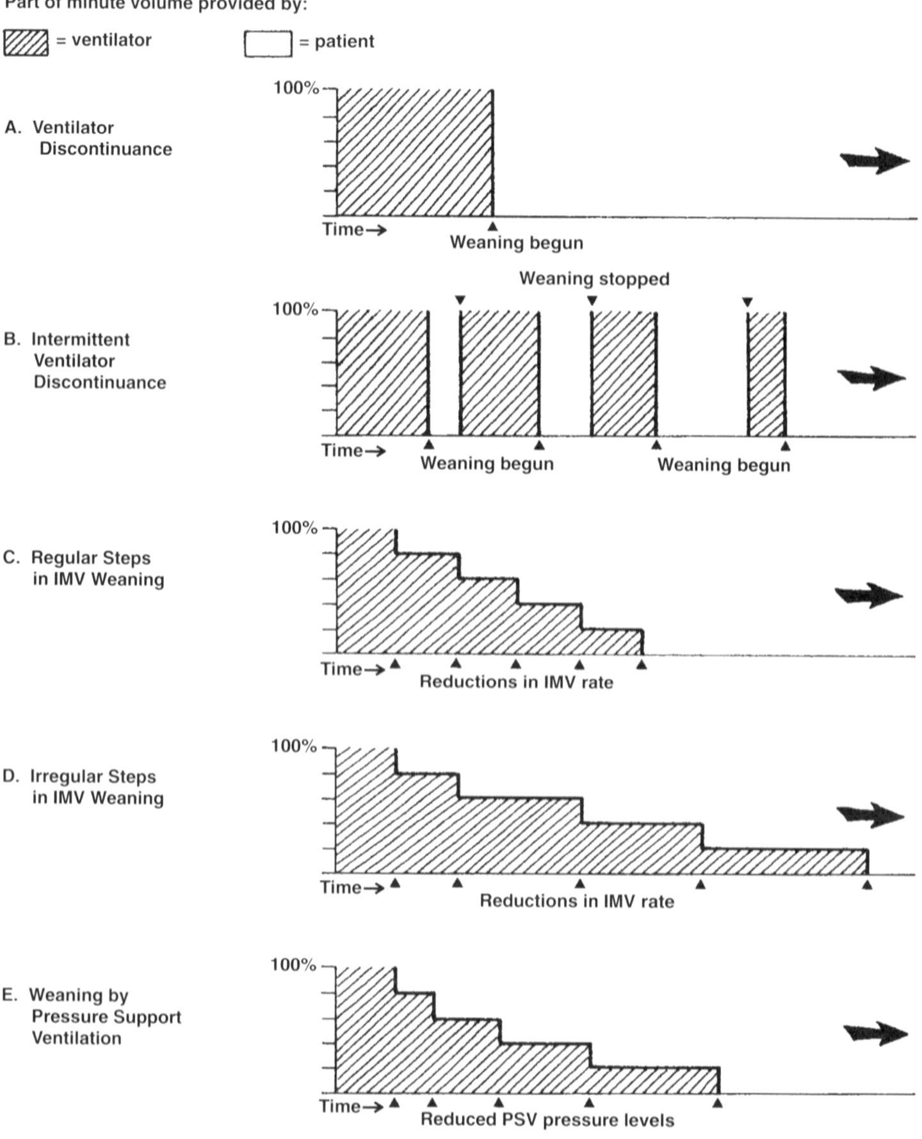

Fig. 14-31 A-E, Options for weaning a patient from a mechanical ventilator.

gas sample should be taken after about 20 minutes. If the blood gas results are acceptable and the patient appears stable, the weaning is continued for an extended period of time.

Intermittent Ventilator Discontinuance

This is the second method used to originally wean patients who had been ventilated by the assist/control mode. It is commonly used after the previously mentioned method proves less than successful. The patient is started on a schedule of intermittent weaning periods and rest periods on the ventilator (Fig. 14-31,B). The method shown has a cycle of lengthening weaning periods and shortening rest periods. This would go on until the patient is weaning for an extended period, as discussed earlier. Another method involves a cycle of set rest periods (commonly one-half to 1 hour) and lengthening weaning periods as the patient becomes a stronger. Again, an arterial blood gas sample should be taken after about 20 minutes of weaning. The weaning period can be extended as long as the patient is stable.

Regular Steps in IMV Weaning

Regular steps are one of two IMV weaning methods. As discussed earlier, IMV/SIMV was originally developed as a ventilating mode and has since become a widely used weaning mode. It allows the patient a more gradual transition toward totally providing all of the work of breathing. IMV seems to work especially well in weaning patients who have been ventilator dependent for an extended period. By gradually taking over more of the work of breathing, the patient reconditions respiratory muscles that may have atrophied through lack of use. The patient is also gaining self-confidence that complete weaning will occur. An additional benefit is that all ventilator alarm systems are functional and the patient does not need to be watched as closely as in the two previously mentioned weaning methods.

This particular IMV weaning pattern can be applied to a patient who is stable and making rapid progress (Fig. 14-31,C). The weaning pattern might involve the IMV rate being reduced in increments of about 2 per minute on a set time schedule. For example, every hour the rate is reduced by 2 per minute. About 20 minutes after reducing the IMV rate, an arterial blood gas sample is taken. The patient's respiratory mechanics are monitored closely. It is important to calculate the patient's spontaneous minute volume (rate × tidal volume). It should be approximately the same volume as was subtracted from the ventilator-delivered minute volume. The process continues as long as the patient tolerates each decrease in the IMV rate. The stable, strong patient can be rather quickly weaned down to an IMV rate of 2 to 4 times/min. The decision is often made at this point to either use a Brigg's adapter, as discussed earlier, or to extubate the airway.

Irregular Steps in IMV Weaning

Irregular steps are the second method of IMV weaning. All of the advantages of IMV as a weaning method that were discussed earlier apply here as well. This method is applied when the regular IMV method is less than successful. Often the patient starts out on a cycle of regular reductions in the IMV rate. This goes on until a point is reached where the patient has a setback and cannot tolerate any further reductions in the IMV rate. The rate may be kept at that level for an extended period (as shown) until the patient is ready for a further decrease (Fig. 13-34,D). Further drops in the IMV rate proceed as the patient tolerates them. No attempt is made to set up a regular pattern of reducing the rate.

It may be necessary to increase the rate to higher previous levels if the patient has a serious setback. Eventually the IMV rate is reduced to a level of 2 to 4 times/min. Frequently these weaker patients find this level of support to be as low as they can go. One possible cause of their being unable to go any lower is the resistance to breathing through the demand-valve and breathing circuit. A trial on a Brigg's adapter (which offers no resistance) may prove to be the final step in weaning. If the patient fails this, the reason is probably the resistance caused by the endotracheal tube. The following weaning method should then be tried on the patient.

Weaning by Pressure Support Ventilation

The PSV mode is available on most modern electrically powered and microprocessor ventilators. It can be used as the newest weaning method. PSV was discussed earlier and is shown in Fig. 14-31,E. When used as a weaning method, the pressure support level is gradually reduced. Decreasing pressure support steps of 2 to 5 cm H_2O are commonly made. The patient has to gradually increase the work of breathing to inspire a tidal volume. Blood gas values and respiratory mechanics should be evaluated after each drop in the pressure support level. A modest pressure support level of 2 to 5 cm H_2O is maintained to overcome any resistance of the endotracheal tube. If the patient does well during an extended trial of minimal pressure support, extubation is performed unless the endotracheal tube is needed for other reasons.

The criteria listed in Table 14-4 can be used in evaluating any patient being weaned by any of these methods. General signs that the patient is not tolerating weaning include anxiety, agitation, a large increase or decrease in the respiratory rate, angina, tachycardia, an increase in premature ventricular contractions or other serious dysrhythmias, bradycardia, hypertension, hypotension, cyanosis, hypoxemia, and hypercarbia with acidemia. The patient probably will not exhibit all of these signs. Some tend to be seen together because they relate to the patient's work of breathing. Others would appear to give conflicting signals of success or failure. It is the practitioner's responsibility to evaluate the patient's condition to determine whether weaning should be continued or ventilatory support resumed.

BIBLIOGRAPHY

AARC Clinical Practice Guideline: Humidification during mechanical ventilation. *Respir Care* 1992;37:887-890.

AARC Clinical Practice Guideline: Patient-ventilator system checks. *Respir Care* 1992;37:882-886.

American College of Chest Physicians' Consensus Conference: Mechanical ventilation. *Respir Care* 1993;38;1389-1417.

Aloan CA: *Respiratory Care of the Newborn*. Philadelphia, Lippincott, 1987.

Banner MJ, Lampotang S: Clinical use of inspiratory and expiratory waveforms, in Kacmarek RM, Stoller JK (eds): *Current Respiratory Care*. Philadelphia, Decker, 1988.

Barnes TA: Mechanical ventilation, in Barnes TA (ed): *Respiratory Care Practice*. Chicago, Mosby, 1988.

Bone RC: Acute respiratory failure: classification, differential diagnosis and introduction to management, in Burton GG, Hodgkin JE (eds): *Respiratory Care*, ed 2. Philadelphia, Lippincott, 1984.

Bone RC: Pressure-volume measurements in detection of bronchospasm and mucous plugging in acute respiratory failure. *Respir Care* 1976;21:620-626.

Bone RC: Monitoring ventilatory mechanics in acute respiratory failure. *Respir Care* 1983;28:597-604.

Boysen PG, McGough E: Pressure-control and pressure-support ventilation: flow patterns, inspiratory time, and gas distribution. *Respir Care* 1988;33:126-134.

Chatburn RL, Lough MD: Mechanical ventilation, in Lough MD, Doershuk CF, Stern RC (eds): *Pediatric Respiratory Therapy*, ed 3. Chicago, Mosby, 1985.

Desautels DA, Blanch PB: Mechanical ventilation, in Burton GG, Hodgkin JE, Ward JJ (eds): *Respiratory Care*, ed 3. Philadelphia, Lippincott, 1991.

DesJardins TR: Cardiopulmonary anatomy and physiology, essentials for respiratory care. Albany, NY, Delmar, 1988.

Eubanks DH, Bone RC: *Comprehensive Respiratory Care*, ed 2. St Louis, Mosby, 1990.

Gurevitch MJ: Selection of the inspiratory: expiratory ratio, in Kacmarek RM, Stoller JK (eds): *Current Respiratory Care*. Philadelphia, Decker, 1988.

Hess DR, Hodgkin JE, Burton GG: Mechanical ventilation: initiation, management, and weaning, in Burton GG, Hodgkin JE, Ward JJ (eds): *Respiratory Care*, ed 3. Philadelphia, Lippincott, 1991.

Hodgkin JE, Gray LS, Burton GG: Techniques in ventilatory weaning, in Burton GG, Hodgkin JE (eds): *Respiratory Care*, ed 2. Philadelphia, Lippincott, 1984.

Kacmarek RM: The role of pressure support ventilation in reducing imposed work of breathing. *Respir Care* 1988;33:99-120.

Kacmarek RM: Systematic modification of ventilatory support, in Barnes TA (ed): *Respiratory Care Practice*. Chicago, Mosby, 1988.

Kacmarek RM, Mack CW, Dimas S: *The Essentials of Respiratory Therapy*, ed 2. Mosby, Chicago, 1985.

Kirby RR: Modes of mechanical ventilation, in Kacmarek RM, Stoller JK (eds): *Current Respiratory Care*. Philadelphia, Decker, 1988.

Kirby RR, Smith RA, Desautels DA: Mechanical ventilation, in Burton GG, Hodgkin JE (eds): *Respiratory Care*, ed 2. Philadelphia, Lippincott, 1984.

Koff PB, Eitzman DV, Neu J: *Neonatal and Pediatric Respiratory Care*. St. Louis, Mosby, 1988.

MacIntyre NR: Respiratory function during pressure support ventilation. *Chest* 1986;89:677-683.

MacIntyre NR: Pressure support: Inspiratory assist, in Kacmarek RM, Stoller JK (eds): *Current Respiratory Care*. Philadelphia, Decker, 1988.

MacIntyre NR: Weaning from mechanical ventilatory support: Volume-assisting intermittent breaths versus pressure-supporting every breath. *Respir Care* 1988;33:121-125.

Martz KV, Joiner JW, Rodger MS: *Management of the Patient-Ventilator System, a Team Approach*, ed 2. St Louis, Mosby, 1984.

McPherson SP: *Respiratory Therapy Equipment*, ed 3. St Louis, Mosby, 1985.

McPherson SP: *Respiratory Therapy Equipment*, ed 4. St Louis, Mosby, 1990.

Pilbeam SP: *Mechanical Ventilation: Physiological and Clinical Applications*. St Louis, Mosby, 1986.

Rarey KP, Youtsey JW: *Respiratory Patient Care*. Englewood Cliffs, NJ, Prentice-Hall, 1981.

Register SD, Downs JB: F_{IO_2} and PEEP, in Kacmarek RM, Stoller JK (eds): *Current Respiratory Care*. Philadelphia, Decker, 1988.

Scanlan CL: Physics and physiology of ventilatory support, in Scanlan CL, Spearman CB, Sheldon RL (eds): *Egan's Fundamentals of Respiratory Care*, ed 5. St Louis, Mosby, 1990.

Scanlan CL: Respiratory failure and the need for ventilatory support, in Scanlan CL, Spearman CB, Sheldon RL (eds): *Egan's Fundamentals of Respiratory Care*, ed 5. St Louis, Mosby, 1990.

Scanlan CL: Selection and application of ventilatory support devices, in Scanlan CL, Spearman CB, Sheldon RL (Eds): *Egan's Fundamentals of Respiratory Care*, ed 5. St Louis, Mosby, 1990.

Schussler NC, Scanlan CL: Neonatal and pediatric intensive care, in Scanlan CL, Spearman CB, Sheldon RL (eds): *Egan's Fundamentals of Respiratory Care,* ed 5. St Louis, Mosby, 1990.

Shapiro BA, Harrison RA, Kacmarek RM, et al: *Clinical Application of Respiratory Care,* ed 3. Chicago, Mosby, 1985.

Spearman CB: Appropriate ventilator selection, in Kacmarek RM, Stoller JK (eds): *Current Respiratory Care.* Philadelphia, Decker, 1988.

Spearman CB, Sheldon RL, Egan DE (eds): *Egan's Fundamentals of Respiratory Care,* ed 4. St Louis, Mosby, 1982.

Vandine JD: Mechanical ventilators, in Barnes TA (ed): *Respiratory Care Practice.* Chicago, Mosby, 1988.

SELF-STUDY QUESTIONS

1. A 40-year-old patient is brought to the emergency room after being in an automobile accident. She has broken ribs on her right side and a right-sided pneumothorax. With which of the following ventilators would you recommend that she be treated?
   A. PR-II
   B. Bird Mark 7
   C. AP-5
   D. Servo 900C
   E. Bird Mark 14

2. Your patient needs to be placed on a ventilator. His body weight is 190 lb. The most appropriate uncorrected ventilator tidal volume would be:
   A. 800 ml
   B. 950 ml
   C. 1350 ml
   D. 500 ml
   E. 190 ml

3. Two patients are brought into the emergency room simultaneously. One has taken an accidental overdose of sleeping pills and has respiratory center depression. The other has pneumonia and bronchitis and is coughing up large amounts of viscous, yellow secretions. The airways of both are intubated, and they will undergo mechanical ventilation. You have available only a Bird Mark 7 and a Puritan-Bennett 7200. Which would you recommend for the patient who has taken the overdose of sleeping pills?
   A. Bird Mark 7.
   B. Bennett 7200.
   C. Either is acceptable for either patient.
   D. Neither is acceptable.

4. Which of the following weaning parameters are acceptable?
   I. Spontaneous tidal volume of 7 ml/kg of ideal body weight
   II. Dead space/tidal volume ratio of 0.4
   III. Intrapulmonary shunt of 10%
   IV. Vital capacity of 9 ml/kg of ideal body weight
   V. Maximum inspiratory pressure of -15 cm H_2O
   A. I, II
   B. III, IV, V
   C. I, II, III

D. II, III, IV
E. I, II, III, IV, V

5. The physician asks your opinion on what weaning method would be most successful in the patient with the previously listed weaning parameters. The patient is on the assist/control mode with a ventilator tidal volume of 800 ml and backup rate of 12 times/min. Her spontaneous tidal volume is 400 ml. You would recommend which of the following methods?
   A. Ventilator discontinuance
   B. Intermittent ventilator discontinuance
   C. Regular steps in IMV weaning
   D. Irregular steps in IMV weaning
   E. Pressure support ventilation

6. Your patient has the desire to breathe spontaneously and has a tidal volume that is 4 ml/kg of ideal body weight. Because of facial trauma from an automobile accident, she has an endotracheal tube that is smaller than the ideal size. She also suffered lung contusions in the crash. Her Pao_2 level is 63 mm Hg on 55% oxygen. What ventilator mode would you recommend for her?
   A. Control
   B. Pressure support ventilation with PEEP
   C. Continuous positive airway pressure (CPAP)
   D. SIMV with pressure support and PEEP
   E. SIMV with pressure support

7. Your patient is recovering from ARDS and is receiving 10 cm H_2O CPAP and 40% oxygen. In evaluating the patient after 1 hour, you notice the following: his Spo_2 has dropped from 95% to 90%, his respiratory rate has increased from 14 to 23 breaths/min, and he is complaining of tiredness. You would recommend which of the following?
   A. Continue for another hour and reevaluate.
   B. Raise the CPAP level to 13 cm H_2O because the Spo_2 value has decreased.
   C. Decrease the CPAP level to 7 cm H_2O because the patient is becoming tired at the present level.
   D. Extubate because the endotracheal tube is increasing his work of breathing.
   E. Initiate SIMV with 10 cm PEEP.

8. Your patient has a heat-moisture exchanger (HME) in place for humidification purposes. You notice that the peak pressure has increased by 10 cm H_2O in the last hour. The nurse reported to you that the patient's secretions were difficult to suction out the last time because they were rather thick. You would recommend which of the following?
   A. Continue to use the HME.
   B. Switch the HME for a cool passover-type humidifier.
   C. Switch to a heated cascade-type humidifier.
   D. Have the nurse instill a few milliliters of normal saline solution before suctioning.
   E. Turn up the temperature on the HME.

9. Your ventilated patient has the following blood gas values on 40% oxygen: Pao_2, 75 mm Hg; $Paco_2$, 28 mm Hg; and pH 7.51. She is on the assist/control mode with a backup rate of 10 and is assisting at a rate of 18 times/min. Her spontaneous tidal volume is 300 ml. What would you suggest?
   A. Start her on SIMV therapy.
   B. Add 200 ml of mechanical dead space.
   C. Sedate her so that she does not assist.
   D. Start her on CPAP therapy.
   E. Increase the backup rate to 18 times/min so that she will not assist.

10. Your male patient has a body surface area of 2.1 m^2. What would be his predicted minute ventilation to maintain a normal Pa_{CO_2} level?
    A. 10 L
    B. 8.4 L
    C. 7.35 L
    D. 1.9 L
    E. 1.67 L

11. The sensitivity control should be set at what level when the patient is being ventilated on the assist/control mode?
    A. 0 cm H_2O
    B. −1 to −2 cm H_2O
    C. −5 cm H_2O
    D. 5 cm H_2O
    E. 1 to 2 cm H_2O

12. In preparing for a mode change from Assist/Control to SIMV, the following must be done:
    I. Turn the sensitivity control off.
    II. Inform the patient of the change in ventilator function.
    III. Turn off the ventilator's sigh control.
    IV. Add 5 cm of therapeutic PEEP to reduce the work of breathing.
    V. Remove any mechanical dead space from the patient's breathing circuit.
    A. I, III, IV
    B. III, IV
    C. I, III, IV, V
    D. IV, V
    E. II, III, V

13. Which of the following indicate that the patient is not tolerating PEEP?
    I. Increased static lung compliance (C_{st})
    II. Decreased static lung compliance (C_{st})
    III. Increased intrapulmonary shunt
    IV. Stable heart rate
    V. Decreasing blood pressure
    A. I, III, V
    B. II, III
    C. I, IV, V
    D. III, IV
    E. II, III, V

Your ventilated patient has an exhaled tidal volume of 800 ml. Because of refractory hypoxemia, 8 cm of PEEP therapy is started. The peak pressure is 40 cm H_2O and the static or plateau pressure is 30 cm H_2O. The compliance factor has been determined to be 3 ml/cm H_2O.

14. The corrected tidal volume for this patient is:
    A. 800 ml
    B. 760 ml
    C. 770 ml
    D. 704 ml
    E. 680 ml

15. Calculate the static compliance (C_{st}) for this patient.
    A. 22 ml/cm H_2O
    B. 33 ml/cm H_2O
    C. 23 ml/cm H_2O

D. 27 ml/cm H_2O
E. 17 ml/cm H_2O

16. Calculate the dynamic compliance (C_{dyn}) for this patient.
A. 17 ml/cm H_2O
B. 32 ml/cm H_2O
C. 20 ml/cm H_2O
D. 25 ml/cm H_2O
E. 22 ml/cm H_2O

Answer Key:

1. D; 2. B; 3. A; 4. C; 5. D; 6. D; 7. E; 8. C; 9. A; 10. B; 11. B; 12. E; 13. E; 14. D; 15. B; 16. E.

Posttest: Practice Entry Level Examination

Instructions

Select the best answer to each question. No calculators or notes may be used. The test must be finished within 3 hours. See the answer key and explanations at the end of the test to evaluate your performance.

Note: This examination is modeled on actual retired entry level examinations given by the National Board of Respiratory Care (NBRC). The same styles of questions are used. It is made up of the same mix of questions that have historically been seen on the actual entry level examinations. (See "Relative Weights of the Various Tested Areas on the Entry Level Examination" in the front matter.) However, no claim is made that the actual NBRC examination will match this practice examination.

1. You need to go into the room of a patient know to have tuberculosis. It is necessary to add water to the nebulizer of his 35% oxygen with aerosol mask. All of the following are infection control procedures that should be followed *except:*
   A. Close the door after you leave.
   B. Wash your hands on leaving the room.
   C. Cover gown over your uniform.
   D. Wear a HEPA filtered mask.

2. A 60-year-old comatose patient needs to have nasotracheal suctioning performed because of pneumonia. Which of the following would be done to ensure a safe procedure?
   I. Coat the tip of the catheter with a water-soluble lubricant
   II. Hyperoxygenate the patient
   III. Apply suction continuously for as long as necessary to remove all of the secretions with only one pass of the catheter
   IV. Insert a pharyngotracheal airway as a catheter guide
   V. Advance the catheter into the trachea only when the patient inspires.
   A. II, III
   B. IV, V
   C. II, III, IV
   D. I, II, IV, V

3. Measuring a patient's maximum inspiratory pressure (MIP) at the bedside will give valuable information on:
   A. Strength of the expiratory muscles of respiration
   B. Lung compliance

C. Airway resistance
D. Strength of the inspiratory muscles of respiration

4. A patient is improving, and the physician wants to begin weaning procedures. Originally she was on assist/control with a rate of 12 times/minute and a tidal volume of 700 ml. Now she is ordered to be placed on pressure support ventilation (PSV). The pressure support level is set at 10 cm H_2O. At first the patient seems comfortable on PSV, but after 45 minutes she complains of it getting difficult to breathe. What would you initially recommend to take care of her complaint?
   A. Give her 10 mg of Valium for anxiety.
   B. Put her back on the assist/control mode.
   C. Increase the pressure support level to 15 cm H_2O.
   D. Add 5 cm of PEEP.

5. After a patient's airway has been intubated during a resuscitation attempt, a chest x-ray film is taken. It is important to inspect the x-ray film to observe:
   A. That the tip of the endotracheal tube is centered in the middle of the trachea
   B. If this chest x-ray film is different from the previous ones
   C. If the heart was damaged by chest compressions
   D. If the cuff is inflated

6. When asking a patient if she knows what hospital she is in and what day of the week it is, you are trying to assess the patient's:
   A. Orientation to place and time
   B. Reaction to chronic illness
   C. Understanding of the English language
   D. Cooperation

7. A Bennett PR-II with a cascade humidifier and modified IPPB circuit are being used to temporarily ventilate a patient in the recovery room. When you come up to check the patient and ventilator, you notice that the inspiratory time is longer than first charted and the machine does not cycle off until the patient blows out. What would you do to correct the problem?
   I. Tighten the cascade jar and lid.
   II. Increase the control pressure.
   III. Tighten the medication nebulizer jar and manifold.
   IV. Pull the air dilution knob out of the body of the machine.
   A. I, II
   B. I, III
   C. II, IV
   D. II, III

8. What should be done if a patient tells you that she cannot feel any gas coming out of the nasal cannula? The flowmeter indicates 5 L/min is being delivered.
   A. Tell her to inhale more slowly.
   B. Make sure that all equipment connections are tight.
   C. Increase the flow to 7 L/min and ask if she can feel it now.
   D. Replace the cannula.

9. All of the following could be the cause of a patient's peak pressure increasing from 35 to 45 cm H_2O *except:*
   A. Bronchospasm.
   B. Resolving pulmonary edema.
   C. The patient is biting on the endotracheal tube.
   D. Secretions in the airway.

10. A 12-year-old patient is admitted through the emergency room with bilateral wheezing. Which of the following would be best to treat this problem?
    A. Aerosolized cromolyn sodium
    B. Aerosolized normal saline solution
    C. 28% oxygen by air entrainment mask
    D. An aerosolized bronchodilator

11. A patient has been receiving aerosolized bronchodilators through a hand-held nebulizer for the last day. Which of the following would you recommend to minimize the risk of her getting a nosocomial infection?
    I. Add a broad-spectrum antibiotic to the nebulizer with each treatment.
    II. Change the small-volume nebulizer and mouthpiece every 24 hours.
    III. Make sure that the medications and saline solution are dated and discarded 24 hours after opening.
    IV. Respiratory care practitioners should wash their hands before giving her a treatment.
    A. I, II
    B. II, III, IV
    C. III, IV
    D. I, II, III, IV

12. A patient tells you that he has been coughing out white sputum. Based on this it is most likely that the patient has:
    A. Chronic bronchitis
    B. Asthma
    C. Pulmonary edema
    D. Cystic fibrosis

13. Toward the end of a small-volume nebulizer treatment to deliver a bronchodilator, the patient complains of tingling fingers and muscle tremors. It is important to note the following information in the patient's chart:
    I. The type of nebulizer that was used
    II. The type of medication in the nebulizer
    III. The patient's vital signs and complaints
    IV. The oxygen flow through the nebulizer
    A. I, II
    B. I, III, IV
    C. II, IV
    D. II, III

14. Your patient has status asthmaticus and is being managed on a volume-cycled ventilator. It is important in this case to set a proper inspiratory flow and inspiratory/expiratory ratio so that:
    A. The tidal volume is evenly distributed.
    B. The patient does not feel dyspnea.
    C. The patient has enough time to completely exhale.
    D. The tidal volume is delivered.

15. While working with a mechanically ventilated patient, you notice that the peak pressure has increased 10 cm H_2O over the last hour. The plateau pressure has not changed. You also notice that the patient has significant wheezing in both lungs that was not present earlier. Based on this you would recommend:
    A. Nebulizing a sympathomimetic bronchodilator.
    B. Nebulizing a corticosteroid.
    C. Suctioning the patient.
    D. Increasing the tidal volume 100 ml to see if it stops the wheezing.

16. On performing a chest assessment, you hear high-pitched wheezes over both lower lobes. This could be caused by all of the following *except:*
    A. Laryngospasm
    B. Emphysema
    C. Airway tumor
    D. Asthma

17. About how many hours will an H cylinder of oxygen last if it has 1100 psig and is emptying at a flow of 8 L/min?
    A. .6
    B. 8.2
    C. 7.2
    D. .7

18. You are working with a 55-year-old male patient who weighs 82 kg (180 lb). He is on a mechanical ventilator with the following settings:

Tidal volume	1000 ml
Rate	12 times/min
Flow	50 L/min
Oxygen	40%
Mode	assist/control

He has the following blood gas values on these settings:

Pao_2	56 mm Hg
$Paco_2$	35 mm Hg
pH	7.44
Bicarbonate	23 mEq/L

The physician wants to know what you would now recommend:
    A. Increase the oxygen to 45%.
    B. Change to SIMV.
    C. Add 150 ml of mechanical dead space.
    D. Increase the respiratory rate to 16 breaths/min.

19. Orientation to time and place can best be determined by which of the following?
    A. The patient knows who her physician is.
    B. The patient knows she is in the hospital on her son's birthday.
    C. The patient can follow your instructions for performing a treatment.
    D. The patient knows that she is in the intensive care unit.

20. You are assisting with the oral intubation of an adult patient's airway. After the tube has been placed, you listen to the breath sounds. You notice that they are decreased on the left compared with the right lung. The most likely cause of this is:
    A. The tip of the endotracheal tube has been inserted into the right mainstem bronchus.
    B. The cuff of the endotracheal tube has been overinflated.
    C. The endotracheal tube has been inserted into the esophagus.
    D. The tip of the endotracheal tube has been inserted into the left mainstem bronchus.

21. A 35-year-old patient is being mechanically ventilated with the SIMV and these settings: backup rate 12 times/min, tidal volume 850 ml, and 45% oxygen. He is not breathing spontaneously. Based on these settings, he has the following blood gas results:

Pa_{O_2}	94 mm Hg
Pa_{CO_2}	29 mm Hg
pH	7.50
Bicarbonate	23 mEq/L

The physician is not pleased with these values. What would you recommend to correct them?
A. Decrease the oxygen percentage.
B. Add mechanical dead space.
C. Decrease the SIMV rate.
D. Give intravenous sodium bicarbonate.

22. A patient with pneumonia is sitting up in bed. Her respiratory rate is regular and 30 times/min. Accessory muscles of ventilation are being used. She is demonstrating which of the following?
A. Kussmaul respiration
B. Cheyne-Stokes respiration
C. Tachypnea
D. Eupnea

23. When will an air entrainment mask deliver a higher oxygen percentage than it is designed to?
A. The air entrainment ports are covered.
B. The oxygen flow is set 1 L/min less than recommended.
C. The ports on the mask are enlarged.
D. Aerosol tubing is added between the mask and air entrainment adapter.

24. The ideal ratio of rescue breaths to chest compressions that should be given by a single rescuer during a CPR attempt on an adult is:
A. 1:5
B. 15:2
C. 2:15
D. 5:1

25. While assisting an anesthesiologist with a difficult intubation, she asks for a curved laryngoscope blade. You would give her a:
A. Shiley blade
B. Miller blade
C. Ballard blade
D. MacIntosh blade

26. While assessing a patient's carotid pulse, it is noted that some beats are stronger than others and some beats are missing. What would most likely cause this?
A. Hypertension
B. Hypotension
C. Cardiac dysrhythmia
D. Cheyne-Stokes breathing

27. A 40-year-old patient is admitted with a diagnosis of pneumonia. He is placed on a 40% air-entrainment mask. After 30 minutes an arterial blood sample is drawn and analyzed with these results:

Pa_{O_2}	53 mm Hg
Pa_{CO_2}	32 mm Hg

pH	7.43
Bicarbonate	24 mEq/L

The physician makes a decision to implement mechanical ventilation. The patient weighs 82 kg (180 lb). Which of the following would be the best set of parameters to start with?

	Rate (times/min)	Tidal Volume (ml)	Oxygen (%)
A.	14	750	40
B.	20	1100	60
C.	8	1300	90
D.	12	1050	50

28. The main reason that respiratory care equipment is cleaned and sterilized between patients is:
    A. To protect the respiratory care practitioners from infection
    B. To prevent cross-contamination between patients
    C. To help control inventory
    D. To repair any damage before it goes to the next patient

29. During a successful CPR attempt, a patient's airway is intubated, and the patient is placed on a mechanical ventilator. You notice that during each inspiration, air is felt to escape from the patient's mouth. What should be done?
    A. Have a nasogastric tube placed to remove air from the patient's stomach.
    B. Put more air into the cuff.
    C. Get a chest x-ray film.
    D. Have another endotracheal tube placed into the patient.

30. Before giving an asthmatic a breathing treatment with an aerosolized bronchodilator, you notice that the breath sounds are diminished bilaterally. After inhaling the medication you notice that the patient's breath sounds reveal wheezing in all lung fields. Based on this you would conclude:
    A. The patient has worsened.
    B. The patient has a pneumothorax and should have a chest tube inserted.
    C. Pulmonary edema has started.
    D. The patient has better airflow.

31. A patient is instructed to inhale as deeply as possible and blow out all his air as quickly as possible until empty. What test is being performed?
    A. FVC
    B. IC
    C. TLC
    D. MVV

32. Your 47-year-old patient tells you that over the last 3 years he has gotten a productive cough in December that lasts until March. This fits symptoms that suggest that he has:
    A. Laryngotracheobronchitis
    B. Cystic fibrosis
    C. Chronic bronchitis
    D. Asthma

33. If a patient is ordered to receive a cromolyn sodium (Intal) capsule three times daily, the best method for dispensing it would be:
    A. Small-volume nebulizer

B. Spinhaler
C. Ultrasonic nebulizer
D. Freon-powered metered dose inhaler

34. Heart failure is usually associated with:
A. Asymmetric chest movement
B. Peripheral edema
C. Clubbing of the fingers
D. Nasal flaring

35. While making routine equipment rounds, the respiratory care practitioner hears a high-pitched sound coming from the pressure relief valve on a patient's bubble-type humidifier. Gas can be felt to escape from the valve. Which of the following could cause this problem?
I. The oxygen tubing is obstructed.
II. Too much oxygen is flowing through the humidifier.
III. The water reservoir jar is screwed too *tightly* into the lid of the humidifier.
IV. The water reservoir jar is screwed too *loosely* into the lid of the humidifier.
A. I, III
B. II, IV
C. I, IV
D. I, II

36. While working in the intensive care unit, you notice the following airway pressures on your adult patient:

Time	Plateau Pressure (cm H_2O)	Peak Pressure (cm H_2O)
0900	25	35
1000	29	40
1100	35	46

Through out this time the patient's ventilator settings have not been changed. What is the most likely cause of these values?
A. Endotracheal suctioning is needed.
B. The patient's lungs are becoming more compliant
C. The patient is developing pneumonia.
D. The patient is performing a Valsalva maneuver.

37. When you palpate a patient's chest, vibrations are felt over the left lung. After the patient coughs, the vibrations are gone. Based on this, you would conclude:
A. Secretions were present in the left lung's airways.
B. The patient has chronic bronchitis.
C. Secretions were present in the right lung's airways.
D. The patient has COPD.

38. A patient with a tracheostomy has 40% oxygen and aerosol delivered by a tracheostomy mask. If the patient develops an *Escherichia coli* infection of the stoma and airways, the most likely source is:
A. Improper sterilization of the tracheostomy mask by the manufacturer
B. Nebulizer water that has been used past its expiration date
C. Inadequate hand washing by the health care workers
D. The patient's own upper airway bacteria

39. Your patient is being maintained on a BEAR 5 ventilator. After endotracheal suctioning, which of the following would show that airway resistance has been decreased?
    A. Lower peak pressure
    B. Larger tidal volume
    C. Lower plateau pressure
    D. Decreased inspiratory time

40. An arterial puncture has been performed to obtain blood for analysis of oxygen, carbon dioxide, and pH. What is the best way to care for the blood sample?
    A. Warm the sample to keep it at body temperature.
    B. Place it into a mix of ice and water.
    C. Put a cap over the needle.
    D. Shake the sample to hemolyse the blood.

41. A patient in congestive heart failure with pulmonary edema should be placed in which of the following positions to minimize hypoxemia?
    A. Trendelenburg
    B. Supine
    C. Semi-Fowler's
    D. Right lateral

42. All of the following medications could be used in the prevention or treatment of asthma *except:*
    A. Beclomethasone dipropionate (Vanceril)
    B. Acetylcysteine (Mucomyst)
    C. Metaproterenol (Alupent)
    D. Cromolyn sodium (Intal)

43. The most effective way to communicate with other members of the health care team about a patient's condition is by:
    A. Discussing the information during patient rounds with the attending physician
    B. Telling the shift supervisor who will tell the other staff members
    C. Paperclipping a note on the front of the patient's chart
    D. Writing the information in the patient's chart

44. A nurse calls you over to the nursing station to confirm a new order. The physician has ordered a patient to receive 5 ml of isoetharine (Bronkosol) and 0.4 ml of normal saline solution by IPPB. What is the best thing to do?
    A. Call the physician to have the order changed.
    B. Change the order to 0.5 ml of Bronkosol because that is the correct dose.
    C. Give the treatment as ordered.
    D. Give the patient 0.5 ml of Bronkosol and 4 ml of normal saline solution by hand-held nebulizer.

45. An infant is placed on CPAP for treatment of atelectasis and pneumonia with hypoxemia. The initial level is 6 cm H_2O. After the patient is placed on the system, you notice that the pressure falls to 2 cm with each inspiration. What should be done to correct the problem?
    A. Tell the patient to relax and breathe more slowly.
    B. Sedate the patient with Valium.
    C. Increase the CPAP level to 8 cm H_2O to make up the difference.
    D. Increase the flow through the system.

46. You are working with a 55-year-old patient who had open heart surgery to replace his aortic valve yesterday. He is awake, has stable vital signs, and has the following weaning

parameters: tidal volume 600 ml, vital capacity 2300 ml, and maximum inspiratory pressure −35 cm H_2O. After breathing spontaneously on a Briggs adapter for 40 minutes, he starts to bleed heavily through his mediastinal chest tube. The nurse checks his vital signs and determines that his blood pressure is 90/50, heart rate is 130 beats/min, and respiratory rate 28 breaths/min. She asks for any suggestions about his care. You would recommend:

A. Let him breathe on the Briggs adapter for 20 more minutes and then let him rest on the ventilator as was previously planned.
B. Draw an arterial blood gas sample to find out if he is hypoxic.
C. He should be placed back on the ventilator.
D. Put him back on the ventilator but change the mode from assist/control to SIMV.

47. A 40-year-old comatose man is found to have a respiratory rate that varies from 8 to 40 times/min. His tidal volume is measured between 200 and 1100 ml and changes unpredictably. His breathing would best be described as:
A. Kussmaul's respiration
B. Biot's respiration
C. Cheyne-Stokes respiration
D. Obstructed inspiration

48. When performing routine equipment rounds, the respiratory care practitioner notices that a patient wearing an aerosol mask is having "puffs" of aerosol delivered instead of a continuous aerosol stream. What could be causing this?
A. Water has collected at a low point in the aerosol tubing.
B. The patient is inhaling at the same rate as the "puffs."
C. The oxygen flowmeter is turned down too low.
D. More water needs to be added to the reservoir.

49. A 2-year-old patient with an upper airway infection demonstrates a high-pitched sound over the larynx when breathing in. Lung sounds are present and normal over all lung fields. What should be recorded in the patient's chart?
A. The patient has normal breath sounds.
B. Both lungs are expanding normally during inspiration.
C. The patient has inspiratory stridor.
D. The patient has bacterial pneumonia.

50. After a patient has been inhaling an aerosol from an ultrasonic nebulizer for 10 minutes, he begins to wheeze. What should be done at this time?
A. Give the patient epinephrine by the intravenous line.
B. Discontinue the treatment, monitor the patient, and notify the physician of the incident.
C. Add 0.5 ml of albuterol to the ultrasonic nebulizer.
D. Power the aerosol with 100% oxygen.

51. The physician has ordered that a 35-year-old patient receive postural drainage therapy of the posterior basal segment of the right lower lobe. To do this, you would:
I. elevate the foot of the bed 30 degrees
II. have the patient lie on his left side
III. have the patient lie prone
IV. elevate the foot of the bed 15 degrees
V. keep the bed flat but put a pillow under the patient's hips
A. II, IV
B. III, V
C. I, III
D. I, II

52. An 18-hour-old, 29-week gestational age neonate is being maintained in an oxygen hood with an F_{IO_2} of 0.5. The neonatologist believes that the patient has IRDS. The following blood gas results are from an umbilical artery sample:

Pa_{O_2}	49 mm Hg
Pa_{CO_2}	37 mm Hg
pH	7.35
Bicaronate	25 mEq/L

Based on this information, what would you recommend?
A. Give 100% oxygen in the oxygen hood.
B. Put the neonate on a Sechrist ventilator.
C. Get a chest x-ray film to look for a pneumothorax.
D. Start 5 cm H_2O CPAP.

53. A patient is admitted through the emergency room with a diagnosis of carbon monoxide poisoning. Arterial blood gases are drawn with her breathing room air and show:

Pa_{O_2}	85 mm Hg
Pa_{CO_2}	32 mm Hg
pH	7.31

Based on this, what change would you recommend for the patient's respiratory care plan?
A. Give the patient 100% oxygen by a non-rebreathing mask.
B. Institute mechanical ventilation with 50% oxygen.
C. Give the patient 28% oxygen by an air entrainment mask.
D. Discharge her because she is not hypoxemic.

54. You notice that your patient is using accessory muscles of respiration. The most likely cause of this is:
A. Breathing is normal.
B. Lung compliance is increased.
C. Airway resistance is increased.
D. Work of breathing is decreased.

55. A 60-kg (132-lb) patient is being ventilated in the assist/control mode. Her tidal volume is 600 ml, rate of 14 times/min, and F_{IO_2} 0.4. Her arterial blood gas results are as follows:

Pa_{O_2}	85 mm Hg
Pa_{CO_2}	29 mm Hg
pH	7.51
HCO_3^-	24 mEq/L

What would you recommend be done?
A. Add mechanical dead space.
B. Increase the tidal volume.
C. Decrease the inspired oxygen percentage.
D. Increase the sigh volume and frequency.

56. Your patient is wearing a non-rebreathing mask receiving 7 L of oxygen/min. You notice that the reservoir bag collapses when the patient inspires. What should be done first?
A. Tell the patient to not breathe so fast.
B. Switch the patient to a nasal cannula at 7 L/min.
C. Increased the oxygen flow.
D. Take the flaps off of the face mask.

57. Your patient refuses to be tipped into a head-down position for postural drainage therapy. She tells you that she becomes too short of breath when she has to lie flat or with her head down. You would note in the chart that the patient refused therapy because of:
    A. Lack of cooperation
    B. Disorientation
    C. Hyperpnea
    D. Orthopnea

58. A 50-year-old man is admitted with a diagnosis of pneumonia. Twenty minutes after the patient is given 40% by mask an arterial blood sample is obtained. Its analysis shows:

Pao_2	70 mm Hg
$Paco_2$	28 mm Hg
pH	7.46
HCO_3^-	22 mEq/L
base excess	−2

Based on the previous information, which of the following statements are true?
    I. The patient has hypoxemia.
    II. He is hyperventilating.
    III. His $P(A - a)o_2$ is increased.
    IV. He has a respiratory alkalosis.
    A. II, III, IV
    B. I, II
    C. II, IV
    D. I, III

59. Before giving your patient a breathing treatment with racemic epinephrine for laryngeal edema, you check his vital signs. His heart rate is 85 beats/min and respiratory rate is 16 breaths/min. Half way into the treatment, his pulse rate is 115 beats/min and respiratory rate is 22 breaths/min. What should be done?
    A. Continue the treatment to completion.
    B. Substitute isoetharine (Bronkosol) for the racemic epinephrine and continue the treatment.
    C. Stop the treatment. Inform the physician and ask for further guidance.
    D. Stop the treatment. Ask the nurse to take the rest of the medication from the nebulizer and give it intravenously.

60. A patient with an intubated airway is ordered to have 35% oxygen delivered to his Brigg's adapter. Currently his equipment consists of an air entrainment (jet) large-volume nebulizer, aerosol tubing, and Briggs adapter. The physician has expressed concern that the patient is not getting enough humidity and less than the ordered oxygen percentage. Which of the following should be done to correct these problems?
    A. Add 100 ml of aerosol tubing to the open end of Brigg's adapter
    B. Adjust the jet nebulizer to deliver 40% oxygen.
    C. Add tubing to have the gas go from the nebulizer to an ultrasonic unit before it goes to the patient.
    D. Substitute a cascade-type humidifier for the large-volume nebulizer.

61. To protect yourself from contamination by a patient who coughs violently during endotracheal suctioning, which of the following should be done?
    I. Wear a mask.
    II. Wear goggles.
    III. Restrain the patient.
    IV. Wear gloves.

V. Suction the patient only when he or she is asleep.
A. I, II, IV
B. I, V
C. I, II, III, IV, V
D. III, IV

62. An alert patient with emphysema and an elevated carbon dioxide level is given 40% oxygen by an air entrainment mask. One hour later the nurse calls you to evaluate the patient. He is now very sleepy and slow to respond. Which of the following is the most likely cause of this?
A. He is simply tired.
B. He is hypoxic.
C. His blood pressure is low.
D. He has oxygen-induced hypoventilation.

63. On entering a room to check on a patient' oxygen mask, you notice her roommate laughing at a television program while eating dinner. Suddenly she stops laughing, cannot speak, and makes urgent motions with her hands to her mouth. You should:
A. Lean her forward and strike her several times between the shoulder blades
B. Perform the Heimlich maneuver (abdominal thrusts) on her
C. Check for a carotid pulse and begin CPR
D. Lay her back in bed and strike her several times over the sternum

64. Inspiratory stridor would be found with:
A. Asthma
B. Pulmonary edema
C. Pneumonia
D. Acute laryngotracheobronchitis

65. After giving an aerosolized medication by a small-volume nebulizer, you proceed to remove the oxygen flowmeter from the wall outlet. Immediately a large rush of gas leaves the outlet. What is the first thing that you should do?
A. Put an air flowmeter into the outlet.
B. Find the zone valve in the hall and turn it off.
C. Put the oxygen flowmeter back into the outlet.
D. Move the patient out of the room and into the hall.

66. During the performance of a respiratory care procedure the patient's pulse increases from 85 to 135 beats/min. Based on this, the best thing to do is:
A. Stop the treatment and inform the patient's physician of the pulse rate change.
B. Continue the treatment to its conclusion and then tell the patient's physician of the pulse rate change.
C. Continue the treatment and then ask your shift supervisor if the treatment should be performed when next scheduled.
D. Stop the treatment now and check the pulse rate before giving it the next time.

67. After a patient's airway has been orally intubated, the best way to determine if the tube has been properly positioned is to:
A. Look in the patient's mouth
B. Find out if the cuff will seal at 20 cm H_2O
C. Have a neck x-ray film taken
D. Have a chest x-ray film taken

68. Near the end of an IPPB treatment to give Alupent and Mucomyst to a patient with bronchitis, she complains of dizziness. After having her stop the treatment, she also

says that her fingers and toes feel "tingly." What is the most likely cause of these conditions?
A. She has hyperventilated.
B. She has had an adverse reaction to the Alupent.
C. She has hyperoxygenated.
D. She has had an adverse reaction to the Mucomyst.

69. A patient with broken ribs and a tension pneumothorax from an automobile accident would most likely demonstrate what emotional state?
A. Euphoria
B. Depression
C. Resentment
D. Panic

70. The nurse calls you over to look at the arterial blood gas results of a 50-kg (110-lb) patient who is being mechanically ventilated. Currently the patient has a tidal volume of 500 ml, rate of 10 times/min, and 35% oxygen. Her blood gas results are as follows:

Pao_2	73 mm Hg
$Paco_2$	48 mm Hg
pH	7.31
HCO_3^-	23 mEq/L
Sao_2	93%

Based on these values, what would you recommend?
A. Increase her tidal volume but decrease her rate to keep the same minute volume.
B. Give her 40% oxygen.
C. Keep the current settings and get another blood gas in 1 hour.
D. Increase her minute volume.

71. Which of the following are needed to calculate the set minute volume for a patient on a volume-cycled ventilator?
I. I/E ratio
II. Rate per minute
III. Tidal volume
IV. Flow
A. II, III
B. I, III
C. I, II, IV
D. I, II, III, IV

72. To determine if the patient's diaphragm moves with each breath, the respiratory care practitioner should:
A. Look for the use of the sternocleidomastoid muscles with each inspiration.
B. Observe chest wall movement with each breath.
C. Observe that the patient's abdomen rises with each inspiration.
D. Note that the trapezius muscles are used with each expiration.

73. After getting a new order to start postural drainage therapy with percussion and vibration, it is important to first:
A. Describe the treatment to the patient.
B. Review pertinent areas of the patient's chart.
C. Auscultate the patient's breath sounds.
D. Get a mechanical percussor.

74. Your 4-year-old patient is being mechanically ventilated with a tidal volume of 200 ml, rate of 20 times/min, and I/E ratio of 1:2. Based on these settings, what is the patient's inspiratory time?
    A. 1 second
    B. 1.5 seconds
    C. 2 seconds
    D. 3 seconds

75. When calibrating a galvanic fuel cell oxygen analyzer, you notice that it reaches 90% when exposed to 100 oxygen. You should proceed to:
    A. Replace the blue crystals with ones that are pink.
    B. Replace the battery.
    C. Replace the pink crystals with blue ones.
    D. Replace the fuel cell.

76. A Bird Mark 8 is being used for IPPB and is being powered by 100% oxygen as the source gas. If the air-mix knob is pulled out, what will happen?
    A. Pure oxygen will be delivered to the patient.
    B. Between 60% and 90% oxygen will be delivered to the patient.
    C. The unit will not cycle off.
    D. The venturi jets will not work properly.

77. A hypotensive patient is spontaneously breathing room air when an arterial blood gas sample is taken for analysis. The following values are found:

Pao_2	105 mm Hg
$Paco_2$	25 mm Hg
pH	7.27
Bicarbonate	12 mEq/L
Base excess	−10

    Based on this information, what best describes the patient's condition?
    A. Partially compensated respiratory alkalosis
    B. Uncompensated hyperventilation
    C. Combined respiratory and metabolic acidosis
    D. Partially compensated metabolic acidosis

78. After giving a patient an aerosolized bronchodilator, followed by postural drainage therapy, he coughs productively. You look at the sputum sample and note that it is foul smelling and green. Based on this, you would suspect that the patient has:
    A. Pulmonary edema
    B. A pulmonary infection with *Mycobacterium tuberculosis*
    C. A pulmonary infection with a fungal organism
    D. A pulmonary infection with *Pseudomonas aeruginosa*

79. You are called to help in the care of a patient admitted with severe pulmonary edema. While starting an intravenous line, the physician tells you to give the patient oxygen. You would start the following:
    A. A non-rebreathing mask
    B. A nasal cannula at 4 L/min
    C. A simple face mask at 4 L/min
    D. A 28% air entrainment mask

80. A physician asks you for a recommendation on how to provide humidity to a newborn in an oxyhood. You suggest the use of a heated cascade-type humidifier for the following reasons:
    I. The aerosol particles are smaller than from a large-volume nebulizer.
    II. It is very quiet.
    III. The aerosol particles are of a uniform size.
    IV. Contamination of the warmed and humidified gas is unlikely.
    A. I, III
    B. I, II
    C. III, IV
    D. II, IV

81. A patient is transported by ambulance to the emergency room. She is very short of breath, and the physician suspects that she has had a heart attack. Her breath sounds reveal moist rales in both bases. Her cough produces a large amount of pink, frothy secretions. The paramedics have placed a simple oxygen mask on her, and it is delivering 4 L of oxygen/min. After you have evaluated her, what would be the best treatment?
    A. Leave the simple mask on her at 4 L/min.
    B. IPPB powered by 100% oxygen.
    C. Intubate her airway and put her on a volume-cycled ventilator.
    D. Suction her to remove the secretions.

82. A patient with pulmonary edema will cough out sputum with the following characteristics:
    I. Pink tint
    II. Foul odor
    III. Frothy
    IV. Watery
    A. I, II
    B. III
    C. I, III, IV
    D. II, IV

83. While performing a maximum expiratory pressure (MEP) test, the patient blows out against the manometer. However, no value is registered. What should be checked?
    A. Make sure the spirometer is turned on.
    B. Make sure the one-way valve is set so air moves from the manometer to the patient.
    C. Make sure the one-way valve is set so air moves from the patient to the manometer.
    D. Both A and B.

84. When you crack open an E cylinder, you hear a loud hissing sound and can feel gas leaking from the area of the regulator. This is despite the flowmeter being turned off. What can be done to correct this problem?
    I. Replace the washer between the regulator and cylinder valve stem.
    II. Turn on the flowmeter.
    III. Tighten the regulator onto the cylinder valve stem.
    IV. Change the type of regulator.
    A. II
    B. I, III
    C. IV
    D. I, II, III

85. You receive an order to perform postural drainage, percussion, and vibration on an 18-year-old female patient. Chest x-ray film and auscultation indicate that the superior and inferior

segments of the left ligula have secretions within them. You would proceed to do all of the following except:
A. Tip the patient's head down 15 degrees
B. Tell her why the treatment is important
C. Rotate her one-fourth turn up from supine
D. Percuss and vibrate in the ideal location

86. Which of the following questions should be asked to find out if a patient has orthopnea?
I. Does blood come up when you cough?
II. Can you lie flat in bed without getting short of breath?
III. How many flights of stairs can you climb?
IV. How many pillows do you use when sleeping?
V. Do any foods you eat seem to make it easier to cough out your secretions?
A. II, IV
B. I
C. III, V
D. I, V

87. A patient is admitted with a diagnosis of bronchiectasis. On evaluating her, you find that she has coarse expiratory crackles in her left lower lobe. Her chest x-ray film shows infiltrates in the same area. What would you recommend to treat her?
A. Metered dose inhaler treatments with terbutaline (Brethaire) qid
B. Postural drainage and percussion
C. Incentive spirometry
D. 28% oxygen by air entrainment mask

88. Your patient is receiving aerosolized bronchodilators to treat her asthma. What is the best way to determine if the medication is having a positive affect?
A. Measure the patient's vital capacity.
B. Measure the patient's maximum inspiratory pressure after the medication has been delivered.
C. Measure a before and after bronchodilator $FEV_{1\%}$.
D. Calculate the patient's minute alveolar ventilation.

89. A 35-year-old patient is suspected of having carbon monoxide poisoning, what is the best way to determine his oxygenation?
A. Pulse oximetry for Spo_2.
B. Blood gas analyzer for Pao_2.
C. CO oximetry for measurement of Sao_2.
D. Transcutaneous Po_2.

90. During a bedside patient assessment, the respiratory care practitioner hears vesicular breath sounds over all lung areas. A note should be put into the chart that this represents:
A. A sound caused by laryngeal edema
B. Normal breath sounds
C. Secretions in the large airways
D. Decreased breath sounds

91. While performing a blood gas analysis on a patient breathing room air, the following values are displayed:

Pao_2	110 mm Hg
$Paco_2$	47 mm Hg
pH	7.43

The patient's blood gas results should be:
A. Phoned to the unit clerk to report to the attending physician.
B. Phoned to the patient's nurse to be shared with the respiratory care practitioner.
C. Discarded because they are not physiologically possible.
D. Phoned to both the attending physician and respiratory care practitioner.

92. Which of the following would be used during a CPR attempt to deliver the highest possible inspired oxygen percentage to the victim?
A. Mouth-to-mouth breathing with the rescuer breathing in oxygen from a flowmeter set on flush
B. A mouth-to-valve mask resuscitator with 5 L/min of oxygen
C. A non-rebreathing mask with 8 L/min of oxygen
D. A manual resuscitator with oxygen reservoir and 10 L/min of oxygen

93. The following bedside spirometry values are measured on a 35-year-old woman:

Tidal volume	450 ml
Dead space	160 ml
Vital capacity	3,900 ml
Respiratory rate	14 breaths/min
Inspiratory capacity	3100 ml

Based on this information, this patient's minute ventilation is:
A. 6300 ml
B. 4060 ml
C. 2240 ml
D. 37.1 L

94. Based on the information presented in question 93, what is this patient's minute alveolar ventilation?
A. 6300 ml
B. 4060 ml
C. 43.4 L
D. 11,200 ml

95. An 18-year-old woman gives birth to a 29-week gestational-age neonate. When evaluating the newborn, you hear an expiratory grunt sound. Why would the neonate do this?
A. To decrease the $Paco_2$ value
B. To prevent atelectasis
C. To help clear out secretions
D. To close the ductus arteriosus

96. On entering a patient's room, you notice that her face and hands are blue-gray. What is the most likely cause of this?
A. Hypoxemia
B. Advanced age
C. The artificial lighting in the room
D. Peripheral edema

97. All of the following can lead to an incorrect or misleading pulse oximetry reading *except:*
A. Black nail polish on the finger being used
B. Strong pulse at the site being used
C. Too much exposure to outside light
D. Presence of carboxyhemoglobin

98. The physician wants to deliver a known inspired oxygen concentration to a patient. This is to help with interpreting the patient's arterial blood gas results. Which of the following devices would you recommend?
   A. Air entrainment mask
   B. Nasal cannula
   C. Simple oxygen mask
   D. Partial rebreathing mask

99. A 10-year-old patient is being mechanically ventilated on the assist/control mode on a Puritan-Bennett 7200 ventilator with a heat-moisture exchanger being used for humidification purposes. The patient's spontaneous tidal volume is 250 ml and mechanical tidal volume is 350 ml, with a backup rate of 20 times/min. Thirty-five percent oxygen is being delivered. Over the course of 6 hours, it is noticed that the peak pressure has increased by 10 cm H_2O and the plateau pressure is unchanged. It also has become more difficult to suction out the endotracheal secretions. What should be done at this time?
   A. Start SIMV.
   B. Change to a cascade-type heated humidifier.
   C. Instill normal saline solution whether suctioning is needed.
   D. Use a larger catheter when suctioning.

100. A 35-year-old man has been mechanically ventilated in the assist/control mode for the last 2 days after his bowel was resected. He is breathing 50% oxygen and has the following arterial blood gas values:

Pao_2	65 mm Hg
$Paco_2$	38 mm Hg
pH	7.41
Bicarbonate	24 mEq/L

The patient is now awake, restless and "fighting" against the ventilator. However, the physician believes that he is not ready to wean off and also should not be sedated. Based on this, what would you recommend?
   A. Give him morphine for pain relief.
   B. Increase the respiratory rate by 5 times/minute.
   C. Begin SIMV.
   D. Begin SIMV and 10 cm H_2O PEEP.

101. A mechanically ventilated patient develops a *Staphylococcus aureus* pneumonia. The most likely cause of the infection is:
   A. The suction catheters are contaminated.
   B. The patient has a urinary tract infection that has led to a blood-born infection.
   C. An infected intravenous catheter site has led to a septicemia and the pneumonia.
   D. Health care workers in the intensive care unit are not washing their hands properly or wearing gloves.

102. The following arterial blood gas results are from a patient who was spontaneously breathing room air:

Pao_2	55 mm Hg
$Paco_2$	58 mm Hg
pH	7.36
Bicarbonate	32 mEq/L
Base excess	+8

Which of the following best describes this patient's condition?
A. Compensated acute respiratory acidosis
B. Uncompensated metabolic acidosis
C. Uncompensated metabolic alkalosis
D. Compensated chronic respiratory acidosis

103. When setting up an oxygen hood on a newborn, all of the following are important considerations *except:*
A. A good fit around the neck
B. Warming the oxygen to body temperature
C. Using a low noise level humidifier
D. The infant's sense of claustrophobia

104. A patient who suddenly experiences an upper airway obstruction will show all of the following *except:*
A. Panic
B. Inspiratory stridor
C. Depression
D. Cyanosis

105. A 10-year-old patient with cystic fibrosis is admitted to the hospital. She has very viscous secretions and wheezing in both lower lobes. Because of the physician's concern that she has a lung infection, a sputum specimen for culture and sensitivity is ordered. The physician asks what medications you would recommend to help with her breathing problems. You would recommend:
I. 0.4 ml of albuterol (Ventolin)
II. 3 ml of normal saline solution
III. 3 ml of 20% acetylcysteine (Mucomyst)
IV. 3 ml of 1.8% saline solution
V. 200 μg of triamcinolone acetonide (Azmacort)
A. V
B. I, IV
C. II, III
D. I, III

106. Which of the following would cause a humidifier to not bubble?
A. The reservoir jar is loose from the lid.
B. The pop-off valve is open.
C. The delivery tube is obstructed.
D. The diffuser head is missing.

107. While performing bedside spirometry on a 40-year-old man a peak flow of 2.5 L/sec is obtained. The most likely reason for this is:
A. He has increased lung compliance.
B. Air is poorly distributed through out his lungs.
C. He has obstruction of his inspiratory air flow.
D. He has obstruction of his expiratory air flow.

108. The use of therapeutic oxygen will help with all of the following *except:*
A. Treating a carbon monoxide poisoning patient
B. Expiration of carbon dioxide
C. Decrease myocardial work
D. Decrease the patient's work of breathing

109. Which of the following best describe how to instruct a patient to cough effectively?
   A. Sit back comfortably. Take in an easy breath, and huff out several times.
   B. Lie back in bed. Hold onto your stomach. Take in a deep breath. Cough it out hard.
   C. Lie on your side. Bend your knees. Hold a pillow over your stomach area. Take in a deep breath and huff out several times.
   D. Sit up straight. Take in a deep breath. Hold it and then blast it out as hard as you can.

110. Your patient had her spleen remove 2 days ago and is still reluctant to take a deep breath. The physician asks for your recommendation to prevent the development of atelectasis. You would suggest which of the following:
   A. Small-volume nebulizer with a bronchodilator
   B. Incentive spirometry
   C. Intermittent positive pressure breathing
   D. Bedside spirometry

111. You are giving an IPPB treatment to a patient using a Bennett PR-II unit. The treatment is progressing normally until you hear a "pop" sound. It is followed by a continuous high-pitched noise and the patient complains that the machine does not shut off as usual. What could be done to correct the problem?
   A. Increase the terminal flow.
   B. Tighten the high pressure oxygen hose on the machine.
   C. Reattach the nebulizer hose to the nebulizer.
   D. Put nose clips on the patient.

112. An adult patient is being changed over from the assist/control mode with a backup rate of 12 times/min and 5 cm PEEP to the SIMV mode with a backup rate of 10 times/min and 5 cm PEEP. When making the change over, which alarm is most important to ensure patient safety?
   A. High pressure
   B. Low pressure
   C. Oxygen percentage
   D. High minute volume

113. Your patient is ordered to start breathing treatments with pentamidine (Pentam). To minimize the possibility of medication being released into the air, you should use which of the following?
   A. Place a heat and moisture exchanger between the nebulizer and the patient's mouthpiece
   B. Use a metered dose inhaler with a spacer
   C. Use a small-volume nebulizer with a scavenging system
   D. Use a small-particle aerosol generator (SPAG) with a high-efficiency particulate air (HEPA) filter

114. You are following the manufacturer's guidelines in setting up a 35% air entrainment mask by running 6 L of oxygen/min through it. The physician wants to know the total flow of gas through the mask. You would calculate the total flow as:
   A. 36 L/min.
   B. 24 L/min.
   C. 66 L/min.
   D. There is not enough information to make the calculation.

115. A patient can be weaned from mechanical ventilation by all of the following methods *except:*
   A. Briggs (T-piece) adapter with reservoir
   B. Intermittent mandatory ventilation (IMV)

C. Control mode
D. SIMV

116. For incentive spirometry to be most effective, the following should be done:
A. The patient should exhale maximally and hold it for several seconds.
B. The patient should inhale and hold a vital capacity for 10 seconds.
C. A maximum inspiratory capacity breath should be held for several seconds.
D. Maximum inspiratory and expiratory efforts should be performed for 10 to 15 seconds.

117. To determine if mouth-to-mouth breathing is effective during a CPR attempt, watch the patient's:
A. Skin color for cyanosis
B. Chest rise when a breath is given
C. Heart rate return to normal
D. Pupils react to light

118. While assisting with the intubation of a neonate's airway, what is the first thing that can be assessed to determine if the tube has been placed into the trachea?
A. Palpate the larynx as the tube is being inserted.
B. Listen for a change in the sound of the neonate's cry.
C. Listen for bilateral lung sounds.
D. Feel for the chest to rise when a breath is delivered by manual resuscitator.

119. Your mechanically ventilated patient needs to be suctioned. He has an appropriately sized oral endotracheal tube. Suctioning should be done
A. Quickly so that the entire procedure takes no longer than 15 seconds
B. Until all of the secretions are removed
C. Quickly so that the entire procedure takes no longer than 30 seconds
D. Until his Spo_2 level drops below 90%

120. You are working with an elderly patient who has atelectasis and is ordered to receive an aerosolized bronchodilator for bronchospasm. He is confused and uncooperative. What would you recommend to the physician?
A. Give a hand-held nebulizer treatment.
B. Use a Freon-powered metered dose inhaler (MDI).
C. Use an incentive spirometer and an MDI.
D. Start IPPB therapy.

121. An adult patient has ARDS and the physician wants to calculate her static lung compliance. She has the following patient settings and monitoring data:

Tidal volume	900 ml
Rate	14 times/min
Peak pressure	50 cm H_2O
Plateau pressure	35 cm H_2O
PEEP	10 cm H_2O
Mechanical dead space	100 ml

The patient's static lung compliance calculates to:
A. 18 ml/cm H_2O
B. 26 ml/cm H_2O
C. 22 ml/cm H_2O
D. 36 ml/cm H_2O

122. A 17-year-old patient has been admitted through the emergency room to the intensive care unit. He is in a coma after taking an overdose of a sedative. His chest x-ray film indicates bilateral atelectasis. To correct this problem, you would recommend all of the following *except:*
   A. Give a tidal volume that is about 15 ml/kg of body weight
   B. Set the inspiratory flow and I/E ratio so that he has at least 4 seconds of expiratory time
   C. Give a large sigh volume
   D. Give a sigh breath about every 5 minutes

123. While you are performing percussion on the superior segment of a patient's left lower lobe, he coughs vigorously. The sputum is mixed with a large amount of bright red blood. You would proceed to:
   A. Stop the treatment and inform the physician.
   B. Continue the treatment and make a note of the sputum in the chart.
   C. Give the patient oxygen by simple mask and continue the treatment.
   D. Quickly discard the sputum sample so that the patient does not see it and become upset.

124. You are called to the emergency room to aid in the care of a car accident victim. The patient is 45 years old and has suffered severe facial trauma to the mouth and nose. She is having difficulty breathing because of bleeding and tissue edema. What would you recommend to help her?
   A. A small nasotracheal tube should be placed.
   B. A small oral endotracheal tube should be placed.
   C. A tracheostomy should be performed.
   D. A nasopharyngeal airway should be placed.

125. You are paged to the recovery room by the nurse to check on a patient that was started on a Bennett MA-1 ventilator about 1 hour ago. At that time the machine and patient were stable. When you arrive, you notice that the patient's breathing is not synchronized with the ventilator. The spirometer bellows rises during the machine's inspiratory phase. What would you do to correct this problem?
   A. Increase the tidal volume.
   B. Put more air into the cuff to the patient's endotracheal tube.
   C. Tell the patient to breathe more slowly and relax.
   D. Reconnect the small-bore tubing to the exhalation valve.

126. You are asked to evaluate a home patient with a nasal CPAP mask for treatment of obstructive sleep apnea. The patient's wife states that he has been snoring more loudly lately and having periods of apnea. After observing the patient's sleeping and breathing patterns for 2 hours, you find that this is the case. What would you do first to try to correct the problem?
   A. Wake the patient and have him go to his physician.
   B. Adjust the nasal mask for a better fit.
   C. Put him on his home mechanical ventilator.
   D. Insert an oropharyngeal airway.

127. Which of the following would be appropriate ways to prevent hypoxemia while suctioning a mechanically ventilated patient?
   I. Select a catheter that is about two thirds the inner diameter of the endotracheal tube.
   II. Give the patient 100% oxygen before suctioning the patient.
   III. Use a catheter that is no more than one half the inner diameter of the endotracheal tube.

IV. Give the patient 100% oxygen after the suctioning has been completed.
V. Increase the patient's inspired oxygen by 10% to 15% before the procedure.
A. I, IV, V
B. II, III, IV
C. I, II
D. III, V

128. A patient requiring mechanical ventilation has her PEEP increased from 10 to 15 cm H_2O. Within 20 minutes her blood pressure has decreased and heart rate has increased. What would you recommend be done?
A. Increase the oxygen percentage.
B. Increase the patient's intravenous fluids.
C. Remove the PEEP completely.
D. Decrease the PEEP back to 10 cm H_2O.

129. An adult's readiness to wean from a ventilator would be supported by all of the following *except:*
A. Vital capacity of 2500 ml
B. Maximum inspiratory pressure of −15 cm H_2O
C. Blood pressure 115/75 mm Hg
D. Intrapulmonary shunt of 7%

130. An order is received to suction a patient's oral secretions as often as necessary. To do this, you would gather all of the following *except:*
A. Vacuum tubing
B. Portable vacuum system
C. Luken's trap
D. Yankauer suction catheter

131. An adult patient is developing ARDS after inhaling smoke from a house fire. The physician anticipates the need to make many changes in the ventilator. He wants to be able to gather as much data on the patient's pulmonary condition as possible. Which ventilator would you recommend for the patient?
A. Siemens Servo 900C
B. Bird Mark 14
C. Puritan-Bennett 7200
D. BEAR 1

132. When starting a new IPPB treatment on a patient, you notice that at first the manometer needle on the Bird Mark 7 is in the negative range. It moves into the positive range later during inspiration just before the machine cycles off. What would you do to correct this problem?
A. Increase the flow rate.
B. Increase the pressure setting.
C. Push the air-mix knob in.
D. Tell the patient to inhale faster.

133. Your patient is admitted with atelectasis and a small functional residual capacity (FRC). Because of this he is hypoxic. What would you recommend to help correct the atelectasis and small FRC?
A. Add therapeutic PEEP
B. Increase the oxygen percentage
C. Suction the patient more frequently
D. Start pressure support ventilation

Directions: Following are two situation sets consisting of a clinical event and a series of questions related to it. Study the situation closely and then choose the best answer to the questions after it. (Past versions of the entry level examination have always had two situation sets. Presumably, this will continue on future versions of the examination.)

Questions 134-136

While performing equipment rounds, you enter a patient's room and find her lying on the floor by her bed. She is cyanotic and does not respond to your trying to awaken her.

134. The first thing that you should do is:
   A. Call out for help.
   B. Check her carotid pulse.
   C. Go to the nurse's station to ask the patient's nurse to help you.
   D. Have the nursing assistant call for an electrocardiogram (ECG) as soon as possible.

135. After determining that the patient is apneic, you should:
   A. Insert an oral endotracheal tube.
   B. Suction any secretions out of the mouth.
   C. Begin rescue breathing.
   D. Insert an oral airway.

136. To begin cardiac compressions you would:
   A. Put her into her bed
   B. Put her onto a stretcher
   C. Put a back board under her
   D. Leave her on the floor

Questions 137-140

A 48-year-old man has just returned from open heart surgery to repair his mitral valve. He has a history of smoking and is about 40 lb overweight. The anesthesiologist orders you to place him on a Servo 900 C ventilator.

137. Initial ventilator orders should include all of the following *except:*
   A. Inspired oxygen
   B. Minute volume
   C. A sigh volume and frequency
   D. Respiratory rate

138. The next day, after the circuit has been changed, you notice that the inspiratory tidal volume is set at 800 ml, as ordered, whereas the expiratory tidal volume is 650 ml. The low-volume alarm is going off. What would you do?
   A. Increase the inspiratory tidal volume until the expiratory volume reaches 800 ml.
   B. Turn off the alarm and chart the tidal volume at 650 ml.
   C. Call the physician for approval to change the tidal volume to 650 ml.
   D. Tighten all of the tubing and humidifier connections and recheck the expiratory tidal volume.

139. Later in the day you notice that the patient's peak pressure has increased from 30 to 45 cm H_2O. The plateau pressure has remained stable at 14 cm H_2O and the mean airway pressure has increased from 12 to 17 cm H_2O. What could be the cause of these pressure changes?
   I. Bronchial secretions
   II. His being overweight

III. Bronchospasm
IV. Heart failure
A. I, III
B. II, IV
C. I, IV
D. II, III

140. Before beginning to wean him off of the ventilation, you would monitor all of the following *except* his:
A. Bronchial secretions
B. Urine electrolytes
C. Vital signs
D. Vital capacity

Answer Key:

1. C;
2. D;
3. D;
4. C;
5. A;
6. A;
7. B;
8. B;
9. B;
10. D;
11. B;
12. B;
13. D;
14. C;
15. A;
16. A;
17. C;
18. A;
19. B;
20. A;
21. C;
22. C;
23. A;
24. C;
25. D;
26. C;
27. D;
28. B;
29. B;
30. D;
31. A;
32. C;
33. B;
34. B;
35. D;
36. C;
37. A;
38. C;
39. A;
40. B;
41. C;
42. B;
43. D;
44. A;
45. D;
46. C;
47. B;
48. A;
49. C;
50. B;
51. C;
52. D;
53. A;
54. C;
55. A;
56. C;
57. D;
58. A;
59. C;
60. A;
61. A;
62. D;
63. B;
64. D;
65. C;
66. A;
67. D;
68. A;
69. D;
70. D;
71. A;
72. C;
73. B;
74. A;
75. D;
76. B;
77. D;
78. D;
79. A;
80. D;
81. B;
82. C;
83. B;
84. B;
85. D;
86. A;
87. B;
88. C;
89. C;
90. B;
91. C;
92. D;
93. A;
94. B;
95. B;
96. A;
97. B;
98. A;
99. B;
100. C;
101. D;
102. D;
103. D;
104. C;
105. D;
106. C;
107. D;
108. B;
109. D;
110. B;
111. C;
112. B;
113. C;
114. A;
115. C;
116. C;
117. B;
118. A;
119. A;
120. D;
121. D;
122. B;
123. A;
124. C;
125. D;
126. B;
127. B;
128. D;
129. B;
130. C;
131. C;
132. A;
133. A.
134. A;
135. C;
136. D;
137. C;
138. D;
139. A;
140. B;

Explanations for the Practice Entry Level Examination

Code: c = Correct
a = Acceptable but not best
u = Unsatisfactory
h = Potentially harmful

Interpretation of the Final Score

The NBRC has set a minimum pass level of 75% for the Entry Level Examination. However, a raw score of 105 correct out of 140 questions may not be the minimum passing score. This is because each question is individually weighted based on its difficulty. For example, Recall questions are less valuable than Analysis questions. A multiplier for the examination is determined based on the total mix of questions. Historically, this has resulted in the examinee needing a raw score only in the lower 70% range to pass the examination.

It is not possible to develop a multiplier for this practice examination. Use 105 correct answers for the minimum pass level. The student or examinee who takes this practice examination should not feel overly encouraged or discouraged by either passing or failing it. Instead, use it to help you identify areas that may need to be improved upon. Study further so that you are better prepared to pass the actual NBRC examination.

1. Explanations:
u A. The door should be closed.
u B. You should wash your hands when finished.
c C. A cover gown is not needed because you will not be working that closely with the patient.
u D. Wearing a mask should help to protect you from airborn droplets if the patient is coughing vigorously.

2. Explanations:
h A. Suctioning should be applied for no longer than 15 seconds at a time.
a B. See D.
h C. See A and D.
c D. All of these steps are important when performing nasotracheal suctioning.

3. Explanations:
u A. Maximum expiratory pressure (MEP) would give information on the strength of the expiratory muscles of respiration.
u B. MIP has no strong relationship to lung compliance.
u C. MIP has no strong relationship to airway resistance.
c D. Measuring the MIP is the best way to determine the strength of the inspiratory muscles of respiration.

4. Explanations:
h A. She should not be given a sedative because she has to initiate each breath in the PSV mode.
u B. This would be a setback. Try increasing the PSV level before going back to the original settings.
c C. Try increasing the pressure support level to see if that helps her overcome the resistance of the endotracheal tube.
h D. There is no indication that the patient is hypoxic and needs PEEP. PEEP can cause serious complications and should not be used without a clear need.

5. Explanations:

c A. Tube position should always be checked after intubation. This is the proper position for the endotracheal tube.

a B. The chest x-ray film will look different now because of the addition of the endotracheal tube. Option A is the better answer.

u C. Usually heart damage cannot be determined by a chest x-ray film.

u D. Measuring the cuff pressure will show you that it is inflated.

6. Explanations:

c A. Knowing what hospital the patient is in shows an orientation to place and what day of the week it is shows orientation to time.

u B. Finding the patient's reaction to chronic illness deals with emotional state.

u C. A non-English-speaking patient could answer these questions through a translator to show orientation the place and time.

u D. Having the patient follow instructions for a task would show cooperation.

7. Explanations:

u A. Increasing the control pressure may help to restore a larger tidal volume when the leak is small. However, it will also increase the inspiratory time. This is not the best solution for a leak problem.

c B. Tightening the cascade and medication nebulizer jar should help to seal the leaks. If leaks are not the source of the problem, the machine will likely have to be replaced.

u C. See A. Giving 100% oxygen will not correct the leak. However, it will help to alleviate hypoxemia.

u D. See A.

8. Explanations:

u A. Changing her inspiratory flow rate will not affect the equipment.

c B. Probably something is loose. Tightening everything should cause the oxygen to exit through the prongs.

h C. Oxygen is considered to be a medication. You cannot change the flow without a physician's order.

a D. Tighten all connections first. Replace a cannula if it is the problem.

9. Explanations:

u A. Bronchospasm will result in a higher airway resistance and an increased peak pressure.

c B. Resolving pulmonary edema would make the lungs more compliant. That would result in a lower peak pressure to deliver the tidal volume.

u C. Biting the endotracheal tube will result in a higher airway resistance and an increased peak pressure.

u D. Bronchial secretions will result in a higher airway resistance and an increased peak pressure.

10. Explanations:

u A. Cromolyn sodium should be used only to prevent an asthma attack.

u B. Inhaling normal saline solution may worsen existing wheezing.

u C. Supplemental oxygen will not affect wheezing.

c D. Inhaling an aerosolized bronchodilator should help reduce the wheezing.

11. Explanations:

u A. An antibiotic should be given to a patient only after an infection has been shown to exist.

c B. Hand washing and replacing equipment and unused medications every 24 hours are two of the best ways to prevent the spread of infection.
a C. See B.
u D. See A and B.

12. Explanations:
u A. Patients with chronic bronchitis usually have viscous yellow or green secretions.
c B. Asthmatic patients without infection tend to have clear or white secretions.
u C. Pulmonary edema secretions are often pink and frothy.
u D. Same as A.

13. Explanations:
u A. The type of nebulizer would have no impact on the patient's problems.
u B. The type of nebulizer and oxygen flow would have no impact on the patient's symptoms.
u C. The oxygen flow would not cause the patient's symptoms.
c D. The type of medication and patient's vital signs and complaints are important to chart.

14. Explanations:
u A. The patient's asthmatic condition will probably prevent even distribution of the tidal volume no matter how low the flow is.
u B. This patient will experience dyspnea until the bronchospasm is relieved.
c C. It is very important that the patient have a long expiratory time to completely exhale. A short inspiratory time will allow for a longer expiratory time.
u D. The tidal volume should be delivered with a volume-cycled ventilator.

15. Explanations:
c A. This is the best medication to treat acute bronchospasm.
a B. Nebulizing a corticosteroid will reduce bronchospasm. However, it is rather slow in doing so.
h C. Suctioning could irritate the airways and cause more wheezing.
h D. Increasing the tidal volume could result in air trapping and barotrauma.

16. Explanations:
c A. Laryngospasm would be demonstrated by inspiratory stridor.
u B. Wheezing is often found with emphysema.
u C. Wheezing is often found over the site of an airway tumor.
u D. Wheezing is often found during an asthma attack.

17. Explanations:
u A. See C.
u B. See C.
c C. The duration is calculate as follows:

$$\text{Minutes of flow} = \frac{\text{gauge pressure in psig} \times \text{cylinder factor}}{\text{Liter flow}}$$

$$= \frac{1100 \times 3.14}{8}$$

$$= 432$$

$$\text{Hours of flow} = \frac{432}{60} = 7.2$$

u D. See C.

18. Explanations:
c A. Increasing the inspired oxygen percentage is the most direct and least hazardous way to increase the $Pa{O_2}$ level.
u B. Changing to SIMV will not increase the patient's oxygen level.
u C. Adding mechanical dead space will not increase the patient's oxygen level and may actually cause it to drop some. In addition, the $Pa{CO_2}$ is not dangerously low.
h D. Increasing the rate from 12 to 16 times/min will likely cause serious hyperventilation and a very alkalotic pH.

19. Explanations:
u A. This would show orientation to person.
c B. This shows orientation to time (her son's birthday) and place (in the hospital).
u C. This shows that the patient is able to cooperate.
u D. This shows orientation to place only.

20. Explanations:
c A. If the endotracheal tube has been inserted into the right bronchus, no air will enter the left lung, and the breath sounds there will be diminished or absent.
u B. Overinflation of the cuff could result in blockage of the tip of the endotracheal tube. Breath sounds would be decreased to both lungs.
u C. Insertion of the endotracheal tube into the esophagus would result in breath sounds being absent in both lungs and air movement sounds being heard over the stomach area.
u D. If the endotracheal tube has been inserted into the left bronchus, no air will enter the right lung, and the breath sounds there will be diminished or absent.

21. Explanations:
u A. The inspired oxygen percentage could be lowered to a safer lever (about 40%) without risking hypoxemia. However, the patient's real problem is hyperventilation and respiratory alkalosis.
u B. Mechanical dead space is not usually added to the circuit when a patient is using the SIMV mode.
c C. Decreasing the SIMV rate will correct the hyperventilation.
h D. Intravenous sodium bicarbonate is contraindicated because it will increase the patient's alkalemia.

22. Explanations:
u A. Kussmaul respiration is seen in patients with diabetic acidosis.
u B. Cheyne-Stokes respiration is cyclical in depth and often rate. It is usually seen in patients with either cerebral edema or pulmonary edema.
c C. These findings are typical of tachypnea.
u D. Eupnea is normal, resting breathing.

23. Explanations:
c A. Covering the air entrainment ports prevents room air from being added to dilute the oxygen flow.
u B. A small decrease in the oxygen flow will not affect the oxygen percentage because there will be a proportionate decrease in the entrained room air.
u C. The ports on the face mask are there to allow excess gas to escape. Enlarging the ports will not affect the oxygen percentage.
u D. Aerosol tubing is commonly added between the mask and air entrainment adapter and will not affect the oxygen percentage.

24. Explanations:
u A. This would be the proper ratio of rescue breaths to chest compressions given by *two* rescuers during a CPR attempt on an adult.
u B. See C.
c C. This is the ideal ratio of rescue breaths to chest compressions for a single rescuer to deliver during a CPR attempt on an adult.
u D. See C.

25. Explanations:
u A. There is no such blade.
u B. The Miller blade is straight.
u C. There is no such blade.
c D. The MacIntosh blade is curved.

26. Explanations:
u A. This would result in a bounding pulse.
u B. This would result in a uniformly faint pulse.
c C. Dysrhythmias such as atrial fibrillation or premature ventricular contractions cause a variable cardiac output and pulses.
u D. Cheyne-Stokes breathing results in variable breathing rate and/or depth.

27. Explanations:
u A. A 750-ml tidal volume is too small at less than 10 ml/kg of body weight.
u B. A rate of 20/min is too fast for an adult. Sixty percent oxygen is more oxygen than needed because the patient is not severely hypoxemic.
u C. A 1300-ml tidal volume is too large at more than 15 ml/kg of body weight. The patient does not need 90% oxygen.
c D. These parameters are appropriate for this adult patient.

28. Explanations:
a A. Although practitioners can become infected from patient equipment other patients are far more susceptible.
c B. Patients are likely to become infected from contaminated equipment because of their weakened condition or other preexisting infections.
u C. Inventory control is a secondary concern after decontamination.
u D. Repairs of damage is a secondary concern after decontamination.

29. Explanations:
u A. Air in the stomach would not be expelled like this with each breath.
c B. Putting more air into the cuff will probably seal the leak. If not, you will know that the tube needs replacing.
u C. A chest x-ray film will not be able to show if there is a problem with the cuff.
h D. It is potentially dangerous to replace a tube on a critically ill patient without knowing if it is really necessary.

30. Explanations:
u A. Wheezing is an improvement over diminished breath sounds.
h B. Placing a chest tube into a patient without a pneumothorax is dangerous.
u C. Rales is the term often used to describe the sound of pulmonary edema.
c D. Wheezing shows that there is improved airflow compared with diminished breath sounds.

31. Explanations:
- c A. These instructions are for a forced vital capacity (FVC) test.
- u B. Inspiratory capacity (IC) is the inspiratory volume measured from the end of exhalation to total lung capacity.
- u C. Total lung capacity (TLC) must be calculated by adding the FVC and residual volume.
- u D. Maximum voluntary ventilation (MVV) is a measurement of how much air the patient can breathe in and out in a set time period.

32. Explanations:
- u A. Laryngotracheobronchitis (croup) is a pediatric condition. The airway infection does not last for months at a time.
- u B. Patients with cystic fibrosis develop a chronic productive cough and other symptoms in early childhood. Most do not live beyond early adulthood.
- c C. Chronic bronchitis is confirmed by a productive cough for at least 3 months for at least 3 years.
- u D. Patients with asthma will have a productive cough during an attack and will be symptom free between attacks. However, this patient does not have the major problem of bronchospasm. Also, asthma attacks do not last for 3 consecutive months.

33. Explanations:
- u A. See B. There is a form of cromolyn sodium that can be given by small-volume nebulizer. However, the capsule form cannot.
- c B. The spinhaler is the only way to dispense cromolyn sodium from a capsule.
- u C. See B.
- u D. See B.

34. Explanations:
- u A. Heart failure is not associated with asymmetric chest movement.
- c B. Peripheral edema is commonly seen in patients with heart failure.
- u C. Clubbing of the fingers is found with a number of lung conditions that cause chronic hypoxemia.
- u D. Nasal flairing is a general sign of labored breathing.

35. Explanations:
- u A. The reservoir jar and lid should be screwed tightly together to prevent a leak.
- u B. A loosely screwed reservoir jar and lid will result in a leak at that point. However, the leak is known to be at the pressure relief valve.
- u C. Same as B.
- c D. Both obstructed oxygen tubing and too high an oxygen flow will cause backpressure and pressure relief valve to pop open.

36. Explanations:
- u A. Tracheal secretions are a common cause of an increased peak pressure but will not cause any change in the plateau pressure.
- u B. If the patient's lungs were becoming more compliant, both the peak and plateau pressures would be lower, not higher.
- c C. A patient who is developing pneumonia will have an increase in the plateau pressure, reflecting the stiffer lungs. The peak pressure will also be forced higher by the higher plateau pressure.
- u D. A Valsalva maneuver could briefly increase the peak pressure. This maneuver is a tightening of the abdominal muscles and closing of the glottis. It is most commonly performed during a bowel movement and would not last for 2 hours.

37. Explanations:
c A. Palpable rhonchi indicate secretions.
u B. A diagnosis of chronic bronchitis cannot be made only on secretions clearing after a cough.
u C. Lack of a vibration in the right lung would indicate that there were no secretions there.
u D. A diagnosis of COPD cannot be made only on secretions clearing after a cough.

38. Explanations:
u A. It is unlikely that this organism would survive the manufacturer's sterilization process.
u B. It is unlikely that sterile water would grow this organism even it has been used after its expiration date.
c C. This organism is found in the lower intestine. It is often spread from improper hand washing after use of the toilet.
u D. This organism is not normally found in the upper airway.

39. Explanations:
c A. A lower peak pressure would show that the airway resistance has decreased after secretions have been suctioned out.
u B. There would be no change in tidal volume on this volume cycled ventilator.
u C. The plateau pressure would be unchanged after suctioning because it reflects only changes in lung compliance.
u D. Inspiratory time is determined by inspiratory gas flow and tidal volume, not airway resistance.

40. Explanations:
u A. Warming will increase the consumption of oxygen by the blood and lower the oxygen pressure.
c B. Placing the blood sample into ice water will prevent the blood from consuming the oxygen within the sample.
u C. Capping the needle is now discouraged to avoid accidental punctures. It is recommended that the needle be pushed into a rubber cube or somehow covered in a safe manner.
u D. If hemolysis is to be done, it should be in the laboratory as the analysis is performed.

41. Explanations:
h A. This will worsen the patient's breathing.
h B. This may worsen the patient's breathing.
c C. Raising the head and chest above the legs should help to reduce some of the blood flow to the heart. This may help to reduce hypoxemia in a patient with congestive heart failure.
h D. This may worsen the patient's breathing.

42. Explanations:
u A. Vanceril is an inhaled corticosteroid.
c B. Mucomyst is a mucolytic that can be very irritating to the airways. It can cause bronchospasm.
u C. Alupent is a sympathomimetic bronchodilator.
u D. Intal is a prophylactic medication against asthma.

43. Explanations:
u A. This will not share the information with anyone besides those doing patient rounds.
u B. There is not way to ensure that the shift supervisor will tell the correct information to all of the staff members.

u C. This is not a secure way to get information into the patient's chart.
c D. This will ensure that anyone with access to the chart will see the information.

44. Explanations:
c A. The physician needs to revise the order to be 0.5 ml of Bronkosol and 4 ml of normal saline solution. Neither you nor the nurse can make this change in this situation.
u B. See A.
h C. Giving 5 ml of Bronkosol is too much and puts the patient at risk of a drug reaction.
u D. See A.

45. Explanations:
u A. An infant probably will not understand what you are saying or be able to cooperate.
u B. Sedation should be considered only after all other possible solutions have been tried and ruled out.
h C. CPAP should not be increased without careful consideration of its possible side effects. The physician has to give the order to make the change. In addition, the CPAP level is supposed to be stable throughout the breathing cycle.
c D. Increasing the flow should meet the patient's inspiratory flow needs. The CPAP level should stabilize at the ordered 6 cm H_2O.

46. Explanations:
u A. It is unwise and may be unsafe to make him breathe spontaneously for 20 more minutes just because it was previously planned.
u B. This patient is unstable and should be put back on the ventilator. It would be helpful to have blood gas data, but the patient's safety must be the first priority.
c C. Put the patient back on the ventilator for his safety. He may be weaned again when the bleeding is stopped if he is ready.
u D. It cannot be said that he failed at breathing on his own. Once ready to try again, he should be given the chance. If he fails because of pulmonary problems, the SIMV mode could be tried as a weaning method.

47. Explanations:
u A. Kussmaul's respiration shows a consistently large tidal volume with a rapid respiratory rate.
c B. Biot's respiration shows an inconsistent tidal volume and rate.
u C. Cheyne-Stokes respiration shows a cyclical increase and decrease in tidal volume. Sometimes the rate varies.
u D. Obstructed inspiration would show a slow inspiration and normal expiration.

48. Explanations:
c A. Water has condensed at a low point in the tubing. Draining it out will restore the continuous aerosol stream.
u B. The patient's breathing pattern can have no affect on the equipment.
u C. Running the oxygen flowmeter too low will reduce the total amount of aerosol that is produced but will not cause aerosol puffing.
u D. If the reservoir were empty, no aerosol would be produced.

49. Explanations:
u A. The patient does have normal breath sounds. However, the laryngeal sounds are abnormal and should be charted as such.
u B. True, however, the laryngeal sounds are abnormal and should be charted as such.
c C. The problem of inspiratory stridor is significant and should be charted.
u D. There is no way to make a diagnosis of bacterial pneumonia based on the limited information of inspiratory stridor.

50. Explanations:
h A. It is improper to give this medication without a physician's order.
c B. Wheezing indicates an adverse reaction. Stop the treatment, monitor the patient, and notify the physician.
h C. It is improper to give this medication without a physician's order.
u D. Oxygen will not stop the wheezing.

51. Explanations:
u A. This position would help to drain the lateral and medial segments of the right middle lobe. Ideally, the patient should be rotated one-fourth turn up from back down on the bed.
u B. This position would drain the superior segments of both lower lobes.
c C. The posterior basal segment of the right (and left) lower lobe would be drained by this position.
u D. This position would help to drain the lateral basal segment of the right lower lobe. Ideally, the patient should lie one-fourth turn up from prone.

52. Explanations:
u A. Pure oxygen is not indicated at this time.
u B. Mechanical ventilation is not indicated by the blood gas results. The neonate has a normal carbon dioxide level.
u C. There is no clinical indication that a pneumothorax is present.
c D. CPAP should improve the Pao_2 level adequately. It is indicated based on the low oxygen level and normal carbon dioxide level.

53. Explanations:
c A. This is appropriate. The Pao_2 level of 85 mm Hg is misleading because it represents only a plasma value. The patient could have significant carbon monoxide poisoning.
u B. Mechanical ventilation is unnecessary because the patient is able to breath adequately.
a C. It is appropriate to give the patient supplemental oxygen. However, giving 100% oxygen will drive the carbon monoxide off of the hemoglobin much faster.
h D. A patient with carbon monoxide poisoning must be admitted for careful observation and supplemental oxygen.

54. Explanations:
u A. Accessory muscles would not be used during normal, resting breathing.
u B. Accessory muscles would not be needed if lung compliance is increased.
c C. Increased airway resistance would increase the patient's work of breathing. Accessory muscles would be needed to aid in breathing.
u D. Accessory muscles would not be needed if work of breathing was decreased.

55. Explanations:
c A. Adding mechanical dead space will make the patient rebreathe some of her own carbon dioxide and correct the hyperventilation problem.
h B. Increasing the tidal volume will hyperventilate the patient even more and make the patient dangerously alkalotic.
u C. The inspired oxygen percentage and Pao_2 level do not justify any adjustments.
h D. See B.

56. Explanations:
u A. The patient is breathing at the rate that he or she feels is necessary.
h B. A nasal cannula will probably deliver a lower oxygen percentage to the patient than the nonrebreather mask.

c C. Increase the oxygen flow until the reservoir bag loses no more than one half of its volume on inspiration.
h D. Removing the flaps will result in the patient inhaling room air and reducing the oxygen percentage.

57. Explanations:
u A. The patient's complaint does not indicate a lack of cooperation.
u B. The patient seems oriented based on what she has said about her situation.
u C. Hyperpnea would be demonstrated by a large tidal volume.
c D. Orthopnea is the inability to lie flat without becoming short of breath.

58. Explanations:
c A. The low carbon dioxide level indicates hyperventilation and is the cause of the respiratory alkalosis with the elevated pH. The $P(A\text{-}a)O_2$ is increased because the patient is inspiring 40% oxygen and has a PaO_2 of only 70 mm Hg.
u B. His PaO_2 level of 70 mm Hg is low but does not indicate hypoxemia.
a C. See A.
u D. See A and B.

59. Explanations:
h A. The patient's vital signs have increased by more than 20%. It may be harmful to give the other half of the medication.
h B. Bronchosol will have no affect on the laryngeal edema. You cannot change medications without a physician's approval.
c C. It is best to stop the treatment, inform the physician of the changes in vital signs, and ask for further instructions.
h D. You cannot give a medication by another route without a physician's approval. Besides, racemic epinephrine is most effective for laryngeal edema when it is inhaled.

60. Explanations:
c A. This 100 ml of aerosol tubing will act as a reservoir of oxygen and aerosol.
u B. This cannot be done without the physician's approval. It will not do anything to increase the amount of aerosol the patient is receiving.
u C. This will increase the humidity level but not increase the oxygen up to the ordered 35%.
u D. Same as C.

61. Explanations:
c A. Wearing a mask, goggles, and gloves will protect you from secretions coughed out by the patient.
h B. A patient should not be suctioned without his or her knowledge. The patient who is suctioned while sleeping will be suddenly awakened and may hurt himself or herself when induced to cough.
h C. Coughing is not an indication to restrain the patient. See the statement in B.
u D. Coughing is not an indication to restrain the patient.

62. Explanations:
u A. A tired person should respond properly when awake.
a B. This is possible but not as likely as option D.
a C. Same as B.
c D. Too much oxygen in a hypercarbic emphysema patient can blunt the hypoxic drive to breathe. Then, the carbon dioxide level rises even higher. The person can become drowsy or even unconscious.

63. Explanations:
- u A. Back blows are only performed on infants with an airway obstruction problem.
- c B. The Heimlich maneuver (abdominal thrusts) is the best way to try to clear on airway obstruction.
- u C. This is not appropriate at this time.
- h D. Striking the patient several times over the sternum may harm the patient.

64. Explanations:
- u A. Wheezing is usually heard during an asthma attack.
- u B. Rales or crackles are often used to describe the sound heard with pulmonary edema.
- u C. There is no specific sound associated with pneumonia. Secretions in airways are referred to as rhonchi.
- c D. Inspiratory stridor is a high-pitched sound on inspiration. It is often heard with acute laryngotracheobronchitis.

65. Explanations:
- u A. An air flowmeter will not fit in to an oxygen outlet.
- a B. This should be done only if the leak cannot be controlled in the room. Option C should be done first.
- c C. Replacing the oxygen flowmeter into the outlet should stop the leak. Contact the maintenance department to correct the problem.
- a D. This should be done if option C did not work and there is a fire hazard in the room.

66. Explanations:
- c A. This is a dangerous increase in pulse rate. The treatment should be stopped and physician informed.
- h B. Continuing the treatment may lead to the patient being harmed. It should be stopped.
- h C. Same as B
- u D. The physician should be the one to decide whether the treatment should be continued or not.

67. Explanations:
- u A. Looking in the mouth will not show you if the tip of the endotracheal tube has been inserted into the trachea.
- u B. Whether or not the cuff seals at 20 cm H_2O does not inform you if the tube is properly inserted into the trachea.
- u C. The neck x-ray film on an adult will not show if the tube tip is within the trachea.
- c D. The best way to determine if the tip of the endotracheal tube is properly placed within the trachea is by looking at it on the patient's chest x-ray film.

68. Explanations:
- c A. These symptoms are seen with hyperventilation (reduced carbon dioxide level).
- u B. These symptoms are not seen with Alupent.
- u C. These symptoms are not caused by an increased oxygen level.
- u D. These symptoms are not seen with Mucomyst.

69. Explanations:
- u A. Euphoria is extreme joy.
- u B. Depression is long-term sadness.
- u C. Resentment is a sense of anger over unfairness or being insulted.
- c D. Panic would be expected of a patient in pain and having great difficulty in breathing.

70. Explanations:
u A. This may result in some increase in the patient's oxygen level but will not correct the elevated carbon dioxide level.
u B. Same as A.
u C. It is unlikely that the blood gas results will be very different in 1 hour.
c D. Increasing her minute volume will decrease the $Paco_2$ level and also increase her Pao_2 level.

71. Explanations:
c A. Minute volume = rate per minute × tidal volume
u B. See A.
u C. See A.
u D. See A.

72. Explanations:
u A. These are accessory muscles of inspiration (See Fig. 1-12).
u B. Although the chest wall should move with each breath, this is not the best way to observe movement of the diaphragm.
c C. This is the best way to note movement of the diaphragm (see Fig. 1-7).
u D. The trapezius muscles are accessory muscles of *inspiration* (see Fig. 1-12).

73. Explanations:
a A. Although important, it is not the first thing to do.
c B. The chart should be reviewed when a new order is received before going to the patient.
a C. Same as A.
u D. There is no reason to presume that a mechanical percussor is indicated.

74. Explanations:
c A. These steps are needed to calculate the inspiratory time:
1. Determine the cycle time by dividing the rate into 60 seconds.

$$\text{Cycle time} = \frac{60}{20} = 3 \text{ seconds}$$

2. Determine the inspiratory time by dividing the sum of the ratio parts (1:2) into the cycle time.

$$\text{Inspiratory time} = \frac{3 \text{ seconds}}{1 + 2} = \frac{3 \text{ seconds}}{3} = 1 \text{ second}$$

u B. See A.
u C. See A.
u D. See A.

75. Explanations:
u A. Humidity does not need to be added to this system for accuracy.
u B. A weak battery would not cause the problem that was found.
u C. Humidity does not need to be removed from this system for accuracy.
c D. Failure to reach 100% is a sign that the electrolyte in the fuel cell is almost gone. The fuel cell must be replaced.

76. Explanations:
u A. Pure oxygen is delivered if the air-mix knob is pushed in.
c B. Between 60% and 90% oxygen is delivered when the air-mix knob is pulled out.

u C. The air-mix knob has no affect on the machine's cycling.
u D. The venturi will work if the air-mix knob is pulled out.

77. Explanations:
u A. Although possible, this is an unlikely finding. Hypotension leads to low perfusion and metabolic acidosis.
u B. This is not a standard description for how to interpret these blood gases. See A.
u C. The low carbon dioxide level would cause a respiratory alkalosis if not for the low bicarbonate level.
c D. The low bicarbonate, base excess, and pH indicate a serious acidosis. This fits the clinical finding of the patient being hypotensive. The low $Paco_2$ value is the result of the patient hyperventilating in an attempt to correct the low pH.

78. Explanations:
u A. Pulmonary edema may result in pink, frothy secretions.
u B. *M. tuberculosis* does not cause green, foul-smelling secretions.
u C. Fungal organisms do not cause green, foul-smelling secretions.
c D. Green, foul-smelling secretions are commonly found in patients with a *Pseudomonas* pulmonary infection.

79. Explanations:
c A. In this situation the patient should receive as much oxygen as possible. A nonrebreathing mask can deliver 80% oxygen or more.
u B. This nasal cannula flow might deliver about 36% oxygen.
u C. This sample mask flow might deliver about 40% oxygen.
u D. 28% oxygen is probably not enough for this patient.

80. Explanations:
u A. A cascade-type humidifier produces water vapor, not aerosol particles.
u B. See A.
u C. See A.
c D. A cascade-type humidifier is very quiet. This is important so as not to damage the newborn's hearing. Contamination of the gas is unlikely because water vapor is molecular water and far too small for any microorganisms to "catch a ride."

81. Explanations:
u A. The simple oxygen mask will not deliver enough oxygen to her.
c B. IPPB will give her 100% oxygen, and the positive pressure may help to limit her pulmonary edema.
u C. This aggressive procedure is not indicated yet.
u D. As long as she is able to cough effectively, suctioning is not indicated.

82. Explanations:
u A. Pulmonary edema sputum is not associated with a foul odor.
a B. Pulmonary edema sputum is also pink and watery.
c C. Sputum that has a pink tint, is frothy, and watery is associated with pulmonary edema.
u D. See answer A.

83. Explanations:
u A. No spirometer is needed in this test.
c B. This is the proper one-way valve placement for a maximum inspiratory pressure test.
u C. This is the proper one-way valve placement for a maximum expiratory pressure test.
u D. See A.

84. Explanations:
- u A. Turning on the flowmeter will allow gas to escape through it. However, it will not stop the original leak.
- c B. After turning off the cylinder, replace the worn washer and tighten the regulator to stop the leak.
- u C. Changing the regulator will not stop the leak if the washer is worn.
- u D. See A.

85. Explanations:
- u A. This would be the appropriate angle to tip the patient in the bed.
- u B. Always inform a patient why a treatment is needed.
- u C. This is the proper position to drain the affected segments.
- c D. She would find it uncomfortable to have percussion and vibration performed on her breast.

86. Explanations:
- c A. Using extra pillows and being unable to sleep flat in bed are signs of orthopnea.
- u B. Hemoptysis is not directly related to orthopnea.
- u C. Climbing stairs is related to exercise level. Some patients find certain foods aid in making secretions less viscous. Neither is directly related to orthopnea.
- u D. See the explanations for answers B and C.

87. Explanations:
- u A. Brethaire is not a mucolytic.
- c B. Postural drainage and percussion should help to mobilize the secretions so that they can be coughed out.
- a C. Incentive spirometry will help to generate a deep breath. That, followed by a strong cough, may help to mobilize the secretions. However, incentive spirometry is not the most effective therapy against bronchial secretions.
- u D. The patient may need supplemental oxygen because of hypoxemia. But, increasing the inspired oxygen will not treat the secretion problem.

88. Explanations:
- a A. Often the vital capacity will increase if the bronchodilator is effective. However, measuring a before and after bronchodilator $FEV_{1\%}$ is better.
- u B. The MIP is a measurement of strength and is not a good indicator of bronchodilator effectiveness.
- c C. A 15% to 20% increase in the $FEV_{1\%}$ after a bronchodilator is given is a good indication that the medication has had a positive effect.
- u D. The minute alveolar ventilation might change after a bronchodilator is given. However, it is not a good indicator of the effectiveness of the medication.

89. Explanations:
- u A. Pulse oximetry should not be used on a patient with carbon monoxide poisoning. It will give a falsely high reading for Spo_2.
- u B. A regular blood gas analyzer will give a Pao_2 value from the patient's blood plasma. This value may be high despite the fact that the patient's hemoglobin is occupied by carbon monoxide. The patient could actually be dangerously hypoxic.
- c C. A CO oximeter is able to measure a true Sao_2 to show how much hemoglobin is able to carry oxygen.
- u D. Transcutaneous Po_2 is a measure of oxygen in the tissues and does not match the Pao_2 or Sao_2 value.

90. Explanations:
- u A. Inspiratory stridor would be heard in a patient with laryngeal edema.

c B. Vesicular breath sounds are normally heard over all lung fields.
u C. Crackles or rhonchi are terms used to label the sound made by secretions in the large airways.
u D. Decreased breath sounds would be abnormal over the lung fields.

91. Explanations:
u A. See C.
u B. See C.
c C. A person breathing room air cannot have a Pao_2 level this high without hyperventilating. Either the $Paco_2$, Pao_2, or both values are inaccurate. Check the oxygen and carbon dioxide electrodes for an error. Fix it and reanalyze the blood sample.
u D. See C.

92. Explanations:
h A. This will probably deliver the lowest percentage of oxygen to the patient of the options A, B, and D. It is possible that the rescuer could be injured by the high flow of gas going into the mouth.
a B. A mouth-to-valve mask resuscitator will effectively ventilate a patient if a manual resuscitator with oxygen reservoir is not available. It should be your second choice.
u C. This will deliver up to 80% to 100% oxygen to a spontaneously breathing patient. However, a CPR victim will likely be apneic, so this will be useless.
c D. This will deliver the highest possible inspired oxygen percentage of the choices offered.

93. Explanations:
c A. Minute volume is found by multiplying respiratory rate × tidal volume: 14 breaths/min × 450 ml = 6300 ml
u B. See A.
u C. See A.
u D. See A.

94. Explanations:
u A. See B.
c B. Minute alveolar ventilation is found by multiplying the respiratory rate × tidal volume − dead space:

$$14 \text{ breaths/min} \times (450 \text{ ml} - 160 \text{ ml}) = 4060 \text{ ml}$$

u C. See B.
u D. See B.

95. Explanations:
u A. Grunting is not done to change the carbon dioxide level.
c B. An expiratory grunt sound is produced as the epiglottis is closed over the trachea at the end of exhalation. This has the effect of keeping extra air in the alveoli to prevent atelectasis.
u C. Grunting will not help to clear out secretions.
u D. Grunting will not help to close the ductus arteriosus.

96. Explanations:
c A. Hypoxemia is a common cause of cyanosis.
u B. Advanced age is not associated with a change in color to blue-gray.
u C. Neither artificial nor natural light should cause a person to look blue-gray.
u D. People in heart failure may have both peripheral edema and cyanosis. However, peripheral edema is not a cause of cyanosis.

97. Explanations:
u A. Black nail polish can block the pulse oximetry light waves.
c B. A strong pulse at the measurement site should result in an accurate reading.
u C. Outside light interference can result in an incorrect pulse oximetry reading.
u D. Pulse oximeters cannot measure the level of carboxyhemoglobin. They will report only the oxygen saturation of the remaining normal hemoglobin. This will result in a misunderstanding of the patient's true oxygenation and amount of functional hemoglobin.

98. Explanations:
c A. Only an air entrainment mask delivers precise and adjustable oxygen percentages.
u B. See A.
u C. See A.
u D. See A.

99. Explanations:
u A. The SIMV mode will do nothing to make the secretions easier to remove.
c B. A cascade-type heated humidifier will do a better job at humidifying the patient's airway than a heat-moisture exchanger. This should result in the secretions becoming less viscous and easier to suction out.
a C. Instilling normal saline solution will help to make the secretions easier to suction out. However, switching to a cascade-type heated humidifier will, overall, be more effective.
u D. Using a larger catheter may help in removing secretions. Remember that it is unsafe to use a catheter that is more than one half the inner diameter of the endotracheal tube. If the secretions are too viscous, a large catheter will not really help.

100. Explanations:
u A. Although morphine is given for pain relief, it also has sedating affects. Normally, you would want to have the patient as alert as possible.
u B. Increasing the respiratory rate would probably result in the patient being hyperventilated.
c C. SIMV will allow the patient to do some breathing on his own so that he does not fight against the ventilator.
u D. It is not clearly established that the patient needs PEEP. Even if he does need it, 10 cm H_2O is too much to start with.

101. Explanations:
u A. This is unlikely because they are sterilized by the manufacturer.
u B. This is an unlikely source for this type of pneumonia.
a C. Although this is a possible source of the infection, it is less likely than answer D.
c D. *Staphylococcus aureus* is a bacteria found on the skin of almost everyone. It is most likely that a health care worker accidentally spread the organism to the patient.

102. Explanations:
u A. See D.
u B. See D.
u C. See D.
c D. Respiratory acidosis is shown by the elevated Pa_{CO_2} level and the acidotic pH. The increased bicarbonate and base excess have pushed the pH close to the normal range. In this way the body compensates for the chronically high carbon dioxide level.

103. Explanations:
u A. A good fit of the hood around the neck will help to keep the oxygen percentage where it is supposed to be.

u B. The inspired oxygen should be warmed to the newborn's body temperature.
u C. Minimizing noise will protect the infant from hearing damage.
c D. It is doubtful if a clear plexiglass hood will cause a newborn to feel claustrophobia (fear of enclosed spaces).

104. Explanations:
u A. Panic is likely to be felt by a suffocating person.
u B. Inspiratory stridor would indicate a partial airway obstruction.
c C. Depression is an unlikely emotion for a suffocating person.
u D. Cyanosis would be found in a hypoxic suffocating patient.

105. Explanations:
u A. An inhaled corticosteroid will not be helpful in this patient with many viscous secretions.
u B. The Ventolin would be helpful to treat her bronchospasm. However, hypertonic saline solution can cause bronchospasm, will tend to impact only in the larger airways, and will inhibit the growth of any bacteria found in a sputum sample.
u C. Both normal saline solution and Mucomyst should help to reduce the viscosity of her secretions. However, the patient is wheezing, and Mucomyst often worsens this problem. See D.
c D. The Ventolin would be helpful to treat her bronchospasm. In addition, the Mucomyst will help to decrease the viscosity of her secretions. The Ventolin will also help to block any bronchospasm that might be induced by the Mucomyst.

106. Explanations:
u A. It should still bubble even though the oxygen will leak out.
u B. Same as A.
c C. No oxygen can be delivered to bubble through the water if the tube is blocked.
u D. The oxygen will still bubble through the water without a diffuser head.

107. Explanations:
u A. Lung compliance cannot be measured by a peak flow test.
u B. Air distribution cannot be measured by a peak flow test.
u C. Peak *inspiratory* flow is not usually measured at the bedside. To measure it, a flow/volume loop test should be performed in the pulmonary function laboratory.
c D. A peak flow of 2.5 L/sec in an adult is low and indicates obstructed expiratory air flow.

108. Explanations:
u A. Pure oxygen is given to drive carbon monoxide off of the hemoglobin.
c B. In normal people the inspired oxygen level has nothing to do with the expiration of carbon dioxide. Oxygen-induced hypoventilation is a concern in patients with hypercarbia who are breathing on hypoxic drive. But, this is because the respiratory center is not functioning properly.
u C. The heart will not have to beat as often to deliver oxygen to the tissues if the oxygen level of the blood is increased.
u D. The patient will not have to breathe as often to meet his or her needs if more oxygen is inspired.

109. Explanations:
u A. See D.
u B. See D.
u C. See D.
c D. This is the best procedure for most patients. Modifications may have to be made with some patients such as those with postoperative pain.

110. Explanations:
u A. An aerosolized bronchodilator will have little, if any, impact on atelectasis.
c B. When incentive spirometry is done properly with a sustained maximal inspiration, it helps to prevent and/or treat atelectasis.
a C. IPPB will help to prevent or treat atelectasis. However, because it is more expensive and complicated, it is not recommended unless the patient cannot perform incentive spirometry.
u D. Bedside spirometry tests have little, if any, effect on atelectasis.

111. Explanations:
u A. Although increasing the terminal flow will allow the unit to cycle off if there is a small leak, it will not fix the problem and stop a massive leak.
u B. If the high-pressure oxygen hose were disconnected from the unit, no gas would enter it, and it would not operate.
c C. Reattaching the nebulizer hose to the unit will take care of the leak.
u D. A minor leak through a patient's nose will not cause all of the described problems.

112. Explanations:
u A. See B.
c B. The low-pressure alarm is the most important. This is because the alarm would sound if the patient became disconnected from the circuit or a major leak developed. Loss of mechanical ventilation can result in severe hypoventilation and even death.
u C. See B.
u D. See D.

113. Explanations:
u A. Placing a heat and moisture exchanger between the nebulizer and the patient will cause all of the aerosol to be filtered out before reaching the patient.
u B. Pentamidine is not available in a metered dose inhaler.
c C. The scavenging system will capture any exhaled aerosol droplets so that they do not enter the room air.
u D. A SPAG system is used only to nebulize ribavirin (Virazol).

114. Explanations:
c A. The air/oxygen ratio in a 35% air entrainment mask is 5:1. That gives a total of the ratio parts of 6. Multiply this times the oxygen flow rate for the answer. (6×6 L/min = 36 L/min total)
u B. See A.
u C. See A.
u D. See A.

115. Explanations:
u A. Brigg's adapter with reservoir is often used to wean patients who have required mechanical ventilation for only a short time.
u B. IMV is often used to wean patients who have required mechanical ventilation for a prolonged time.
c C. The control mode cannot be used for weaning because the patient is prevented from triggering any assisted breaths on the ventilator.
u D. Same as B.

116. Explanations:
h A. This may actually cause more atelectasis.
u B. It is not necessary to perform a vital capacity maneuver or hold it for 10 seconds.

c C. Holding a maximum inspiratory capacity breath for several seconds should help to open up atelectatic areas.
u D. This maneuver describes a maximum voluntary ventilation effort.

117. Explanations:
u A. Cyanosis is the result of having at least 5 vol % of desaturated hemoglobin. It could be present during a CPR attempt even if rescue breathing is being done properly.
c B. Seeing the chest rise during the delivery of a breath confirms that the airway is open and the breath is filling the lungs.
u C. The heart rate may or may not return to normal during CPR even when rescue breathing is being done properly.
u D. When the brain is well oxygenated, the pupils will react to light by constricting. Cardiac output, oxygen content of the blood, and rescue breathing all have an impact on how much oxygen gets to the brain. This is not the best way to evaluate mouth-to-mouth breathing.

118. Explanations:
c A. Palpation of the larynx during the insertion of the endotracheal tube is an immediate and easy way to tell if the trachea has been intubated.
u B. This would not work if the neonate was not crying.
a C. This would indicate tracheal intubation but is not the first sign.
a D. Same as C.

119. Explanations:
c A. This is the correct time frame for suctioning.
u B. While the goal is to remove all of the secretions, this will likely take several passes of the catheter. Each suctioning episode should last no longer than 15 seconds.
u C. Thirty seconds is too long to perform suctioning.
h D. It is dangerous to have the Spo_2 level drop below 90%.

120. Explanations:
u A. A hand-held nebulizer will be ineffective for delivering the medication if the patient cannot coordinate his breathing properly. It will do nothing for atelectasis.
u B. Same as A.
u C. Incentive spirometry and MDI both require patient cooperation.
c D. IPPB will both deliver the medication and help to open up the atelectatic areas.

121. Explanations:
u A. See the calculation in D.
u B. See the calculation in D.
u C. See the calculation in D.
c D.

$$\text{Static compliance} = \frac{\text{tidal volume}}{\text{plateau pressure} - \text{PEEP}}$$

$$= \frac{900 \text{ ml}}{35 - 10}$$

$$= \frac{900 \text{ ml}}{25}$$

$$= 36 \text{ ml/cm } H_2O$$

122. Explanations:

u A. This tidal volume is at the high end of the normal range. This will help correct the atelectasis.

c B. Inspiratory flow and I/E ratio would have little impact on opening up atelectatic areas.

u C. A large sigh would help to open up areas of atelectasis.

u D. Frequent sigh breaths would help to open up areas of atelectasis.

123. Explanations:

c A. The physician should be informed of new hemoptysis. He or she will decide if the procedure should be continued.

h B. The treatment should not be continued. Hemoptysis indicates an injury that should be evaluated first.

h C. Oxygen should not be given without a physician's approval. See B.

u D. This is not a professional way to act. The patient needs to know that the physician will be informed of the situation.

124. Explanations:

u A. This is not appropriate because of the nasal trauma.

u B. This is not appropriate because of the oral trauma.

c C. This will assure an airway now and later when surgery is performed to correct her facial injuries.

u D. This will not assure a patient airway.

125. Explanations:

u A. Increasing the tidal volume will only cause more gas to be vented through the circuit to the bellows.

u B. Overinflating the cuff will not stop the leak in the ventilator circuit.

u C. The patient is breathing as he is because the machine's tidal volume is not being delivered to him.

c D. A disconnection of the small-bore tubing to the exhalation valve will prevent the valve from closing during inspiration. The gas will bypass the patient and enter the spirometer bellows. Simply reconnect the tubing.

126. Explanations:

u A. This is disruptive of the patient's sleep. It is unlikely that the patient could quickly go to his doctor.

c B. Adjusting the nasal mask to fit better will stop the leak. The CPAP will be restored and the airway obstruction will be opened.

u C. This may have to be done but only after step B is tried.

u D. An oropharyngeal airway is not well tolerated in a patient who is not comatose.

127. Explanations:

h A. See B. These choices would likely cause the patient to become hypoxic.

c B. It is best to give the patient 100% oxygen before and after the suctioning procedure and to use a catheter that is no more than one half the inner diameter of the endotracheal tube.

h C. See B. These choices would likely cause the patient to become hypoxic.

h D. See B. These choices would likely cause the patient to become hypoxic.

128. Explanations:

u A. Increasing the oxygen percentage is not likely to change her vital signs in this situation.

u B. There is no clear indication that the patient needs more intravenous fluid.

h C. Removing the PEEP completely could result in dangerous hypoxemia.
c D. Putting the PEEP back to the previous level should result in the patient's vital signs returning to normal. Remember that PEEP can cause a decrease in venous return to the heart and that results in a decrease in cardiac output.

129. Explanations:
u A. This is an acceptable vital capacity.
c B. The maximum inspiratory pressure should be at least −20 to −25 cm H_2O to wean successfully.
u C. This is an acceptable blood pressure.
u D. This is an acceptable shunt fraction.

130. Explanations:
u A. This is necessary.
u B. This is necessary.
c C. Luken's trap is for collecting a sample of sputum from the lungs to send to the laboratory for culturing of any infectious organisms.
u D. This is necessary.

131. Explanations:
u A. The Siemens Servo 900C is a widely used adult ventilator that does offer information on peak, mean, and plateau pressures. However, it does not offer as much patient data as the Puritan-Bennett 7200.
u B. The Bird Mark 14 offers no patient data other than peak pressure.
c C. The Puritan-Bennett 7200 is a microprocessor ventilator. It has software that provide patient data on peak, mean, and plateau pressures. In addition, a software package and the add-on video monitor allow pressure, volume, and flow graphics to be looked at. Bedside spirometry can also be performed on it.
u D. The BEAR 1 offers no patient data other than peak and plateau pressures.

132. Explanations:
c A. Increasing the flow rate will deliver more gas to the patient initially. This should meet the patient's needs, and the pressure manometer needle will not be drawn into the negative range.
u B. Increasing the pressure will not deliver the gas to the patient any faster.
u C. Pushing the air-mix knob into the unit will decrease the flow.
u D. If the patient inhales faster, the problem will be worsened. The manometer needle will deflect even more into the negative range.

133. Explanations:
c A. Therapeutic PEEP on the ventilator will increase the FRC, should help to correct the atelectasis, and will increase the patient's oxygen level.
u B. Increasing the oxygen percentage should help improve the patient's oxygen level but will not correct the small FRC or atelectasis.
u C. Suctioning will only help to remove secretions.
u D. Pressure support ventilation will not help to correct the small FRC or atelectasis.

134. Explanations:
c A. Calling for help is the appropriate next step after finding that the patient is cyanotic and unresponsive.
u B. The carotid pulse should be checked only after the patient has been ventilated.
u C. It is a waste of time to leave the patient to seek help.
u D. It is completely inappropriate to call for an ECG at this time.

135. Explanations:
- u A. It is too early to intubate the patient's airway.
- u B. Ventilation should be tried first. If the airway is obstructed, it will then need to be cleared.
- c C. It is appropriate to begin rescue breathing after opening the airway and finding out that the patient is apneic.
- u D. An oral airway may need to be inserted if the patient is resuscitated successfully. It would be used to keep the tongue from blocking the back of the throat.

136. Explanations:
- h A. This is a waste of time and will result in poor compression results because of the soft mattress.
- h B. Same as A.
- u C. A back board would not be needed if she were left on the hard floor.
- c D. Leaving her on the hard floor will result in the best cardiac output from the chest compressions.

137. Explanations:
- u A. It is necessary to have an order for the oxygen percentage.
- u B. It is necessary to have an order for the minute volume on this ventilator.
- c C. Sign volume and frequency are fixed on this unit in the assist/control mode.
- u D. It is necessary to have an order for the respiratory rate.

138. Explanations:
- u A. This will increase the patient's tidal volume but does not correct the problem.
- h B. It is dangerous to turn off a low-volume alarm. Also, you will be charting the wrong tidal volume as the correct one.
- u C. This does not fix the problem of unequal volumes. Even if the physician agrees to the change, it is not good respiratory care.
- c D. Tighten all of the connections to determine if a leak caused the unequal volumes. If true, you have corrected the problem.

139. Explanations:
- c A. Both bronchial secretions and bronchospasm will result in more airway resistance. This will result in a higher peak pressure and stable plateau pressure.
- u B. His weight is stable and will not cause the sudden increase in peak pressure.
- u C. Heart failure could result in pulmonary edema but would show itself as an increase in the plateau pressure.
- u D. See B and C.

140. Explanations:
- u A. Secretions should be evaluated before weaning.
- c B. Urine electrolyte values will have little, if any, impact on ability to successfully wean from the ventilator.
- u C. Vital signs should be evaluated before weaning.
- u D. Vital capacity should be evaluated because it relates to the patient's ability to take a deep breath and cough.

INDEX